Infectious Diseases:
In Context

Infectious Diseases: In Context

Brenda Wilmoth Lerner & K. Lee Lerner, Editors

VOLUME 2

MALARIA TO ZOONOSES

THOMSON

GALE

Detroit • New York • San Francisco • New Haven, Conn. • Waterville, Maine • London

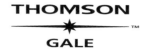

Infectious Diseases: In Context

Brenda Wilmoth Lerner and K. Lee Lerner, Editors

Project Editor
Madeline S. Harris

Editorial
Kathleen Edgar, Debra Kirby, Kristine Krapp, Paul Lewon, Elizabeth Manar, Kimberley McGrath, Jennifer Stock

Production Technology
Paul Lewon

Indexing Services
Factiva, Inc.

Rights and Acquisitions
Lisa Kincade, Ronald Montgomery, Tracie Richardson, Robyn Young

Imaging and Multimedia
Lezlie Light

Product Design
Jennifer Wahi

Product Management
Janet Witalec

Composition
Evi Seoud, Mary Beth Trimper

Manufacturing
Wendy Blurton, Dorothy Maki

LIBRARY OF CONGRESS CATALOGING-IN-PUBLICATION DATA

Infectious diseases: in context / Brenda Wilmoth Lerner & K. Lee Lerner, editors.
  p. cm.
  Includes bibliographical references and index.
  ISBN-13: 978-1-4144-2960-1 (set hardcover)–
  ISBN-13: 978-1-4144-2961-8 (vol. 1 hardcover)–
  ISBN-13: 978-1-4144-2962-5 (vol. 2 hardcover)–
  ISBN-13: 978-1-4144-2963-2 (set ebook)
  1. Communicable diseases–Encyclopedias.
  I. Lerner, Brenda Wilmoth. II. Lerner, K. Lee.
  RC111.I516 2008
  616.003–dc22
                                                        2007019024

This title is also available as an e-book.
ISBN 978-1-4144-2963-2
Contact your Gale sales representative for ordering information.

Printed in Canada
10 9 8 7 6 5 4 3 2 1

Contents

VOLUME 1

Contents

VOLUME 2

Contents

Advisors and Contributors

While compiling this volume, the editors relied upon the expertise and contributions of the following scientists, scholars, and researchers, who served as advisors and/or contributors for *Infectious Diseases: In Context*:

Susan Aldridge, Ph.D.
Independent scholar and writer
London, United Kingdom

William Arthur Atkins, M.S.
Independent scholar and writer
Normal, Illinois

Stephen A. Berger, M.D.
Director, Geographic Medicine
Tel Aviv Medical Center
Tel Aviv, Israel

L.S. Clements, M.D., Ph.D.
Assistant Professor of Pediatrics
University of South Alabama
College of Medicine
Mobile, Alabama

Bryan Davies, L.L.B.
Writer and journalist
Ontario, Canada

Paul Davies, Ph.D.
Director, Science Research Institute
Adjunct Professor Université
Paris - La Sorbonne.
Paris, France

Antonio Farina, M.D., Ph.D.
Department of Embryology, Obstetrics, and Gynecology
University of Bologna
Bologna, Italy

Larry Gilman, Ph.D.
Independent scholar and journalist
Sharon, Vermont

Tony Hawas, M.A.
Writer and journalist
Brisbane, Australia

Brian D. Hoyle, Ph.D.
Microbiologist
Nova Scotia, Canada

Kenneth T. LaPensee, Ph.D., MPH
Epidemiologist and Medical Policy Specialist
Hampton, New Jersey

Agnieszka Lichanska, Ph.D.
Institute for Molecular Sciences
University of Queensland
Brisbane, Australia

Adrienne Wilmoth Lerner, J.D.
Independent scholar
Jacksonville, Florida

Eric v.d. Luft, Ph.D., M.L.S.
Adjunct Lecturer, Center for Bioethics and Humanities
SUNY Upstate Medical University
Syracuse, New York

Caryn Neumann, Ph.D.
Visiting Assistant Professor
Denison University
Granville, Ohio

Anna Marie Roos, Ph.D.
Research Associate, Wellcome Unit for the History of Medicine
University of Oxford
Oxford, United Kingdom

Constance K. Stein, Ph.D.
Director of Cytogenetics, Associate Professor
SUNY Upstate Medical University
Syracuse, New York

Jack Woodall, Ph.D.
Director, Nucleus for the Investigation of Emerging Infectious Diseases
Institute of Medical Biochemistry, Center for Health Sciences
Federal University of Rio de Janeiro
Rio de Janeiro, Brazil

Melanie Barton Zoltán, M.S.
Independent scholar
Amherst, Massachusetts

Acknowledgments

The editors are grateful to the truly global group of scholars, researchers, and writers who contributed to *Infectious Diseases: In Context*.

The editors also wish to thank copyeditors Christine Jeryan, Kate Kretchmann, and Alicia Cafferty Lerner, whose keen eyes and sound judgments greatly enhanced the quality and readability of the text.

The editors gratefully acknowledge and extend thanks to Janet Witalec and Debra Kirby at the Gale Group for their faith in the project and for their sound content advice and guidance. Without the able guidance and efforts of talented teams in IT, rights and acquisition management, and imaging at the Gale Group, this book would not have been possible. The editors are especially indebted to Kim McGrath, Elizabeth Manar, Kathleen Edgar, Kristine Krapp, and Jennifer Stock for their invaluable help in correcting copy. The editors also wish to acknowledge the contributions of Marcia Schiff at the Associated Press for her help in securing archival images.

Deep and sincere thanks and appreciation are due to Project Manager Madeline Harris who, despite a myriad of publishing hurdles and woes, managed miracles with skill, grace, and humor.

Introduction

Humanity shares a common ancestry with all living things on Earth. We often share especially close intimacies with the microbial world. In fact, only a small percentage of the cells in the human body are human at all. "We" are vastly outnumbered, even within our bodies, by microbial life that can only be counted on the same scale as the vast numbers of stars in the universe. This is also an essential relationship, because humanity could not survive without an array of microflora that both nourish us and that provide needed enzymes for life processes.

Yet, the common biology and biochemistry that unites us also makes us susceptible to contracting and transmitting infectious disease.

Throughout history, microorganisms have spread deadly diseases and caused widespread epidemics that have threatened and altered human civilization. In the modern era, civic sanitation, water purification, immunization, and antibiotics have dramatically reduced the overall morbidity and the mortality rates of infectious disease in more developed nations. Yet, much of the world is still ravaged by disease and epidemics; new threats constantly appear to challenge the most advanced medical and public health systems.

Although specific diseases may be statistically associated with particular regions or other demographics, disease does not recognize social class or political boundary. In our intimately connected global village, an outbreak of disease in a remote area may quickly transform into a global threat. Given the opportunity, the agents of disease may spread across the globe at the speed of modern travel, and also leap from animals to humans.

The articles presented in these volumes, written by some of the world's leading experts, are designed to be readable and to instruct, challenge, and excite a range of student and reader interests while, at the same time, providing a solid foundation and reference for more advanced students and readers. It speaks both to the seriousness of their dedication to combating infectious disease and to the authors' great credit that the interests of younger students and lay readers were put forefront in preparation of these entries.

The editors are especially pleased to have contributions and original primary source essays within the volumes by experts that are currently in the forefront of international infectious disease research and policy. Jack Woodall, Ph.D., recounts memories of belonging to a team that identified and determined the cause of Machupo hemorrhagic fever in "Virus Hunters" and of his association with the developer of the yellow fever vaccine in "Yellow Fever." He also explains "ProMED," a disease-reporting system (of which Woodall is a founder) that allows scientists around the world, whether in the hospital, laboratory, or the field, to share real-time information about outbreaks of emerging infectious diseases. Jack Woodall now serves as the director of the Nucleus for the Investigation of Emerging Infectious Diseases at the Federal University of Rio de Janeiro in Brazil.

Stephen A. Berger, M.D., Ph.D., Director of Geographic Medicine at Tel Aviv Medical Center in Tel Aviv, Israel, served as a contributing advisor for *Infectious Diseases: In Context* and was the developer of GIDEON (Global Infectious Disease and Epidemiology Network), the world's premier global infectious diseases database. Dr. Berger explains the Web-based tool that helps physicians worldwide diagnose infectious diseases. Dr. Berger also contributes "Travel and Infectious Disease" and a special introduction. Dr. Berger's contributions reflect a dedication to teaching that has five times earned him the New York Medical College Teaching Award. Dr. Berger, author of numerous articles and books, including *Introduction to Infectious Diseases, The Healthy Tourist*, and *Exotic Viral Diseases: A Global Guide,* was gracious with his time, writing, and advice.

The editors are indebted to both of these distinguished scientists for their generous contributions of time and compelling material.

Readers interests were are also well-served by Anthony S. Fauci, M.D., Director of the National Institutes of Allergy and Infectious Diseases, for what was, at the time *Infectious Diseases: In Context* went to press, a preview of his latest version of the map of emerging and re-emerging infectious diseases, and also by L. Scott Clements, M.D., Ph.D., for his advice and articles, including "Childhood Infectious Diseases: Immunization Impacts."

Space limitations of this volume force the editors to include only those infectious diseases that directly affect human health. It is important to note, however, that diseases affecting plants and animals can have a significant indirect impact on the lives of humans. The 2001 outbreak of foot and mouth disease in the United Kingdom, for example, resulted in the slaughter of over six million pigs, sheep, and cattle, crippling farmers, tourism, and other commerce, and ultimately costing an estimated four billion dollars to the U.K. economy. At press time, the cocoa industry in Ghana is threatened by the Cocoa Swollen Shoot Virus, where farmers are reluctant to cut down their infected mature cocoa trees and plant healthy seedlings. Ghana is among the leading exporters worldwide of cocoa for chocolate. Scientists are also concerned about a lack of forthcoming information from the Chinese government concerning an epidemic virus among pigs in China that is contributing to a pork shortage and the strongest inflation in China in a decade. Although these diseases cannot inflict illness in humans, they can ultimately affect the nutritional, social, economic, and political status of a nation and its people.

Despite the profound and fundamental advances in science and medicine during the last fifty years, there has never been a greater need for a book that explains the wide-ranging impacts of infectious disease. It is hubris to assume that science alone will conquer infectious diseases. Globally, deaths due to malaria alone may double over the next twenty years and ominous social and political implications cannot be ignored when death continues to cast a longer shadow over the poorest nations.

The fight against infectious disease depends on far more than advances in science and public health. The hope that threats and devastation of infectious diseases could be eliminated for all humankind have long since been dashed upon the hard realities that health care is disproportionately available, and cavernous gaps still exist between health care in wealthier nations as opposed to poorer nations. Victory in the "war" against infectious disease will require advances in science and advances in our understanding of our fragile environment and common humanity.

K. Lee Lerner & Brenda Wilmoth Lerner, editors

DUBLIN, IRELAND, JULY 2007

Brenda Wilmoth Lerner and K. Lee Lerner were members of the International Society for Infectious Disease and delegates to the 12th International Congress on Infectious Disease in Lisbon, Portugal, in June 2006. Primarily based in London and Paris, the Lerner & Lerner portfolio includes more than two dozen books and films that focus on science and science-related issues.

"...any man's death diminishes me, because I am involved in mankind, and therefore never send to know for whom the bells tolls; it tolls for thee." —John Donne, 1624 (published) *Devotions upon Emergent Occasions*, no. 17 (Meditation)

The book is respectfully dedicated to Dr. Carlo Urbani and those who risk—and far too often sacrifice—their lives in an attempt to lessen the toll of infectious diseases.

A Special Introduction by Stephen A. Berger, M.D.

The Burden of Infectious Disease in Our Changing, Globalizing World

As we move into the twenty-first century, we continue to exist in a sea of ancient, hostile adversaries that threaten our very existence—both as individuals, and as a race of medium-sized mammals. The good news is that modern technology allows us to understand, diagnose, and treat an expanding number of infectious diseases. The bad news is that this same modern technology increasingly places us at risk for those same diseases.

For the purpose of clarity, I will classify the infectious diseases of humans into six broad categories: traditional, new, emerging, re-emerging, disappearing, and extinct. The latter category is depressingly small, and in fact contains only a single disease. The last case of smallpox was reported in Somalia in 1977, and the viral agent hibernates (as far as we know) in secure freezers located in the United States and Russian Federation. The few disappearing diseases include measles, leprosy, guinea worm, and poliomyelitis—conditions whose numbers have decreased in recent years, but which could suddenly blossom into outbreaks when the political and social climate permits.

One must distinguish between "new diseases" and "newly discovered" diseases. The former category includes conditions that had never before affected mankind: AIDS, SARS, Ebola. In contrast, Legionnaire's disease, Chlamydial infection, and Lyme disease appear to have affected man for many centuries, but were only "discovered" when appropriate technology permitted.

Emerging diseases such as West Nile fever and Dengue are certainly not new, but expand both geographically and numerically with the advent of mass tourism and the dispersal of mosquitoes in suitable animals or other vehicles. As the term implies, "re-emerging" diseases such as malaria repopulate areas from which they had been eliminated, often as the result of man-made alteration of the environment, elimination of natural predators, global warming, deforestation, and crowding. The best-known disease in this category is influenza, which is caused by a virus that seems to evolve and mutate continually into agents that are not recognized by the human host. Even this phenomenon is largely driven by the practice of some human populations to raise swine and ducks in crowded, unsanitary conditions that promote interchange of viral material.

The vast majority of infectious diseases might be classified as "traditional," forever with us and largely unchanged: the common cold, chickenpox, urinary tract infection, pneumonia, typhoid, gonorrhea, meningitis, and hundreds of others. In some cases, vaccines have altered the incidence of some traditional diseases among select populations. In other cases, increasing life span and advances in medical and surgical intervention have actually created a favorable ecological niche for heretofore non-pathogenic microbes.

Sadly, several new and distressing disease patterns have been the direct result of advances in managing the infection itself. Tuberculosis has been a largely treatable disease since the 1940's; but as of 2007, strains of the causative agent are increasingly resistant to all known drugs. Highly resistant microbes are now commonplace in cases of AIDS, malaria, and gonorrhea, as well as many of the traditional bacteria for which antibiotics were primarily developed: staphylococci, pneumococci and *E. coli*.

Hopefully, the seemingly self-destructive aspect of mankind will be overtaken by continued advances in the treatment, prevention, and understanding of the microbes that share our world.

Stephen A. Berger, M.D.
Director of Geographic Medicine
Tel Aviv Medical Center
Tel Aviv, Israel

About the *In Context* Series

Written by a global array of experts yet aimed primarily at high school students and an interested general readership, the *In Context* series serves as an authoritative reference guide to essential concepts of science, the impacts of recent changes in scientific consensus, and the effects of science on social, political, and legal issues.

Cross-curricular in nature, *In Context* books align with, and support, national science standards and high school science curriculums across subjects in science and the humanities, and facilitate science understanding important to higher achievement in the No Child Left Behind (NCLB) science testing. Inclusion of original essays written by leading experts and primary source documents serve the requirements of an increasing number of high school and international baccalaureate programs, and are designed to provide additional insights on leading social issues, as well as spur critical thinking about the profound cultural connections of science.

In Context books also give special coverage to the impact of science on daily life, commerce, travel, and the future of industrialized and impoverished nations.

Each book in the series features entries with extensively developed words-to-know sections designed to facilitate understanding and increase both reading retention and the ability of students to understand reading in context without being overwhelmed by scientific terminology.

Entries are further designed to include standardized subheads that are specifically designed to present information related to the main focus of the book. Entries also include a listing of further resources (books, periodicals, Web sites, audio and visual media) and references to related entries.

In addition to maps, charts, tables and graphs, each *In Context* title has approximately 300 topic-related images that visually enrich the content. Each *In Context* title will also contain topic-specific timelines (a chronology of major events), a topic-specific glossary, a bibliography, and an index especially prepared to coordinate with the volume topic.

About This Book

The goal of *Infectious Diseases: In Context* is to help high-school and early college-age students understand the essential facts and deeper cultural connections of topics and issues related to the scientific study of infectious disease.

The relationship of science to complex ethical and social considerations is evident, for example, when considering the general rise of infectious diseases that sometimes occurs as an unintended side effect of the otherwise beneficial use of medications. Nearly half the world's population is infected with the bacterium causing tuberculosis (TB); although for most people the infection is inactive, yet the organism causing some new cases of TB is evolving toward a greater resistance to the antibiotics that were once effective in treating TB. Such statistics also take on added social dimension when considering that TB disproportionately impacts certain social groups (the elderly, minority groups, and people infected with HIV).

In an attempt to enrich the reader's understanding of the mutually impacting relationship between science and culture, as space allows we have included primary sources that enhance the content of *In Context* entries. In keeping with the philosophy that much of the benefit from using primary sources derives from the reader's own process of inquiry, the contextual material introducing each primary source provides an unobtrusive introduction and springboard to critical thought.

General Structure

Infectious Diseases: In Context is a collection of 250 entries that provide insight into increasingly important and urgent topics associated with the study of infectious disease.

The articles in the book are meant to be understandable by anyone with a curiosity about topics related to infectious disease, and the first edition of *Infectious Diseases: In Context* has been designed with ready reference in mind:

- Entries are arranged alphabetically, rather than by chronology or scientific subfield.
- The **chronology** (timeline) includes many of the most significant events in the history of infectious disease and advances of science. Where appropriate, related scientific advances are included to offer additional context.
- An extensive glossary section provides readers with a ready reference for content-related terminology. In addition to defining terms within entries, specific Words-to-Know sidebars are placed within each entry.
- A bibliography section (citations of books, periodicals, websites, and audio and visual material) offers additional resources to those resources cited within each entry.
- A **comprehensive general index** guides the reader to topics and persons mentioned in the book.

Entry Structure

In Context entries are designed so that readers may navigate entries with ease. Toward that goal, entries are divided into easy-to-access sections:

- **Introduction**: A opening section designed to clearly identify the topic.
- **Words-to-know** sidebar: Essential terms that enhance readability and critical understanding of entry content.
- Established but flexible **rubrics** customize content presentation and identify each section, enabling the reader to navigate entries with ease. Inside *Infectious Diseases: In Context* entries readers will find two key schemes of organization. Most entries contain internal discussions of **Disease History, Characteristics, and Transmission**, followed by **Scope and Distribution**, then a summary of **Treatment and Prevention**. General social or science topics may have a simpler structure discussing, for example, **History and Scientific Foundations**. Regardless, the goal of *In Context* entries is a consistent, content-appropriate, and easy-to-follow presentation.
- **Impacts and Issues**: Key scientific, political, or social considerations related to the entry topic.
- **Bibliography:** Citations of books, periodicals, web sites, and audio and visual material used in preparation of the entry or that provide a stepping stone to further study.
- **"See also" references** clearly identify other content-related entries.

Infectious Diseases: In Context special style notes

Please note the following with regard to topics and entries included in *Infectious Diseases: In Context*:

- Primary source selection and the composition of sidebars are not attributed to authors of signed entries to which the sidebars may be associated. In all cases, the sources for sidebars containing external content (e.g., a CDC policy position or medical recommendation) are clearly indicated.
- The Centers for Disease Control and Prevention (CDC) includes parasitic diseases with infectious diseases, and the editors have adopted this scheme.
- Equations are, of course, often the most accurate and preferred language of science, and are essential to epidemiologists and medical statisticians. To better serve the intended audience of *Infectious Diseases: In Context*, however, the editors attempted to minimize the inclusion of equations in favor of describing the elegance of thought or essential results such equations yield.
- A detailed understanding of biology and chemistry is neither assumed nor required for *Infectious Diseases: In Context*. Accordingly, students and other readers should not be intimidated or deterred by the sometimes complex names of chemical molecules or biological classification. Where necessary, sufficient information regarding chemical structure or species classification is provided. If desired, more information can easily be obtained from any basic chemistry or biology reference.

Bibliography citation formats (How to cite articles and sources)

In Context titles adopt the following citation format:

Books

Magill, Gerard, ed. *Genetics and Ethics: An Interdisciplinary Study*. New York: Fordham University Press, 2003.

Verlinsky, Yury, and Anver Kuliev. *Practical Preimplantation Genetic Diagnosis*. New York: Springer, 2005.

Web Sites

ADEAR. Alzheimer's Disease Education and Referral Center. National Institute on Aging. <http://www.alzheimers.org/generalinfo.htm> (accessed January 23, 2006).

Genetics and Public Policy Center. <http://dnapolicy.org/index.jhtml.html> (accessed January 23, 2006).

Human Genetics in the Public Interest. The Center for Genetics and Society. <http://www.genetics-and-society.org> (accessed January 26, 2006).

PGD: Preimplantation Genetic Diagnosis. "Discussion by the Genetics and Public Policy Center." <http://dnapolicy.org/downloads/pdfs/policy_pgd.pdf> (accessed January 23, 2006).

Alternative citation formats

There are, however, alternative citation formats that may be useful to readers and examples of how to cite articles in often used alternative formats are shown below.

APA Style

Books: Kübler-Ross, Elizabeth. (1969) *On Death and Dying.* New York: Macmillan. Excerpted in K. Lee Lerner and Brenda Wilmoth Lerner, eds. (2006) *Medicine, Health, and Bioethics: Essential Primary Sources,* Farmington Hills, Mich.: Thomson Gale.

Periodicals: Venter, J. Craig, et al. (2001, February 16). "The Sequence of the Human Genome." *Science,* vol. 291, no. 5507, pp. 1304–51. Excerpted in K. Lee Lerner and Brenda Wilmoth Lerner, eds. (2006) *Medicine, Health, and Bioethics: Essential Primary Sources,* Farmington Hills, Mich.: Thomson Gale.

Web Sites: Johns Hopkins Hospital and Health System. "Patient Rights and Responsibilities." Retrieved January 14, 2006 from Http://www.hopkinsmedicine.org/patients/JHH/patient_rights.html. Excerpted in K. Lee Lerner and Brenda Wilmoth Lerner, eds. (2006) *Medicine, Health, and Bioethics: Essential Primary Sources,* Farmington Hills, Mich.: Thomson Gale.

Chicago Style

Books: Kübler-Ross, Elizabeth. *On Death and Dying.* New York: Macmillan, 1969. Excerpted in K. Lee Lerner and Brenda Wilmoth Lerner, eds. *Medicine, Health, and Bioethics: Essential Primary Sources,* Farmington Hills, MI: Thomson Gale, 2006.

Periodicals: Venter, J. Craig, et al. "The Sequence of the Human Genome." *Science* (2001): 291, 5507, 1304–1351. Excerpted in K. Lee Lerner and Brenda Wilmoth Lerner, eds. *Medicine, Health, and Bioethics: Essential Primary Sources,* Farmington Hills, MI: Thomson Gale, 2006.

Web Sites: *Johns Hopkins Hospital and Health System.* "Patient Rights and Responsibilities." <http://www.hopkinsmedicine.org/patients/JHH/patient_rights.html.> (accessed January 14, 2006). Excerpted in K. Lee Lerner and Brenda Wilmoth Lerner, eds. *Medicine, Health, and Bioethics: Essential Primary Sources,* Farmington Hills, MI: Thomson Gale, 2006.

MLA Style

Books: Kübler-Ross, Elizabeth. *On Death and Dying,* New York: Macmillan, 1969. Excerpted in K. Lee Lerner and Brenda Wilmoth Lerner, eds. *Medicine, Health, and Bioethics: Essential Primary Sources,* Farmington Hills, Mich.: Thomson Gale, 2006.

Periodicals: Venter, J. Craig, et al. "The Sequence of the Human Genome." *Science,* 291 (16 February 2001): 5507, 1304–51. Excerpted in K. Lee Lerner and Brenda Wilmoth Lerner, eds. *Terrorism: Essential Primary Sources,* Farmington Hills, Mich.: Thomson Gale, 2006.

Web Sites: "Patient's Rights and Responsibilities." Johns Hopkins Hospital and Health System. 14 January 2006. <http://www.hopkinsmedicine.org/patients/JHH/patient_rights.html.> Excerpted in K. Lee Lerner and Brenda Wilmoth Lerner, eds. *Terrorism: Essential Primary Sources*, Farmington Hills, Mich.: Thomson Gale, 2006.

Turabian Style (Natural and Social Sciences)

Books: Kübler-Ross, Elizabeth. *On Death and Dying*, (New York: Macmillan, 1969). Excerpted in K. Lee Lerner and Brenda Wilmoth Lerner, eds. *Medicine, Health, and Bioethics: Essential Primary Sources*, (Farmington Hills, Mich.: Thomson Gale, 2006).

Periodicals: Venter, J. Craig, et al. "The Sequence of the Human Genome." *Science*, 291 (16 February 2001): 5507, 1304–1351. Excerpted in K. Lee Lerner and Brenda Wilmoth Lerner, eds. *Medicine, Health, and Bioethics: Essential Primary Sources*, (Farmington Hills, Mich.: Thomson Gale, 2006).

Web Sites: Johns Hopkins Hospital and Health System."Patient's Rights and Responsibilities." available from http://www.hopkinsmedicine.org/patients/JHH/patient_rights.html; accessed14 January 2006. Excerpted in K. Lee Lerner and Brenda Wilmoth Lerner, eds. *Medicine, Health, and Bioethics: Essential Primary Sources*, (Farmington Hills, Mich.: Thomson Gale, 2006).

Using Primary Sources

The definition of what constitutes a primary source is often the subject of scholarly debate and interpretation. Although primary sources come from a wide spectrum of resources, they are united by the fact that they individually provide insight into the historical *milieu* (context and environment) during which they were produced. Primary sources include materials such as newspaper articles, press dispatches, autobiographies, essays, letters, diaries, speeches, song lyrics, posters, works of art—and in the twenty-first century, web logs—that offer direct, first-hand insight or witness to events of their day.

Categories of primary sources include:

- Documents containing firsthand accounts of historic events by witnesses and participants. This category includes diary or journal entries, letters, email, newspaper articles, interviews, memoirs, and testimony in legal proceedings.
- Documents or works representing the official views of both government leaders and leaders of other organizations. These include primary sources such as policy statements, speeches, interviews, press releases, government reports, and legislation.
- Works of art, including (but certainly not limited to) photographs, poems, and songs, including advertisements and reviews of those works that help establish an understanding of the cultural milieu (the cultural environment with regard to attitudes and perceptions of events).
- Secondary sources. In some cases, secondary sources or tertiary sources may be treated as primary sources. For example, if an entry written many years after an event, or to summarize an event, includes quotes, recollections, or retrospectives (accounts of the past) written by participants in the earlier event, the source can be considered a primary source.

Analysis of primary sources

The primary material collected in this volume is not intended to provide a comprehensive or balanced overview of a topic or event. Rather, the primary sources are intended to generate interest and lay a foundation for further inquiry and study.

In order to properly analyze a primary source, readers should remain skeptical and develop probing questions about the source. Using historical documents requires that readers analyze them carefully and extract specific information. However, readers must also read "beyond the text" to garner larger clues about the social impact of the primary source.

In addition to providing information about their topics, primary sources may also supply a wealth of insight into their creator's viewpoint. For example, when reading a news article about an outbreak of disease, consider whether the reporter's words also indicate something about his or her origin, bias (an irrational disposition in favor of someone or something), prejudices (an irrational disposition against someone or something), or intended audience.

Students should remember that primary sources often contain information later proven to be false, or contain viewpoints and terms unacceptable to future generations. It is important to view the primary source within the historical and social context existing at its creation. If for example, a newspaper article is written within hours or days of an event, later developments may reveal some assertions in the original article as false or misleading.

Test new conclusions and ideas

Whatever opinion or working hypothesis the reader forms, it is critical that they then test that hypothesis against other facts and sources related to the incident. For example, it might be wrong to conclude that factual mistakes are deliberate unless evidence can be produced of a pattern and practice of such mistakes with an intent to promote a false idea.

The difference between sound reasoning and preposterous conspiracy theories (or the birth of urban legends) lies in the willingness to test new ideas against other sources, rather than rest on one piece of evidence such as a single primary source that may contain errors. Sound reasoning requires that arguments and assertions guard against argument fallacies that utilize the following:

- false dilemmas (only two choices are given when in fact there are three or more options);
- arguments from ignorance (*argumentum ad ignorantiam*; because something is not known to be true, it is assumed to be false);
- possibilist fallacies (a favorite among conspiracy theorists who attempt to demonstrate that a factual statement is true or false by establishing the possibility of its truth or falsity. An argument where "it could be" is usually followed by an unearned "therefore, it is.");
- slippery slope arguments or fallacies (a series of increasingly dramatic consequences is drawn from an initial fact or idea);
- begging the question (the truth of the conclusion is assumed by the premises);
- straw man arguments (the arguer mischaracterizes an argument or theory and then attacks the merits of their own false representations);
- appeals to pity or force (the argument attempts to persuade people to agree by sympathy or force);
- prejudicial language (values or moral goodness, good and bad, are attached to certain arguments or facts);
- personal attacks (*ad hominem*; an attack on a person's character or circumstances);
- anecdotal or testimonial evidence (stories that are unsupported by impartial observation or data that is not reproducible);
- *post hoc* (after the fact) fallacies (because one thing follows another, it is held to cause the other);
- the fallacy of the appeal to authority (the argument rests upon the credentials of a person, not the evidence).

Despite the fact that some primary sources can contain false information or lead readers to false conclusions based on the "facts" presented, they remain an invaluable resource regarding past events. Primary sources allow readers and researchers to come as close as possible to understanding the perceptions and context of events and thus to more fully appreciate how and why misconceptions occur.

Glossary

A

ABIOGENESIS: Also known as spontaneous generation; the incorrect theory that living things can be generated from nonliving things.

ABIOTIC: A term used to describe the portion of an ecosystem that is not living, such as water or soil.

ABSCESS: An abscess is a pus-filled sore, usually caused by a bacterial infection. It results from the body's defensive reaction to foreign material. Abscesses are often found in the soft tissue under the skin in areas such as the armpit or the groin. However, they may develop in any organ, and they are commonly found in the breast and gums. If they are located in deep organs such as the lung, liver, or brain, abscesses are far more serious and call for more specific treatment.

ACARACIDES: Chemicals that kill mites and ticks are acaracides.

ACQUIRED (ADAPTIVE) IMMUNITY: Immunity is the ability to resist infection and is subdivided into innate immunity, which an individual is born with, and acquired, or adaptive, immunity, which develops according to circumstances and is targeted to a specific pathogen. There are two types of acquired immunity, known as active and passive. Active immunity is either humoral, involving production of antibody molecules against a bacterium or virus, or cell-mediated, where T-cells are mobilized against infected cells. Infection and immunization can both induce acquired immunity. Passive immunity is induced by injection of the serum of a person who is already immune to a particular infection.

ACQUIRED IMMUNODEFICIENCY SYNDROME (AIDS): A disease of the immune system caused by the human immunodeficiency virus (HIV). It is characterized by the destruction of a particular type of white blood cell and increased susceptibility to infection and other diseases.

ACTIVE INFECTION: An active infection is one that is currently producing symptoms or in which the infective agent is multiplying rapidly. In contrast, a latent infection is one in which the infective agent is present, but not causing symptoms or damage to the body nor reproducing at a significant rate.

ADAPTIVE IMMUNITY: Adaptive immunity is another term for acquired immunity, referring to the resistance to infection that develops through life and is targeted to a specific pathogen. There are two types of adaptive immunity, known as active and passive. Active immunity is either humoral, involving production of antibody molecules against a bacterium or virus, or cell-mediated, in which T-cells are mobilized against infected cells. Infection and immunization can both induce acquired immunity.

ADHESION: Physical attraction between different types of molecules.

AEROBES: Aerobic microorganisms require the presence of oxygen for growth. Molecular oxygen functions in the respiratory pathway of the microbes to produce the energy necessary for life. Bacteria, yeasts, fungi, and algae are capable of aerobic growth.

AEROSOL: Particles of liquid or solid dispersed as a suspension in gas.

AGGREGATIONS: When blood clots (becomes solid, usually in response to injury), cells called platelets form clumps called aggregations. An instrument called an aggregometer measures the degree of platelet aggregation in blood.

AIDS (ACQUIRED IMMUNODEFICIENCY SYNDROME): A disease of the immune system caused by the human immunodeficiency virus (HIV). It is characterized by the destruction of a particular type of white blood cell and increased susceptibility to infection and other diseases.

AIRBORNE PRECAUTIONS: Airborne precautions are procedures that are designed to reduce the chance that certain disease-causing (pathogenic) microorganisms will be transmitted through the air.

AIRBORNE TRANSMISSION: Airborne transmission refers to the ability of a disease-causing (pathogenic) microorganism to be spread through the air by droplets expelled during sneezing or coughing.

ALLELE: Any of two or more alternative forms of a gene that occupy the same location on a chromosome.

ALLERGIES: An allergy is an excessive or hypersensitive response of the immune system to substances (allergens) in the environment. Instead of fighting off a disease-causing foreign substance, the immune system launches a complex series of actions against the particular irritating allergen. The immune response may be accompanied by a number of stressful symptoms, ranging from mild to life threatening. In rare cases, an allergic reaction leads to anaphylactic shock—a condition characterized by a sudden drop in blood pressure, difficulty in breathing, skin irritation, collapse, and possible death.

ALVEOLI: An alveolus (alveoli is plural) is a tiny air sac located within the lungs. The exchange of oxygen and carbon dioxide takes place within these sacs.

AMEBIC DYSENTERY: Amebic (or amoebic) dysentery, which is also referred to as amebiasis or amoebiasis, is an inflammation of the intestine caused by the parasite *Entamoeba histolytica*. The severe form of the malady is characterized by the formation of localized lesions (ulcers) in the intestine, especially in the region known as the colon; abscesses in the liver and the brain; vomiting; severe diarrhea with fluid loss leading to dehydration; and abdominal pain.

AMERICAN TYPE CULTURE COLLECTION: The American Type Culture Collection (ATCC) is a not-for-profit bioscience organization that maintains the world's largest and most diverse collection of microbiological life. Many laboratories and institutions maintain their own stockpile of microorganisms, usually those that are in frequent use in the facility. Some large culture collections are housed and maintained by universities or private enterprises, but none of these rivals the ATCC in terms of size.

AMPLIFICATION: A process by which something is made larger or the quantity increased.

ANADROMOUS: Fish that migrate from ocean (salt) water to fresh water, such as salmon, are termed anadromous.

ANAEROBIC BACTERIA: Bacteria that grow without oxygen, also called anaerobic bacteria or anaerobes. Anaerobic bacteria can infect deep wounds, deep tissues, and internal organs where there is little oxygen. These infections are characterized by abscess formation, foul-smelling pus, and tissue destruction.

ANTHRAX: Anthrax refers to a disease that is caused by the bacterium *Bacillus anthracis*. The bacterium can enter the body via a wound in the skin (cutaneous anthrax), via contaminated food or liquid (gastrointestinal anthrax), or can be inhaled (inhalation anthrax).

ANTIBACTERIAL: A substance that reduces or kills germs (bacteria and other microorganisms but not viruses). Also often a term used to describe a drug used to treat bacterial infections.

ANTIBIOTIC: A drug, such as penicillin, used to fight infections caused by bacteria. Antibiotics act only on bacteria and are not effective against viruses.

ANTIBIOTIC RESISTANCE: The ability of bacteria to resist the actions of antibiotic drugs.

ANTIBIOTIC SENSITIVITY: Antibiotic sensitivity refers to the susceptibility of a bacterium to an antibiotic. Each type of bacteria can be killed by some types of antibiotics and not be affected by other types. Different types of bacteria exhibit different patterns of antibiotic sensitivity.

ANTIBODIES: Antibodies, or Y-shaped immunoglobulins, are proteins found in the blood that help to fight against foreign substances called antigens. Antigens, which are usually proteins or polysaccharides, stimulate the immune system to produce antibodies. The antibodies inactivate the antigen and help to remove it from the body. While antigens can be the source of infections from pathogenic bacteria and viruses, organic molecules detrimental to the body from internal or environmental sources also act as antigens. Genetic engineering and the use of various mutational mechanisms allow the construction of a vast array of antibodies (each with a unique genetic sequence).

ANTIBODY RESPONSE: The specific immune response that utilizes B cells to kill certain kinds of antigens.

ANTIBODY-ANTIGEN BINDING: Antibodies are produced by the immune system in response to antigens (material perceived as foreign). The antibody response to a particular antigen is highly specific and often involves a physical association between the two molecules. Biochemical and molecular forces govern this association.

ANTIFUNGAL: Antifungals (also called antifungal drugs) are medicines used to fight fungal infections. They are of two kinds, systemic and topical. Systemic antifungal drugs are medicines taken by mouth or by injection to treat infections caused by a fungus. Topical antifungal drugs are medicines applied to the skin to treat skin infections caused by a fungus.

ANTIGEN: Antigens, which are usually proteins or polysaccharides, stimulate the immune system to produce antibodies. The antibodies inactivate the antigen and help to remove it from the body. While antigens can be the source of infections from pathogenic bacteria and viruses, organic molecules detrimental to the body from internal or environmental sources also act as antigens. Genetic engineering and the use of various mutational mechanisms allow the construction of a vast array of antibodies (each with a unique genetic sequence).

ANTIGENIC DRIFT: Antigenic drift describes the gradual accumulation of mutations in genes (e.g., in genes coding for surface proteins) over a period of time.

ANTIGENIC SHIFT: Antigenic shift describes an abrupt and major genetic change (e.g., in genes coding for surface proteins of a virus).

ANTIHELMINTHIC: Antihelminthic drugs are medicines that rid the body of parasitic worms.

ANTIMICROBIAL: An antimicrobial material slows the growth of bacteria or is able to kill bacteria. Antimicrobial materials include antibiotics (which can be used inside the body) and disinfectants (which can only be used outside the body).

ANTIRETROVIRAL (ARV) DRUGS: Antiretroviral (ARV) drugs prevent the reproduction of a type of virus called a retrovirus. The human immunodefiency virus (HIV), which causes acquired immune deficiency syndrome (AIDS, also cited as acquired immune deficiency syndrome), is a retrovirus. These ARV drugs are therefore used to treat HIV infections. These medicines cannot prevent or cure HIV infection, but they help to keep the virus in check.

ANTIRETROVIRAL (ARV) THERAPY: Treatment with antiretroviral (ARV) drugs prevents the reproduction of a type of virus called a retrovirus. The human immunodeficiency virus (HIV), which causes acquired immu-

nodeficiency syndrome (AIDS, also cited as acquired immune deficiency syndrome), is a retrovirus. ARV drugs are therefore used to treat HIV infections. These medicines cannot prevent or cure HIV infection, but they help to keep the virus in check.

ANTISENSE DRUG: An antisense drug binds to mRNA, thereby blocking gene activity. Some viruses have mRNA as their genetic material, so an antisense drug could inhibit their replication.

ANTISEPTIC: A substance that prevents or stops the growth and multiplication of microorganisms in or on living tissue.

ANTITOXIN: An antidote to a toxin that neutralizes its poisonous effects.

ANTIVIRAL DRUGS: Antiviral drugs are compounds that are used to prevent or treat viral infections, via the disruption of an infectious mechanism used by the virus, or to treat the symptoms of an infection.

ARBOVIRUS: An arbovirus is a virus that is typically spread by blood-sucking insects, most commonly mosquitoes. Over 100 types of arboviruses cause disease in humans. Yellow fever and dengue fever are two examples.

ARENAVIRUS: An arenavirus is a virus that belongs in a viral family known as Arenaviridae. The name arenavirus derives from the appearance of the spherical virus particles when cut into thin sections and viewed using a transmission electron microscope. The interior of the particles is grainy or sandy in appearance, due to the presence of ribosomes that have been acquired from the host cell. The Latin designation *arena* means "sandy."

ARTHROPOD: A member of the largest single animal phylum, consisting of organisms with segmented bodies, jointed legs or wings, and exoskeletons.

ARTHROPOD-BORNE DISEASE: A disease caused by one of a phylum of organisms characterized by exoskeletons and segmented bodies.

ARTHROPOD-BORNE VIRUS: A virus caused by one of a phylum of organisms characterized by exoskeletons and segmented bodies.

ASEPSIS: Asepsis means without germs, more specifically without microorganisms.

ASPIRATION: Aspiration is the drawing out of fluid from a part of the body; it can cause pneumonia when stomach contents are transferred to the lungs through vomiting.

ASSAY: A determination of an amount of a particular compound in a sample (e.g., to make chemical tests to determine the relative amount of a particular substance in a sample). A method used to quantify a biological compound.

ASYMPTOMATIC: A state in which an individual does not exhibit or experience symptoms of a disease.

ATAXIA: Ataxia is an unsteadiness in walking or standing that is associated with brain diseases such as kuru or Creutzfeldt-Jakob disease.

ATOPY: Atopy is an inherited tendency towards hypersensitivity towards immunoglobulin E, a key component of the immune system, which plays an important role in asthma, eczema, and hay fever.

ATROPHY: Decreasing in size or wasting away of a body part or tissue.

ATTENUATED: An attenuated bacterium or virus has been weakened and is often used as the basis of a vaccine against the specific disease caused by the bacterium or virus.

ATTENUATED STRAIN: A specific strain of bacteria that has been killed or weakened, often used as the basis of a vaccine against the specific disease caused by the bacterium.

AUTOCLAVE: An autoclave is a device that is designed to kill microorganisms on solid items and in liquids by exposure to steam at a high pressure.

AUTOIMMUNE DISEASE: A disease in which the body's defense system attacks its own tissues and organs.

AUTOINFECTION: Autoinfection is the reinfection of the body by a disease organism already in the body, such as eggs left by a parasitic worm.

B

B CELL: Also known as B lymphocyte; a kind of cell produced in bone marrow that secretes antibodies.

BABESIOSIS: An infection of the red blood cells caused by *Babesia microti*, a form of parasite (parasitic sporozoan).

BACILLUS ANTHRACIS: The bacterium that causes anthrax.

BACTEREMIA: Bacteremia occurs when bacteria enter the bloodstream. This condition may occur through a wound or infection or through a surgical procedure or injection. Bacteremia may cause no symptoms and resolve without treatment, or it may produce fever and other symptoms of infection. In some cases, bacteremia leads to septic shock, a potentially life-threatening condition.

BACTERIA: Single-celled microorganisms that live in soil, water, plants, and animals, and whose activities range from the development of disease to fermentation. They play a key role in the decay of organic matter and the cycling of nutrients. Bacteria exist in various shapes, including spherical, rod-shaped, and spiral. Some bacteria are agents of disease. Different types of bacteria cause many sexually transmitted diseases, including syphilis, gonorrhea, and chlamydia. Bacteria also cause diseases such as typhoid, dysentery, and tetanus. Bacterium is the singular form of bacteria.

BACTERIOCIDAL: Bacteriocidal is a term that refers to the treatment of a bacterium such that the organism is killed. A bacteriocidal treatment is always lethal and is also referred to as sterilization.

BACTERIOLOGICAL STRAIN: A bacterial subclass of a particular tribe and genus.

BACTERIOPHAGE: A bacteriophage is a virus that infects bacteria. When a bacteriophage that carries the diphtheria toxin gene infects diphtheria bacteria, the bacteria produce diphtheria toxin.

BACTERIOSTATIC: Bacteriostatic refers to a treatment that restricts the ability of the bacterium to grow.

BACTERIUM: Singular form of the term bacteria—single-celled microorganisms—bacterium refers to an individual microorganism.

BASIDIOSPORE: A fungal spore of Basidomycetes. Basidomycetes are classified under the Fungi kingdom as belonging to the phylum Mycota (i.e., Basidomycota or Basidiomycota), class Mycetes (i.e., Basidiomycetes). Fungi are frequently parasites that decompose organic material from their hosts, such as the parasites that grow on rotten wood, although some may cause serious plant diseases such as smuts (Ustomycetes) and rusts (Teliomycetes). Some live in a symbiotic relationship with plant roots (Mycorrhizae). A cell type termed basidium is responsible for sexual spore formation in Basidomycetes, through nuclear fusion followed by meiosis, thus forming haploid basidiospores.

BED NETS: A type of netting that provides protection from diseases caused by insects such as flies and mosquitoes. It is often used when sleeping to allow air to flow through its mesh structure while preventing insects from biting.

BIFURCATED NEEDLE: A bifurcated needle is a needle that has two prongs with a wire suspended between them. The wire is designed to hold a certain amount of vaccine. Development of the bifurcated needle was a major advance in vaccination against smallpox.

BIOFILM: A biofilm is a population of microorganisms that forms following the adhesion of bacteria, algae, yeast, or fungi to a surface. These surface growths can be found in natural settings such as on rocks in streams and in infections such as can occur on catheters. Microorganisms can colonize living and inert natural and synthetic surfaces.

BIOINFORMATICS: Bioinformatics, or computational biology, refers to the development of new database methods to store genomic information (information related to genes and the genetic sequence), computational software programs, and methods to extract, process, and evaluate this information. Bioinformatics also refers to the refinement of existing techniques to acquire the genomic data. Finding genes and determining their function, predicting the structure of proteins and sequence of ribonucleic acid (RNA) from the available sequence of deoxyribonucleic acid (DNA), and determining the evolutionary relationship of proteins and DNA sequences are aspects of bioinformatics.

BIOLOGICAL WARFARE: Biological warfare, as defined by The United Nations, is the use of any living organism (e.g., bacterium, virus) or an infective component (e.g., toxin), to cause disease or death in humans, animals, or plants. In contrast to bioterrorism, biological warfare is defined as the "state-sanctioned" use of biological weapons on an opposing military force or civilian population.

BIOLOGICAL WEAPON: A weapon that contains or disperses a biological toxin, disease-causing microorganism, or other biological agent intended to harm or kill plants, animals, or humans.

BIOMAGNIFICATION: The increasing concentration of compounds at a higher trophic level or the tendency of organisms to accumulate certain chemicals to a concentration larger than that occurring in their inorganic, non-living environment, such as soil or water, or, in the case of animals, larger than in their food.

BIOMODULATOR: A biomodulator, short for biologic response modulator, is an agent that modifies some characteristic of the immune system, which may help in the fight against infection.

BIOSAFETY LABORATORY: A laboratory that deals with all aspects of potentially infectious agents or biohazards.

BIOSAFETY LEVEL 4 FACILITY: A specialized biosafety laboratory that deals with dangerous or exotic infectious agents or biohazards that are considered high risks for spreading life-threatening diseases, either because the disease is spread through aerosols or because there is no therapy or vaccine to counter the disease.

BIOSHIELD PROJECT: A joint effort between the U.S. Department of Homeland Security and the Department of Health and Human Services, Project Bio-Shield is tasked to improve treatment of diseases caused by biological, chemical, and radiological weapons.

BIOSPHERE: The sum total of all life-forms on Earth and the interaction among those life-forms.

BIOTECHNOLOGY: Use of biological organisms, systems, or processes to make or modify products.

BIOWEAPON: A weapon that uses bacteria, viruses, or poisonous substances made by bacteria or viruses.

BLOODBORNE PATHOGENS: Disease-causing agents carried or transported in the blood. Bloodborne infections are those in which the infectious agent is transmitted from one person to another via contaminated blood.

BLOODBORNE ROUTE: Via the blood. For example, bloodborne pathogens are pathogens (disease-causing agents) carried or transported in the blood. Bloodborne infections are those in which the infectious agent is transmitted from one person to another via contaminated blood. Infections of the blood can occur as a result of the spread of an ongoing infection caused by bacteria such as *Yersinia pestis, Haemophilus influenzae,* or *Staphylococcus aureus.*

BOTULINUM TOXIN: Botulinum toxin is among the most poisonous substances known. The toxin, which can be ingested or inhaled, and which disrupts transmission of nerve impulses to muscles, is naturally produced by the bacterium *Clostridium botulinum.* Certain strains of *C. baratii* and *C. butyricum* can also be capable of producing the toxin.

BOTULISM: Botulism is an illness produced by a toxin that is released by the soil bacterium *Clostridium botulinum.* One type of toxin is also produced by *Clostridium baratii.* The toxins affect nerves and can produce paralysis. The paralysis can affect the functioning of organs and tissues that are vital to life.

BROAD-SPECTRUM: The term "broad-spectrum" refers to a series of objects or ideas with great variety between them. In medicine, the term is often applied to drugs, which act on a large number of different disease-causing agents.

BROAD-SPECTRUM ANTIBIOTICS: Broad-spectrum antibiotics are drugs that kill a wide range of bacteria rather than just those from a specific family. For example, Amoxicillin is a broad-spectrum antibiotic that is used against many common illnesses such as ear infections.

BRONCHIOLITIS: Bronciolitis is an inflammation (-itis) of the bronchioles, the small air passages in the lungs that enter the alveoli (air sacs).

BUBO: A swollen lymph gland, usually in the groin or armpit, characteristic of infection with bubonic plague.

BUSH MEAT: The meat of terrestrial wild and exotic animals, typically those that live in parts of Africa, Asia, and the Americas; also known as wild meat.

C

CADAVER: The body of a deceased human, especially one designated for scientific dissection or other research.

CAMPYLOBACTERIOSIS: Campylobacteriosis is a bacterial infection of the intestinal tract of humans. The infection, which typically results in diarrhea, is caused by members of the genus *Campylobacter*. In particular, *Campylobacter jejuni* is the most common cause of bacterial diarrhea in the United States, with more occurrences than salmonella (another prominent disease-causing bacteria associated with food poisoning). Worldwide, approximately 5 to 14% of all diarrhea may be the result of campylobacteriosis.

CAPSID: The protein shell surrounding a virus particle.

CARBOLIC ACID: An acidic compound that, when diluted with water, is used as an antiseptic and disinfectant.

CARCINOGEN: A carcinogen is any biological, chemical, or physical substance or agent that can cause cancer. There are over one hundred different types of cancer, which can be distinguished by the type of cell or organ that is affected, the treatment plan employed, and the cause of the cancer. Most of the carcinogens that are commonly discussed come from chemical sources artificially produced by humans. Some of the better-known carcinogens are the pesticide DDT (dichlorodiphenyltrichloroethane), asbestos, and the carcinogens produced when tobacco is smoked.

CASE FATALITY RATE: The rate of patients suffering disease or injury that die as a result of that disease or injury during a specific period of time.

CASE FATALITY RATIO: A ratio indicating the amount of persons who die as a result of a particular disease, usually expressed as a percentage or as the number of deaths per 1,000 cases.

CATALYST: Substance that speeds up a chemical process without actually changing the products of reaction.

CD4+ T CELLS: CD4 cells are a type of T cell found in the immune system that are characterized by the presence of a CD4 antigen protein on their surface. These are the cells most often destroyed as a result of HIV infection.

CELL CYCLE AND CELL DIVISION: The series of stages that a cell undergoes while progressing to division is known as cell cycle. In order for an organism to grow and develop, the organism's cells must be able to duplicate themselves. Three basic events must take place to achieve this duplication: the deoxyribonucleic acid (DNA), which makes up the individual chromosomes within the cell's nucleus must be duplicated; the two sets of DNA must be packaged up into two separate nuclei; and the cell's cytoplasm must divide itself to create two separate cells, each complete with its own nucleus. The two new cells—products of the single original cell—are known as daughter cells.

CELL MEMBRANE: The cell is bound by an outer membrane that, as described by a membrane model termed the fluid mosaic model, is comprised of a phospholipid lipid bilayer with proteins—molecules that also act as receptor sites—interspersed within the phospholipid bilayer. Varieties of channels exist within the membrane. In eukaryotes (cells with a true nucleus) there are a number of internal cellular membranes that can partition regions within the cells' interior. Some of these membranes ultimately become continuous with the nuclear membrane. Bacteria and viruses do not have inner membranes.

CENTERS FOR DISEASE CONTROL AND PREVENTION (CDC): The Centers for Disease Control and Prevention (CDC) is one of the primary public health institutions in the world. CDC is headquartered in Atlanta, Georgia, with facilities at nine other sites in the United States. The centers are the focus of U.S. government efforts to develop and implement prevention and control strategies for diseases, including those of microbiological origin.

CESTODE: A class of worms characterized by flat, segmented bodies, commonly known as tapeworms.

CHAGAS DISEASE: Chagas disease is a human infection that is caused by a microorganism that establishes a parasitic relationship with a human host as part of its life cycle. The disease is named for the Brazilian physician Carlos Chagas, who in 1909 described the involvement of the flagellated protozoan known as *Trypanosoma cruzi* in a prevalent disease in South America.

CHAIN OF TRANSMISSION: Chain of transmission refers to the route by which an infection is spread from its source to a susceptible host. An example of a chain of transmission is the spread of malaria from an infected animal to humans via mosquitoes.

CHANCRE: A sore that occurs in the first stage of syphilis at the place where the infection entered the body.

CHEMILUMINESCENT SIGNAL: A chemiluminescent signal is the production of light that results from a chemical reaction. A variety of tests to detect infectious organisms or target components of the organisms rely on the binding of a chemical-containing probe to the target and the subsequent development of light following the addition of a reactive compound.

CHEMOTHERAPY: Chemotherapy is the treatment of a disease, infection, or condition with chemicals that have a specific effect on its cause, such as a microorganism or cancer cell. The first modern therapeutic chemical was derived from a synthetic dye. The sulfonamide drugs developed in the 1930s, penicillin and other antibiotics of the 1940s, hormones in the 1950s, and more recent drugs that interfere with cancer cell metabolism and reproduction have all been part of the chemotherapeutic arsenal.

CHICKENPOX: Chickenpox (also called varicella disease and sometimes spelled chicken pox) is a common and extremely infectious childhood disease that can also affect adults. It produces an itchy, blistery rash that typically lasts about a week and is sometimes accompanied by a fever.

CHILDBED FEVER: A bacterial infection occurring in women following childbirth, causing fever and, in some cases, blood poisoning and possible death.

CHLORINATION: Chlorination refers to a chemical process that is used primarily to disinfect drinking water and spills of microorganisms. The active agent in chlorination is the element chlorine, or a derivative of chlorine (e.g., chlorine dioxide). Chlorination is a swift and economical means of destroying many, but not all, microorganisms that are a health-threat in fluids such as drinking water.

CHRONIC: Chronic infections persist for prolonged periods of time—months or even years—in the host. This lengthy persistence is due to a number of factors, which can include masking of the disease-causing agent (e.g., bacteria) from the immune system, invasion of host cells, and the establishment of an infection that is resistant to antibacterial agents.

CHRONIC FATIGUE SYNDROME: Chronic fatigue syndrome (CFS) is a condition that causes extreme tiredness. People with CFS have debilitating fatigue that lasts for six months or longer. They also have many other symptoms. Some of these symptoms are pain in the joints and muscles, headache, and sore throat. CFS appears to result from a combination of factors.

CILIA: Cilia are specialized arrangements of microtubules and have two general functions. They propel certain unicellular organisms, such as paramecium, through the water. In multicellular organisms, if cilia extend from stationary cells that are part of a tissue layer, they move fluid over the surface of the tissue.

CIRRHOSIS: Cirrhosis is a chronic, degenerative, irreversible liver disease in which normal liver cells are damaged and are then replaced by scar tissue. Cirrhosis changes the structure of the liver and the blood vessels that nourish it. The disease reduces the liver's ability to manufacture proteins and process hormones, nutrients, medications, and poisons.

CLINICAL TRIALS: According to the National Institutes of Health, a clinical trial is "a research study to answer specific questions about vaccines or new therapies or new ways of using known treatments." These studies allow researchers to determine whether new drugs or treatments are safe and effective. When conducted carefully, clinical trials can provide fast and safe answers to these questions.

CLOACA: The cavity into which the intestinal, genital, and urinary tracts open in vertebrates such as fish, reptiles, birds, and some primitive mammals.

CLUSTER: In epidemiology, cluster refers to a grouping of individuals contracting an infectious disease or foodborne illness very close in time or place.

COCCIDIUM: Any single-celled animal (protozoan) belonging to the sub-class Coccidia. Some coccidia species can infest the digestive tract, causing coccidiosis.

COHORT: A cohort is a group of people (or any species) sharing a common characteristic. Cohorts are identified and grouped in cohort studies to determine the frequency of diseases or the kinds of disease outcomes over time.

COHORTING: Cohorting is the practice of grouping persons with similar infections or symptoms together, in order to reduce transmission to others.

COLONIZATION: Colonization is the process of occupation and increase in number of microorganisms at a specific site.

COLONIZE: Colonize refers to the process in which a microorganism is able to persist and grow at a given location.

COMMUNITY-ACQUIRED INFECTION: Community-acquired infection is an infection that develops outside of a hospital, in the general community. It differs from hospital-acquired infections in that those who are infected are typically in better health than hospitalized people.

CONGENITAL: Existing at the time of birth.

CONJUNCTIVITIS: Conjunctivitis (also called pink eye) is an inflammation or redness of the lining of the white part of the eye and the underside of the eyelid (conjunctiva) that can be caused by infection, allergic reaction, or physical agents like infrared or ultraviolet light. Conjunctivitis is one of the most common eye infections in children and adults in the United States. Luckily, it is also one of the most treatable infections. Because it is so common in the United States and around the world, and is often not reported to health organizations, accurate statistics are not available for conjunctivitis.

CONTACT PRECAUTIONS: Contact precautions are actions developed to minimize the transfer of microorganisms directly by physical contact and indirectly by touching a contaminated surface.

CONTAGIOUS: A disease that is easily spread among a population, usually by casual person-to-person contact.

CONTAMINATED: The unwanted presence of a microorganism or compound in a particular environment. That environment can be in the laboratory setting, for example, in a medium being used for the growth of a species of bacteria during an experiment. Another environment can be the human body, where contamination by bacteria can produce an infection. Contamination by bacteria and viruses can occur on several levels and their presence can adversely influence the results of experiments. Outside the laboratory, bacteria and viruses can contaminate drinking water supplies, foodstuffs, and products, thus causing illness.

COWPOX: Cowpox refers to a disease that is caused by the cowpox or catpox virus. The virus is a member of the orthopoxvirus family. Other viruses in this family include the smallpox and vaccinia viruses. Cowpox is a rare disease and is mostly noteworthy as the basis of the formulation, over 200 years ago, of an injection by Edward Jenner that proved successful in curing smallpox.

CREPITANT: A crackling sound that accompanies breathing, a common symptom of pneumonia or other diseases of the lungs.

CREUTZFELDT-JAKOB DISEASE (CJD): Creutzfeldt-Jakob disease (CJD) is a transmissible, rapidly progressing, fatal neurodegenerative disorder related to bovine spongiform encephalopathy (BSE), commonly called mad cow disease.

CULL: A cull is the selection, often for destruction, of a part of an animal population. Often done just to reduce numbers, a widespread cull was carried out during the epidemic of bovine spongiform encephalopathy (BSE or mad cow disease) in the United Kingdom during the 1980s.

CULTURE: A culture is a single species of microorganism that is isolated and grown under controlled conditions. The German bacteriologist Robert Koch first developed culturing techniques in the late 1870s. Following Koch's initial discovery, medical scientists quickly sought to identify other pathogens. Today bacteria cultures are used as basic tools in microbiology and medicine.

CULTURE AND SENSITIVITY: Culture and sensitivity refer to laboratory tests that are used to identify the type of microorganism causing an infection and the compounds to which the identified organism is sensitive and resistant. In the case of bacteria, this approach permits the selection of antibiotics that will be most effective in dealing with the infection.

CUTANEOUS: Pertaining to the skin.

CYST: Refers to either a closed cavity or sac or the stage of life during which some parasites live inside an enclosed area. In a protozoan's life, it is a stage when it is covered by a tough outer shell and has become dormant.

CYTOKINE: Cytokines are a family of small proteins that mediate an organism's response to injury or infection. Cytokines operate by transmitting signals between cells in an organism. Minute quantities of cytokines are secreted, each by a single cell type, and regulate functions in other cells by binding with specific receptors. Their interactions with the receptors produce secondary signals that inhibit or enhance the action of certain genes within the cell. Unlike endocrine hormones, which can act throughout the body, most cytokines act locally near the cells that produced them.

CYTOTOXIC: A cytotoxic agent is one that kills cells. Cytotoxic drugs kill cancer cells but may also have application in killing bacteria.

D

DEBRIDEMENT: Debridement is the medical process of removing dead, damaged, or infected tissue from pressure ulcers, burns, and other wounds, in order to speed healing of the surrounding healthy tissue.

DEFINITIVE HOST: The organism in which a parasite reaches reproductive maturity.

DEGRADATION (CELLULAR): Degradation means breakdown and refers to the destruction of host cell components, such as DNA, by infective agents such as bacteria and viruses.

DEHYDRATION: Dehydration is the loss of water and salts essential for normal bodily function. It occurs when the body loses more fluid than it takes in. Water is very important to the human body because it makes up about 70% of the muscles, around 75% of the brain, and approximately 92% of the blood. A person who weights about 150 pounds (68 kilograms) will contain about 80 quarts (just over 75 liters) of water. About two cups of water are lost each day just from regular breathing. If the body sweats more and breathes more heavily than normal, the human body loses even more water. Dehydration occurs when that lost water is not replenished.

DEMENTIA: Dementia, which is from the Latin word *dement* meaning "away mind," is a progressive deterioration and eventual loss of mental ability that is severe enough to interfere with normal activities of daily living; lasts more than six months; has not been present since birth; and is not associated with a loss or alteration of consciousness. Dementia is a group of symptoms caused by gradual death of brain cells. Dementia is usually caused by degeneration in the cerebral cortex, the part of the brain responsible for thoughts, memories, actions, and personality. Death of brain cells in this region leads to the cognitive impairment that characterizes dementia.

DEMOGRAPHICS: The characteristics of human populations or specific parts of human populations, most often reported through statistics.

DEOXYRIBONUCLEIC ACID (DNA): Deoxyribonucleic acid (DNA) is a double-stranded, helical molecule that forms the molecular basis for heredity in most organisms.

DERMATOPHYTE: A dermatophyte is a parasitic fungus that feeds off keratin, a protein which is abundant in skin, nails, and hair and therefore often causes infection of these body parts.

DIAGNOSIS: Identification of a disease or disorder.

DIARRHEA: To most individuals, diarrhea means an increased frequency or decreased consistency of bowel movements; however, the medical definition is more exact than this explanation. In many developed countries, the average number of bowel movements is three per day. However, researchers have found that diarrhea, which is not a disease, best correlates with an increase in stool weight; a stool weight above 10.5 ounces (300 grams) per day generally indicates diarrhea. This is mainly due to excess water, which normally makes up 60 to 85% of fecal matter. In this way, true diarrhea is distinguished from diseases that cause only an increase in the number of bowel movements (hyperdefecation) or incontinence (involuntary loss of bowel contents). Diarrhea is also classified by physicians into acute, which lasts one to two weeks, and chronic, which continues for longer than four weeks. Viral and bacterial infections are the most common causes of acute diarrhea.

DIATOM: Algae are a diverse group of simple, nucleated, plant-like aquatic organisms that are primary producers. Primary producers are able to utilize photosynthesis to create organic molecules from sunlight, water, and carbon dioxide. Ecologically vital, algae account for roughly half of the photosynthetic production of organic material on Earth in both freshwater and marine environments. Algae exist either as single cells or as multicellular organizations. Diatoms are microscopic, single-celled algae that have intricate glass-like outer cell walls partially composed of silicon. Different species of diatom can be identified based upon the structure of these walls. Many diatom species are planktonic, suspended in the water column moving at the mercy of water currents. Others remain attached to submerged surfaces. One bucketful of water may contain millions of diatoms. Their abundance makes them important food sources in aquatic ecosystems.

DIMORPHIC: This refers to the occurrence of two different shapes or color forms within the species, usually occurring as sexual dimorphism between males and females.

DINOFLAGELLATE: Dinoflagellates are microorganisms that are regarded as algae. Their wide array of exotic shapes and, sometimes, armored appearance, is distinct from other algae. The closest microorganisms in appearance are the diatoms.

DIPHTHERIA: Diphtheria is a potentially fatal, contagious bacterial disease that usually involves the nose, throat, and air passages, but may also infect the skin. Its most striking feature is the formation of a grayish membrane covering the tonsils and upper part of the throat.

DISINFECTANT: Disinfection and the use of chemical disinfectants is one key strategy of infection control. Disinfectants reduce the number of living microorganisms, usually to a level that is considered to be safe for the particular environment. Typically, this entails the destruction of those microbes that are capable of causing disease.

DISSEMINATED: Disseminated refers to the previous distribution of a disease-causing microorganism over a larger area.

DISSEMINATION: The spreading of a disease in a population, or of disease organisms in the body, is dissemination. A disease that occurs over a large geographic area.

DISTAL: Distal comes from the same root word as "distant," and is the medical word for distant from some agreed-on point of reference. For example, the hand is at the distal end of the arm from the trunk.

DNA: Deoxyribonucleic acid, a double-stranded, helical molecule that is found in almost all living cells and that determines the characteristics of each organism.

DNA FINGERPRINTING: DNA fingerprinting is the term applied to a range of techniques that are used to show similarities and dissimilarities between the DNA present in different individuals (or organisms).

DNA PROBES: Substances (agents) that bind directly to a predefined specific sequence of nucleic acids in DNA.

DORMANT: Inactive, but still alive. A resting, nonactive state.

DROPLET: A droplet is a small airborne drop or particle—less than 5 microns (a millionth of a meter) in diameter—of fluid, such as may be expelled by sneezing or coughing.

DROPLET TRANSMISSION: Droplet transmission is the spread of microorganisms from one space to another (including from person to person) via droplets that are larger than 5 microns in diameter. Drop-lets are typically expelled into the air by coughing and sneezing.

DRUG RESISTANCE: Drug resistance develops when an infective agent, such as a bacterium, fungus, or virus, develops a lack of sensitivity to a drug that would normally be able to control or even kill it. This tends to occur with overuse of anti-infective agents, which selects out populations of microbes most able to resist them, while killing off those organisms that are most sensitive. The next time the anti-infective agent is used, it will be less effective, leading to the eventual development of resistance.

DYSENTERY: Dysentery is an infectious disease that has ravaged armies, refugee camps, and prisoner-of-war camps throughout history. The disease is still a major problem in developing countries with primitive sanitary facilities.

DYSPLASIA: Abnormal changes in tissue or cell development.

E

ECTOPARASITES: Parasites that cling to the outside of their host, rather than their host's intestines. Common points of attachment are the gills, fins, or skin of fish.

ELBOW BUMP: The elbow bump is a personal greeting that can be used as an alternative to the handshake: the two people greeting each other bump elbows. It is recommended by the World Health Organization for use by researchers handling highly infectious organisms, such as Ebola virus.

ELECTROLYTES: Compounds that ionize in a solution; electrolytes dissolved in the blood play an important role in maintaining the proper functioning of the body.

ELECTRON: A fundamental particle of matter carrying a single unit of negative electrical charge.

EMBRYONATED: When an embryo has been implanted in a female animal, that animal is said to be embryonated.

EMERGING DISEASE: New infectious diseases such as SARS and West Nile virus, as well as previously known diseases such as malaria, tuberculosis, and bacterial pneumonias that are appearing in forms resistant to drug treatments are termed emerging infectious diseases.

ENCEPHALITIS: A type of acute brain inflammation, most often due to infection by a virus.

ENCEPHALOMYELITIS: Simultaneous inflammation of the brain and spinal cord is encephalomyelitis.

ENCEPHALOPATHY: Any abnormality in the structure or function of the brain.

ENCYSTED LARVAE: Encysted larvae are larvae that are not actively growing and dividing and are more resistant to environmental conditions.

ENDEMIC: Present in a particular area or among a particular group of people.

ENDOCYTOSIS: Endocytosis is a process by which host cells allow the entry of outside substances, including viruses, through their cell membranes.

ENTERIC: Involving the intestinal tract or relating to the intestines.

ENTEROBACTERIAL INFECTIONS: Enterobacterial infections are caused by a group of bacteria that dwell in the intestinal tract of humans and other warm-blooded animals. The bacteria are all Gram-negative and rod-shaped. As a group they are termed Enterobacteriaceae. A prominent member of this group is *Escherichia coli*. Other members are the various species in the genera *Salmonella, Shigella, Klebsiella, Enterobacter, Serratia, Proteus*, and *Yersinia*.

ENTEROPATHOGEN: An enteropathogen is a virus or pathogen that invades the large or small intestine, causing disease.

ENTEROTOXIN: Enterotoxin and exotoxin are two classes of toxin that are produced by bacteria.

ENTEROVIRUS: Enteroviruses are a group of viruses that contain ribonucleic acid as their genetic material. They are members of the picornavirus family. The various types of enteroviruses that infect humans are referred to as serotypes, in recognition of their different antigenic patterns. The different immune response is important, as infection with one type of enterovirus does not necessarily confer protection to infection by a different type of enterovirus. There are 64 different enterovirus serotypes. The serotypes include polio viruses, coxsackie A and B viruses, echo-viruses, and a large number of what are referred to as non-polio enteroviruses.

ENZYME: Enzymes are molecules that act as critical catalysts in biological systems. Catalysts are substances that increase the rate of chemical reactions without being consumed in the reaction. Without enzymes, many reactions would require higher levels of energy and higher temperatures than exist in biological systems. Enzymes are proteins that possess specific binding sites for other molecules (substrates).

A series of weak binding interactions allows enzymes to accelerate reaction rates. Enzyme kinetics is the study of enzymatic reactions and mechanisms. Enzyme inhibitor studies have allowed researchers to develop therapies for the treatment of diseases, including AIDS.

EPIDEMIC: *Epidemic*, from the Greek meaning prevalent among the people, is most commonly used to describe an outbreak of an illness or disease in which the number of individual cases significantly exceeds the usual or expected number of cases in any given population.

EPIDEMIOLOGIST: Epidemiologists study the various factors that influence the occurrence, distribution, prevention, and control of disease, injury, and other health-related events in a defined human population. By the application of various analytical techniques, including mathematical analysis of the data, the probable cause of an infectious outbreak can be pinpointed.

EPIDEMIOLOGY: Epidemiology is the study of the various factors that influence the occurrence, distribution, prevention, and control of disease, injury, and other health-related events in a defined human population. By the application of various analytical techniques, including mathematical analysis of the data, the probable cause of an infectious outbreak can be pinpointed.

EPIZOOTIC: The abnormally high occurrence of a specific disease in animals in a particular area, similar to a human epidemic.

EPSTEIN-BARR VIRUS (EBV): Epstein-Barr virus (EBV) is part of the family of human herpes viruses. Infectious mononucleosis (IM) is the most common disease manifestation of this virus, which, once established in the host, can never be completely eradicated. Very little can be done to treat EBV; most methods can only alleviate resultant symptoms.

ERADICATE: To get rid of; the permanent reduction to zero of global incidence of a particular infection.

ERADICATION: The process of destroying or eliminating a microorganism or disease.

ERYTHEMA: Erythema is skin redness due to excess blood in capillaries (small blood vessels) in the skin.

ESCHAR: Any scab or crust forming on the skin as a result of a burn or disease is an eschar. Scabs from cuts or scrapes are not eschars.

ETIOLOGY: The study of the cause or origin of a disease or disorder.

EX SITU: A Latin term meaning "from the place" or removed from its original place.

EXECUTIVE ORDER: Presidential orders that implement or interpret a federal statute, administrative policy, or treaty.

EXOTOXIN: A toxic protein produced during bacterial growth and metabolism and released into the environment.

EYE DROPS: Eye drops are saline-containing fluid that is added to the eye to cleanse the eye or is a solution used to administer antibiotics or other medication.

F

FASCIA: Fascia is a type of connective tissue made up of a network of fibers. It is best thought of as being the packing material of the body. Fascia surrounds muscles, bones, and joints and lies between the layers of skin. It functions to hold these structures together, protecting these structures and defining the shape of the body. When surrounding a muscle, fascia helps prevent a contracting muscle from catching or causing excessive friction on neighboring muscles.

FECAL-ORAL TRANSMISSION: The spread of disease through the transmission of minute particles of fecal material from one organism to the mouth of another organism. This can occur by drinking contaminated water, eating food that was exposed to animal or human feces (perhaps by watering plants with unclean water), or by the poor hygiene practices of those preparing food.

FIBROBLAST: A cell type that gives rise to connective tissue.

FILOVIRUS: A filovirus is any RNA virus that belongs to the family *Filoviridae*. Filoviruses infect primates. Marburg virus and Ebola virus are filoviruses.

FLEA: A flea is any parasitic insect of the order *Siphonaptera*. Fleas can infest many mammals, including humans, and can act as carriers (vectors) of disease.

FLORA: In microbiology, flora refers to the collective microorganisms that normally inhabit an organism or system. Human intestines, for example, contain bacteria that aid in digestion and are considered normal flora.

FOCI: In medicine, a focus is a primary center of some disease process (for example, a cluster of abnormal cells). Foci is plural for focus (more than one focus).

FOMITE: A fomite is an object or a surface to which infectious microorganisms such as bacteria or viruses can adhere and be transmitted. Papers, clothing, dishes, and other objects can all act as fomites. Transmission is often by touch.

FOOD PRESERVATION: The term food preservation refers to any one of a number of techniques used to prevent food from spoiling. It includes methods such as canning, pickling, drying and freeze-drying, irradiation, pasteurization, smoking, and the addition of chemical additives. Food preservation has become an increasingly important component of the food industry as fewer people eat foods produced on their own lands, and as consumers expect to be able to purchase and consume foods that are out of season.

FULMINANT: A fulminant infection is an infection that appears suddenly and whose symptoms are immediately severe.

G

GAMETOCYTE: A germ cell with the ability to divide for the purpose of producing gametes, either male gametes called spermatocytes or female gametes called oocytes.

GAMMA GLOBULIN: Gamma globulin is a term referring to a group of soluble proteins in the blood, most of which are antibodies that can mount a direct attack upon pathogens and can be used to treat various infections.

GANGRENE: Gangrene is the destruction of body tissue by a bacteria called *Clostridium perfringens* or a combination of streptococci and staphylococci bacteria. *C. perfringens* is widespread; it is found in soil and the intestinal tracts of humans and animals. It becomes dangerous only when its spores germinate, producing toxins and destructive enzymes, and germination occurs only in an anaerobic environment (one almost totally devoid of oxygen). While gangrene can develop in any part of the body, it is most common in fingers, toes, hands, feet, arms, and legs, the parts of the body most susceptible to restricted blood flow. Even a slight injury in such an area is at high risk of causing gangrene. Early treatment with antibiotics, such as penicillin, and surgery to remove the dead tissue will often reduce the need for amputation. If left untreated, gangrene results in amputation or death.

GASTROENTERITIS: Gastroenteritis is an inflammation of the stomach and the intestines. More commonly, gastroenteritis is called the stomach flu.

GENE: A gene is the fundamental physical and functional unit of heredity. Whether in a microorganism or in a human cell, a gene is an individual element of an organism's genome and determines a trait or characteristic by regulating biochemical structure or metabolic process.

GENE THERAPY: Gene therapy is the name applied to the treatment of inherited diseases by corrective genetic engineering of the dysfunctional genes. It is part of a broader field called genetic medicine, which involves the screening, diagnosis, prevention, and treatment of hereditary conditions in humans. The results of genetic screening can pinpoint a potential problem to which gene therapy can sometimes offer a solution. Genetic defects are significant in the total field of medicine, with up to 15 out of every 100 newborn infants having a hereditary disorder of greater or lesser severity. More than 2,000 genetically distinct inherited defects have been classified so far, including diabetes, cystic fibrosis, hemophilia, sickle-call anemia, phenylketonuria, Down syndrome, and cancer.

GENETIC ENGINEERING: Genetic engineering is the altering of the genetic material of living cells in order to make them capable of producing new substances or performing new functions. When the genetic material within the living cells (i.e., genes) is working properly, the human body can develop and function smoothly. However, should a single gene—even a tiny segment of a gene go awry—the effect can be dramatic: deformities, disease, and even death are possible.

GENOME: All of the genetic information for a cell or organism. The complete sequence of genes within a cell or virus.

GENOTYPE: The genetic information that a living thing inherits from its parents that affects its makeup, appearance, and function.

GEOGRAPHIC FOCALITY: The physical location of a disease pattern, epidemic, or outbreak; the characteristics of a location created by interconnections with other places.

GEOGRAPHIC INFORMATION SYSTEM (GIS): A system for archiving, retrieving, and manipulating data that has been stored and indexed according to the geographic coordinates of its elements. The system generally can utilize a variety of data types, such as imagery, maps, tables, etc.

GEOGRAPHIC MEDICINE: Geographic medicine, also called geomedicine, is the study of how human health is affected by climate and environment.

GERM THEORY OF DISEASE: The germ theory is a fundamental tenet of medicine that states that microorganisms, which are too small to be seen without the aid of a microscope, can invade the body and cause disease.

GLOBAL OUTBREAK ALERT AND RESPONSE NETWORK (GOARN): A collaboration of resources for the rapid identification, confirmation, and response to outbreaks of international importance.

GLOBALIZATION: The integration of national and local systems into a global economy through increased trade, manufacturing, communications, and migration.

GLOMERULONEPHRITIS: Glomerulonephritis is inflammation of the kidneys. Mostly it affects the glomeruli, the small capsules in the kidney where blood flowing through capillaries transfers body wastes to urine.

GRAM NEGATIVE BACTERIA: Gram-negative bacteria are bacteria whose cell walls are comprised of an inner and outer membrane that are separated from one another by a region called the periplasm. The periplasm also contains a thin but rigid layer called the peptidoglycan.

GRANULOCYTE: Any cell containing granules (small, grain-like objects) is a granulocyte. The term is often used to refer to a type of white blood cell (leukocyte).

GROUP A STREPTOCOCCUS (GAS): A type (specifically a serotype) of the streptococcus bacteria, based on the antigen contained in the cell wall.

H

HARM-REDUCTION STRATEGY: In public health, a harm-reduction strategy is a public-policy scheme for reducing the amount of harm caused by a substance such as alcohol or tobacco. The phrase may refer to any medical strategy directed at reducing the harm caused by a disease, substance, or toxic medication.

HELMINTH: A representative of various phyla of worm-like animals.

HELMINTHIC DISEASE: Helminths are parasitic worms such as hookworms or flatworms. Helminthic disease by such worms is infectious. A synonym for helminthic is verminous.

HELSINKI DECLARATION: A set of ethical principles governing medical and scientific experimentation on human subjects; it was drafted by the World Medical Association and originally adopted in 1964.

HEMAGGLUTININ: Often abbreviated as HA, hemagglutinin is a glycoprotein, a protein that contains a short chain of sugar as part of its structure.

HEMOLYSIS: The destruction of blood cells, an abnormal rate of which may lead to lowered levels of these cells. For example, Hemolytic anemia is caused by destruction of red blood cells at a rate faster than they can be produced.

HEMORRHAGE: Very severe, massive bleeding that is difficult to control.

HEMORRHAGIC FEVER: A hemorrhagic fever is caused by viral infection and features a high fever and copious (high volume of) bleeding. The bleeding is caused by the formation of tiny blood clots throughout the bloodstream. These blood clots—also called microthrombi—deplete platelets and fibrinogen in the bloodstream. When bleeding begins, the factors needed for the clotting of the blood are scarce. Thus, uncontrolled bleeding (hemorrhage) ensues.

HEPA FILTER: A HEPA (high efficiency particulate air) filter is a filter that is designed to nearly totally remove airborne particles that are 0.3 microns (millionth of a meter) in diameter or larger. Such small particles can penetrate deeply into the lungs if inhaled.

HEPADNAVIRUSES: Hepadnaviridae is a family of hepadnaviruses comprised by two genera, *Avihepadnavirus* and *Orthohepadnavirus*. Hepadnaviruses have partially double-stranded DNA and they replicate their genome in the host cells using an enzyme called reverse transcriptase. Because of this, they are also termed retroviruses. The viruses invade liver cells (hepatocytes) of vertebrates. When hepadna retroviruses invade a cell, a complete viral double-stranded (ds) DNA is made before it randomly inserts in one of the host's chromosomes. Once part of the chromosomal DNA, the viral DNA is then transcribed into an intermediate messenger RNA (mRNA) in the hosts' nucleus. The viral mRNA then leaves the nucleus and undergoes reverse transcription, which is mediated by the viral reverse transcriptase.

HEPATITIS AND HEPATITIS VIRUSES: Hepatitis is an inflammation of the liver, a potentially life-threatening disease most frequently caused by viral infections but which may also result from liver damage caused by toxic substances such as alcohol and certain drugs. There are six major types of hepatitis viruses: hepatitis A (HAV), hepatitis B (HBV), hepatitis C (HCV), hepatitis D (HDV), hepatitis E (HEV), and hepatitis G (HGV).

HERD IMMUNITY: Herd immunity is a resistance to disease that occurs in a population when a proportion of them have been immunized against it. The theory is that it is less likely that an infectious disease will spread in a group where some individuals are unlikely to contract it.

HERPESVIRUS: Herpesvirus is a family of viruses, many of which cause disease in humans. The *herpes simplex*-1 and *herpes simplex*-2 viruses cause infection in the mouth or on the genitals. Other common types of herpesvirus include chickenpox, Epstien-Barr virus, and cytomegalovirus. Herpesvirus is notable for its ability to remain latent, or inactive, in nerve cells near the area of infection, and to reactivate long after the initial infection. *Herpes simplex*-1 and -2, along with chickenpox, cause familiar skin sores. Epstein-Barr virus causes mononucleosis. Cytomegalovirus also causes a like-like infection, but it can be dangerous to the elderly, infants, and those with weakened immune systems.

HETEROPHILE ANTIBODY: A heterophile antibody is an antibody that is found in the blood of someone with infectious mononucleosis, also known as glandular fever.

HIGH-LEVEL DISINFECTION: High-level disinfection is a process that uses a chemical solution to kill all bacteria, viruses, and other disease-causing agents except for bacterial endospores and prions. High-level disinfection should be distinguished from sterilization, which removes endospores (a bacterial structure that is resistant to radiation, drying, lack of food, and other things that would be lethal to the bacteria) and prions (misshapen proteins that can cause disease) as well.

HIGHLY ACTIVE ANTIRETROVIRAL THERAPY (HAART): Highly active antiretroviral therapy (HAART) is the name given to the combination of drugs given to people with human immunodeficiency virus (HIV) infection to slow or stop the progression of their condition to AIDS (acquired human immunodeficiency syndrome). HIV is a retrovirus and the various components of HAART block its replication by different mechanisms.

HISTAMINE: Histamine is a hormone that is chemically similar to the hormones serotonine, epinephrine, and norepinephrine. A hormone is generally defined as a chemical produced by a certain cell or tissue that causes a specific biological change or activity to occur in another cell or tissue located elsewhere in the body. Specifically, histamine plays a role in localized immune responses and in allergic reactions.

HISTOCOMPATIBILITY: The histocompatibility molecules (proteins) on the cell surfaces of one individual of a species are unique. Thus, if the cell is transplanted into another person, the cell will be recognized by the immune system as being foreign. The histocompatibility molecules act as antigens in the recipient and so can also be called histocompatibility antigens or transplantation antigens. This is the basis of the rejection of transplanted material.

HISTOPATHOLOGY: Histopathology is the study of diseased tissues. A synonym for histopathology is pathologic histology.

HIV (HUMAN IMMUNODEFICIENCY VIRUS): The virus that causes AIDS (acquired immunodeficiency syndrome).

HOMOZYGOUS: A condition in which two alleles for a given gene are the same.

HORIZONTAL GENE TRANSFER: Horizontal gene transfer is a major mechanism by which antibiotic resistance genes get passed between bacteria. It accounts for many hospital-acquired infections.

HORIZONTAL TRANSMISSION: Horizontal transmission refers to the transmission of a disease-causing microorganism from one person to another, unrelated person by direct or indirect contact.

HOST: An organism that serves as the habitat for a parasite or possibly for a symbiont. A host may provide nutrition to the parasite or symbiont, or it may simply provide a place in which to live.

HOST FOCALITY: Host focality refers to the tendency of some animal hosts, such as rodents carrying hantavirus and other viruses, to exist in groups in specific geographical locations and act as a local reservoir of infection.

HUMAN GROWTH HORMONE: Human growth hormone is a protein that is made and released from the pituitary gland, which increases growth and manufacture of new cells.

HUMAN IMMUNODEFICIENCY VIRUS (HIV): The human immunodeficiency virus (HIV) belongs to a class of viruses known as the retroviruses. These viruses are known as RNA viruses because they have RNA (ribonucleic acid) as their basic genetic material instead of DNA (deoxyribonucleic acid).

HUMAN T-CELL LEUKEMIA VIRUS: Two types of human T-cell leukemia virus (HTLV) are known. They are also known as human T-cell lymphotrophic viruses. HTLV-I often is carried by a person with no obvious symptoms. However, HTLV-I is capable of causing a number of maladies. These include abnormalities of the T cells and B cells, a chronic infection

of the myelin covering of nerves that causes a degeneration of the nervous system, sores on the skin, and an inflammation of the inside of the eye. HTLV-II infection usually does not produce any symptoms. However, in some people a cancer of the blood known as hairy cell leukemia can develop.

HYBRIDIZATION: A process of combining two or more different molecules or organisms to create a new molecule or organism (oftentimes called a hybrid organism).

HYGIENE: Hygiene refers to the health practices that minimize the spread of infectious microorganisms between people or between other living things and people. Inanimate objects and surfaces such as contaminated cutlery or a cutting board may be a secondary part of this process.

HYPERENDEMIC: A disease that is endemic (commonly present) in all age groups of a population is hyperendemic. A related term is holoendemic, meaning a disease that is present more in children than in adults.

HYPERINFECTION: A hyperinfection is an infection that is caused by a very high number of disease-causing microorganisms. The infection results from an abnormality in the immune system that allows the infecting cells to grow and divide more easily than would normally be the case.

I

IATROGENIC: Any infection, injury, or other disease condition caused by medical treatment is iatrogenic (pronounced eye-at-roh-GEN-ik).

IMMUNITY HUMORAL REGULATION: One way in which the immune system responds to pathogens is by producing soluble proteins called antibodies. This is known as the humoral response and involves the activation of a special set of cells known as the B lymphocytes, because they originate in the bone marrow. The humoral immune response helps in the control and removal of pathogens such as bacteria, viruses, fungi, and parasites before they enter host cells. The antibodies produced by the B cells are the mediators of this response.

IMMIGRATION: The relocation of people to a different region or country from their native lands; also refers to the movement of organisms into an area in which they were previously absent.

IMMUNE GLOBULIN: Globulins are a type of protein found in blood. The immune globulins (also called immunoglobulins) are Y-shaped globulins that act as antibodies, attaching themselves to invasive cells or materials in the body so that they can be identified and attacked by the immune system. There are five immune globulins, designated IgM, IgG, IgA, IgD, and IgE.

IMMUNE RESPONSE: The body's production of antibodies or some types of white blood cells in response to foreign substances.

IMMUNE SYNAPSE: Before they can help other immune cells respond to a foreign protein or pathogenic organism, helper T cells must first become activated. This process occurs when an antigen-presenting cell submits a fragment of a foreign protein, bound to a Class II MHC molecule (virus-derived fragments are bound to Class I MHC molecules), to the helper T cell. Antigen-presenting cells are derived from bone marrow, and include both dendritic cells and Langerhans cells, as well as other specialized cells. Because T cell responses depend upon direct contact with their target cells, their antigen receptors, unlike antibodies made by B cells, exist bound to the membrane only. In the intercellular gap between the T cell and the antigen-presenting cell, a special pattern of various receptors and complementary ligands forms that is several microns in size.

IMMUNE SYSTEM: The body's natural defense system that guards against foreign invaders and that includes lymphocytes and antibodies.

IMMUNO-BASED TEST: An immuno-based test is a medical technology that tests for the presence of a disease by looking for a reaction between disease organisms that may be present in a tissue or fluid sample and antibodies contained in the test kit.

IMMUNOCOMPROMISED: A reduction of the ability of the immune system to recognize and respond to the presence of foreign material.

IMMUNODEFICIENCY: In immunodeficiency disorders, part of the body's immune system is missing or defective, thus impairing the body's ability to fight infections. As a result, the person with an immunodeficiency disorder will have frequent infections that are generally more severe and last longer than usual.

IMMUNOGENICITY: Immunogenicity is the capacity of a host to produce an immune response to protect itself against infectious disease.

IMMUNOLOGY: Immunology is the study of how the body responds to foreign substances and fights off infection and other disease. Immunologists study the molecules, cells, and organs of the human body that participate in this response.

IMMUNOSUPPRESSION: A reduction of the ability of the immune system to recognize and respond to the presence of foreign material.

IMPETIGO: Impetigo refers to a very localized bacterial infection of the skin. It tends to afflict primarily children, but can occur in people of any age. Impetigo caused by the bacteria *Staphylococcus aureus* (or staph) affects children of all ages, while impetigo caused by the bacteria called group A streptococci (Streptoccus pyogenes or strep) is most common in children ages two to five years.

IMPORTED CASE OF DISEASE: Imported cases of disease happen when an infected person who is not yet showing symptoms travels from his home country to another country and develops symptoms of his disease there.

IN SITU: A Latin term meaning "in place" or in the body or natural system.

INACTIVATED VACCINE: An inactivated vaccine is a vaccine that is made from disease-causing microorganisms that have been killed or made incapable of causing the infection. The immune system can still respond to the presence of the microorganisms.

INACTIVATED VIRUS: An inactivated virus is incapable of causing disease but still stimulates the immune system to respond by forming antibodies.

INCIDENCE: The number of new cases of a disease or injury that occur in a population during a specified period of time.

INCUBATION PERIOD: Incubation period refers to the time between exposure to a disease-causing virus or bacteria and the appearance of symptoms of the infection. Depending on the microorganism, the incubation time can range from a few hours (for example, food poisoning due to *Salmonella*) to a decade or more (for example, acquired immunodeficiency syndrome, or AIDS).

INFECTION CONTROL: Infection control refers to policies and procedures used to minimize the risk of spreading infections, especially in hospitals and health care facilities.

INFECTION CONTROL PROFESSIONAL (ICP): Infection control professionals are a group of nurses, doctors, laboratory workers, microbiologists, public health officials, and others who have specialized training in the prevention and control of infectious disease. Infection control professionals develop methods to control infection and instruct others in their use. These methods include proper handwashing; correct wearing of protective masks, eye-guards, gloves, and other specialized clothing; vaccination; monitoring for infection; and investigating ways to treat and prevent infection. Courses and certifications are available for those wishing to become infection control professionals.

INFORMED CONSENT: An ethical and informational process in which a person learns about a procedure or clinical trial, including potential risks or benefits, before deciding to voluntarily participate in a study or undergo a particular procedure.

INNATE IMMUNITY: Innate immunity is the resistance against disease that an individual is born with, as distinct from acquired immunity, which develops with exposure to infectious agents.

INOCULUM: An inoculum is a substance such as virus, bacterial toxin, or a viral or bacterial component that is added to the body to stimulate the immune system, which then provides protection from an infection by the particular microorganism.

INPATIENT: A patient who is admitted to a hospital or clinic for treatment, typically requiring the patient to stay overnight.

INSECTICIDE: A chemical substance used to kill insects.

INTERMEDIATE HOST: An organism infected by a parasite while the parasite is in a developmental form, not sexually mature.

INTERMEDIATE-LEVEL DISINFECTION: Intermediate-level disinfection is a form of disinfection that kills bacteria, most viruses, and mycobacteria.

INTERNATIONAL HEALTH REGULATIONS: International regulations introduced by the World Health Organization (WHO) that aim to control, monitor, prevent, protect against, and respond to the spread of disease across national borders while avoiding unnecessary interference with international movement and trade.

INTERTRIGO: Intertrigo, sometimes called eczema intertrigo, is a skin rash, often occurring in obese persons on parts of the body symmetrically opposite each other. It is caused by irritation of skin trapped under hanging folds of flesh such as pendulous breasts.

INTRAVENOUS: In the vein. For example, the insertion of a hypodermic needle into a vein to instill a fluid, withdraw or transfuse blood, or start an intravenous feeding.

IONIZING RADIATION: Any electromagnetic or particulate radiation capable of direct or indirect ion production in its passage through matter. In general use: Radiation that can cause tissue damage or death.

IRRADIATION: A method of preservation that treats food with low doses of radiation to deactivate enzymes and to kill microorganisms and insects.

ISOLATION: Isolation, within the health community, refers to the precautions that are taken in the hospital to prevent the spread of an infectious agent from an infected or colonized patient to susceptible persons. Isolation practices are designed to minimize the transmission of infection.

ISOLATION AND QUARANTINE: Public health authorities rely on isolation and quarantine as two important tools among the many they use to fight disease outbreaks. Isolation is the practice of keeping a disease victim away from other people, sometimes by treating them in their homes or by the use of elaborate isolation systems in hospitals. Quarantine separates people who have been exposed to a disease but have not yet developed symptoms from the general population. Both isolation and quarantine can be entered voluntarily by patients when public health authorities request it, or it can be compelled by state governments or by the federal Centers for Disease Control and Prevention.

J

JAUNDICE: Jaundice is a condition in which a person's skin and the whites of the eyes are discolored a shade of yellow due to an increased level of bile pigments in the blood as a result of liver disease. Jaundice is sometimes called icterus, from a Greek word for the condition.

K

KERITITIS: Keratitis, sometimes called corneal ulcers, is an inflammation of the cornea, the transparent membrane that covers the colored part of the eye (iris) and pupil of the eye.

KOCH'S POSTULATES: Koch's postulates are a series of conditions that must be met for a microorganism to be considered the cause of a disease. German microbiologist Robert Koch (1843–1910) proposed the postulates in 1890.

KOPLIK'S SPOTS: Koplik's spots, named after American pediatrician Henry Koplik (1858-1927) and also called Koplik's sign, are red spots with a small blue-white speck in the center found on the tongue and the insides of the cheeks during the early stages of measles.

L

LARVAE: Immature forms (wormlike in insects; fishlike in amphibians) of an organism capable of surviving on its own. Larvae do not resemble the parent and must go through metamorphosis, or change, to reach the adult stage.

LATENT: A condition that is potential or dormant, not yet manifest or active, is latent.

LATENT INFECTION: An infection already established in the body but not yet causing symptoms, or having ceased to cause symptoms after an active period, is a latent infection.

LATENT VIRUS: Latent viruses are those viruses that can incorporate their genetic material into the genetic material of the infected host cell. Because the viral genetic material can then be replicated along with the host material, the virus becomes effectively "silent" with respect to detection by the host. Latent viruses usually contain the information necessary to reverse the latent state. The viral genetic material can leave the host genome to begin the manufacture of new virus particles.

LEGIONNAIRES' DISEASE: Legionnaires' disease is a type of pneumonia caused by *Legionella* bacteria. The bacterial species responsible for Legionnaires' disease is *L. pneumophila*. Major symptoms include fever, chills, muscle aches, and a cough that is initially nonproductive. Definitive diagnosis relies on specific laboratory tests for the bacteria, bacterial antigens, or antibodies produced by the body's immune system. As with other types of pneumonia, Legionnaires' disease poses the greatest threat to people who are elderly, ill, or immunocompromised.

LENS: An almost clear, biconvex structure in the eye that, along with the cornea, helps to focus light onto the retina. It can become infected, causing inflammation, for example, when contact lenses are improperly used.

LEPTOSPIRE: Also called a leptospira, a leptospire is any bacterial species of the genus *Leptospira*. Infection with leptospires causes leptospirosis.

LESION: The tissue disruption or the loss of function caused by a particular disease process.

LIPOPOLYSACCHARIDE (LPS): Lipopolysaccharide (LPS) is a molecule that is a constituent of the outer membrane of Gram-negative bacteria. The molecule can also be referred to as endotoxin. LPS can help protect the bacterium from host defenses and can contribute to illness in the host.

LIVE VACCINE: A live vaccine uses a virus or bacteria that has been weakened (attenuated) to cause an immune response in the body without causing disease. Live vaccines are preferred to killed vaccines, which use a dead virus or bacteria, because they cause a stronger and longer-lasting immune response.

LOW-LEVEL DISINFECTION: Low-level disinfection is a form of disinfection that is capable of killing some viruses and some bacteria.

LYMPHADENOPATHY: Any disease of the lymph nodes (gland-like bodies that filter the clear intercellular fluid called lymph to remove impurities) is lymphadenopathy.

LYMPHATIC SYSTEM: The lymphatic system is the body's network of organs, ducts, and tissues that filters harmful substances out of the fluid that surrounds body tissues. Lymphatic organs include the bone marrow, thymus, spleen, appendix, tonsils, adenoids, lymph nodes, and Peyer's patches (in the small intestine). The thymus and bone marrow are called primary lymphatic organs, because lymphocytes are produced in them. The other lymphatic organs are called secondary lymphatic organs. The lymphatic system is a complex network of thin vessels, capillaries, valves, ducts, nodes, and organs that runs throughout the body, helping protect and maintain the internal fluids system of the entire body by both producing and filtering lymph and by producing various blood cells. The three main purposes of the lymphatic system are to drain fluid back into the bloodstream from the tissues, to filter lymph, and to fight infections.

LYMPHOCYTE: A type of white blood cell; includes B and T lymphocytes. A type of white blood cell that functions as part of the lymphatic and immune systems by stimulating antibody formation to attack specific invading substances.

M

M PROTEIN: M protein is an antibody found in unusually large amounts in the blood or urine of patients with multiple myeloma, a form of cancer that arises in the white blood cells that produce antibodies.

MACAQUE: A macaque is any short-tailed monkey of the genus *Macaca*. Macaques, including rhesus monkeys, are often used as subjects in medical research because they are relatively affordable and resemble humans in many ways.

MACULOPAPULAR: A macule is any discolored skin spot that is flush or level with the surrounding skin surface: a papule is a small, solid bump on the skin. A maculopapular skin disturbance is one that combines macules and papules.

MAJOR HISTOCOMPATIBILITY COMPLEX (MHC): The proteins that protrude from the surface of a cell that identify the cell as "self." In humans, the proteins coded by the genes of the major histocompatibility complex (MHC) include human leukocyte antigens (HLA), as well as other proteins. HLA proteins are present on the surface of most of the body's cells and are important in helping the immune system distinguish "self" from "non-self" molecules, cells, and other objects.

MALAISE: Malaise is a general or nonspecific feeling of unease or discomfort, often the first sign of disease infection.

MALIGNANT: A general term for cells that can dislodge from the original tumor, then invade and destroy other tissues and organs.

MATERIEL: A French-derived word for equipment, supplies, or hardware.

MEASLES: Measles is an infectious disease caused by a virus of the paramyxovirus group. It infects only humans, and the infection results in life-long immunity to the disease. It is one of several exanthematous (rash-producing) diseases of childhood, the others being rubella (German measles), chickenpox, and the now rare scarlet fever. The disease is particularly common in both preschool and young school children.

MENINGITIS: Meningitis is an inflammation of the meninges—the three layers of protective membranes that line the spinal cord and the brain. Meningitis can occur when there is an infection near the brain or spinal cord, such as a respiratory infection in the sinuses, the mastoids, or the cavities around the ear. Disease organisms can also travel to the meninges through the bloodstream. The first signs may be a severe headache and neck stiffness followed by fever, vomiting, a rash, and, then, convulsions leading to loss of consciousness. Meningitis generally involves two types: non-bacterial meningitis, which is often called aseptic meningitis, and bacterial meningitis, which is referred to as purulent meningitis.

MENINGITIS BELT: The Meningitis Belt is an area of Africa south of the Sahara Desert, stretching from the Atlantic to the Pacific coast, where meningococcal meningitis is common.

MEROZOITE: The motile, infective stage of malaria, responsible for disease symptoms.

MESSENGER RIBONUCLEIC ACID (MRNA): A molecule of RNA that carries the genetic information for producing one or more proteins; mRNA is produced by copying one strand of DNA, but in eukaryotes it is able to move from the nucleus to the cytoplasm (where protein synthesis takes place).

MICROBICIDE: A microbicide is a compound that kills microorganisms such as bacteria, fungi, and protozoa.

MICROFILIAE: Live offspring produced by adult nematodes within the host's body.

MICROORGANISM: Microorganisms are minute organisms. With only a single currently known exception (i.e., *Epulopiscium fishelsonia*, a bacterium that is billions of times larger than the bacteria in the human intestine and is large enough to view without a microscope), microorganisms are minute organisms that require microscopic magnification to view. To be seen, they must be magnified by an optical or electron microscope. The most common types of microorganisms are viruses, bacteria, blue-green bacteria, some algae, some fungi, yeasts, and protozoans.

MIGRATION: In medicine, migration is the movement of a disease symptom from one part of the body to another, apparently without cause.

MIMICKED: In biology, mimicry is the imitation of another organism, often for evolutionary advantage. A disease that resembles another (for whatever reason) is sometimes said to have mimicked the other. Pathomimicry is the faking of symptoms by a patient, also called malingering.

MINIMAL INHIBITORY CONCENTRATION (MIC): The minimal inhibitory concentration (MIC) refers to the lowest level of an antibiotic that prevents growth of the particular type of bacteria in a liquid food source after a certain amount of time. Growth is detected by clouding of the food source. The MIC is the lowest concentration of the antibiotic at which the no cloudiness occurs.

MITE: A mite is a tiny arthropod (insect-like creature) of the order *Acarina*. Mites may inhabit the surface of the body without causing harm, or may cause various skin ailments by burrowing under the skin. The droppings of mites living in house dust are a common source of allergic reactions.

MMR VACCINE: MMR (measles, mumps, rubella) vaccine is a vaccine that is given to protect someone from measles, mumps, and rubella. The vaccine is made up of viruses that cause the three diseases. The viruses are incapable of causing the diseases but can still stimulate the immune system.

MONO SPOT TEST: The mononucleosis (mono) spot test is a blood test used to check for infection with the Epstein-Barr virus, which causes mononucleosis.

MONOCLONAL ANTIBODIES: Antibodies produced from a single cell line that are used in medical testing and, increasingly, in the treatment of some cancers.

MONONUCLEAR LEUKOCYTE: A mononuclear leukocyte is a type of white blood cell active in the immune system.

MONOVALENT VACCINE: A monovalent vaccine is one that is active against just one strain of a virus, such as the one that is in common use against the poliovirus.

MORBIDITY: The term "morbidity" comes from the Latin word *morbus*, which means sick. In medicine it refers not just to the state of being ill, but also to the severity of the illness. A serious disease is said to have a high morbidity.

MORPHOLOGY: The study of form and structure of animals and plants. The outward physical form possessed by an organism.

MORTALITY: Mortality is the condition of being susceptible to death. The term mortality comes from the Latin word *mors*, which means death. Mortality can also refer to the rate of deaths caused by an illness or injury, i.e., rabies has a high mortality rate.

MOSQUITO COILS: Mosquito coils are spirals of inflammable paste that, when burned, steadily release insect repellent into the air. They are often used in Asia, where many coils release octachlorodipropyl ether, which can cause lung cancer.

MOSQUITO NETTING: Fine meshes or nets hung around occupied spaces, especially beds, to keep out disease-carrying mosquitoes. Mosquito netting is a cost-effective way of preventing malaria.

MRSA: Methicillin-resistant *Staphylococcus aureus* are bacteria resistant to most penicillin-type antibiotics, including methicillin.

MULTIBACILLARY: The more severe form of leprosy (Hansen's disease) is called multibacillary leprosy. It is defined as the presence of more than 5 skin lesions on the patient with a positive skin-smear test. The less severe form of leprosy is called paucibacillary leprosy.

MULTI-DRUG RESISTANCE: Multi-drug resistance is a phenomenon that occurs when an infective agent loses its sensitivity against two or more of the drugs that are used against it.

MULTI-DRUG THERAPY: Multi-drug therapy is the use of a combination of drugs against infection, each of which attacks the infective agent in a different way. This strategy can help overcome resistance to anti-infective drugs.

MUTABLE VIRUS: A mutable virus is one whose DNA changes rapidly so that drugs and vaccines against it may not be effective.

MUTATION: A mutation is a change in an organism's DNA that occurs over time and may render it less sensitive to the drugs that are used against it.

MYALGIA: Muscular aches and pain.

MYCOBACTERIA: *Mycobacteria* is a genus of bacteria that contains the bacteria causing leprosy and tuberculosis. The bacteria have unusual cell walls that are harder to dissolve than the cell walls of other bacteria.

MYCOTIC: Mycotic means having to do with or caused by a fungus. Any medical condition caused by a fungus is a mycotic condition, also called a mycosis.

MYCOTIC DISEASE: Mycotic disease is a disease caused by fungal infection.

N

NATIONAL ELECTRONIC TELECOMMUNICATIONS SYSTEM FOR SURVEILLANCE (NETSS): A computerized public health surveillance information system that provides the Centers for Disease Control and Prevention (CDC) with weekly data regarding cases of nationally notifiable diseases.

NECROPSY: A necropsy is a medical examination of a dead body: also called an autopsy.

NECROTIC: Necrotic tissue is dead tissue in an otherwise living body. Tissue death is called necrosis.

NEEDLESTICK INJURY: Any accidental breakage or puncture of the skin by an unsterilized medical needle (syringe) is a needlestick injury. Health-care providers are at particular risk for needlestick injuries (which may transmit disease) because of the large number of needles they handle.

NEGLECTED TROPICAL DISEASE: Many tropical diseases are considered to be neglected because, despite their prevalence in less-developed areas, new vaccines and treatments are not being developed for them.

Malaria was once considered to be a neglected tropical disease, but recently a great deal of research and money have been devoted to its treatment and cure.

NEMATODES: Also known as roundworms; a type of helminth characterized by long, cylindrical bodies.

NEURAMINIDASE: Also abbreviated (NA), neuraminidase is a glycoprotein, a protein that contains a short chain of sugar as part of its structure.

NEUROTOXIN: A poison that interferes with nerve function, usually by affecting the flow of ions through the cell membrane.

NEUTROPHIL: An immune cell that releases a bacteria-killing chemical; neutrophils are prominent in the inflammatory response. A type of white blood cell that phagocytizes foreign microorganisms. It also releases lysozyme.

NOBEL PEACE PRIZE: An annual prize bequeathed by Swedish inventor Alfred Nobel (1833–1896) and awarded by the Norwegian Nobel Committee to an individual or organization that has "done the most or the best work for fraternity between the nations, for the abolition or reduction of standing armies and for the holding and promotion of peace congresses."

NODULE: A nodule is a small, roundish lump on the surface of the skin or of an internal organ.

NON-GOVERNMENTAL ORGANIZATION (NGO): A voluntary organization that is not part of any government; often organized to address a specific issue or perform a humanitarian function.

NORMAL FLORA: The bacteria that normally inhabit some part of the body, such as the mouth or intestines, are normal flora. Normal flora are essential to health.

NOROVIRUS: Norovirus is a type of virus that contains ribonucleic acid as the genetic material and causes an intestinal infection known as gastroenteritis. A well-known example is Norwalk-like virus.

NOSOCOMIAL INFECTION: A nosocomial infection is an infection that is acquired in a hospital. More precisely, the Centers for Disease Control in Atlanta, Georgia, defines a nosocomial infection as a localized infection or an infection that is widely spread throughout the body that results from an adverse reaction to an infectious microorganism or toxin that was not present at the time of admission to the hospital.

NOTIFIABLE DISEASES: Diseases that the law requires must be reported to health officials when diagnosed, including active tuberculosis and several sexually transmitted diseases; also called reportable diseases.

NUCLEOTIDE: The basic unit of a nucleic acid. It consists of a simple sugar, a phosphate group, and a nitrogen–containing base.

NUCLEOTIDE SEQUENCE: A particular ordering of the chain structure of nucleic acid that provides the necessary information for a specific amino acid.

NUCLEUS, CELL: Membrane–enclosed structure within a cell that contains the cell's genetic material and controls its growth and reproduction. (Plural: nuclei.)

NUTRITIONAL SUPPLEMENTS: Nutritional supplements are substances necessary to health, such as calcium or protein, that are taken in concentrated form to compensate for dietary insufficiency, poor absorption, unusually high demand for that nutrient, or other reasons.

NYMPH: In aquatic insects, the larval stage.

O

ONCOGENIC VIRUS: An oncogenic virus is a virus that is capable of changing the cells it infects so that the cells begin to grow and divide uncontrollably.

OOCYST: An oocyst is a spore phase of certain infectious organisms that can survive for a long time outside the organism and so continue to cause infection and resist treatment.

OOPHORITIS: Oophoritis is an inflammation of the ovary, which happens in certain sexually transmitted diseases.

OPPORTUNISTIC INFECTION: An opportunistic infection is so named because it occurs in people whose immune systems are diminished or not functioning normally; such infections are opportunistic insofar as the infectious agents take advantage of their hosts' compromised immune systems and invade to cause disease.

OPTIC SOLUTION: Any liquid solution of a medication that can be applied directly to the eye is an optic solution.

ORAL REHYDRATION THERAPY: Patients who have lost excessive water from their tissues are said to be dehydrated. Restoring body water levels by giving the patient fluids through the mouth (orally) is oral rehydration therapy. Often, a special mixture of water, glucose, and electrolytes called oral rehydration solution is given.

ORCHITIS: Orchitis is inflammation of one or both testicles. Swelling and pain are typical symptoms. Orchitis may be caused by various sexually transmitted diseases or escape of sperm cells into the tissues of the testicle.

OUTBREAK: The appearance of new cases of a disease in numbers greater than the established incidence rate, or the appearance of even one case of an emergent or rare disease in an area.

OUTPATIENT: A person who receives health care services without being admitted to a hospital or clinic for an overnight stay.

OVA: Mature female sex cells produced in the ovaries. (Singular: ovum.)

OVIPOSITION: Ovum is Latin for "egg." To oviposition is to position or lay eggs, especially when done by an insect.

P

PANCREATITIS: Pancreatitis is an inflammation of the pancreas, an organ that is important in digestion. Pancreatitis can be acute (beginning suddenly, usually with the patient recovering fully) or chronic (progressing slowly with continued, permanent injury to the pancreas).

PANDEMIC: Pandemic, which means all the people, describes an epidemic that occurs in more than one country or population simultaneously.

PAPULAR: A papule is a small, solid bump on the skin; papular means pertaining to or resembling a papule.

PAPULE: A papule is a small, solid bump on the skin.

PARAMYXOVIRUS: Paramyxovirus is a type of virus that contains ribonucleic acid as the genetic material and has proteins on its surface that clump red blood cells and assist in the release of newly made viruses from the infected cells. Measles virus and mumps virus are two types of paramyxoviruses.

PARASITE: An organism that lives in or on a host organism and that gets its nourishment from that host. The parasite usually gains all the benefits of this relationship, while the host may suffer from various diseases and discomforts, or show no signs of the infection. The life cycle of a typical parasite usually includes several developmental stages and morphological changes as the parasite lives and moves through the environment

and one or more hosts. Parasites that remain on a host's body surface to feed are called ectoparasites, while those that live inside a host's body are called endoparasites. Parasitism is a highly successful biological adaptation. There are more known parasitic species than nonparasitic ones, and parasites affect just about every form of life, including most all animals, plants, and even bacteria.

PAROTITIS: Parotitis is inflammation of the parotid gland. There are two parotid glands, one on each side of the jaw, at the back. Their function is to secret saliva into the mouth.

PAROXYSM: In medicine, a paroxysm may be a fit, convulsion, or seizure. It may also be a sudden worsening or recurrence of disease symptoms.

PASTEURIZATION: Pasteurization is a process where fluids such as wine and milk are heated for a predetermined time at a temperature that is below the boiling point of the liquid. The treatment kills any microorganisms that are in the fluid but does not alter the taste, appearance, or nutritive value of the fluid.

PATHOGEN: A disease-causing agent, such as a bacteria, virus, fungus, etc.

PATHOGENIC: Something causing or capable of causing disease.

PATHOGENS: Agents or microorganisms causing or capable of causing disease.

PAUCIBACILLARY: Paucibacillary refers to an infectious condition, such as a certain form of leprosy, characterized by few, rather than many, bacilli, which are a rod-shaped type of bacterium.

PCR (POLYMERASE CHAIN REACTION): The polymerase chain reaction, or PCR, refers to a widely used technique in molecular biology involving the amplification of specific sequences of genomic DNA.

PERSISTENCE: Persistence is the length of time a disease remains in a patient. Disease persistence can vary from a few days to life-long.

PESTICIDE: Substances used to reduce the abundance of pests, any living thing that causes injury or disease to crops.

PHAGOCYTOSIS: The process by which certain cells engulf and digest microorganisms and consume debris and foreign bodies in the blood.

PHENOTYPE: The visible characteristics or physical shape produced by a living thing's genotype.

PLAGUE: A contagious disease that spreads rapidly through a population and results in a high rate of death.

PLASMID: A circular piece of DNA that exists outside of the bacterial chromosome and copies itself independently. Scientists often use bacterial plasmids in genetic engineering to carry genes into other organisms.

PLEURAL CAVITY: The lungs are surrounded by two membranous coverings, the pleura. One of the pleura is attached to the lung, the other to the ribcage. The space between the two pleura, the pleural cavity, is normally filled with a clear lubricating fluid called pleural fluid.

PNEUMONIA: Pneumonia is inflammation of the lung accompanied by filling of some air sacs with fluid (consolidation). It can be caused by a number of infectious agents, including bacteria, viruses, and fungi.

POSTEXPOSURE PROPHYLAXIS: Postexposure prophylaxis is treatment with drugs immediately after exposure to an infectious microorganism. The aim of this approach is to prevent an infection from becoming established.

POSTHERPETIC NEURALGIA: Neuralgia is pain arising in a nerve that is not the result of any injury. Postherpetic neuralgia is neuralgia experienced after infection with a herpesvirus, namely *Herpes simplex* or *Herpes zoster.*

POTABLE: Water that is clean enough to drink safely is potable water.

PREVALENCE: The actual number of cases of disease (or injury) that exist in a population.

PRIMARY HOST: The primary host is an organism that provides food and shelter for a parasite while allowing it to become sexually mature, while a secondary host is one occupied by a parasite during the larval or asexual stages of its life cycle.

PRIONS: Prions are proteins that are infectious. Indeed, the name prion is derived from "proteinaceous infectious particles." The discovery of prions and confirmation of their infectious nature overturned a central dogma that infections were caused only by intact organisms, particularly microorganisms such as bacteria, fungi, parasites, or viruses. Since prions lack genetic material, the prevailing attitude was that a protein could not cause disease.

PRODROMAL SYMPTOMS: Prodromal symptoms are the earliest symptoms of a disease.

PRODROME: A prodrome of a disease is a symptom indicating the disease's onset; it may also be called a prodroma. For example, painful swallowing is often a prodrome of infection with a cold virus.

PROPHYLAXIS: Pre-exposure treatments (e.g., immunization) that prevents or reduces severity of disease or symptoms upon exposure to the causative agent.

PROSTRATION: A condition marked by nausea, disorientation, dizziness, and weakness caused by dehydration and prolonged exposure to high temperatures; also called heat exhaustion or hyperthermia.

PROTOZOA: Single-celled animal-like microscopic organisms that live by taking in food rather than making it by photosynthesis and must live in the presence of water. (Singular: protozoan.) Protozoa are a diverse group of single-celled organisms, with more than 50,000 different types represented. The vast majority are microscopic, many measuring less than 5 one-thousandth of an inch (0.005 millimeters), but some, such as the freshwater Spirostomun, may reach 0.17 inches (3 millimeters) in length, large enough to enable it to be seen with the naked eye.

PRURITIS: Pruritis is the medical term for itchiness.

PRURULENT: Containing, discharging, or producing pus.

PUERPERAL: An interval of time around childbirth, from the onset of labor through the immediate recovery period after delivery.

PUERPERAL FEVER: Puerperal fever is a bacterial infection present in the blood (septicemia) that follows childbirth. The Latin word *puer* meaning boy or child, is the root of this term. Puerperal fever was much more common before the advent of modern aseptic practices, but infections still occur. Louis Pasteur showed that puerperal fever is most often caused by *Streptococcus* bacteria, which is now treated with antibiotics.

PULMONARY: Having to do with the lungs or respiratory system. The pulmonary circulatory system delivers deoxygenated blood from the right ventricle of the heart to the lungs, and returns oxygenated blood from the lungs to the left atrium of the heart. At its most minute level, the alveolar capillary bed, the pulmonary circulatory system is the principle point of gas exchange between blood and air that moves in and out of the lungs during respiration.

PURULENT: Any part of the body that contains or releases pus is said to be purulent. Pus is a fluid produced by inflamed, infected tissues and is made up of white blood cells, fragments of dead cells, and a liquid containing various proteins.

PUSTULES: A pustule is a reservoir of pus visible just beneath the skin. It is usually sore to the touch and surrounded by inflamed tissue.

PYELONEPHRITIS: Inflammation caused by bacterial infection of the kidney and associated blood vessels is termed pyelonephritis.

PYROGENIC: A substance that causes fever is pyrogenic. The word "pyrogenic" comes from the Greek word *pyr* meaning fire.

Q

QUANTITATED: An act of determining the quantity of something, such as the number or concentration of bacteria in an infectious disease.

QUARANTINE: Quarantine is the practice of separating people who have been exposed to an infectious agent but have not yet developed symptoms from the general population. This can be done voluntarily or involuntarily by the authority of states and the federal Centers for Disease Control and Prevention.

R

RALES: French term for a rattling sound in the throat or chest.

RASH: A rash is a change in appearance or texture of the skin. A rash is the popular term for a group of spots or red, inflamed skin that is usually a symptom of an underlying condition or disorder. Often temporary, a rash is only rarely a sign of a serious problem.

REASSORTMENT: A condition resulting when two or more different types of viruses exchange genetic material to form a new, genetically different virus.

RECEPTOR: Protein molecules on a cell's surface that acts as a "signal receiver" and allow communication between cells.

RECOMBINANT DNA: DNA that is cut using specific enzymes so that a gene or DNA sequence can be inserted.

RECOMBINATION: Recombination is a process during which genetic material is shuffled during reproduction to form new combinations. This mixing is important from an evolutionary standpoint because it allows the expression of different traits between generations. The process involves a physical exchange of nucleotides between duplicate strands of deoxyribonucleic acid (DNA).

RED TIDE: Red tides are a marine phenomenon in which water is stained a red, brown, or yellowish color because of the temporary abundance of a particular species of pigmented dinoflagellate (these events are known as "blooms"). Also called phytoplankton, or planktonic algae, these single-celled organisms of the class Dinophyceae move using a tail-like structure called a flagellum. They also photosynthesize, and it is their photosynthetic pigments that can tint the water during blooms. Dinoflagellates are common and widespread. Under appropriate environmental conditions, various species can grow very rapidly, causing red tides. Red tides occur in all marine regions with a temperate or warmer climate.

RE-EMERGING INFECTIOUS DISEASE: Re-emerging infectious diseases are illnesses such as malaria, diphtheria, tuberculosis, and polio that were once nearly absent from the world but are starting to cause greater numbers of infections once again. These illnesses are reappearing for many reasons. Malaria and other mosquito-borne illnesses increase when mosquito-control measures decrease. Other diseases are spreading because people have stopped being vaccinated, as happened with diphtheria after the collapse of the Soviet Union. A few diseases are re-emerging because drugs to treat them have become less available or drug-resistant strains have developed.

REHYDRATION: Dehydration is excessive loss of water from the body; rehydration is the restoration of water after dehydration.

REITER'S SYNDROME: Reiter's syndrome (also called Reiter syndrome, Reiter disease, or reactive arthritis), named after German doctor Hans Reiter (1881-1969), is a form of arthritis (joint inflammation) that appears in response to bacterial infection in some other part of the body.

RELAPSE: Relapse is a return of symptoms after the patient has apparently recovered from a disease.

REPLICATE: To replicate is to duplicate something or make a copy of it. All reproduction of living things depends on the replication of DNA molecules or, in a few cases, RNA molecules. Replication may be used to refer to the reproduction of entire viruses and other microorganisms.

REPLICATION: A process of reproducing, duplicating, copying, or repeating something, such as the duplication of DNA or the recreation of characteristics of an infectious disease in a laboratory setting.

REPORTABLE DISEASE: By law, occurrences of some diseases must be reported to government authorities when observed by health-care professionals. Such diseases are called reportable diseases or notifiable diseases. Cholera and yellow fever are examples of reportable diseases.

RESERVOIR: The animal or organism in which the virus or parasite normally resides.

RESISTANCE: Immunity developed within a species (especially bacteria) via evolution to an antibiotic or other drug. For example, in bacteria, the acquisition of genetic mutations that render the bacteria invulnerable to the action of antibiotics.

RESISTANT BACTERIA: Resistant bacteria are microbes that have lost their sensitivity to one or more antibiotic drugs through mutation.

RESISTANT ORGANISM: An organism that has developed the ability to counter something trying to harm it. Within infectious diseases, the organism, such as a bacterium, has developed a resistance to drugs, such as antibiotics.

RESPIRATOR: A respirator is any device that assists a patient in breathing or takes over breathing entirely for them.

RESTRICTION ENZYME: A special type of protein that can recognize and cut DNA at certain sequences of bases to help scientists separate out a specific gene. Restriction enzymes recognize certain sequences of DNA and cleave the DNA at those sites. The enzymes are used to generate fragments of DNA that can be subsequently joined together to create new stretches of DNA.

RETROVIRUS: Retroviruses are viruses in which the genetic material consists of ribonucleic acid (RNA) instead of the usual deoxyribonucleic acid (DNA). Retroviruses produce an enzyme known as reverse transcriptase that can transform RNA into DNA, which can then be permanently integrated into the DNA of the infected host cells.

REVERSE TRANSCRIPTASE: An enzyme that makes it possible for a retrovirus to produce DNA (deoxyribonucleic acid) from RNA (ribonucleic acid).

RHINITIS: An inflammation of the mucous lining of the nose. A nonspecific term that covers infections, allergies, and other disorders whose common feature is the location of their symptoms. These symptoms include infected or irritated mucous membranes, producing a discharge, congestion, and swelling of the tissues of the nasal passages. The most widespread form of infectious rhinitis is the common cold.

RIBONUCLEIC ACID (RNA): Any of a group of nucleic acids that carry out several important tasks in the synthesis of proteins. Unlike DNA (deoxyribonucleic acid), it has only a single strand. Nucleic acids are complex molecules that contain a cell's genetic information and the instructions for carrying out cellular processes. In eukaryotic cells, the two nucleic acids, ribonucleic acid (RNA) and deoxyribonucleic acid (DNA), work together to direct protein synthesis. Although it is DNA that contains the instructions for directing the synthesis of specific structural and enzymatic proteins, several types of RNA actually carry out the processes required to produce these proteins. These include messenger RNA (mRNA), ribosomal RNA (rRNA), and transfer RNA (tRNA). Further processing of the various RNAs is carried out by another type of RNA called small nuclear RNA (snRNA). The structure of RNA is very similar to that of DNA, however, instead of the base thymine, RNA contains the base uricil in its place.

RING VACCINATION: Ring vaccination is the vaccination of all susceptible people in an area surrounding a case of an infectious disease. Since vaccination makes people immune to the disease, the hope is that the disease will not spread from the known case to other people. Ring vaccination was used in eliminating the smallpox virus.

RNA VIRUS: An RNA virus is one whose genetic material consists of either single- or double-stranded ribonucleic acid (RNA) rather than deoxyribonucleic acid (DNA).

ROUNDWORM: Also known as nematodes; a type of helminth characterized by long, cylindrical bodies. Roundworm infections are diseases of the digestive tract and other organ systems that are caused by roundworms. Roundworm infections are widespread throughout the world, and humans acquire most types of roundworm infection from contaminated food or by touching the mouth with unwashed hands that have come into contact with the parasite larva. The severity of infection varies considerably from person to person. Children are more likely to have heavy infestations and are also more likely to suffer from malabsorption and malnutrition than adults.

ROUS SARCOMA VIRUS: Rous sarcoma virus, named after American doctor Francis Peyton Rous (1879-1970), is a virus that can cause cancer in some birds, including chickens. It was the first virus known to be able to cause cancer.

RUMINANTS: Cud-chewing animals with a four-chambered stomachs and even-toed hooves.

S

SANITATION: Sanitation is the use of hygienic recycling and disposal measures that prevent disease and promote health through sewage disposal, solid waste disposal, waste material recycling, and food processing and preparation.

SCHISTOSOMES: Blood flukes that infect an estimated 200 million people.

SEIZURE: A seizure is a sudden disruption of the brain's normal electrical activity accompanied by altered consciousness and/or other neurological and behavioral abnormalities. Epilepsy is a condition characterized by recurrent seizures that may include repetitive muscle jerking called convulsions. Seizures are traditionally divided into two major categories: generalized seizures and focal seizures. Within each major category, however, there are many different types of seizures. Generalized seizures come about due to abnormal neuronal activity on both sides of the brain, while focal seizures, also named partial seizures, occur in only one part of the brain.

SELECTION: Process which favors one feature of organisms in a population over another feature found in the population. This occurs through differential reproduction—those with the favored feature produce more offspring than those with the other feature, such that they become a greater percentage of the population in the next generation.

SELECTION PRESSURE: Selection pressure refers to factors that influence the evolution of an organism. An example is the overuse of antibiotics, which provides a selection pressure for the development of antibiotic resistance in bacteria.

SELECTIVE PRESSURE: Selective pressure refers to the tendency of an organism that has a certain characteristic to be eliminated from an environment or to increase in numbers. An example is the increased prevalence of bacteria that are resistant to multiple kinds of antibiotics.

SENTINEL: A sentinel is a guard or watcher; in medicine, a sentinel node is a lymph node near the breast in which cancer cells from a breast tumor are likely to be found at an early stage of the cancer's spreading (metastasization).

SENTINEL SURVEILLANCE: Sentinel surveillance is a method in epidemiology where a subset of the population is surveyed for the presence of communicable diseases. Also, a sentinel is an animal used to indicate the presence of disease within an area.

SEPSIS: Sepsis refers to a bacterial infection in the bloodstream or body tissues. This is a very broad term covering the presence of many types of microscopic disease-causing organisms. Sepsis is also called bacteremia. Closely related terms include septicemia and septic syndrome. According to the Society of Critical Care Medicine, severe sepsis affects about 750,000 people in the United States each year. However, it is predicted to rapidly rise to one million people by 2010 due to the aging U.S. population. Over the decade of the 1990s, the incident rate of sepsis increased over 91%.

SEPTIC: The term "septic" refers to the state of being infected with bacteria, particularly in the bloodstream.

SEPTICEMIA: Prolonged fever, chills, anorexia, and anemia in conjunction with tissue lesions.

SEQUENCING: Finding the order of chemical bases in a section of DNA.

SEROCONVERSION: The development in the blood of antibodies to an infectious organism or agent. Typically, seroconversion is associated with infections caused by bacteria, viruses, and protozoans. But seroconversion also occurs after the deliberate inoculation with an antigen in the process of vaccination. In the case of infections, the development of detectable levels of antibodies can occur quickly, in the case of an active infection, or can be prolonged, in the case of a latent infection. Seroconversion typically heralds the development of the symptoms of the particular infection.

SEROTYPES: Serotypes or serovars are classes of microorganisms based on the types of molecules (antigens) that they present on their surfaces. Even a single species may have thousands of serotypes, which may have medically quite distinct behaviors.

SEXUALLY TRANSMITTED DISEASE (STD): Sexually transmitted diseases (STDs) vary in their susceptibility to treatment, their signs and symptoms, and the consequences if they are left untreated. Some are caused by bacteria. These usually can be treated and cured. Others are caused by viruses and can typically be treated but not cured. More than 15 million new cases of STDs are diagnosed annually in the United States.

SHED: To shed is to cast off or release. In medicine, the release of eggs or live organisms from an individual infected with parasites is often referred to as shedding.

SHOCK: Shock is a medical emergency in which the organs and tissues of the body are not receiving an adequate flow of blood. This condition deprives the organs and tissues of oxygen (carried in the blood) and allows the buildup of waste products. Shock can result in serious damage or even death.

SOCIOECONOMIC: Concerning both social and economic factors.

SOUTHERN BLOT ANALYSIS: Southern blot refers to an electrophoresis technique in which pieces of deoxyribonucleic acid (DNA) that have resulted from enzyme digestion are separated from one another on the basis of size, followed by the transfer of the DNA fragments to a flexible membrane. The membrane can then be exposed to various probes to identify target regions of the genetic material.

SPECIAL PATHOGENS BRANCH: A group within the U.S. Centers for Disease Control and Prevention (CDC) whose goal is to study highly infectious viruses that produce diseases within humans.

SPIROCHETE: A bacterium shaped like a spiral. Spiral-shaped bacteria, which live in contaminated water, sewage, soil, and decaying organic matter, as well as inside humans and animals.

SPONGIFORM: Spongiform is the clinical name for the appearance of brain tissue affected by prion diseases, such as Creutzfeld-Jakob disease or bovine spongiform encephalopathy (mad cow disease). The disease process leads to the formation of tiny holes in brain tissue, giving it a spongy appearance.

SPONTANEOUS GENERATION: Also known as abiogenesis; the incorrect and discarded assumption that living things can be generated from nonliving things.

SPORE: A dormant form assumed by some bacteria, such as anthrax, that enables the bacterium to survive high temperatures, dryness, and lack of nourishment for long periods of time. Under proper conditions, the spore may revert to the actively multiplying form of the bacteria.

SPOROZOAN: The fifth Phylum of the Protist Kingdom, known as Apicomplexa, comprises several species of obligate intracellular protozoan parasites classified as Sporozoa or Sporozoans, because they form reproductive cells known as spores. Many sporozoans are parasitic and pathogenic species, such as *Plasmodium falciparum, P. malariae, P. vivax, Toxoplasma gondii, Pneumocysts carinii, Cryptosporidum parvum* and *Cryptosporidum muris.* The Sporozoa reproduction cycle has both asexual and sexual phases. The asexual phase is termed schizogony (from the Greek, meaning generation through division), in which merozoites (daughter cells) are produced through multiple nuclear fissions. The sexual phase is known as sporogony (i.e., generation of spores) and is followed by gametogony or the production of sexually reproductive cells termed gamonts.

SPOROZOITE: Developmental stage of a protozoan (e.g., a malaria protozoan) during which it is transferred from vector (with malaria, a mosquito) to a human host.

STAINING: Staining refers to the use of chemicals to identify target components of microorganisms.

STANDARD PRECAUTIONS: Standard precautions are the safety measures taken to prevent the transmission of disease-causing bacteria. These include proper handwashing; wearing gloves, goggles, and other protective clothing; proper handling of needles; and sterilization of equipment.

STERILIZATION: Sterilization is a term that refers to the complete killing or elimination of living organisms in the sample being treated. Sterilization is absolute. After the treatment the sample is either devoid of life or the possibility of life (as from the subsequent germination and growth of bacterial spores) or it is not considered sterile.

STRAIN: A subclass or a specific genetic variation of an organism.

STREP THROAT: Streptococcal sore throat, or strep throat as it is more commonly called, is an infection caused by group A *Streptococcus* bacteria. The main target of the infection is the mucous membranes lining the pharynx. Sometimes the tonsils are also infected (tonsillitis). If left untreated, the infection can develop into rheumatic fever or other serious conditions.

STREPTOCOCCUS: A genus of bacteria that includes species such as *Streptococci pyogenes*, a species of bacteria that causes strep throat.

SUPERINFECTION: When a new infection occurs in a patient who already has some other infection, it is called a superinfection. For example, a bacterial infection appearing in a person who already had viral pneumonia would be a superinfection.

SURVEILLANCE: The systematic analysis, collection, evaluation, interpretation, and dissemination of data. In public health, it assists in the identification of health threats and the planning, implementation, and evaluation of responses to those threats.

SYLVATIC: Sylvatic means pertaining to the woods and refers to diseases such as plague that are spread by animals such as ground squirrels and other wild rodents.

SYSTEMIC: Any medical condition that affects the whole body (i.e., the whole system) is systemic.

T

T CELL: Immune-system white blood cells that enable antibody production, suppress antibody production, or kill other cells. When a vertebrate encounters substances that are capable of causing it harm, a protective system known as the immune system comes into play. This system is a network of many different organs that work together to recognize foreign substances and destroy them. The immune system can respond to the presence of a disease-causing agent (pathogen) in two ways. In cell-mediated immunity, immune cells known as the T cells produce special chemicals that can specifically isolate the pathogen and destroy it. The other branch of immunity is called humoral immunity, in which immune cells called B cells can produce soluble proteins (antibodies) that can accurately target and kill the pathogen.

TAPEWORM: Tapeworms are parasitic flatworms of class *Cestoidea*, phylum *Platyhelminthes*, that live inside the intestine. Tapeworms have no digestive system, but absorb predigested nutrients directly from their surroundings.

T-CELL VACCINE: A T-cell vaccine is one that relies on eliciting cellular immunity, rather than humoral antibody-based immunity, against infection. T cell vaccines are being developed against the human immunodeficiency virus (HIV) and hepatitis C.

TICK: A tick is any blood-sucking parasitic insect of suborder *Ixodides*, superfamily *Ixodoidea*. Ticks can transmit a number of diseases, including Lyme disease and Rocky Mountain spotted fever.

TOGAVIRUS: Togaviruses are a type of virus. Rubella is caused by a type of togavirus.

TOPICAL: Any medication that is applied directly to a particular part of the body's surface is termed topical; for example, a topical ointment.

TOXIC: Something that is poisonous and that can cause illness or death.

TOXIN: A poison that is produced by a living organism.

TOXOID: A toxoid is a bacterial toxin that has been altered chemically to make it incapable of causing damage, but is still capable of stimulating an immune response. Toxoids are used to stimulate antibody production, which is protective in the event of exposure to the active toxin.

TRANSFUSION-TRANSMISSIBLE INFECTIONS: Any infection that can be transmitted to a person by a blood transfusion (addition of stored whole blood or blood fractions to a person's own blood) is a transfusion-transmissible infection. Some diseases that can be transmitted in this way are AIDS, hepatitis B, hepatitis C, syphilis, malaria, and Chagas disease.

TRANSMISSION: Microorganisms that cause disease in humans and other species are known as pathogens. The transmission of pathogens to a human or other host can occur in a number of ways, depending upon the microorganism.

TREMATODES: Trematodes, also called flukes, are a type of parasitic flatworm. In humans, flukes can infest the liver, lung, and other tissues.

TRICLOSAN: A chemical that kills bacteria. Most antibacterial soaps use this chemical.

TRISMUS: Trismus is the medical term for lockjaw, a condition often associated with tetanus, infection by the *Clostridium tetani* bacillus. In trismus or lockjaw, the major muscles of the jaw contract involuntarily.

TROPHOZOITE: The amoeboid, vegetative stage of the malaria protozoa.

TYPHUS: A disease caused by various species of *Rickettsia*, characterized by fever, rash, and delirium. Insects such as lice and chiggers transmit typhus. Two forms of typhus, epidemic typhus and scrub typhus, are fatal if untreated.

U

UNIVERSAL PRECAUTION: Universal precaution refers to an infection control strategy in which all human blood and other material is assumed to be potentially infectious, specifically with organisms such as human immunodeficiency virus (HIV) and hepatitis B virus. The precautions are aimed at preventing contact with blood or the other materials.

V

VACCINATION: Vaccination is the inoculation, or use of vaccines, to prevent specific diseases within humans and animals by producing immunity to such diseases. It is the introduction of weakened or dead viruses or microorganisms into the body to create immunity by the production of specific antibodies.

VACCINE: A substance that is introduced to stimulate antibody production and thus provide immunity to a particular disease.

VACCINIA VIRUS: The vaccinia virus is a usually harmless virus that is closely related to the virus that causes smallpox, a dangerous disease. Infection with the vaccinia virus confers immunity against smallpox, so vaccinia virus has been used as a vaccine against smallpox.

VARICELLA ZOSTER IMMUNE GLOBULIN (VZIG): Varicella zoster immune globulin is a preparation that can give people temporary protection against chickenpox after exposure to the Varicella virus. It is used for children and adults who are at risk of complications of the disease or who are susceptible to infection because they have weakened immunity.

VARICELLA ZOSTER VIRUS (VZV): Varicella zoster virus is a member of the alpha herpes virus group and is the cause of both chickenpox (also known as varicella) and shingles (herpes zoster).

VARIOLA VIRUS: Variola virus (or variola major virus) is the virus that causes smallpox. The virus is one of the members of the poxvirus group (Family Poxviridae). The virus particle is brick shaped and contains a double strand of deoxyribonucleic acid. The variola virus is among the most dangerous of all the potential biological weapons.

VARIOLATION: Variolation was the pre-modern practice of deliberately infecting a person with smallpox in order to make them immune to a more serious form of the disease. It was dangerous, but did confer immunity on survivors.

VECTOR: Any agent that carries and transmits parasites and diseases. Also, an organism or chemical used to transport a gene into a new host cell.

VECTOR-BORNE DISEASE: A vector-borne disease is one in which the pathogenic microorganism is transmitted from an infected individual to another individual by an arthropod or other agent, sometimes with other animals serving as intermediary hosts. The transmission depends upon the attributes and requirements of at least three different living organisms: the pathologic agent, either a virus, protozoa, bacteria, or helminth (worm); the vector, commonly arthropods such as ticks or mosquitoes; and the human host.

VENEREAL DISEASE: Venereal diseases are diseases that are transmitted by sexual contact. They are named after Venus, the Roman goddess of female sexuality.

VESICLE: A membrane-bound sphere that contains a variety of substances in cells.

VIRAL SHEDDING: Viral shedding refers to the movement of the herpes virus from the nerves to the surface of the skin. During shedding, the virus can be passed on through skin-to-skin contact.

VIRION: A virion is a mature virus particle, consisting of a core of ribonucleic acid (RNA) or deoxyribonucleic acid (DNA) surrounded by a protein coat. This is the form in which a virus exists outside of its host cell.

VIRULENCE: Virulence is the ability of a disease organism to cause disease: a more virulent organism is more infective and liable to produce more serious disease.

VIRUS: Viruses are essentially nonliving repositories of nucleic acid that require the presence of a living prokaryotic or eukaryotic cell for the replication of the nucleic acid. There are a number of different viruses that challenge the human immune system and that may produce disease in humans. A virus is a small, infectious agent that consists of a core of genetic material—either deoxyribonucleic acid (DNA) or ribonucleic acid (RNA)—surrounded by a shell of protein. Very simple microorganisms, viruses are much smaller than bacteria that enter and multiply within cells. Viruses often exchange or transfer their genetic material (DNA or RNA) to cells and can cause diseases such as chickenpox, hepatitis, measles, and mumps.

VISCERAL: Visceral means pertaining to the viscera. The viscera are the large organs contained in the main cavities of the body, especially the thorax and abdomen, for example, the lungs, stomach, intestines, kidneys, or liver.

W

WATER-BORNE DISEASE: Water-borne disease refers to diseases that are caused by exposure to contaminated water. The exposure can occur by drinking the water or having the water come in contact with the body. Examples of water-borne diseases are cholera and typhoid fever.

WAVELENGTH: A distance of one cycle of a wave; for instance, the distance between the peaks on adjoining waves that have the same phase.

WEAPONIZATION: The use of any bacterium, virus, or other disease-causing organism as a weapon of war. Among other terms, it is also called germ warfare, biological weaponry, and biological warfare.

WEIL'S DISEASE: Weil's disease, named after German doctor Adolf Weil (1848-1916), is a severe form of leptospirosis or seven-day fever, a disease caused by infection with the corkscrew-shaped bacillus *Leptospira interrogans*.

WILD VIRUS: Wild- or wild-type virus is a genetic description referring to the original form of a virus, first observed in nature. It may remain the most common form in existence but mutated forms develop over time and sometimes become the new wild type virus.

Z

ZOONOTIC: A zoonotic disease is a disease that can be transmitted between animals and humans. Examples of zoonotic diseases are anthrax, plague, and Q-fever.

Chronology

c.2500 The characteristic symptoms of malaria are first described in Chinese medical writings.

c.1000 Hindu physicians exhibit broad clinical knowledge of tuberculosis. In India, the Laws of Manu consider it to be an unclean, incurable disease and an impediment to marriage.

c.430 Plague of Athens caused by unknown infectious agent. One third of the population (increased by those fleeing the Spartan army) die.

c.400 Hippocrates (460–370 BC), Greek physician, and his disciples found their medical practice based on reason and experiment. They attribute disease to natural causes and use diet and medication to restore the body's balance of humors.

c.400 Hippocratic texts recommend irrigation with fresh water as a treatment for septic wounds.

c.300 A medical school is set up in Alexandria where the first accurate anatomical observations using dissection are made. The principal exponents of the school are Greek physician Herophilus (c.335–c.280 BC) and Greek physician Erasistratus (c.304–c.250 BC).

c.300 Herophilus, Greek anatomist, establishes himself as the first systemic anatomist and the first to perform human dissections.

91 Greek scientific medicine takes hold in Rome when the physician Asclepiades (c.130–40 BC) of Bithynia settles in the West.

c.30 Aulus Cornelius Celsus, Roman encyclopedist, writes his influential book *De Re Medicina*. This work *On Medicine* contains descriptions of many conditions and operations, and is probably drawn mostly from the collection of writings of the school of Hippocrates. It is rediscovered during the fifteenth century and becomes highly influential. (See 1426)

c.75 Dioscorides, Greek physician, writes the first systematic pharmocopoeia. His *De Materia Medica* in five volumes provides accurate botanical and pharmacological information. It is preserved by the Arabs and, when translated into Latin and printed in 1478, becomes a standard botanical reference.

150 Cladius Galen says that pus formation is required for wound healing. This proves to be incorrect and hinders the treatment of wounds for centuries.

c.160 Bubonic plague (termed "barbarian boils") sweeps China.

c.160 Galen (c.130-c.200), Greek physician, in his *De Usu Partium* describes the pineal gland as a secretory organ that is important to thinking. He names it the pineal because it resembles a pine cone.

c.166 Plague in Rome (possibly smallpox or bubonic plague) eventually kills millions throughout the weakening Roman empire.

167 Stabiae, a popular health resort for tuberculosis sufferers, is established near Naples,

Italy. It is believed that the fumes from nearby Mt. Vesuvius are beneficial for lung ulcers.

170 Galen, the Greek physician, first describes gonorrhea.

c.200 Galen describes internal inflammations as caused by personal factors.

c.370 Basil of Caesarea (330–379) founds and organizes a large hospital at Caesarea (near Palestine).

c.400 Fabiola, a Christian noblewoman, founds the first nosocomium or hospital in Western Europe. After establishing the first hospital in Rome, she founds a hospice for pilgrims in Porto, Italy.

430 Earliest recorded plague in Europe is an epidemic that breaks out in Athens, Greece.

c.500 During this century, the "plague of Justinian" kills about one million people.

529 Benedict of Nursia founds the monastery at Monte Cassino in central Italy. It becomes, if not an actual medical school, at least an important center of scholarship in which medicine played a great part. It also acquires great fame throughout the West and its medical teachings are spread by the Benedictines to their monasteries scattered all over Europe.

610 In China, Ch'ao Yuan-fang writes a treatise on the causes and symptoms of diseases. Medical knowledge spreads from China to Japan via the Korean peninsula.

644 Rotharus, King of Lombardy also called Rothari, issues his edict ordering the segregation of all lepers.

c.700 Benedictus Crispus, archbishop of Milan from 681 to about 730, writes his *Commentarium Medicinale*, an elementary practical manual in verse. It describes the use of medicinal plants for curing illnesses.

c.850 Christian physician Sabur ibn Sahl of Jundishapur compiles a twenty-two volume work on antidotes that dominates Islamic pharmacopeia for the next 400 years.

c.850 Islamic philosopher al-Kindi (813–873) writes his *De Medicinarum Compositarum Gradibus*, which attempts to base dosages of medicine on mathematical measurements.

c.875 Bertharius, the abbot of Montcasino from 857 to 884, writes two treatises, *De Innu-*

meris Remediorum Utilitatibus and *De Innumeris Morbis* that give insight into the kind of medicine practiced in the monasteries.

896 Abu Bakr al-Razi (also known as Rhazes (c.845-c.930), Persian physician and alchemist, distinguishes between the specific characteristics of measles and smallpox. He is also believed to be the first to classify all substances into the great classification of animal, vegetable, and mineral. (See 918)

c.900 First medical books written in Anglo-Saxon appear. *Lacnunga* and the *Leech Book of Bald* appear and have some botanical sections.

c.955 Jewish "prince of medicine," Isaac Israeli, dies. He writes classic works on fever and uroscopy, as well as a *Guide of the Physicians*.

c.980 Abu Al–Qasim Al–Zahravi (Abucasis) creates a system and method of human dissection along with the first formal specific surgical techniques.

c.1000 Ibn Sina, or Avicenna, publishes *Al-Quanun*, or Canon of Medicine, where he held that medicines could be discovered and tried by experiment or by reasoning.

1137 St. Bartholomew's hospital is founded in London.

1140 Bologna, Italy, begins to develop as a major European medical center. In the next century, the Italian physician Taddeo Alderotti (c.1233–1303) opens a school of medicine there.

1200 Physicians in Italy begin to write case-histories that describe symptoms and observable pathology of diseases.

c.1267 Roger Bacon (1214–1292), English philosopher and scientist, asserts that natural phenomena should be studied empirically.

1302 First formally recorded post-mortem or judicial autopsy is performed in Bologna, Italy, by Italian physician Bartolomeo da Varignana. A postmortem is ordered by the court in a case of suspected poisoning.

1333 Public botanical garden is established in Venice, Italy, to grow herbs that have medical uses.

1345 First apothecary shop or drug store opens in London, England.

1348 The beginning of a three-year epidemic caused by *Yersinia pestis* kills almost one-third of the population of urban Europe. In the aftermath of the epidemic, measures are introduced by the Italian government to improve public sanitation, marking the origin of public health.

1374 As the plague spreads, the Republic of Ragusa places the first quarantines on crews of ships thought to be infected.

1388 Richard II (1367–1400), king of England, establishes the first sanitary laws in England.

1489 Typhus is first brought to Europe by soldiers who had been fighting in Cyprus.

1491 First anatomical book to contain printed illustrations is German physician Johannes de Ketham's *Fasciculus Medicinae*.

1492 Venereal diseases, smallpox, and influenza are brought by the Columbus expedition (and subsequent European explorers) to the New World. Millions of native peoples eventually die from these diseases because of a lack of prior exposure to stimulate immunity. In some regions, whole villages succumb, and across broader regions up to 95% of the native population dies.

1525 Gonzalo Hernandez de Oviedo y Valdes (1478–1557) of Spain publishes the first systematic description of the medicinal plants of Central America.

1525 Paracelsus (1493–1541), Swiss physician and alchemist, begins the use of mineral substances as medicines.

1527 Paracelsus (1493–1541), Swiss physician and alchemist, publicly burns the writings of Galen at Basel. He rejects the traditional medical methods as irrational, and he founds iatrochemistry, asserting that the body is linked in some way to the laws of chemistry.

1528 The Italian physician Fracastorius describes an epidemic of typhus among French troops invading Naples.

1530 Girolamo Fracastoro (1478–1553), Italian physician and poet, writes his poem called "Syphilis" (*Syphilis sive Morbus Gallici*), which gives the definitive name to the sexually transmitted disease that is spreading throughout Europe.

1536 Paracelsus (1493–1541), Swiss physician and alchemist, publishes his surgical treatise, *Chirurgia Magna*.

1543 Andreas Vesalius (1514–1564), Dutch anatomist, publishes his *De Corporis Humani Corporis Fabrica*, the first accurate book on human anatomy. Its illustrations are of the highest level of both realism and art, and the result revolutionizes biology.

1546 Girolamo Fracastoro (1478–1553), Italian physician, writes his *De Contagione et Contagiosis Morbis*, which contains new ideas on the transmission of contagious diseases and is considered as the scientific beginning of that study.

1563 Epidemic cholera is described by Garcia del Huerto, working in Goa, India.

1567 A book on miner's tuberculosis by Swiss physician and alchemist Paracelsus (1493–1541) is posthumously published.

1602 Felix Platter (1536–1614), Swiss anatomist, publishes his *Praxis Medica*, which is the first modern attempt at the classification of diseases.

1621 Johannes Baptista van Helmont (1577–1635), Dutch physician and alchemist, writes his *Ortus Medicinae* in which he becomes one of the founders of modern pathology. He studies the anatomical changes that occur in disease.

1624 Adriaan van den Spigelius (1578–1625), Dutch anatomist, publishes the first account of malaria.

1640 Juan del Vigo introduces cinchona into Spain. Native to the Andes, the bark of this tree is processed to obtain quinine, used in the treatment of malaria.

1642 First treatise on the use of cinchona bark (quinine powder) for treating malaria is written by Spanish physician Pedro Barba (1608–1671).

1648 René Descartes (1596–1650), French philosopher and mathematician, writes *De Homine*, the first European textbook on physiology. He considers the body to be a material machine and offers his mechanist theory of life.

1648 Willem Piso (1611–1678), Dutch physician and botanist (also called Le Pois), points out the effectiveness of ipecac against dysentery in his book *De Medicina Brasiliensi*. He is among the first to become acquainted with tropical diseases, and he distinguishes between yaws and syphilis.

1660 The Royal Society of London is founded in England with Henry Oldenburg (c.1618–1677) Secretary and Robert Hooke (1635–1702) Curator of Experiments. Two years later (1662), King Charles II (1630–1685) grants it a royal charter, and it becomes known as the "Royal Society of London for the Promotion of Natural Knowledge."

1665 Bubonic plague epidemic in London kills 75,000 people. It is during this scourge that English scientist and mathematician Isaac Newton (1642–1727) leaves school in London and stays at his mother' farm in the country. There he formulates his laws of motion.

1665 First drawing of the cell is made by Robert Hooke (1635–1703), English physicist. While observing a sliver of cork under a microscope, Hooke notices it is composed of a pattern of tiny rectangular holes he calls "cells" because each looks like a small, empty room. Although he does not observe living cells, the name is retained.

1665 Robert Hooke (1635–1703), English physicist, publishes his landmark book on microscopy called *Micrographia*. Containing some of the most beautiful drawings of microscopic observations ever made, his book led to many discoveries in related fields.

1666 Robert Boyle (1627–1691), English physicist and chemist, publishes *The Origine of Formes and Qualities* in which he begins to explain all chemical reactions and physical properties through the existence of small, indivisible particles or atoms.

1668 Francesco Redi (1626–1697), Italian physician, conducts experiments to disprove spontaneous generation and shows that maggots are not born spontaneously, but come from eggs laid by flies. He publishes his *Esperienze Intorno all Generazione degli Insetti*.

1671 Michael Ettmüller (1644–1683), German physician, attributes the contagiousness of tuberculosis to sputum.

1672 French physician Le Gras introduces ipecac into Europe as he brings it to Paris this year. The root of the Brazilian plant ipecacuanha is used to cure dysentery. (See 1625)

1674 Antoni van Leeuwenhoek (1632–1723), Dutch biologist and microscopist, observes "animacules" in lake water viewed through a ground glass lens. This observation of what will eventually be known as bacteria represents the start of the formal study of microbiology.

1675 John Josselyn, English botanist, publishes an account of the plants and animals he encounters while living in America and indicates that tuberculosis existed among the Native Americans before the coming of the Europeans.

1677 Antoni van Leeuwenhoek (1632–1723), Dutch biologist and microscopist, discovers spermatozoa and describes them in a letter he publishes in *Philosophical Transactions* in 1679. In the same year, Johan Ham also sees them microscopically, but the semen he observes comes from a patient suffering from gonorrhea, and Ham concludes that spermatozoa are a consequence of the disease.

1700 Bernardino Ramazzini (1633–1714), Italian physician, publishes the first systematic treatment on occupational diseases. His book, *De Morbis Artificum*, opens up an entirely new department of modern medicine—diseases of trade or occupation and industrial hygiene.

1721 The word "antiseptic" first appears in print.

1730 George Martine performs the first tracheostomy on a patient with diphtheria.

1735 Botulism first described.

1748 John Fothergill describes diphtheria in "Account of the Putrid Sore Throat."

1762 Marcus Anton von Plenciz, Sr. (1705–1786), Austrian physician, expresses the idea that all infectious diseases are caused by living organisms and that there is a specific organism for each disease.

1767 William Heberden demonstrates that chicken-pox is not a mild form of smallpox, but a different disease.

1780 George Adams (1750–1795), English engineer, devises the first microtome. This mechanical instrument cuts thin slices for examination under a microscope, thus replacing the imprecise procedure of cutting by hand-held razor.

1789 Polio is first described by Michael Underwood in England.

1796 Edward Jenner (1749–1823) uses cowpox virus to develop a smallpox vaccine. By modern standards, this was human experimentation as Jenner injected healthy eight-year-old James Phillips with cowpox and then after a period of months with smallpox.

1798 Government legislation is passed to establish hospitals in the United States devoted to the care of ill mariners. This initiative leads to the establishment of a Hygenic Laboratory that eventually grows to become the National Institutes of Health.

1800 Marie-François-Xavier Bichat publishes his first major work, *Treatise on Tissues,* which establishes histology as a new scientific discipline. Bichat distinguishes 21 kinds of tissue and relates particular diseases to particular tissues.

1801 A hospital is established in London, England, to treat the victims of typhus.

1802 John Dalton introduces modern atomic theory into the science of chemistry.

1814 The Royal Hospital for Diseases of the Chest is founded in London, England, in an attempt to keep consumptive patients (people with tuberculosis) segregated.

1816 The stethoscope, which is an important tool for diagnosing pneumonia, is introduced by Rene LaËnnec.

1817 Start of first cholera pandemic, which spreads from Bengal to China in the east and to Eygpt in the west.

1818 William Charles Wells suggests the theory of natural selection in an essay dealing with human color variations. He notes that dark-skinned people seem more resistant to tropical diseases than lighter-skinned people. Wells also calls attention to selection carried out by animal breeders. Jerome Lawrence, James Cowles Prichard, and others make similar suggestions, but do not develop their ideas into a coherent and convincing theory of evolution.

1818 Xavier Bichat (1771–1802), French physician, publishes his first major work, *Trait, des membranes en general,* in which he propounds the notion of tissues. This work also founds histology, distinguishing 21 kinds of tissue and relating disease to them.

1820 First United States *Pharmacopoeia* is published.

1824 Start of second cholera pandemic, which penetrates as far as Russia and also reaches England, North America, the Caribbean, and Latin America.

1826 Pierre Bretonneau (1778–1862), French physician, describes and names diptheria in his specification of diseases.

1829 Salicin, the precursor of aspirin, is purified from the bark of the willow tree.

1831 Charles Robert Darwin (1809–1882) begins his historic voyage on the H.M.S. *Beagle* (1831–1836). His observations during the voyage lead to his theory of evolution by means of natural selection.

1835 Jacob Bigelow (1787–1879), American physician, publishes his book *On Self-Limited Diseases* in which he states the commonsense idea that some diseases will simply run their course and subside without the benefit of any treatment from a physician.

1836 Theodor Schwann carries out experiments that refute the theory of the spontaneous generation. He also demonstrates that alcoholic fermentation depends on the action of living yeast cells. The same conclusion is reached independently by Charles Caignard de la Tour.

1837 Pierre-Françs-Olive Rayer (1793–1867), French physician, is the first to describe the disease glanders as found in man and to prove that it is not a form of tuberculosis.

1838 Angelo Dubini (1813–1902), Italian physician, discovers *Ankylostoma duodenale,* the cause of hookworm disease, in the intestinal tract.

1838 Matthias Jakob Schleiden notes that the nucleus first described by Robert Brown is a characteristic of all plant cells. Schleiden describes plants as a community of cells and cell products. He helps establish cell theory and stimulates Theodor Schwann's recognition that animals are also composed of cells and cell products.

1839 Third cholera pandemic begins with entry of British troops in Afghanistan and travels to Persia, Central Asia, Europe, and the Americas.

1841 Friedrich Gustav Jacob Henle (1809–1885), German pathologist and anatomist, publishes his *Allegemeine Anatomie*, which becomes the first systematic textbook of histology (the study of minute tissue structure and includes the first statement of the germ theory of communicable disease).

1842 Edwin Chadwick, a pioneer in sanitary reform, reports that deaths from typhus in 1838 and 1839 in England exceeded those from smallpox.

1842 Oliver Wendell Holmes recommends that surgeons wash their hands using calcium chloride to prevent spread of infection from corpses to patients.

1843 First outbreak of polio in the United States occurs.

1843 Gabriel Andral (1797–1876), French physician, is the first to urge that blood be examined in cases of disease.

1846 American Medical Association establishes a code of ethics for physicians which declares their obligation to treat victims of epidemic diseases even at a risk to their own lives. (See 1912)

1847 A series of yellow fever epidemics sweeps the American Southern states. The epidemics recur for more than thirty years.

1847 The first sexually transmitted disease clinic is opened at the London Docks Hospital.

1849 John Snow (1813–1858), English physician, first states the theory that cholera is a water-borne disease. During a cholera epidemic in London in 1854, Snow breaks the handle of the Broad Street Pump, thereby shutting down the main source of disease transmission during the outbreak.

1849 John Snow publishes the groundbreaking paper "On the Transmission of Cholera."

1855 Third, or Modern, pandemic of plague probably begins in Yunan province, China.

1857 Louis Pasteur demonstrates that lactic acid fermentation is caused by a living organism. Between 1857 and 1880, he performs a series of experiments that refute the doctrine of spontaneous generation. He also introduces vaccines for fowl cholera, anthrax, and rabies, based on attenuated strains of viruses and bacteria.

1858 Rudolf Ludwig Carl Virchow publishes his landmark paper "Cellular Pathology" and establishes the field of cellular pathology. Virchow asserts that all cells arise from pre-existing cells (*Omnis cellula e cellula*). He argues that the cell is the ultimate locus of all disease.

1859 Charles Robert Darwin publishes his landmark book *On the Origin of Species by Means of Natural Selection*.

1861 Carl Gegenbaur confirms Theodor Schwann's suggestion that all vertebrate eggs are single cells.

1862 First demonstration of pasteurization.

1864 Fourth cholera pandemic starts and revisits locations of previous pandemics.

1865 An epidemic of rinderpest kills 500,000 cattle in Great Britain. Government inquiries into the outbreak pave the way for the development of contemporary theories of epidemiology and the germ theory of disease.

1865 French physiologist Claude Bernard publishes *Introduction to the Study of Human Experimentation*, which advocates "Never perform an experiment which might be harmful to the patient even if advantageous to science...."

1866 The Austrian botanist and monk Johann Gregor Mendel (1822–1884) discovers the laws of heredity and writes the first of a series of papers on heredity (1866–1869). The papers formulate the laws of hybridization. Mendel's work is disregarded until 1900, when Hugo de Vries rediscovers it. Unbeknownst to both Darwin and Mendel, Mendelian laws provide the scientific framework for the concepts of gradual evolution and continuous variation.

1867 Joseph Lister publishes a study that implicates microorganisms with infection. Based on this, his use of early disinfectants during surgery markedly reduces post-operative infections and death.

1867 Robert Koch establishes the role of bacteria in anthrax, providing the final piece of evidence in support of the germ theory of disease. Koch goes on to formulate postulates that, when fulfilled, confirm bacteria or viruses as the cause of an infection.

1868 Carl August Wunderlich (1815–1877), German physician, publishes his major work on the relation of animal heat or fever to disease. He is the first to recognize that fever is not itself a disease, but is rather a symptom.

1869 Johann Friedrich Miescher discovers nuclein, a new chemical isolated from the nuclei of pus cells. Two years later, he isolates nuclein from salmon sperm. This material comes to be known as nucleic acid.

1871 Ferdinand Julius Cohn coins the term bacterium.

1871 First U.S. city to use a filter on its public water supply is Poughkeepsie, New York. The evidence mounts that much disease is spread by contaminated drinking water.

1873 Franz Anton Schneider describes cell division in detail. His drawings include both the nucleus and chromosomal strands.

1875 Ferdinand Cohn publishes a classification of bacteria in which the genus name *Bacillus* is used for the first time.

1875 Koch's postulates used for the first time to demonstrate that anthrax is caused by *Bacillus anthracis*, validating the germ theory of disease.

1877 Louis Pasteur (1822–1895), French chemist, first distinguishes between aerobic and anaerobic bacteria.

1877 Paul Erlich recognizes the existence of the mast cells of the immune system.

1877 Robert Koch describes new techniques for fixing, staining, and photographing bacteria.

1877 Wilhelm Friedrich Kühne proposes the term enzyme (meaning "in yeast"). Kühne establishes the critical distinction between enzymes, or "ferments," and the microorganisms that produce them.

1878 Joseph Lister publishes a paper describing the role of a bacterium he names *Bacterium lactis* in the souring of milk.

1878 Robert Koch (1843–1910), German bacteriologist, publishes his landmark findings on the etiology or cause of infectious disease. Koch' postulates state that the causative microorganism must be located in a diseased animal, and that after it is cultured or grown, it must then be capable of causing disease in a healthy animal. Finally, the newly-infected animal must yield the same bacteria as those found in the original animal.

1878 Thomas Burrill demonstrates that a plant disease (pear blight) is caused by a bacterium (*Micrococcus amylophorous*).

1879 Albert Nisser (1855–1916) identifies the bacterium *Neiserria gonorrhoeoe* as the cause of gonorrhea.

1880 C. L. Alphonse Laveran isolates malarial parasites in erythrocytes of infected people and demonstrates that the organism can replicate in the cells.

1880 The first issue of the journal *Science* is published by the American Association for the Advancement of Science.

1881 Fifth cholera pandemic begins and is widespread in China and Japan in the Far East, as well as Germany and Russia in Europe, although the disease does not spread in North America.

1881 *Streptococcus pneumoniae*, a major cause of bacterial pneumonia, is discovered independently by Louis Pasteur and George Sternberg.

1882 Angelina Fannie and Walter Hesse in Koch's laboratory develop agar as a solid grow medium for microorganisms. Agar replaces gelatin as the solid growth medium of choice in microbiology.

1882 Friedrich August Johannes Loffler (1852–1915), German bacteriologist, and F. Schulze discover the bacterium causing glanders, a contagious and destructive disease of animals, especially horses, that can be transmitted to humans.

1883 Edwin Theodore Klebs and Frederich Loeffler independently discover *Corynebacterium diphtheriae*, the bacterium that causes diphtheria.

1883 Robert Koch discovers *V. cholerae* as the causative agent of cholera in Egypt.

1883 Surgical gowns and headgear begin to be used by surgeons.

1884 Elie Metchnikoff discovers the antibacterial activity of white blood cells, which he calls "phagocytes," and formulates the theory of phagocytosis. He also develops the cellular theory of vaccination.

1884 Hans Christian J. Gram develops the Gram stain, a method of categorizing bacteria into one of two groups (gram-positive and gram-negative) based upon the chemical reaction of the bacteria cell walls to a staining procedure.

1884 Louis Pasteur and coworkers publish a paper entitled *A New Communication on Rabies*. Pasteur proves that the causal agent of rabies can be attenuated and the weakened virus can be used as a vaccine to prevent the disease. This work serves as the basis of future work on virus attenuation, vaccine development, and the concept that variation is an inherent characteristic of viruses.

1885 Francis Galton devises a new statistical tool, the correlation table.

1885 French chemist Louis Pasteur (1822–1895) inoculates a boy, Joseph Meister, against rabies. Meister had been bitten by a dog infected with rabies, and the treatment saved his life. This is the first time Pasteur uses an attenuated (weakened) germ on a human being.

1885 Russian hematologist Antonin Filatov makes the first formal description of mononucleosis.

1885 Theodor Escherich identifies a bacterium inhabiting the human intestinal tract that he names *Bacterium coli* and shows that the bacterium causes infant diarrhea and gastroenteritis. The bacterium is subsequently named *Escherichia coli*.

1886 Camillo Golgi describes two forms of malaria, with fever occurring every two and every three days, respectively.

1887 Julius Richard Petri develops a culture dish that has a lid to exclude airborne contaminants. The innovation is subsequently termed the Petri dish.

1888 Francis Galton publishes *Natural Inheritance*, considered a landmark in the establishment of biometry and statistical studies of variation. Galton also proposes the Law of Ancestral Inheritance, a statistical description of the relative contributions to heredity made by previous generations.

1888 Martinus Beijerinck uses a growth medium enriched with certain nutrients to isolate the bacteria *Rhizobium*, demonstrating that nutritionally-tailored growth media are useful in bacterial isolation.

1888 The diphtheria toxin is discovered by Emile Roux and Alexandre Yersin.

1888 The Institute Pasteur is formed in France.

1890 Emil Adolf von Behring (1854–1917), German bacteriologist, uses his new discovery of antitoxins to develop an antitoxin for diphtheria—a disease that usually brought death to the children it attacked.

1891 First child is treated with the diphtheria antitoxin.

1891 Paul Ehrlich (1854–1915), German bacteriologist, discovers that methyl blue dye immobilizes malaria bacterium and begins searching for other, more potent microbial dyes. (See 1904)

1891 Paul Ehrlich proposes that antibodies are responsible for immunity.

1891 Prussian State dictates that even jailed prisoners must give consent prior to treatment (for tuberculosis).

1891 Robert Koch proposes the concept of delayed type hypersensitivity.

1892 Dmitri Ivanowski demonstrates that filterable material causes tobacco mosaic disease. The infectious agent is subsequently showed to be the tobacco mosaic virus. Ivanowski's discovery heralds the field of virology.

1892 First vaccine for diphtheria becomes available.

1892 Albert Neisser, the discoverer of gonorrhea bacteria, injects human subjects with syphilis, prompting debate and leading to regulations on human experimentation.

1892 Richard Pfeiffer discovers *Haemophilius influenzae*, a cause of both pneumonia and influenza.

1894 Alexandre Yersin isolates *Yersinia (Pasteurella) pestis*, the bacterium responsible for bubonic plague.

1894 Wilhelm Konrad Roentgen discovers x-rays.

1895 Heinrich Dreser, working for the Bayer Company in Germany, produces a drug he thought to be as effective an analgesic as morphine, but without its harmful side effects. Bayer begins mass production of diacetylmorphine, and in 1898, markets the new drug under the brand name "heroin" as a cough sedative.

1896   Edmund Beecher Wilson, American zoologist, publishes the first edition of his highly influential treatise *The Cell in Development and Heredity.* Wilson calls attention to the relationship between chromosomes and sex determination.

1896   William Joseph Dibdin (1850–1925), English engineer, and his colleague Schweder improve the sewage disposal systems in England with the introduction of a bacterial system of water purification. These improvements greatly reduce the number of water-borne diseases like cholera and typhoid fever.

1897   American physician William Welch describes and names *Plasmodium falciparum,* a protozoan parasite and cause of malaria.

1898   First state-run sanatorium for tuberculosis in the United States opens in Massachusetts.

1898   Friedrich Loeffler and Paul Frosch publish their *Report on Foot-and-Mouth Disease.* They prove that this animal disease is caused by a filterable virus and suggest that similar agents might cause other diseases.

1898   Martinus Wilhelm Beijerinck (1851–1931), Dutch botanist, discovers and names the causative agent of the tobacco mosaic disease. He describes it as a new type of microscopically-visible organism which eventually comes to be known as a virus.

1898   The First International Congress of Genetics is held in London.

1898   The transmission of plague by flea-infested rodents is shown by French bacteriologist Paul-Louis Simond (1858–1947).

1899   A meeting to organize the Society of American Bacteriologists is held at Yale University. The society will later become the American Society for Microbiology.

1899   George Henry Falkiner Nuttall (1862–1937), American biologist, first summarizes the role of insects, arachnids, and myriapods as transmitters of bacterial and parasitic diseases.

1899   Start of the sixth cholera pandemic, which affects the Far East, apart from sporadic outbreaks in parts of Euorpe.

1900   Karl Landsteiner discovers the blood-agglutination phenomenon and the four major blood types in humans.

1900   Pandemic plague becomes widely disseminated throughout the world, reaching Europe, North and South America, India, the Middle East, Africa, and Australia.

1900   Paul Erlich proposes the theory concerning the formation of antibodies by the immune system.

1900   Walter Reed (1851–1902), American surgeon, discovers that the yellow fever virus is transmitted to humans by a mosquito. This is the first demonstration of a viral cause of a human disease.

1901   Joseph Everett Dutton (1874-1905), English physician, and his colleague J. L. Todd discover the parasite *Trypanosoma gambiense* that is responsible for the African sleeping sickness disease.

1902   Ronald Ross (1857–1932), a British officer with the Indian Medical Service, receives the Nobel Prize for identifying mosquitoes as the transmitter of malaria.

1904   Paul Ehrlich (1854–1915), German bacteriologist, discovers a microbial dye called trypan red that helps destroy the trypanosomes that cause such diseases as sleeping sickness. This is the first such active agent against trypanosomes (parasitic protozoa).

1905   Fritz Richard Schaudinn (1871–1906), German zoologist, discovers *Treponema pallidum,* the organism or parasite causing syphilis. His discovery of this almost invisible parasite is due to his consummate technique and staining methods.

1905   Jules-Jean-Baptiste-Vincent Bordet (1870–1961), Belgian bacteriologist, and his colleague, Octave Gengou, discover the bacillus of whooping cough (*B. pertussis*). Bordet goes on to discover a method of immunization against this dreaded childhood disease.

1906   Charles Nicolle of the Pasteur Institute in Paris shows a link between typhus and lice.

1906   Pure Food and Drugs Act passed in the United States, beginning the organization that would become the FDA (Food and Drug Administration).

1906 Viennese physician Clemens von Pirquet (1874–1929) coins the term allergy to describe the immune reaction to certain compounds.

1907 Alphonse Laveran, a French army surgeon stationed in Algeria, identifies malaria parasites (protozoa) in blood.

1907 Charles Franklin Craig (1872–1950), American physician, and Percy Moreau Ashburn (1872–1940), American surgeon, work in the Phillipines and are the first to prove that dengue fever (also called "breakbone fever") is caused by a virus. (See 1925)

1907 Clemens Peter Pirquet von Cesenatico (1874–1929), Austrian physician, first introduces the cutaneous or skin reaction test for the diagnosis of tuberculosis.

1907 William Bateson urges biologists to adopt the term "genetics" to indicate the importance of the new science of heredity.

1909 Sigurd Orla-Jensen proposes that the physiological reactions of bacteria are primarily important in their classification.

1909 Thomas Hunt Morgan selects the fruit fly *Drosophila* as a model system for the study of genetics. Morgan and his coworkers confirm the chromosome theory of heredity and realize the significance of the fact that certain genes tend to be transmitted together. Morgan postulates the mechanism of "crossing over." His associate, Alfred Henry Sturtevant demonstrates the relationship between crossing over and the rearrangement of genes in 1913.

1909 Walter Reed General Hospital opens in Washington, D.C.

1909 Wilhelm Ludwig Johannsen argues the necessity of distinguishing between the appearance of an organism and its genetic constitution. He invents the terms "gene" (carrier of heredity), "genotype" (an organism's genetic constitution), and "phenotype" (the appearance of the actual organism).

1910 Howard Taylor Ricketts, discoverer of the *Rickettsia* genus of bacteria, dies of the *Rickettsia*-caused disease typhus while investigating an outbreak in Mexico City.

1910 Paul Ehrlich (1854–1915), German bacteriologist, announces his discovery of an effective treatment for syphilis. He names this new drug Salvarsan, and it is now called arsphenamine. His discovery marks the first chemotherapeutic agent for a bacterial disease.

1911 The first known retrovirus, Rous sarcoma virus, is discovered by Peyton Rous, who also showed that the virus could induce cancer.

1912 The United States Public Health Service is established.

1913 Shick designs a skin test which determines immunity to diphtheria.

1914 Frederick William Twort (1877–1950), English bacteriologist, and Felix H. D'Herelle (1873–1949), Canadian-Russian physician, independently discover bacteriophage, viruses which destroy bacteria.

1915 A typhus epidemic in Serbia causes 150,000 deaths.

1915 Stanislaus Prowazek dies of typhus when investigating an outbreak in a Russian prisoner of war camp, having identified *R. prowazekii*, the causative agent.

1915 U.S. Public Health Office allows induction of pellagra in Mississippi prisoners.

1916 Felix Hubert D'Herelle carries out further studies of the agent that destroys bacterial colonies and gives it the name "bacteriophage" (bacteria eating agent). D'Herelle and others unsuccessfully attempted to use bacteriophages as bactericidal therapeutic agents.

1917 D'Arcy Wentworth Thompson publishes *On Growth and Form,* which suggests that the evolution of one species into another occurs as a series of transformations involving the entire organism, rather than a succession of minor changes in parts of the body.

1918 Global influenza pandemic kills more people than numbers of soldiers who died fighting during World War I (1914–1918). By the end of 1918, more than 25 million people die from virulent strain of Spanish influenza.

1918 Thomas Hunt Morgan and coworkers publish *The Physical Basis of Heredity,* a survey of the remarkable development of the new science of genetics.

1919   James Brown uses blood agar to study the destruction of blood cells by the bacterium *Streptococcus*. He observes three reactions that he designates alpha, beta, and gamma.

1919   The Health Organization of the League of Nations was established for the prevention and control of disease around the world.

1920   Data on diphtheria is gathered for the first time in the United States, showing around 13,000 deaths per year.

1920   Sprunt and Evans coined the term infectious mononucleosis, as they described the abnormal mononuclear leukocytes observed in patients with the condition.

1921   Otto Loewi (1873–1961), German-American physiologist, discovers that acetylcholine functions as a neurotransmitter. It is the first such brain chemical to be so identified.

1922   John Stephens describes *P. ovale*.

1924   Albert Jan Kluyver publishes *Unity and Diversity in the Metabolism of Microorganisms*. He demonstrates that different microorganisms have common metabolic pathways of oxidation, fermentation, and synthesis of certain compounds. Kluyver also states that life on Earth depends on microbial activity.

1924   The last urban epidemic of plague in the United States begins in Los Angeles.

1926   James B. Sumner publishes a report on the isolation of the enzyme urease and his proof that the enzyme is a protein. This idea is controversial until 1930 when John Howard Northrop confirms Sumner's ideas by crystallizing pepsin. Sumner, Northrop, and Wendell Meredith Stanley ultimately share the Nobel Prize for chemistry in 1946.

1927   Thomas Rivers publishes a paper that differentiates bacteria from viruses, establishing virology as a field of study that is distinct from bacteriology.

1928   Fred Griffith discovers that certain strains of pneumococci could undergo some kind of transmutation of type. After injecting mice with living R type pneumococci and heat-killed S type, Griffith is able to isolate living virulent bacteria from the infected mice. Griffith suggests that some unknown "principle" had transformed the harmless R strain of the pneumococcus to the virulent S strain.

1928   Philip and Cecil Drinker of Harvard School of Public Health introduce the "iron lung" for treatment of paralytic polio.

1928   Scottish biochemist Alexander Fleming (1881–1955) discovers penicillin. In his published report (1929), Fleming observes that the mold *Penicillium notatum* inhibits the growth of some bacteria. This is the first anti-bacterial, and it opens a new era of "wonder drugs."

1929   Alexander Fleming publishes account of bacteriolytic power of penicillin.

1929   Francis O. Holmes introduces the technique of "local lesion" as a means of measuring the concentration of tobacco mosaic virus. The method becomes extremely important in virus purification.

1929   Willard Myron Allen, American physician, and George Washington Corner, American anatomist, discover progesterone. They demonstrate that it is necessary for the maintenance of pregnancy.

1930   Max Theiler demonstrates the advantages of using mice as experimental animals for research on animal viruses. Theiler uses mice in his studies of the yellow fever virus.

1930   Ronald A. Fisher publishes *Genetical Theory of Natural Selection*, a formal analysis of the mathematics of selection.

1930   United States Food, Drug, and Insecticide Administration is renamed Food and Drug Administration (FDA).

1932   At Tuskegee, Alabama, African-American sharecroppers become unknowing and unwilling subjects of experimentation on the untreated natural course of syphilis. Even after penicillin came into use in the 1940's, the men remained untreated.

1932   William J. Elford and Christopher H. Andrewes develop methods of estimating the sizes of viruses by using a series of membranes as filters. Later studies prove that the viral sizes obtained by this method were comparable to those obtained by electron microscopy.

1933   "Regulation on New Therapy and Experimentation" decreed in Germany.

1934 Discovery of chloroquine is announced by Hans Andersag at Bayer, in Germany

1934 J.B.S. Haldane presents the first calculations of the spontaneous mutation frequency of a human gene.

1934 John Marrack begins a series of studies that leads to the formation of the hypothesis governing the association between an antigen and the corresponding antibody.

1935 Wendall Meredith Stanley (1904–1971), American biochemist, discovers that viruses are partly protein-based. By purifying and crystallizing viruses, he enables scientists to identify the precise molecular structure and propagation modes of several viruses.

1936 George P. Berry and Helen M. Dedrick report that the Shope virus could be "transformed" into myxomatosis/Sanarelli virus. This virological curiosity was variously referred to as "transformation," "recombination," and "multiplicity of reactivation." Subsequent research suggests that it is the first example of genetic interaction between animal viruses, but some scientists warn that the phenomenon might indicate the danger of reactivation of virus particles in vaccines and in cancer research.

1937 American researcher H. R. Cox cultures *Rickettsiae* in the yolks of fertilized hens' eggs, opening the door to research into a vaccine.

1938 Emory L. Ellis and Max Delbrück perform studies on phage replication that mark the beginning of modern phage work. They introduce the "one-step growth" experiment, which demonstrates that after bacteriophages attack bacteria, replication of the virus occurs within the bacterial host during a "latent period," after which viral progeny are released in a "burst."

1939 Ernest Chain and H. W. Florey refine the purification of penicillin, allowing the mass production of the antibiotic.

1939 Paul Müller in Switzerland discovers the insecticidal properties of DDT.

1939 Richard E. Shope reports that the swine influenza virus survived between epidemics in an intermediate host. This discovery is an important step in revealing the role of intermediate hosts in perpetuating specific diseases.

1941 George W. Beadle and Edward L. Tatum publish their classic study on the biochemical genetics entitled Genetic Control of Biochemical Reactions in Neurospora. Beadle and Tatum irradiate red bread mold *Neurospora* and prove that genes produce their effects by regulating particular enzymes. This work leads to the one-gene-one enzyme theory.

1941 Norman M. Gregg of Australia discovers that rubella during pregnancy can cause congenital abnormalities. Children of mothers who had rubella (German measles) during their pregnancy are found to suffer from blindness, deafness, and heart disease.

1941 The term "antibiotic" is coined by Selman Waksman.

1942 Jules Freund and Katherine McDermott identify adjuvants (e.g., paraffin oil) that act to boost antibody production.

1942 Luria and Max Delbrück demonstrate statistically that inheritance of genetic characteristics in bacteria follows the principles of genetic inheritance proposed by Charles Darwin. For their work, the two (along with Alfred Day Hershey) are awarded the 1969 Nobel Prize in Medicine or Physiology.

1942 Neil Hamilton Fairley, the Australian physician, wins a Fellowship of the Royal Society for work on anemia caused by the rupture of red blood cells in malaria.

1943 At University of Cincinnati Hospital experiments are performed using mentally disabled patients.

1943 Penicillin starts to become available as a therapy for Allied troops.

1944 Oswald T. Avery, Colin M. MacLeod, and Maclyn McCarty publish a landmark paper on the pneumococcus transforming principle. The paper is entitled *Studies on the chemical nature of the substance inducing transformation of pneumococcal types*. Avery suggests that the transforming principle seems to be deoxyribonucleic acid (DNA), but contemporary ideas about the structure of nucleic acids suggest that

DNA does not possess the biological specificity of the hypothetical genetic material.

1944 Selman Waksman introduces streptomycin.

1944 To combat battle fatigue during World War II (1939–1945), nearly 200 million amphetamine tablets are issued to American soldiers stationed in Great Britain during the war.

1944 The United States Public Health Service Act is passed.

1944 University of Chicago Medical School professor Dr. Alf Alving conducts malaria experiments on more than 400 Illinois prisoners.

1945 Joshua Lederberg and Edward L. Tatum demonstrate genetic recombination in bacteria.

1946 Felix Bloch and Edward Mills Purcell develop nuclear magnetic resonance (NMR) as viable tool for observation and analysis.

1946 Hermann J. Muller is awarded the Nobel Prize in Medicine or Physiology for his contributions to radiation genetics.

1946 Max Delbrück and W. T. Bailey, Jr. publish a paper entitled *Induced Mutations in Bacterial Viruses.* Despite some confusion about the nature of the phenomenon in question, this paper establishes the fact that genetic recombinations occur during mixed infections with bacterial viruses. Alfred Hershey and R. Rotman make the discovery of genetic recombination in bacteriophage simultaneously and independently. Hershey and his colleagues prove that this phenomenon can be used for genetic analyses. They construct a genetic map of phage particles and show that phage genes can be arranged in a linear fashion.

1946 Nazi physicians and scientists tried by international court at Nuremberg.

1947 Four years after the mass-production and use of penicillin, microbial resistance is detected.

1947 Nuremberg Code issued regarding voluntary consent of human subjects.

1948 Barbara McClintock publishes her research on transposable regulatory elements ("jumping genes") in maize. Her work was not appreciated until similar phenomena were discovered in bacteria and fruit flies in the 1960s

and 1970s. McClintock was awarded the Nobel Prize in physiology or medicine in 1983.

1948 Chloramphenicol and tetracycline are shown to be effective treatments for typhus.

1948 James V. Neel reports evidence that the sickle-cell disease is inherited as a simple Mendelian autosomal recessive trait.

1948 World Health Organization (WHO) is formed. The WHO subsequently becomes the principle international organization managing public health related issues on a global scale. Headquartered in Geneva, the WHO becomes, by 2002, an organization of more than 190 member countries. The organization contributes to international public health in areas including disease prevention and control, promotion of good health, addressing disease outbreaks, initiatives to eliminate diseases (e.g., vaccination programs), and development of treatment and prevention standards.

1949 John F. Endes, Thomas H. Weller, and Frederick C. Robbins publish "Cultivation of Polio Viruses in Cultures of Human Embryonic Tissues." The report by Enders and coworkers is a landmark in establishing techniques for the cultivation of poliovirus in cultures on non-neural tissue and for further virus research. The technique leads to the polio vaccine and other advances in virology.

1949 Macfarlane Burnet and his colleagues begin studies that lead to the immunological tolerance hypothesis and the clonal selection theory. Burnet receives the 1960 Nobel Prize in Physiology or Medicine for this research.

1950 Dr. Joseph Stokes of the University of Pennsylvania infects 200 women prisoners with viral hepatitis.

1950 Robert Hungate develops the roll-tube culture technique, which is the first technique that allows anaerobic bacteria to be grown in culture.

1951 Esther M. Lederberg discovers a lysogenic strain of *Escherichia coli* K12 and isolates a new bacteriophage, called lambda.

1951 Rosalind Franklin obtains sharp x-ray diffraction photographs of deoxyribonucleic acid (DNA).

1951   The eradication of malaria from the United States is announced.

1951   University of Pennsylvania under contract with U.S. Army conducts psychopharmacological experiments on hundreds of Pennsylvania prisoners.

1952   Alfred Hershey and Martha Chase publish their landmark paper "Independent Functions of Viral Protein and Nucleic Acid in Growth of Bacteriophage." The famous "blender experiment" suggests that DNA is the genetic material.

1952   James T. Park and Jack L. Strominger demonstrate that penicillin blocks the synthesis of the peptidoglycan of bacteria. This represents the first demonstration of the action of a natural antibiotic.

1952   Karl Maramorosch demonstrate that some viruses could multiply in both plants and insects. This work leads to new questions about the origins of viruses.

1952   Joshua Lederberg and Esther Lederberg develop the replica plating method that allows for the rapid screening of large numbers of genetic markers. They use the technique to demonstrate that resistance to antibacterial agents such as antibiotics and viruses is not induced by the presence of the antibacterial agent.

1952   Polio peaks in the United States, with 57,268 cases recorded.

1952   Renato Dulbecco develops a practical method for studying animal viruses in cell cultures. His so-called plaque method is comparable to that used in studies of bacterial viruses, and the method proves to be important in genetic studies of viruses. These methods are described in his paper *Production of Plaques in Monolayer Tissue Cultures by Single Particles of an Animal Virus.*

1952   Rosalind Franklin completes a series of x-ray crystallography studies of two forms of DNA. Her colleague, Maurice Wilkins, gives information about her work to James Watson.

1952   Selman Abraham Waksman, Russian-American microbiologist, is awarded the Nobel Prize for Physiology or Medicine for his discovery of streptomycin, the first antibiotic effective against tuberculosis.

1952   William G. Gochenour of the United States demonstrates that pretibial fever (also called Fort Bragg Fever) is not caused by a virus but rather is an infection caused by a microorganism called *Leptospira*.

1952   William Hayes isolates a strain of *E. coli* that produces recombinants thousands of times more frequently than previously observed. The new strain of K12 is named Hfr (high-frequency recombination) by Hayes.

1953   James D. Watson and Francis H. C. Crick publish two landmark papers in the journal *Nature*: "Molecular structure of nucleic acids: a structure for deoxyribonucleic acid," and "Genetical implications of the structure of deoxyribonucleic acid." Watson and Crick propose a double helical model for DNA and call attention to the genetic implications of their model. Their model is based, in part, on the x-ray crystallographic work of Rosalind Franklin and the biochemical work of Erwin Chargaff. Their model explains how the genetic material is transmitted.

1953   Jonas Salk begins testing a polio vaccine comprised of a mixture of killed viruses.

1954   John Enders, Thomas Weller and Frederick Robbins of Harvard School of Public Health receive the Nobel Prize for Physiology or Medicine for their work on poliovirus

1954   John Franklin Enders (1897-1985), American micrologist, and Thomas Peebles, American pediatrician, develop the first vaccine for measles. A truly practical and successful vaccine requires more time. (See 1963)

1954   Jonas Edward Salk, American virologist, produces the first successful anti-poliomyelitis vaccine, which prevents paralytic polio. It is soon (1955) followed by the Polish-American virologist, Albert Bruce Sabin's (1906-1993) development of the first oral vaccine. (See 1959)

1954   Thomas Weller isolated the varicella zoster virus from chickenpox lesions.

1955   Fred L. Schaffer and Carlton E. Schwerdt report on their successful crystallization of the polio virus. Their achievement is the first successful crystallization of an animal virus.

1955   Jonas Salk's inactivated polio vaccine is approved for use.

1955   National Institutes of Health organizes a Division of Biologics Control within FDA, following death from faulty polio vaccine.

1956   Alfred Gierer and Gerhard Schramm demonstrate that naked RNA from tobacco mosaic virus is infectious. Subsequently, infectious RNA preparations are obtained for certain animal viruses.

1956   Niels Kai Jerne, Danish physician, proposes the clonal selection theory of antibody selection to explain how white blood cells are able to produce a large range of antibodies.

1956   Researchers start hepatitis experiments on mentally disabled children at The Willowbrook State School.

1957   Alick Isaacs (1921-1967), Scottish virologist, demonstrates that antibodies act only against bacteria. This means that antibodies are not one of the body's natural forms of defense against viruses. This knowledge leads eventually to the discovery of interferon this same year by Isaacs and his colleague, Jean Lindenmann of Switzerland. They find that the generation of a small amount of protein is the body's first line of defense against a virus. (See c.1968)

1957   Alick Isaacs and Jean Lindenmann publish their pioneering report on the drug interferon, a protein produced by interaction between a virus and an infected cell that can interfere with the multiplication of viruses.

1957   François Jacob and Elie L. Wollman demonstrate that the single linkage group of *Escherichia coli* is circular and suggest that the different linkage groups found in different Hfr strains result from the insertion at different points of a factor in the circular linkage group that determines the rupture of the circle.

1957   The World Health Organization advances the oral polio vaccine developed by Albert Sabin (1906-1993) as a safer alternative to the Salk vaccine.

1958   George W. Beadle, Edward L. Tatum, and Joshua Lederberg were awarded the Nobel Prize in physiology or medicine. Beadle and Tatum were honored for the work in *Neurospora* that led to the one gene-one enzyme theory. Lederberg was honored for discoveries concerning genetic recombination and the organization of the genetic material of bacteria.

1958   Matthew Meselson and Frank W. Stahl publish their landmark paper "The replication of DNA in *Escherichia coli*," which demonstrated that the replication of DNA follow the semiconservative model.

1959   Albert Bruce Sabin (1906-1993), Polish-American virologist, announces successful results from testing live attenuated polio vaccine. His vaccine eventually is preferred over the Salk vaccine, since it can be administered orally and offers protection with a single dose.

1959   English biochemist Rodney Porter begins studies that lead to the discovery of the structure of antibodies. Porter receives the 1972 Nobel Prize in Physiology or Medicine for this research.

1959   Robert L. Sinsheimer reports that bacteriophage ØX174, which infects *Escherichia coli*, contains a single-stranded DNA molecule, rather than the expected double-stranded DNA. This provides the first example of a single-stranded DNA genome.

1959   Sydney Brenner and Robert W. Horne publish a paper entitled *A Negative Staining Method for High Resolution Electron Microscopy of Viruses*. The two researchers develop a method for studying the architecture of viruses at the molecular level using the electron microscope.

1961   Francis Crick, Sydney Brenner, and others propose that a molecule called transfer RNA uses a three base code in the manufacture of proteins.

1961   French pathologist Jacques Miller discovers the role of the thymus in cellular immunity.

1961   Marshall Warren Nirenberg synthesizes a polypeptide using an artificial messenger RNA (a synthetic RNA containing only the base uracil) in a cell-free protein-synthesizing system. The resulting polypeptide only contains the amino acid phenylalanine, indicating that UUU was the codon for phenylalanine. This important step in deciphering the genetic code is described in the landmark paper by Nirenberg and J. Heinrich Matthaei, *The Dependence of Cell-Free Synthesis in E. coli upon Naturally Occurring or Synthetic Polyribonucleotides.* This work establishes the messenger concept and a system that could be used to work out the relationship between the sequence of nucleotides in the genetic material and amino acids in the gene product.

1961   Noel Warner establishes the physiological distinction between the cellular and humoral immune responses.

1962   James D. Watson, Francis Crick, and Maurice Wilkins are awarded the Nobel Prize in physiology or medicine for their work in elucidating the structure of DNA.

1962   United States Congress passes Kefauver-Harris Drug Amendments that shift the burden of proof of clinical safety to drug manufacturers. For the first time, drug manufacturers had to prove their products were safe and effective before they could be sold.

1963   Albert Sabin's live polio vaccine is approved for use.

1964   Michael Epstein and Yvonne Barr discover the Epstein-Barr virus that is the cause of mononucleosis.

1964   Retrovir is developed as a cancer treatment. While not useful for cancer, the drug subsequently becomes the first drug approved for the treatment of AIDS.

1964   World Medical Association adopts Helsinki Declaration.

1965   Anthrax vaccine adsorbed (AVA), is approved for use in the United States.

1965   François Jacob, André Lwoff, and Jacques Monod are awarded the Nobel Prize in physiology or medicine for their discoveries concerning genetic control of enzymes and virus synthesis.

1966   Bruce Ames develops a test to screen for compounds that cause mutations, including those that are cancer causing. The so-called Ames test utilizes the bacterium *Salmonella typhimurium*.

1966   Daniel Carleton Gajdusek, American pediatrician, transfers for the first time a viral disease of the central nervous system from humans to another species. The viral disease kuru is found in New Guinea and is spread by the ritual eating of the deceased's brains.

1966   FDA and National Academy of Sciences begin investigation of effectiveness of drugs previously approved because they were thought safe.

1966   Marshall Nirenberg and Har Gobind Khorana lead teams that decipher the genetic code. All of the 64 possible triplet combinations of the four bases (the codons) and their associated amino acids are determined and described.

1966   Merck, Sharp, and Dohme Laboratories began research into a varicella-zoster vaccine.

1966   *New England Journal of Medicine* article exposes unethical Tuskegee syphilis study.

1966   NIH Office for Protection of Research Subjects ("OPRR") created.

1966   Paul D. Parman and Harry M. Myer, Jr., develop a live-virus rubella vaccine.

1967   A hemorrhagic fever outbreak in Marburg, Germany occurs. The virus responsible is subsequently named the marburg virus, and the disease called marburg hemorrhagic fever.

1967   British physician M. H. Pappworth publishes "Human Guinea Pigs," advising "No doctor has the right to choose martyrs for science or for the general good."

1968   FDA administratively moves to Public Health Service.

1968   Mark Steven Ptashne and Walter Gilbert independently identify the bacteriophage genes that are the repressors of the lac operon.

1968   Robert W. Holley, Har Gobind Khorana, and Marshall W. Nirenberg are awarded the Nobel Prize in physiology or medicine for their interpretation of the genetic code and its function in protein synthesis.

1968   Werner Arber discovers that bacteria defend themselves against viruses by producing DNA-cutting enzymes. These enzymes quickly become important tools for molecular biologists.

1969   By Executive Order, the United States renounces first-use of biological weapons and restricts future weapons research programs to issues concerning defensive responses (e.g., immunization, detection, etc.).

1969 Jonathan R. Beckwith, American molecular biologist, and colleagues isolate a single gene.

1969 Max Delbrück, Alfred D. Hershey, and Salvador E. Luria are awarded the Nobel Prize in physiology or medicine for their discoveries concerning the replication mechanism and the genetic structure of viruses.

1969 United States Surgeon General William Stewart announces: "The time has come to close the book on infectious diseases."

1970 First outbreak of drug-resistant tuberculosis recorded in the United States.

1970 Howard Martin Temin and David Baltimore independently discover reverse transcriptase in viruses. Reverse transcriptase is an enzyme that catalyzes the transcription of RNA into DNA.

1972 Biological and Toxin Weapons Convention first signed. BWC prohibits the offensive weaponization of biological agents (e.g., anthrax spores). The BWC also prohibits the transformation of biological agents with established legitimate and sanctioned purposes into agents of a nature and quality that could be used to effectively induce illness or death.

1972 Introduction of amoxcillin, a drug related to penicillin, which is a treatment of choice for bacterial pneumonia.

1972 Mishiaka Takahashi isolated the varicella virus from a 3-year-old patient and named it Oka, after the patient's name. The isolated virus was later used by Merck to develop a vaccine.

1972 Paul Berg and Herbert Boyer produce the first recombinant DNA molecules.

1972 Recombinant technology emerges as one of the most powerful techniques of molecular biology. Scientists are able to splice together pieces of DNA to form recombinant genes. As the potential uses, therapeutic and industrial, became increasingly clear, scientists and venture capitalists establish biotechnology companies.

1973 Concerns about the possible hazards posed by recombinant DNA technologies, especially work with tumor viruses, leads to the establishment of a meeting at Asilomar, California. The proceedings of this meeting are subsequently published by the Cold Spring Harbor Laboratory as a book entitled *Biohazards in Biological Research*.

1973 Herbert Wayne Boyer and Stanley H. Cohen create recombinant genes by cutting DNA molecules with restriction enzymes. These experiments mark the beginning of genetic engineering.

1974 National Research Act establishes "The Common Rule" for protection of human subjects.

1974 Peter Doherty and Rolf Zinkernagl discover the basis of immune determination of self and non-self.

1975 César Milstein and George Kohler create monoclonal antibodies.

1975 David Baltimore, Renato Dulbecco, and Howard Temin share the Nobel Prize in physiology or medicine for their discoveries concerning the interaction between tumor viruses and the genetic material of the cell and the discovery of reverse transcriptase.

1975 HHS promulgates Title 45 of Federal Regulations titled "Protection of Human Subjects," requiring appointment and utilization of Institutional Review Board (IRB).

1976 First outbreak of Ebola virus observed in Zaire, resulting in more than 300 cases with a 90% death rate.

1976 Swine flu breaks identified in soldiers stationed in New Jersey. Virus identified as H1N1 virus causes concern due to its similarities to H1N1 responsible for Spanish Flu pandemic. President Gerald Ford calls for emergency vaccination program. More than 20 deaths result from Guillain-Barre syndrome related to the vaccine.

1977 Carl R. Woese and George E. Fox publish an account of the discovery of a third major branch of living beings, the Archaea. Woese suggests that an rRNA database could be used to generate phylogenetic trees.

1977 Earliest known AIDS (acquired immunodeficiency syndrome) victims in the United States are two homosexual men in New York who are diagnosed as suffering from Kaposi's sarcoma.

1977   Frederick Sanger develops the chain termination (dideoxy) method for sequencing DNA, and uses the method to sequence the genome of a microorganism.

1977   The first known human fatality from H5N1 avian flu occurs in Hong Kong.

1977   The last reported smallpox case is recorded. Ultimately, the World Health Organization (WHO) declares the disease eradicated.

1979   National Commission issues Belmont Report.

1979   The last case of wild poliovirus infection is recorded in the United States.

1980   Congress passes the Bayh-Dole Act, the Act is amended by the Technology Transfer Act in 1986.

1980   In *Diamond v. Chakrabarty* the U.S. Supreme Court rules that a genetically modified bacterium can be patented.

1980   Researchers successfully introduce a human gene, which codes for the protein interferon, into a bacterium.

1980   The FDA promulgates 21 CFR 50.44 prohibiting use of prisoners as subjects in clinical trials.

1981   AIDS (acquired immunodeficiency syndrome) is officially recognized by the U.S. Center for Disease Control, and the first clinical description of this disease is made. It soon becomes recognized that AIDS is an infectious disease caused by a virus that spreads virtually exclusively by infected blood or body fluids.

1981   First disease-causing human retrovirus, human T-cell leukemia virus, discovered.

1981   The first cases of AIDS are reported among previously healthy young men in Los Angeles, California, and New York presenting with *Pneumocystis carinii* pneumonia and Kaposi's sarcoma.

1982   The U.S. Food and Drug Administration approves the first genetically engineered drug, a form of human insulin produced by bacteria.

1983   *Escherichia coli* O157:H7 is identified as a human pathogen.

1983   Luc Montainer and Robert Gallo discover the human immunodeficiency virus that causes acquired immunodeficiency syndrome.

1984   Niels Kai Jerne, Danish-English immunologist, Georges J. F. Kohler, German immunologist, and Cesar Milstein, Argentinian immunologist, are awarded the Nobel Prize for Physiology or Medicine for theories concerning the specificity in development and control of the immune system and the discovery of the principle for production of monoclonal antibodies.

1984   WHO begins a program to control trypanosomiasis.

1985   Alec Jeffreys develops "genetic fingerprinting," a method of using DNA polymorphisms (unique sequences of DNA) to identify individuals. The method, which has been used in paternity, immigration, and murder cases, is generally referred to as "DNA fingerprinting."

1985   First vaccine for *H. influenzae* type B is licensed for use.

1985   Japanese molecular biologist Susuma Tonegawa discovers the genes that code for immunoglobulins. He receives the 1986 Nobel Prize in Physiology or Medicine for this discovery.

1985   Kary Mullis, who was working at Cetus Corporation, develops the polymerase chain reaction (PCR), a new method of amplifying DNA. This technique quickly becomes one of the most powerful tools of molecular biology. Cetus patents PCR and sells the patent to Hoffman-LaRoche, Inc. in 1991.

1986   Congress passes the National Childhood Vaccine Injury Act, requiring patient information on vaccines and reporting of adverse events after vaccination.

1986   First genetically-engineered vaccine approved for human use is the hepatitis B vaccine. The U.S. Food and Drug Administration gives its approval.

1986   First license to market a living organism that was produced by genetic engineering is granted by the U.S. Department of Agriculture. It allows Biologics Corporation to sell a virus that is used as a vaccine against a herpes disease in pigs.

1986   International Committee on the Taxonomy of Viruses officially names the AIDS virus as HIV (human immunosufficiency virus).

1987 An illness outbreak in Prince Edward Island, Canada, which sickens over 100 people and kills three, leads to the first isolation and identification of domoic acid.

1987 Maynard Olson creates and names yeast artificial chromosomes (YACs), which provided a technique to clone long segments of DNA.

1987 The U.S. Congress charters a Department of Energy advisory committee, the Health and Environmental Research Advisory Committee (HERAC), which recommends a 15-year, multidisciplinary, scientific, and technological undertaking to map and sequence the human genome. DOE designates multidisciplinary human genome centers. National Institute of General Medical Sciences at the National Institutes of Health (NIH NIGMS) began funding genome projects.

1988 First report of vancomycin-resistant enterococci, a type of Streptococcus that is resistant to almost all antiobitics.

1988 The Human Genome Organization (HUGO) is established by scientists in order to coordinate international efforts to sequence the human genome. The Human Genome Project officially adopts the goal of determining the entire sequence of DNA comprising the human chromosomes.

1988 The World Health Organization (WHO) and its partners announce the Global Polio Eradication Initiative.

1989 Ebola-Reston virus is the source of an outbreak at an animal facility in Virginia. The outbreak becomes the basis for the best-selling book "The Hot Zone."

1989 Sidney Altman and Thomas R. Cech are awarded the Nobel Prize in chemistry for their discovery of ribozymes (RNA molecules with catalytic activity). Cech proves that RNA could function as a biocatalyst as well as an information carrier.

1990 Only 24 cases of diphtheria reported in the United States during preceding ten-year period.

1991 Cholera returns to the Western Hemisphere when an outbreak in Peru spreads to other Latin American countries.

1991 World Health Organization announces CIOMS Guidelines (the International Ethical Guidelines for Biomedical Research Involving Human Subjects).

1992 Craig Venter establishes The Institute for Genomic Research (TIGR) in Rockville, Maryland. TIGR later sequences the genome of *Haemophilus influenzae* and many other bacterial genomes.

1993 An international research team, led by Daniel Cohen, of the Center for the Study of Human Polymorphisms in Paris, produces a rough map of all 23 pairs of human chromosomes.

1993 Beginning in April, a five-week contamination of the drinking water supply of Milwaukee, Wisconsin, by *Cryptosporidium parvum* sickens 400,000 people and kills an estimated 104 people.

1993 Hanta virus emerged in the United States in a 1993 outbreak on a "Four Corners" (the juncture of Utah, Colorado, New Mexico, Arizona) area Native American Reservation. The resulting Hanta pulmonary syndrome (HPS) had a 43% mortality rate.

1993 Outbreaks in Moscow and St. Petersburg mark the return of epidemic diphtheria to the Western world.

1994 AZT (zidovudine) approved by the FDA for use in reducing maternal-fetal HIV transmission.

1994 DOE announces the establishment of the Microbial Genome Project as a spin-off of the Human Genome Project.

1994 Ebola-Ivory Coast virus discovered.

1994 Geneticists determine that DNA repair enzymes perform several vital functions, including preserving genetic information and protecting the cell from cancer.

1994 The WHO declares the Americas free of polio.

1994 The WHO reports the start of epidemics of plague in Malawi, Mozambique, and India after 15 years absence.

1995 Edward B. Lewis, Christiane Nüsslein-Volhard, and Eric F. Wieschaus, developmental biologists, shared the Nobel Prize in physiology or medicine to cover discrimination based on genetic information related to illness, disease, or other conditions.

1995 Peter Funch and Reinhardt Moberg Kristensen create a new phylum, Cycliophora, for a novel invertebrate called *Symbion pandora*, which is found living in the mouths of Norwegian lobsters.

1995   Public awareness of potential use of chemical or biological weapons by a terrorist group increases following an Aum Shinrikyo, a Japanese cult, attack, which releases sarin gas in a Tokyo subway, killing a dozen people and sending thousands to the hospital.

1995   The U.S. FDA approved the varicella-zoster vaccine developed by Merck for vaccinations of persons 12 months of age and older.

1995   The Programme Against African Trypanosomiasis (PAAT) is created.

1995   The sequence of *Mycoplasma genitalium* is completed. *M. genitalium*, regarded as the smallest known bacterium, is considered a model of the minimum number of genes needed for independent existence.

1996   FDA approves the antidepressant buproprion (Zyban) and a nicotine nasal spray for the treatment of nicotine dependence.

1996   H5N1 avian flu virus is identified in Guangdong, China.

1996   International participants in the genome project meet in Bermuda and agree to formalize the conditions of data access. The agreement, known as the "Bermuda Principles," calls for the release of sequence data into public databases within 24 hours.

1996   Researchers C. Cheng and L. Olson demonstrate that the spinal cord can be regenerated in adult rats. Experimenting on rats with severed spinal cords, Cheng and Olson use peripheral nerves to connect white matter and gray matter.

1996   Researchers find that abuse and violence can alter a child's brain chemistry, placing him or her at risk for various problems, including drug abuse, cognitive disabilities, and mental illness, later in life.

1996   Scientists discover a link between autoptosis (cellular suicide, a natural process whereby the body eliminates useless cells) gone awry and several neurodegenerative conditions, including Alzheimer's disease.

1996   Scientists report further evidence that individuals with two mutant copies of the CC-CLR-5 gene are generally resistant to HIV infection.

1996   The Health Care Portability and Accountability Act incorporates provisions to prohibit the use of genetic information in certain health-insurance eligibility decisions. The Department of Health and Human Services was charged with the enforcement of health-information privacy provisions.

1996   U.S. Comprehensive Methamphetamine Control Act increases penalties for the manufacture, distribution, and possession of methamphetamines, as well as the reagents and chemicals needed to make it.

1996   William R. Bishai and co-workers report that SigF, a gene in the tuberculosis bacterium, enables the bacterium to enter a dormant stage.

1997   FDA reports and investigates correlation of heart valve disease in patients using phen-fen drug combination for weight loss. Similar reports were reported for patients using only dexfenluramine or fenfluramine. The FDA noted that the combination phen-fen treatment had not received FDA approval.

1997   Institute of Medicine (IOM), a branch of the National Academy of Sciences, publishes the report, *Marijuana: Assessing the Science Base*, which concludes that cannabinoids show significant promise as analgesics, appetite stimulants, and anti-emetics, and that further research into producing these medicines is warranted.

1997   Mickey Selzer, neurologist at the University of Pennsylvania, and co-workers, find that in lampreys, which have a remarkable ability to regenerate a severed spinal cord, neurofilament messenger RNA effects the regeneration process by literally pushing the growing axons and moving them forward.

1997   The DNA sequence of *Escherichia coli* is completed.

1997   While performing a cloning experiment, Christof Niehrs, a researcher at the German Center for Cancer Research, identifies a protein responsible for the creation of the head in a frog embryo.

1997   William Jacobs and Barry Bloom create a biological entity that combines the characteristics of a bacterial virus and a plasmid (a

DNA structure that functions and replicates independently of the chromosomes). This entity is capable of triggering mutations in *Mycobacterium tuberculosis.*

1997 Outbreaks of highly pathogenic H5N1 influenza are reported in poultry at farms and live animal markets in Hong Kong.

1998 A live, orally-administered rotavirus vaccine is approved for use in the United States. Use was discontinued in 1999 due to complications in some vaccinated children.

1998 Craig Venter forms a company (later named Celera), and predicts that the company would decode the entire human genome within three years. Celera plans to use a "whole genome shotgun" method, which would assemble the genome without using maps. Venter says that his company would not follow the Bermuda principles concerning data release.

1998 U.S. Department of Energy (Office of Science) funds bacterial artificial chromosome and sequencing projects.

1998 Scientists find that an adult human's brain can, with certain stimuli, replace cells. This discovery heralds potential breakthroughs in neurology.

1998 Sibutramine (Meridia), introduced as a weight-loss drug. Sibutramine inhibits the reuptake of the brain chemicals norepinephrine, dopamine, and serotonin, but does not promote monoamine release like the amphetamines.

1998 The World Health Organization reports a resurgence in tuberculosis cases worldwide; TB is killing more people than at any other point in history. Recommends Directly Observed Therapy (DOT) treatment, which is 95% effective in curing patients, even in developing nations.

1999 Pharmaceutical research in Japan leads to the discovery of donepezil (Aricept), the first drug intended to help ward off memory loss in Alzheimer's disease and other age-related dementias.

1999 Scientists announce the complete sequencing of the DNA making up human chromosome 22. The first complete human chromosome sequence is published in December 1999.

1999 The National Institutes of Health and the Office for Protection from Research Risks (OPRR) require researchers conducting or overseeing human subjects to ethics training.

1999 The public genome project responds to Craig Venter's challenge with plans to produce a draft genome sequence by 2000. Most of the sequencing is done in five centers, known as the "G5": the Whitehead Institute for Biomedical Research in Cambridge, MA; the Sanger Centre near Cambridge, UK; Baylor College of Medicine in Houston, TX; Washington University in St. Louis, MO; the DOE's Joint Genome Institute (JGI) in Walnut Creek, CA.

2000 On June 26, 2000, leaders of the public genome project and Celera announce the completion of a working draft of the entire human genome sequence. Ari Patrinos of the DOE helps mediate disputes between the two groups so that a fairly amicable joint announcement could be presented at the White House in Washington, D.C.

2000 Office for Protection from Research Risks (OPRR) becomes part of the Department of Health and Human Services, Office of Human Research Protection (OHRP).

2000 The federal government approves irradiation of raw meat, the only technology known to kill *E. coli* O157 bacteria while preserving the integrity of the meat.

2000 The first volume of *Annual Review of Genomics and Human Genetics* is published. Genomics is defined as the new science dealing with the identification and characterization of genes and their arrangement in chromosomes and human genetics as the science devoted to understanding the origin and expression of human individual uniqueness.

2000 The municipal water supply of Walkerton, Ontario, Canada, is contaminated in the summertime by a strain of the bacterium *Escherichia coli* O157:H7, sickening 2,000 people and killing 7.

2000 The WHO declares the Western Pacific region, including China, free of polio.

2001 *American Journal of Psychiatry* publishes studies providing evidence that methamphetamine can cause brain damage that results in slower motor and cognitive functioning—even in users who take the drug for less than a year.

2001   In February, the complete draft sequence of the human genome is published. The public sequence data is published in the British journal *Nature* and the Celera sequence is published in the American journal *Science*. Increased knowledge of the human genome allows greater specificity in pharmacological research and drug interaction studies.

2001   Microbiologists reveal that bacteria possess an internal protein structure similar to that of human cells.

2001   President George W. Bush announces the United States will allow and support limited forms of stem cell research.

2001   Researchers at Eli Lilly in Minneapolis sequence the genome of *Streptoccocus pneumoniae.*

2001   Scientists from the Whitehead Institute announce test results that show patterns of errors in cloned animals that might explain why such animals die early and exhibit a number of developmental problems. The report stimulates new debate on ethical issues related to cloning.

2001   Study entitled *Global Illicit Drug Trends* conducted by the United Nations Office for Drug Control and Crime Prevention (ODCCP), estimates that 14 million people use cocaine worldwide. Although cocaine use leveled off, the United States still maintains the highest levels of cocaine abuse.

2001   Terrorists attack United States on September 11, 2001, and kill thousands by crashing airplanes into buildings.

2001   Letters containing a powdered form of *Bacillus anthracis*, the bacteria that causes anthrax, are mailed to government representatives, members of the news media, and others in the United States. More than 20 cases and five deaths eventually result. As of August 2007, the case remains open and unsolved.

2001   The Chemical and Biological Incident Response Force (CBIRF) sends a 100-member initial response team into the Dirksen Senate Office Building in Washington alongside Environmental Protection Agency (EPA) specialists to detect and remove anthrax. A similar mission was undertaken at the Longworth House Office Building in October, during which time samples were collected from more than 200 office spaces.

2001   The Pan African Trypanosomiasis and Tsetse Eradication campaign (PATTEC) begins operation.

2001   U.S. military endorses the situational temporary usefulness of caffeine, recommending it as a safe and effective stimulant for its soldiers in good health.

2002   A company called DrinkSafe Technology announces the invention of a coaster that can be used to test whether a drink has been drugged by changing color when a drop of the tampered drink is placed on it.

2002   Following September 11, 2001, terrorist attacks on the United States, the Public Health Security and Bioterrorism Preparedness and Response Act of 2002 is passed in an effort to improve the ability to prevent and respond to public health emergencies.

2002   In June 2002, traces of biological and chemical weapon agents are found in Uzbekistan on a military base used by U.S. troops fighting in Afghanistan. Early analysis dates and attributes the source of the contamination to former Soviet Union biological and chemical weapons programs that utilized the base.

2002   In the aftermath of the September 11, 2001, terrorist attacks on the United States, by the first few months of 2002 the United States government dramatically increases funding to stockpile drugs and other agents that could be used to counter a bioterrorist attack.

2002   Scientists found that stockpiled smallpox vaccine doses can be effective if diluted to one-tenth their original concentration, greatly enhancing the number of doses available to respond to an emergency.

2002   Severe acute respiratory syndrome (SARS) virus is found in patients in China, Hong Kong, and other Asian countries. The newly discovered coronavirus is not identified until early 2003. The spread of the virus reaches epidemic proportions in Asia and expands to the rest of the world.

2002   The Best Pharmaceuticals for Children Act passed in an effort to improve safety and efficacy of patented and off-patent medicines for children.

2002 The Defense Advanced Research Projects Agency (DARPA) initiates the Biosensor Technologies program in 2002 to develop fast, sensitive, automatic technologies for the detection and identification of biological warfare agents.

2002 The Pathogen Genomic Sequencing program is initiated by the Defense Advanced Research Project Agency (DARPA) to focus on characterizing the genetic components of pathogens in order to develop novel diagnostics, treatments, and therapies for the diseases they cause.

2002 The planned destruction of stocks of smallpox causing Variola virus at the two remaining depositories in the U.S. and Russia is delayed over fears that large scale production of vaccine might be needed in the event of a bioterrorist action.

2002 The WHO declares the 51 countries of its European region free of polio.

2003 Almost 500,000 civic and health care workers at strategic hospitals, governmental facilities, and research centers across the United States are slated to receive smallpox immunizations as part of a strategic plan for ready response to a biological attack using the smallpox virus.

2003 An international research team funded by NINR found that filters made from old cotton saris cut the number of cholera cases in rural Bangladesh villages almost in half. Other inexpensive cloth should work just as well in other parts of the world where cholera is endemic. Cholera is a waterborne disease that causes severe diarrhea and vomiting, killing thousands of people around the world every year. This simple preventive measure has the potential to make a significant impact on a global health problem.

2003 By early May, WHO officials have confirmed reports of more than 3,000 cases of SARS from 18 different countries with 111 deaths attributed to the disease. United States health officials reported 193 cases with no deaths. Significantly, all but 20 of the U.S. cases are linked to travel to infected areas, and the other 20 cases are accounted

for by secondary transmission from infected patients to family members and health care workers. Health authorities assert that the emergent virus responsible for SARS will remain endemic (part of the natural array of viruses) in many regions of China well after the current outbreak is resolved.

2003 Canadian scientists at the British Columbia Cancer Agency in Vancouver announce the sequence of the genome of the coronavirus most likely to be the cause of SARS. Within days, scientists at the Centers for Disease Control (CDC) in Atlanta, Georgia, offer a genomic map that confirms more than 99% of the Canadian findings.

2003 Differences in outbreaks in Hong Kong between 1997 and 2003 cause investigators to conclude that the H5N1 virus has mutated.

2003 Following approximately five deaths by heart attack correlated to individuals receiving the new smallpox vaccine, U.S. health officials at the Centers for Disease Control (CDC) announce a suspension of administration of the new smallpox vaccine to patients with a history of heart disease until the matter can be fully investigated.

2003 Preliminary trials for a malaria vaccine are scheduled to begin in malaria-endemic African areas, where approximately 3,000 children die from the disease every day.

2003 SARS cases in Hanoi reach 22, as a simultaneous outbreak of the same disease occurs in Hong Kong. The World Health Organization issues a global alert about a new infectious disease of unknown origin in both Vietnam and Hong Kong.

2003 SARS is added to the list of quarantinable diseases in the United States.

2003 Studies indicate that women with a history of some sexually transmitted diseases, including the human papillomavirus, are at increased risk for developing cervical cancer.

2003 Studies show no correlation between immunization schedules and sudden infant death syndrome (SIDS) occurrences.

2003 The first case of an unusually severe pneumonia occurs in Hanoi, Vietnam, and is identified two days later as severe acute respiratory syndrome (SARS) by Italian physician and epidemiologist Carlo

Urbani, who formally identifies SARS as a unique disease and names it. Urbani later dies of SARS.

2003 The first case of bovine spongiform encephalopathy (BSE, mad cow disease) in the United States is found in a cow in Washington state. Investigations later reveal that the cow was imported from a Canadian herd, which included North America's first "home-grown" case of BSE six months earlier.

2003 The World Health Organization (WHO) takes the unusual step of issuing a travel warning that describes SARS as a worldwide health threat. WHO officials announced that SARS cases, and potential cases, had been tracked from China to Singapore, Thailand, Vietnam, Indonesia, Philippines, and Canada.

2003 United States invades Iraq and finds chemical, biological, and nuclear weapons programs, but no actual weapons.

2003 WHO Global Influenza Surveillance Network intensifies work on development of a H5N1 vaccine for humans.

2004 A 35-year-old television producer in the Guangdong province of China is the first person to become ill with SARS since the end of the May 2003, the initial outbreak of the newly-identified disease. Within two weeks, three other persons are suspected of having SARS in the region, and teams from the World Health Organization return to investigate possible human-to-human, animal-to-human, and environmental sources of transmission of the disease.

2004 Chinese health officials in the Guangdong province of China launch a mass slaughter of civet cats, a cousin of the mongoose considered a delicacy and thought to be a vector of SARS, in an attempt to control the spread of the disease.

2004 On December 26, the most powerful earthquake in more than 40 years occurred underwater off the Indonesian island of Sumatra. The tsunami produced a disaster of unprecedented proportion in the modern era. The International Red Cross puts the death toll at over 150,000 lives.

2004 Project BioShield Act of 2004 authorizes U.S. government agencies expedite procedures related to rapid distribution of treatments as countermeasures to chemical, biological, and nuclear attack.

2005 A massive 7.6-magnitude earthquake leaves more than 3 million homeless and without food and basic medical supplies in the Kashmir mountains between India and Pakistan; 80,000 people die.

2005 H5N1 virus, responsible for avian flu moves from Asia to Europe. The World Health Organization attempts to coordinate multinational disaster and containment plans. Some nations begin to stockpile antiviral drugs.

2005 Hurricane Katrina slams into the U.S. Gulf Coast, causing levee breaks and massive flooding to New Orleans. Damage is extensive across the coasts of Louisiana, Mississippi, and Alabama. Federal Emergency Management Agency (FEMA) is widely criticized for a lack of coordination in relief efforts. Three other major hurricanes make landfall in the United States within a two-year period, stressing relief and medical supply efforts. Long-term health studies begin of populations in devastated areas.

2005 The WHO reports outbreaks of plague in the Democratic Republic of Congo.

2005 U.S. FDA Drug Safety Board is founded.

2005 United States president George W. Bush addresses the issue of HIV/AIDS in black women in the United States, acknowledging it as a public health crisis.

2006 European Union bans the importation of avian feathers (non-treated feathers) from countries neighboring or close to Turkey.

2006 Mad cow disease confirmed in an Alabama cow as third reported case in the United States.

2006 More than a dozen people are diagnosed with avian flu in Turkey, but U.N. health experts assure the public that human-to-human transmission is still rare and only suspected in a few cases in Asia.

2006 Researchers begin human trials for vaginal microbicide gels.

2007 Texas governor Rick Perry adds the HPV vaccine to the list of required vaccines for school-age girls.

2007 Four people are hospitalized with botulism poisoning in the United States after more than 90 potentially contaminated meat products, including canned chili, were removed from grocery shelves across the country.

2007 The Centers for Disease Control and Prevention (CDC) issues a rare order for isolation when a New Jersey man infected with a resistant strain of tuberculosis flies on multiple trans-Atlantic commercial flights.

Malaria

■ Introduction

Malaria is the leading cause of death worldwide from parasitic infection. According to the World Health Organization (WHO) there are more than 500 million cases of malaria each year in tropical and subtropical regions of the world, and one to two million deaths, most of which occur in sub-Saharan Africa, with children being disproportionately affected.

The name "malaria" means "bad air" which used to be thought the cause of the disease. However, in the nineteenth century, it was established that malaria is caused by *Plasmodia* which are single-celled parasites that are carried by mosquitoes belonging to the *Anopheles* genus. Four species of *Plasmodia* are involved in malaria: *P. falciparum*, *P. vivax*, *P. ovale* and *P. malariae*. Malaria caused by *P. falciparum* is by far the most serious and the cause of most fatalities. There are several drugs that can be used for both the treatment and prevention of malaria. However, parasites have evolved resistance to one of the main ones, chloroquine, in certain areas.

■ Disease History, Characteristics, and Transmission

What historical accounts of war call "marsh fever," "inter-mittent fever," or "remittent fever," match current descriptions of malaria. One of the earliest recorded cas-ualties of malaria may have been the great military cam-paigner of ancient Greece, Alexander the Great, who died of a fever in 323 BC. Malaria and dysentery also caused much sickness during the Crusades (1095–c.1300). It was also a major cause of disease among European armies on campaigns in tropical regions up to the 1820s, when quinine—extracted from cinchona bark—was found to be useful in both treating and preventing the disease.

However, quinine proved to be only a partial solution to malaria among the military, for it continued to be a problem during World War I (1914–1918) in Macedonia,

Mesopotamia, and East Africa. In 1918, around 90% of British and French troops in Macedonia contracted malaria despite the use of quinine. In the World War II

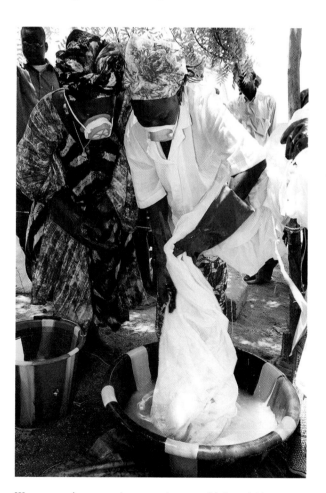

Women are shown treating mosquito nets with insecticides at an overcrowded medical clinic in Senegal in 2004. The insecticides will help prevent malaria, which kills more than one million children in the world each year, especially in Africa south of the Sahara desert.
© *Nic Bothma/epa/Corbis.*

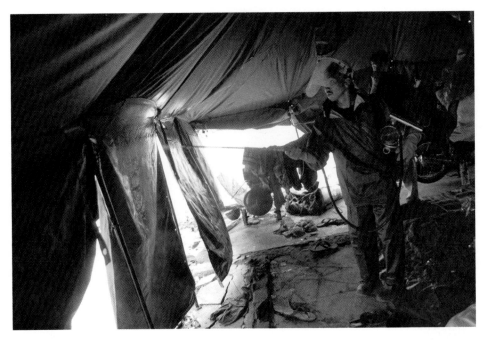

A health worker sprays down a tent to prevent malaria from breaking out in a refugee camp in Banda Aceh, Indonesia, one month after the earthquake and tsunami of December 2004. *Charles Pertwee/Getty Images.*

(1939–1945), quinine supplies were limited, and military commanders had lost their faith in it, so the Allies turned to the synthetic drug mepacrine instead. This was shown to have a dramatic effect in reducing the rate of malaria among Australian troops in New Guinea and among Allied troops in Burma. The insecticide DDT was introduced in 1944 and this was sprayed from the air to protect troops operating in marshy malarious areas of Burma and Italy.

The malaria parasite enters the body through the bite of an infected female *Anopheles* mosquito and travels through the blood to the liver, then back to the blood, undergoing a complex life cycle as it does so. The incubation time of malaria is typically between seven and 30 days. Symptoms occur within a month in 75% of cases, and within two months in 90% of cases. For travelers returning from areas where malaria is endemic, symptoms may, therefore, not start until well after their return home. Sometimes persons are infected with two or more species of *Plasmodium*.

The specific pattern of symptoms experienced in a bout of malaria depends upon which of the four species of Plasmodium is responsible for the disease. High fever with chills, headache, aching limbs, nausea, and diarrhea are common symptoms, however. Often the patient will experience a cycle of shivering and chills followed by flushing, fever, and profuse sweating. This bout of symptoms tends to spike (peak or temporarily worsen) every day or so, and is related to the parasites bursting out of the red blood cells they have infected.

In acute malaria, there may be swollen liver, pallor (paleness), jaundice (yellowing of the skin and eyes), anemia (reduced ability of blood to transport oxygen), and respiratory distress. Complications are most common among children, pregnant women and travelers and are usually caused by *P. falciparum* malaria. Cerebral malaria is the most serious complication of malaria and accounts for 80% of all fatalities from the disease. Around 0.5–1% of *P. falciparum* malaria cases lead to cerebral malaria. The other *Plasmodium* species do not cause cerebral malaria. The symptoms of cerebral malaria include seizures, stupor and coma. The death rate is between 20 and 50%. However, a full recovery without morbidity (disease or disability) is common among many survivors.

Other complications of *P. falciparum* malaria include a swollen spleen, kidney failure, and low blood sugar—the latter occurring because the parasites consume glucose 75 times faster than the red blood cell and therefore deplete its supplies. Death from a ruptured spleen has been reported in *P. ovale* malaria.

The risk of relapse depends upon the type of malaria the patient has. *P. falciparum* malaria, although responsible for most fatalities, does not actually lead to long-term relapse although survivors may suffer flare-ups over the year after the first attack. *P. vivax* causes a relapsing form of the disease, lasting up to five years, because of dormant parasites residing in the liver, as does *P. ovale*, although the latter is far less common. *P. malariae* may produce a low-grade chronic infection characterized by bouts of fever, lasting up to 50 years, although it too is uncommon.

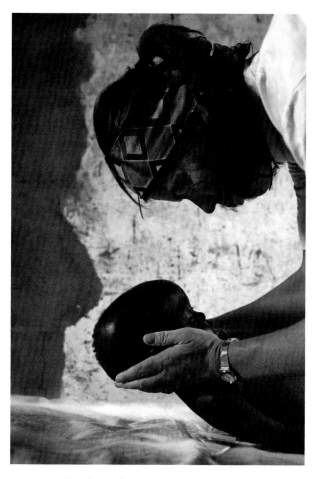

A doctor cradles the head of a one-year-old who is suffering from malaria at the Médecins sans Frontières (Doctors Without Borders) hospital at a camp for the internally displaced in Uganda, June 2005. *AP Images/James Stanmeyer/VII.*

The process by which *Plasmodia* parasites are transmitted begins with the bite of the infected female *Anopheles* mosquito, in order to take a blood meal from the host. The infectious sporozoite form of the parasite is injected into the skin through the mosquito's salivary glands, and travels through the bloodstream to the liver. They then reproduce asexually within liver cells. This process takes one to two weeks, and during this period, the patient will not have any symptoms.

The infected liver cells rupture, releasing parasite forms called merozoites which enter red blood cells, maturing and multiplying. This process takes about 48 hours and then these parasites rupture the red blood cell, releasing more merozoites, which go on to infect further red blood cells. The release of the merozoites causes inflammation and a release of toxins, which causes a spike of fever. This stage can cause a massive increase in the number of parasites, particularly in *P. falciparum* because this species infects all types of red blood cells. It is possible for more than 1% of all the red blood cells in the body to contain *P. falciparum* parasites.

In a further twist to this complex life cycle, some *Plasmodium* merozoites develop within the red blood cells into sexual forms, known as gametocytes. If another mosquito bites, she may take up these parasites in the blood meal and they can mate sexually inside the mosquito to form more sporozoites, ready to complete the cycle from the beginning with the next bite of the same, or another, host.

P. vivax and *P. ovale* have a hepatic form which lies dormant for several weeks, giving rise to relapse symptoms when they are released into the blood. *P. malariae* may be transmitted from person-to-person through blood and organ donations from people who are already infected with the parasite, even though they may not have symptoms. Each stage in the life cycle of each species of *Plasmodium* has a specific morphology, which allows for accurate diagnosis in expert hands.

■ Scope and Distribution

There are around 500 million symptomatic cases of malaria every year around the world. Most of the one to two million deaths occur in Africa and at least half of these occur among children. In the United Kingdom and the United States, there are 1,000 to 2,000 cases of malaria each year, and around ten deaths, mainly occurring in travelers returning from endemic areas, leading to around ten deaths. Around 80% of those affected have returned from traveling in Africa.

Malaria is endemic in tropical and subtropical regions, including sub-Saharan Africa, South East Asia, Papua New Guinea, the Pacific States, Haiti and parts of South America. The parasites require a temperature of at least 68°F (20°C) to complete their lifecycles. Besides temperature, humidity and rainfall are factors affecting the transmission of malaria. The disease is endemic in more than 100 countries and territories, with more than 40% of the world's population being at risk.

Malaria has been known for more than 4,000 years and the disease used to be even more widespread than it is today, for endemic malaria has been eliminated from the United States, Europe, Puerto Rico, Chile, Israel, Lebanon, Taiwan, Singapore, most of the Caribbean, and North Korea. Some Pacific islands do not have malaria, despite favorable climatic factors, because *Anopheles* mosquitoes do not live there. However, despite elimination from some countries, there has been a resurgence in others, such as Sri Lanka.

The four *Plasmodium* parasites have differing geographical distributions. *P. falciparum* has the widest spread, and is found in Central and South America, Haiti, the Dominican Republic, sub-Saharan Africa, India, Pakistan and South East Asia. *P. vivax* occurs in sub-Saharan Africa, Central and South America and Asia. *P. ovale* occurs in sub-Saharan Africa, South East Asia and Papua New Guinea. *P. malariae* is found only in sub-Saharan Africa. There are

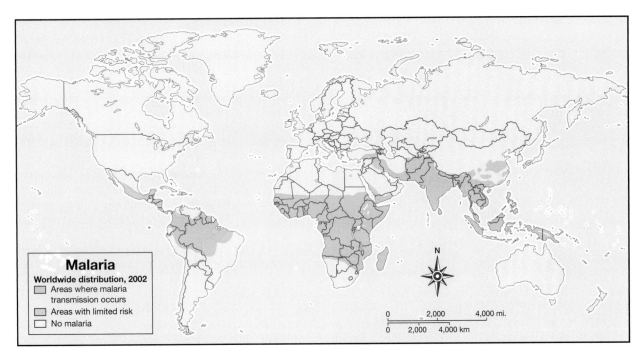

Map depicting worldwide malaria distribution in 2005. *© Copyright World Health Organization (WHO). Reproduced by permission.*

430 species in the *Anopheles* genus and only 30 to 50 transmit malaria. Some prefer to bite non-human animals, other are active inside rather than outside—therefore, risk of contracting malaria depends very much on the nature of the local mosquito population.

Returning travelers are especially at risk of malaria, as are pregnant women. Malaria should always be suspected if someone develops fevers and chills up to one year after return from a malarious area. Malaria in a pregnant woman can cause fetal death or low birth weight. The disease can also be passed on during childbirth, and will cause severe anemia in the newborn.

Malaria has often accompanied military campaigns throughout the course of human history because the disease is encouraged by the conditions of war. The movement of troops or refugees leads to the spread of many kinds of parasites, including *Plasmodia*, and those without immunity are at risk when they travel to areas where the disease is endemic. Moreover, war may damage drainage and irrigation systems, which encourages the breeding of mosquitoes.

■ Treatment and Prevention

There are several drugs which can be used for the treatment and prevention of malaria. These include chloroquine, mefloquine, pyrimethamine, proguanil, primaquine, and artemisinin. The latter is the most recent drug introduced and it comes from the Chinese herbal remedy qinghaosu. Drug resistance has begun to emerge in some areas, with chloroquine resistant *P. falciparum* being a problem in

Africa and elsewhere, and chloroquine resistant *P. vivax* in South East Asia. The WHO recommends the use of artemesinin in combination with another anti-malarial drug as first-line treatment for malaria, but the choice depends upon the *Plasmodium* species involved and the extent of drug resistance in the area where the disease was contracted.

Patients with malaria need close medical attention as well as medication. Often this means supervision in the high dependency or intensive care unit. It is especially important that fluid balance and glucose levels are maintained.

Prevention of malaria involves taking prophylactic medication before, during and after travel to malarious areas. The highest risk is a trip to an area where there is chloroquine-resistant *P. falciparum* where mefloquine, doxycycline or Malarone (a combination of atovaquone-proguanil) is often prescribed for malaria prophylaxis (prevention). Would-be travelers should take advice from the Centers for Disease Control and Prevention (CDC) or their national equivalent on the specific protection they need. Pregnant women, in particular, need prophylaxis. Only chloroquine and proguanil are recommended for use during pregnancy, therefore travel to chloroquine-resistant areas should be avoided.

The other key to prevention is avoiding the bite of the *Anopheles* mosquito. This can be challenging, as it is smaller and less conspicuous than some other mosquito species, and a bite could go unnoticed. *Anopheles* bite primarily between dusk and dawn. Wearing clothes of thick woven material, like cotton, that cover most of the body and sleeping under bed nets impregnated with permethrin insecticide are helpful, along with the use of an insect repellent containing DEET (diethylmethyltoluamide) on exposed areas of skin. Malaria sometimes occurs despite preventive measures, including medication, so those who at risk should still be on the lookout for telltale symptoms like fever.

■ Impacts and Issues

An effective vaccine would be an enormous advance in the global fight against malaria. For 20 years, various agencies of the United Nations, the World Bank and other non-governmental organizations have been searching for a vaccine as a top priority in their tropical disease research programs. Success has, unfortunately, proved elusive. It is hard to grow the malaria parasites in culture, which means the experiments that would help develop a vaccine cannot readily be carried out. The complex lifecycle of the parasites, which are constantly evolving, is also a huge challenge to vaccine researchers. Some people in endemic areas seem to have a natural immunity to malaria. Understanding the biochemical basis of this might open up a route to a vaccine but, so far, this has proved difficult.

Each death from malaria is a tragedy—whether it occurs in a returning traveler to the United States or in a child in Africa. There have been many needless deaths because of wrong or delayed diagnosis. Many doctors in the West are unfamiliar with malaria and may not realize that gastrointestinal symptoms are often prominent in the disease; fever may not be the only symptom. Returning travelers may assume that if they have taken prophylactic medication, then protection is assured. Symptoms setting in several weeks or even months after return from a malarious area may wrongly be assumed to be severe influenza.

The correct diagnosis of malaria depends upon identifying the parasites in a blood smear treated with Giemsa stain. Both thin and thick smears are usually examined. The thin smear preserves the morphology of the parasites so that the species involved can be identified. The thick smear contains more parasites and allows for more rapid diagnosis. Levels of parasites in the blood fall between bouts of fever and the smear may appear negative, even if the person has the disease. Three negative smears, taken at intervals, are required to definitely exclude the disease.

Malaria continues to be a global health problem. The disease has re-emerged in places where it was assumed the disease has been eradicated. For instance, Sri Lanka and India were virtually free of malaria at the end of the 1970s, but from the 1980s, the number of cases began to increase, reaching levels not seen since before World War II by the 1990s. Resistance of the parasites to anti-malarial drugs, and resistance of *Anopheles* mosquitoes to insecticides are the major factors in

> ## WORDS TO KNOW
>
> **ENDEMIC:** Present in a particular area or among a particular group of people.
>
> **GAMETOCYTE:** A germ cell with the ability to divide for the purpose of producing gametes, either male gametes called spermatocytes or female ones called oocytes.
>
> **MEROZOITE:** The motile, infective stage of malaria, responsible for disease symptoms.
>
> **MORBIDITY:** The term "morbidity" comes from the Latin word "morbus," which means sick. In medicine it refers not just to the state of being ill, but also to the severity of the illness. A serious disease is said to have a high morbidity.
>
> **PARASITE:** An organism that lives in or on a host organism and that gets its nourishment from that host. The parasite usually gains all the benefits of this relationship, while the host may suffer from various diseases and discomforts, or show no signs of the infection. The life cycle of a typical parasite usually includes several developmental stages and morphological changes as the parasite lives and moves through the environment and one or more hosts. Parasites that remain on a host's body surface to feed are called ectoparasites, while those that live inside a host's body are called endoparasites. Parasitism is a highly successful biological adaptation. There are more known parasitic species than nonparasitic ones, and parasites affect just about every form of life, including most all animals, plants, and even bacteria.
>
> **PROPHYLAXIS:** Treatment to prevent the onset or recurrence of disease.
>
> **RE-EMERGENT DISEASE:** A disease that has disappeared for a period of time, only to reappear at a later time.
>
> **SPOROZOITE:** Developmental stage of the malaria protozoan during which it is transferred from mosquito to human host.

the resurgence of the disease. Moreover, increased movements by travelers and migrants on a global scale are likely to add to the risk of re-introducing the malaria to countries where it had previously been eradicated.

The Bill and Melinda Gates Foundation supports mosquito-borne disease research and prevention efforts worldwide, including the development of effective and affordable drugs, improvement of existing preventative measures, and vaccine development. In 2005, The Gates Foundation announced three grants totaling $258.3 million for continued research and development of anti-malarial drugs, vaccines, and insecticide-based mosquito control methods. On the eve of the first White House Malaria Summit, the Gates Foundation announced another large grant of $83.5 million to expand access to bednets and treatment in malaria prone regions.

As most scientists agree that the Earth's temperature is rising, it is likely that more areas of the world will become habitats for the *Anopheles* mosquito and its parasites. Therefore, the search for a vaccine and new anti-malarial drugs has never been more urgent.

■ Primary Source Connection

Use of the insecticide DDT in the decades after World War II helped to greatly reduce the incidence of malaria throughout many countries of the world. By the 1970s, agricultural use of DDT was linked to thinning bird egg-shells, and after the populations of many birds plummeted, DDT use was banned in most developed countries by the 1985. A large drop in DDT use in developing countries followed, and by the 1990s, malaria made a resurgence.

In the following speech delivered to the National Press Club in Washington, D.C., in September 2006, Arata Kochi called for the renewed use of DDT in Africa, especially indoors in shelters made of mud and thatch, where it could function as both insect repellent and insecticide. Kochi, a Japanese physician, is the director of the malaria department for the World Health Organization. As of 2007, Kochi's plan of targeted DDT use indoors is being carried out in several sub-Saharan African nations including Zambia, South Africa, Angola, Uganda, Tanzania, and Mozambique.

WHO Malaria Head to Environmentalists: "Help Save African Babies as You Are Helping to Save the Environment."

I am here today with one urgent message to everyone who cares about the environment. Your concern, your activism, your heroics have helped—and continue to help—protect the earth's wildlife and nature.

I am here today to ask you, please: Help save African babies as you are helping to save the environment.

African babies do not have a powerful movement like the environmental movement to champion their well-being. They need your help.

Nearly one year ago, I was asked to take charge of the World Health Organization's Global Malaria Programme. I knew the job would be a challenge. Little progress was being made in controlling malaria, even though WHO had declared—way back in 1998—that rolling back malaria would be one of its greatest priorities.

I asked my staff; I asked malaria experts around the world: "Are we using every possible weapon to fight this disease?" It became apparent that we were not. One powerful weapon against malaria was not being deployed. In a battle to save the lives of nearly one million children ever year—most of them in Africa—the world was reluctant to spray the inside of houses and huts with insecticides; especially with a highly effective insecticide known as *dichlorodiphenyltrichloroethane*, or "DDT."

Even though indoor spraying with DDT and other insecticides had been remarkably effective in preventing malaria sickness and death where used, this strategy seemed to have been abandoned by most countries nearly 30 years ago. By the early 1980s, WHO was no longer actively promoting it.

Some people told me that there was a good reason why its wide scale use had been phased out. I was told the practice was unsafe for humans, birds, fish, and wildlife; that the use of DDT in the United States in the 1950s had led to the near extinction of the bald eagle. I was told that indoor spraying with DDT was "politically unpopular."

But I believe that public health policies must be based on the science and the data, not on conventional wisdom or politics. As we examined the issue, we found that the scientific and programmatic evidence told a different story: We found that:

- One of the best tools we have against malaria is indoor residual house spraying, as it has proven to be just as cost effective as other malaria prevention measures.

- Of the dozen insecticides WHO has approved as safe for house spraying, the most effective is DDT.

- DDT presents no health risk when used properly indoors. Well-managed indoor spraying programmes using DDT pose no harm to wildlife or to humans.

That is why today, after this reevaluation, the World Health Organization is announcing that indoor residual spraying with DDT and other insecticides will again play a major role in its efforts to fight the disease.

WHO is now recommending the use of indoor spraying not only in epidemic areas, but also in areas with constant and high malaria transmission, including throughout Africa.

WHO is calling on all malaria control programmes around the world to develop and issue a clear statement outlining their position on indoor spraying with long lasting insecticides such as DDT, specifying where and how it will be implemented in accordance with WHO guidelines, and how these progammes will provide all possible support to accelerate and manage this intervention effectively.

WHO *will* use every possible and safe method to control malaria.

Help save African babies as you are helping to save the environment. Help us advocate for careful limited use of indoor spraying. Help us set up the appropriate and proper management systems so that DDT is used effectively. And finally, help us raise the necessary funds to research and develop even more effective and affordable interventions.

Arata Kochi

KOCHI, ARATA. "WHO MALARIA HEAD TO ENVIRONMENTALISTS: HELP SAVE AFRICAN BABIES AS YOU ARE HELPING TO SAVE THE ENVIRONMENT." WORLD HEALTH ORGANIZATION PRESS STATEMENT. SEPTEMBER 15, 2006.

■ Primary Source Connection

Malaria is an ancient killer. For thousands of years, no one knew exactly what caused malaria and, therefore, no one could stop it. In 1880, Charles-Louis-Alphonse Laveran, a French military physician serving in Algeria, identified the plasmodium parasite in the blood of a sick artilleryman. Seventeen years later in India, Captain Ronald Ross extracted a plasmodium cyst from a dissected female *Anopheles* mosquito and identified malaria as an insect-borne parasitic disease.

Sir Ronald Ross (1857–1932) studied medicine in London before joining the Indian Medical Service in 1881. Throughout his career he focused with a single-minded intensity on the prevention of malaria, and in 1897 discovered the species of mosquito that spreads the disease. His work won him a Nobel Prize in 1902. Ross spent the remainder of his life conducting studies in the malarial centers of the world, and forming organizations to combat malaria. He directed the Ross Institute and Hospital for Tropical Diseases, established in his honor in 1926, until his death in 1932. In addition to his medical work, Ross was an acclaimed poet, and wrote the following poem shortly after discovering how malaria was transmitted.

This Day Relenting God

This day relenting God
Hath placed within my hand
A wondrous thing; and God
Be praised. At his command,

Seeking his secret deeds
With tears and toiling breath,
I find thy cunning seeds,
O million-murdering Death.

I know this little thing
A myriad men will save,
O Death, where is thy sting?
Thy victory, O Grave?

Ronald Ross

ROSS, RONALD. "THIS DAY RELENTING GOD." IN *MEMOIRS WITH A FULL ACCOUNT OF THE GREAT MALARIA PROBLEM AND ITS SOLUTION* LONDON: JOHN MURRAY, 1923.

SEE ALSO *Climate Change and Infectious Disease; Travel and Infectious Disease; Tropical Infectious Diseases; Vector-borne Disease.*

BIBLIOGRAPHY

Books

Lock, Stephen, John Last, and Georg Dunea. *The Oxford Illustrated Companion to Medicine.* Oxford: Oxford University Press, 2001.

Tan, James. *Expert Guide to Infectious Diseases.* Philadephia: American College of Physicians, 2002.

Wilson, Walter, and Merle A. Sande. *Current Diagnosis & Treatment in Infectious Diseases.* New York: McGraw Hill, 2001.

Web Sites

Centers for Disease Control and Prevention (CDC). "Malaria." <http://www.cdc.gov/malaria> (accessed May 9, 2007).

World Health Organization. "Malaria." May 2007 <http://www.who.int/topics/malaria/en> (accessed May 9, 2007).

Susan Aldridge

Marburg Hemorrhagic Fever

■ Introduction

Marburg hemorrhagic fever is one of a group of severe infections known as hemorrhagic fevers. The term hemorrhagic denotes the ability of these viral diseases to cause massive bleeding (hemorrhaging).

Marburg hemorrhagic fever is caused by a type of virus called a filovirus. The virus contains ribonucleic acid (RNA) as the genetic material. It was the discovery of the agent of Marburg hemorrhagic fever that led to the creation of the filovirus viral group. Other filoviruses identified so far include the four strains (types) of Ebola virus.

■ Disease History, Characteristics, and Transmission

Both Marburg fever and Marburg virus were discovered in 1967. At that time, outbreaks of the fever occurred in three laboratories where scientists were studying the virus. One of these labs was located in the German city of Marburg, from which the name of both the disease and the virus was taken.

Over 30 people became ill during this initial outbreak. The source of the virus was found to be African green monkey tissues that had been imported to the lab from Uganda as part of an effort to develop a polio

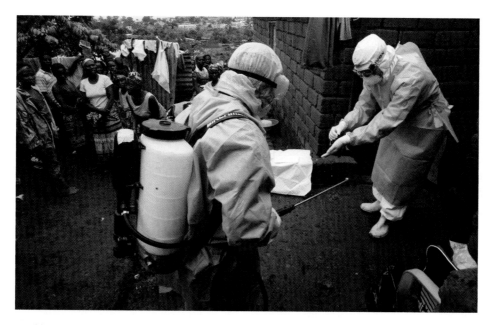

World Health Organization officials examine the home of a suspected Marburg virus victim in the northern Angolan town of Uige in April 2005. More than 200 people died from the disease during the outbreak, with children under the age of five being particularly vulnerable. © *Mike Hutchings/Reuters/Corbis.*

WORDS TO KNOW

ENDEMIC: Present in a particular area or among a particular group of people.

FILOVIRUS: A filovirus is any RNA virus belong to the family *Filoviridae*. Filoviruses infect primates; Marburg virus and Ebola virus are filoviruses

HEMORRHAGIC FEVER: A hemorrhagic fever is caused by viral infection and features a high fever and a high volume of (copious) bleeding. The bleeding is caused by the formation of tiny blood clots throughout the bloodstream. These blood clots—also called micro-thrombi—deplete platelets and fibrinogen in the bloodstream. When bleeding begins, the factors needed for the clotting of the blood are scarce. Thus, uncontrolled bleeding (hemorrhage) ensues.

HOST: Organism that serves as the habitat for a parasite, or possibly for a symbiont. A host may provide nutrition to the parasite or symbiont, or simply a place in which to live.

RESERVOIR: The animal or organism in which the virus or parasite normally resides.

the viral RNA, with that DNA then being used to produce the necessary components for new virus.

The symptoms of Marburg hemorrhagic fever include fever, chills, and headache. Initial symptoms may be mistaken for influenza. Approximately five days later, a rash appears mainly on the chest, stomach, and back. Nausea with vomiting, chest and abdominal pain, and diarrhea can develop. Subsequently, more severe symptoms may appear, including liver dysfunction with jaundice, pancreas inflammation, rapid weight loss, liver failure, and hemorrhaging. At this stage, organ failure often leads to a rapid death.

In the small number of cases known so far, the mortality rate is approximately 25%. Those who recover can display a number of recurring diseases, such as hepatitis.

Scope and Distribution

Marburg hemorrhagic fever is endemic (naturally occurring) in Africa. So far, it has not been discovered to be indigenous to any other continent. As of 2007, the full distribution of the virus in Africa is still unclear, but seems to include western Kenya, Uganda, and possibly Zimbabwe. The only way to determine distribution presently is to wait for the appearance of an outbreak of the disease.

Primates are a suspected natural reservoir of the infection, since the 1967 German outbreak involved African monkeys. However, this assumption has not been proven. This situation is similar to that of the other known filovirus, the Ebola virus. The sporadic and devastating nature of past Ebola and Marburg hemorrhagic fever outbreaks have limited scientists' ability to study the virus and determine its natural reservoir and potential hosts.

Treatment and Prevention

As of 2007, there is no cure or specific treatment for Marburg hemorrhagic fever. Rather, combating the infection involves standard precautions by attending physicians and other caregivers, such as handwashing and changing surgical garb before examining or tending to another patient. In addition, precautions to prevent the spread of the virus include wearing protective gowns, caps, foot covers, and masks equipped with face shields to guard against a spill or spray of blood. Treatment so far has been a catch-up effort designed to try and keep a patient stabilized and, in the worse cases, alive by the maintenance of blood pressure, fluid levels, and the proper concentrations of electrolytes. Also, ensuring that the blood remains capable of clotting can help reduce the loss of blood during hemorrhaging.

Even diagnosing the disease is challenging. In its early stages, the disease displays symptoms that are

vaccine. Victims included not only laboratory staff who were directly exposed to the virus, but also family members and caregivers who contracted the illness from a staff member with the disease. This pattern of transmission helped to establish the contagious nature of the virus.

The next reported case occurred in 1975, and it was determined to have been acquired in Zimbabwe. Another case was reported in 1980, this time in western Kenya. Cases reported in 1987 and 1998 also originated in other African countries.

The exact mechanism of transmission of the virus to humans is unknown. However, it is known that person-to-person transmission is possible, probably via contaminated blood or other body fluids. Other methods of transmission include handling medical equipment or touching surfaces that are contaminated with fluids infected with the virus.

Symptoms appear suddenly 5–10 days after infection. Presumably during this incubation period the virus is commandeering host cell replication machinery so that deoxyribonucleic acid (DNA) can be synthesized from

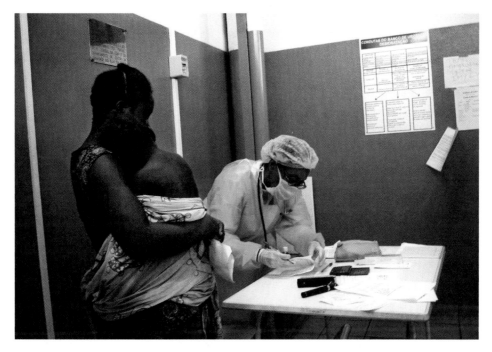

A woman brings her child to the hospital for testing following an outbreak of the deadly Marburg virus in Luanda, Uganda, in April 2005. Medical experts worked around the clock during the outbreak to check for suspected cases of the disease. *Florence Panoussian/AFP/Getty Images.*

similar to influenza, malaria, and typhoid fever. In addition, once symptoms appear the disease can swiftly worsen.

The presence of the viral genetic material can be detected using a number of molecular techniques. This can confirm the presence of the virus just a few days after infection. However, because there have been so few cases to date and since Marburg hemorrhagic fever is not a disease that is easily studied in the laboratory, the diagnostic significance of these molecular advances is unclear.

■ Impacts and Issues

Outbreaks of Marburg hemorrhagic fever are sporadic. This limits the number of people who are affected by the disease. However, this does not diminish the severity of the illness. The rapid onset of the disease and its high death rate can cause panic in communities that are affected.

Despite the rarity of Marburg hemorrhagic fever, outbreaks can occur. A recent example is the outbreak that occurred in 2005 in Uige, Angola, in which at least 270 people became ill. The death rate exceeded 90%. Another large outbreak occurred from 1998–2000 in the Democratic Republic of the Congo, in which 154 people became ill and 128 died.

Investigations of the 2005 Angolan outbreak determined that one cause was the unsafe use of needles to deliver injections in homes, medical clinics, and a pediatric ward. Re-use of the needles, which were intended to be used once and disposed of, facilitated in the spread of the virus. In the aftermath of the outbreak, the World Health Organization (WHO) instituted a safe injection campaign, which has helped reduce the re-use of contaminated needles in the region.

In both outbreaks, the isolated nature of the regions that were affected contributed to the spread of the disease. Medical care was rudimentary and clinics were not always adequately supplied to cope with the infection. Cultural practices, such as the open viewing and touching of the deceased prior to burial, also likely contributed to the spread of the virus. The WHO is working to increase awareness of the disease, especially in rural regions of countries such as Angola. With an increased understanding of the disease and its spread, it is hoped that alterations in behavior and cultural practices may help reduce the potential for future outbreaks.

Perhaps the greatest impact the disease has had is as an example of how diseases may be spreading from their natural, nonhuman hosts to humans. Identification of the natural host of a disease and the regions in which the natural host exists in greater numbers is vital if the disease is to be eradicated. In the case of Marburg hemorrhagic fever, the natural host is thought to be a primate.

Avoiding contact with primates in the wild (including their use as food) reduces the risk of contracting the disease.

The study of Marburg hemorrhagic fever requires a high containment facility called a biosafety type-4 lab, where air flow into and out of laboratories is controlled and stringent precautions regarding the wearing of protective clothing and decontamination following work with the virus are enforced. These steps help ensure that the virus does not escape from the lab and that researchers are protected from infection. Efforts to educate the medical community about Marburg symptomology are also important, since the virus can quickly infect health care workers and has the potential for rapid spread into the community. This potential for rapid person-to-person spread combined with the ferocity of the disease has heightened concerns that the Marburg virus could be used as an agent of bioterrorism.

SEE ALSO *Ebola; Emerging Infectious Diseases; Hemorrhagic Fevers.*

BIBLIOGRAPHY

Books

Drexler, Madeline. *Secret Agents: The Menace of Emerging Infections.* New York: Penguin, 2003.

Powell, Michael, and Oliver Fischer. *101 Diseases You Don't Want to Get.* New York: Thunder's Mouth Press, 2005.

Zimmerman, Barry E., and David J. Zimmerman. *Killer Germs.* New York: McGraw-Hill, 2002.

Web Sites

Centers for Disease Control and Prevention. "Marburg Hemorrhagic Fever." March 3, 2006. <http://www.cdc.gov/ncidod/dvrd/spb/mnpages/dispages/marburg.htm> (accessed May 7, 2007).

Brian Hoyle

Marine Toxins

Introduction

Marine toxins are naturally occurring compounds that can contaminate some types of seafood. The seafood may not show any signs of contamination, but, if eaten, it can cause various human illnesses.

Disease History, Characteristics, and Transmission

Marine toxins have probably existed for thousands of years. Biblical accounts of illnesses match the symptoms of paralytic shellfish poisoning, and the Red Sea may have been named "red" because of the frequent explosive growth of certain algae. Accounts of the consequences of marine toxins date back centuries. For example, a June 17, 1793, entry in a diary kept by the ship's surgeon during Captain George Vancouver's expedition off the West Coast of North America describes the death of a shipmate that is consistent with the effects of eating contaminated mussels.

In the coastal regions of the United States, the illnesses most frequently caused by marine toxins, from most common to least common, are scombrotoxic fish poisoning, ciguatera poisoning, paralytic shellfish poisoning, neurotoxic shellfish poisoning, and amnesic shellfish poisoning.

Scombrotoxic fish poisoning is a bacterial illness caused by the degradation of fish (mainly tuna and bonito). The bacteria degrade fish proteins, and a by-product of the protein decomposition is a group of compounds called histamines. When the spoiled fish is eaten, the high histamine level causes poisoning. Symptoms may begin only a few minutes after eating the seafood or several hours later. The symptoms include the development of a rash, flushing of the skin, sweating, and headache. As the body tries to expel the poison, abdominal pain, vomiting, and diarrhea also can occur. Some people also experience a burning or metallic sensation in the mouth.

The symptoms of scombrotoxic fish poisoning are temporary, and tend to fade after a few hours. Usually no treatment is necessary, although some people do benefit from drugs called antihistamines that counteract the effects produced by the excess histamines, as well as from a drug called epinephrine. Symptoms can be more severe in those who are taking some medications that slow the breakdown of histamine.

The second most common type of illness caused by marine toxins in the United States is ciguatera poisoning. This type of poisoning is due to the contamination of tropical reef fish by tiny marine plants called dinoflagellates. The illness is an example of what is termed biological magnification or biomagnification. In this case, the dinoflagellates are present in fish species that are food for a larger species. That species in turn becomes food for a larger marine animal. This pattern continues, with the concentration of the poison increasing from creature to creature. The animal at the top of this food chain (with ciguatera poisoning, it is often the barracuda) may have a high concentration of the poison. The person who eats that animal ingests the accumulated load of toxin. In addition to the barracuda, other fishes may contain high levels of the dinoflagellate toxin, including grouper, sea bass, snapper, and mullet. These popular sport fishes are found in tropical waters off of Hawaii, the Virgin Islands, Puerto Rico, and islands in the South Pacific.

Symptoms of ciguatera poisoning usually appear within minutes of eating a contaminated fish. The symptoms include nausea with vomiting, abdominal cramps, diarrhea, sweating, headache, muscle aches, dizziness, itchy skin, and general weakness. More usual symptoms are possible, such as alterations in taste and temperature sensations, and nightmares and hallucinations may occur. The symptoms tend to fade in 1–4 weeks.

Paralytic shellfish poisoning is caused by another dinoflagellate that can explode in numbers during an event called a "red tide." The name refers to the appearance of

WORDS TO KNOW

BIOMAGNIFICATION: The increasing concentration of compounds at higher trophic level or the tendency of organisms to accumulate certain chemicals to a concentration larger than that occurring in their inorganic, non-living environment, such as soil or water, or in the case of animals, larger than in their food.

DEGRADATION: Degradation means breakdown and refers to the destruction of host cell components, such as DNA, by infective agents such as bacteria and viruses.

DIATOM: Algae are a diverse group of simple, nucleated, plant-like aquatic organisms that are primary producers. Primary producers are able to utilize photosynthesis to create organic molecules from sunlight, water, and carbon dioxide. Ecologically vital, algae account for roughly half of photosynthetic production of organic material on Earth in both freshwater and marine environments. Algae exist either as single cells or as multicellular organizations. Diatoms are microscopic, single-celled algae that have intricate glass-like outer cell walls partially composed of silicon. Different species of diatom can be identified based upon the structure of these walls. Many diatom species are planktonic, suspended in the water column moving at the mercy of water currents. Others remain attached to submerged surfaces. One bucketful of water may contain millions of diatoms. Their abundance makes them important food sources in aquatic ecosystems.

DINOFLAGELLATE: Dinoflagellates are microorganisms that are regarded as algae. Their wide array of exotic shapes and, sometimes, armored appearance is distinct from other algae. The closest microorganisms in appearance are the diatoms.

HISTAMINE: Histamine is a hormone that is chemically similar to the hormones serotonine, epinephrine, and norepinephrine. A hormone is generally defined as a chemical produced by a certain cell or tissue that causes a specific biological change or activity to occur in another cell or tissue located elsewhere in the body. Specifically, histamine plays a role in localized immune responses and in allergic reactions.

RED TIDE: Red tides are a marine phenomenon in which water is stained a red, brown, or yellowish color because of the temporary abundance of a particular species of pigmented dinoflagellate (these events are known as "blooms"). Also called phytoplankton, or planktonic algae, these single-celled organisms of the class Dinophyceae move using a tail-like structure called a flagellum. They also photosynthesize, and it is their photosynthetic pigments that can tint the water during blooms. Dinoflagellates are common and widespread. Under appropriate environmental conditions, various species can grow very rapidly, causing red tides. Red tides occur in all marine regions with a temperate or warmer climate.

the water, which becomes discolored by the presence of vast numbers of the reddish brown dinoflagellates. The affected marine creatures are often filter-feeders—those that feed by straining sea water to remove tiny nutrients. The toxin-laden dinoflagellates accumulate in mussels, clams, oysters, crabs, and scallops. Lobsters also can become contaminated.

Symptoms of paralytic shellfish poisoning begin within several minutes to several hours of eating contaminated seafood. Initially, the symptoms are mild and include numbness of the face, arms, and legs; more severe symptoms follow, including dizziness, nausea, and loss of coordination. Some people become paralyzed and can die when they become unable to breathe.

Neurotoxic shellfish poisoning is another illness that is caused by a dinoflagellate. Shellfish are involved; they concentrate the toxin during filter-feeding. As with the other illnesses caused by marine toxins, symptoms tend to occur soon after consuming the contaminated seafood. Symptoms include dizziness, numbness, a tingling sensation in the mouth, arms, and legs, and loss of coordination. Recovery occurs within several days.

Finally, amnesic shellfish poisoning is a rare event that is caused by a microscopic plant (diatom) called *Nitzchia pungens*. Concentration of the diatom in shellfish, such as mussels, also concentrates a component of the diatom known as domoic acid. When contaminated mussels are eaten, the domoic acid causes an intestinal upset, dizziness, headache, and loss of orientation. In severe cases, there can be brain damage when domoic acid attaches to chemical receptors in brain cells, disrupting cell function. Permanent loss of memory, paralysis, and death can result.

Scope and Distribution

Marine toxins are found in coastal regions in almost all parts of the globe, except at the higher latitudes of the Arctic and Antarctic. Different illnesses often have different distributions. For example, neurotoxic shellfish poisoning tends to occur in the Gulf of Mexico and along the southern Atlantic Coast of the United States.

Illnesses caused by marine toxins occur in greater numbers in more equatorial regions, since the warmer waters encourage the growth of the microorganisms that produce the toxins. However, outbreaks occur during the warmer months in other regions.

There is no evidence that gender or race influences a person's susceptibility to marine toxins. The elderly and those with a less efficient immune system may be more at risk.

Treatment and Prevention

Treatment typically involves making the patient as comfortable as possible and waiting for the illness to pass. Scombrotoxic fish poisoning can be treated with drugs aimed at neutralizing the effects of the excess histamine.

There are no vaccines that provide protection against poisoning by marine toxins. The best prevention strategy is to use caution when eating seafood. For example, eating raw shellfish is risky and should be avoided. Warnings about algal blooms and reports of seafood-related illnesses should be taken seriously. Seafood from the affected region should be avoided until public health officials have determined that the danger is over.

Impacts and Issues

In the United States, about 30 people are poisoned by the toxins in seafood each year. The consequences of this poisoning can range from a short-term and inconvenient illness to permanent damage, memory loss, and death.

Because coastal areas often attract tourists and tourists often want to sample the local seafood, an outbreak of poisoning by a marine toxin can affect the local economy. For example, in 1987 there was an outbreak of amnesic shellfish poisoning on Prince Edward Island, Canada, which sickened more than 100 people and caused several deaths. In the years following the outbreak, fear over consumption of seafood and a lingering perception that the coast of the province was dangerous caused a marked drop in visitors. This adversely affected the island' economy, which heavily relies on summer tourism.

Periodic outbreaks involving larger numbers of people also occur. In fact, studies by the Woods Hole Oceanographic Institution and the U.S. National Oceanographic and Atmospheric Administration indicate that the frequency of algal blooms has been increasing along the coasts of the

IN CONTEXT: MARINE MICROORGANISMS

Marine microorganisms often inhabit a harsh environment. Ocean temperatures are generally very cold—approximately 37.4° F (about 3° C) on average—and this temperature tends to remain this cold except in shallow areas. About 75% of the oceans of the world are below 3,300 ft (1,000 m) in depth. The pressure on objects like bacteria at increasing depths is enormous.

Some marine bacteria have adapted to the pressure of the ocean depths and require the presence of the extreme pressure in order to function. Such bacteria are barophilic if their requirement for pressure is absolute or barotrophic if they can tolerate both extreme and near-atmospheric pressures. Similarly, many marine bacteria have adapted to the cold growth temperatures. Those which tolerate the temperatures are described as psychrotrophic, while those bacteria that require the cold temperatures are psychrophilic ("cold loving").

Marine microbiology has become the subject of much commercial interest. Compounds with commercial potential as nutritional additives and antimicrobials are being discovered from marine bacteria, actinomycetes and fungi. For example the burgeoning marine nutraceuticals market represents millions of dollars annually, and the industry is still in its infancy. As relatively little is still known of the marine microbial world, as compared to terrestrial microbiology, many more commercial and medically-relevant compounds undoubtedly remain undiscovered.

United States and other countries since the 1970s. While the cause of the increased number of blooms is not absolutely certain, a general consensus among scientists is that the documented warming of the coastal oceans has made conditions more favorable for algal growth. If so, a consequence of global warming could be more algal blooms and more cases of marine toxin-related illness.

In coastal regions of the United States, Canada, and other maritime countries, government agencies monitor ocean catches and aquaculture facilities for the presence of the various toxic species. Detection of these toxic species can lead to the closure of a region to fishing and the sale of commercially raised seafood until the problem is resolved.

The health risk posed by marine toxins has been balanced somewhat by the discovery that some marine toxins can act as anti-cancer drugs. A 2006 University of Wisconsin study reported that marine toxins can bind to a cell component called actin and that this interaction can disable rapidly growing cells, such as cancer cells.

SEE ALSO *Waterborne Disease.*

BIBLIOGRAPHY

Books

Belkin, Shimshon S., and Rita R. Colwell. *Oceans and Health: Pathogens in the Marine Environment.* New York: Springer, 2005.

Sindermann, Carl J. *Coastal Pollution: Effects on Living Resources and Humans.* Boca Raton: CRC, 2005.

Periodicals

Allingham, J. S., et al. "Structures of Microfilament Destabilizing Toxins Bound to Actin Provide Insight into Toxin Design and Activity." *Proceedings of the National Academy of Science* 102 (2005): 14527–14532.

Brian Hoyle

Measles (Rubeola)

■ Introduction

Measles is an acute viral illness that is one of the most common diseases of childhood, along with mumps and German measles (rubella). The clinical name for measles is rubeola, which comes from the Latin word *ruber* meaning red, and is a reference to the pinkish-red rash that is characteristic of the disease. Measles is a highly infectious disease, spread by coughs, sneezes, and person-to-person contact. It will occasionally lead to serious and even potentially fatal complications, such as pneumonia and encephalitis. Once someone has had measles, they are usually immune for life. Vaccination was introduced in the 1960s in the Western world and has led to a dramatic reduction in the number of children contracting measles. Since humans are the only hosts for the

measles virus, it should be possible to eradicate measles, through universal vaccination. This requires a global effort to bring the vaccine to children everywhere.

■ Disease History, Characteristics, and Transmission

Measles is caused by a virus from the Paramyxoviridae family, which also includes the influenza and mumps viruses. It is a single stranded, enveloped, RNA virus—that is, its genetic material is RNA rather than DNA. The incubation time of the measles virus is 9–12 days. The virus first infects the epithelial cells lining the upper respiratory tract and then spreads to the rest of the body.

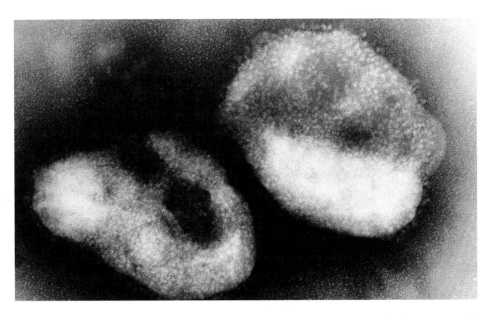

Paramyxoviruses are a group of viruses that include the agents of human measles (rubeola), mumps, and respiratory diseases, as well as canine distemper. © *Visuals Unlimited/Corbis.*

531

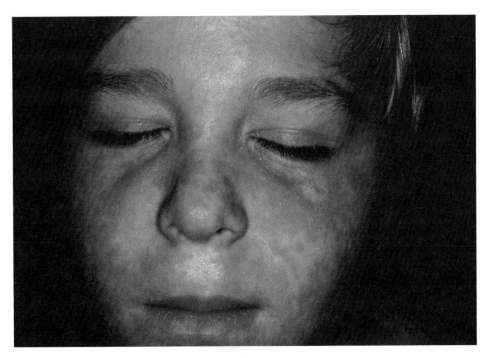

The measles (rubeola) rash as seen on a child's face.   *CNRI/Photo Researchers, Inc.*

In typical or natural measles, the early symptoms are like those of a common cold and include coughing, sneezing, sore throat, and fever. Within a few days, characteristic small white spots called Koplik's spots develop inside the mouth. A day or so later, a rash appears, starting behind the ears and spreading to the face and down the body and lasting for three or four days. Complications occur in up to 30% of cases of measles, and include pneumonia and otitis media, a middle ear infection that can lead to deafness. Encephalitis, an inflammation of the brain, is a complication in around one out of 1,000 cases of measles and has a 10% mortality rate. Mortality (death) from measles complications is highest among infants under two years old and in adults.

There is also a modified form of measles that occurs among those who have been incompletely vaccinated. Modified measles is less severe than typical measles and Koplik's spots may be absent. However, the risk of complications is the same. Rarely, a form of the disease called atypical measles may occur, usually among those who received vaccine in the 1960s. Atypical measles is characterized by sudden onset of fever, muscle pain, abdominal pain, and headache. Koplik's spots are rarely present and pneumonia is a common complication. Subacute sclerosing panencephalitis is an extremely rare degenerative disease of the brain and nervous system that is thought to arise from persistent measles infection in the brain. It occurs at a rate of around one per 100,000 cases and develops several years after measles exposure.

Measles is spread through the aerosol route—that is, through coughs and sneezes—and also by person-to-person contact. It is one of the most infectious diseases known, with around 90% of those being exposed becoming infected. A person is infectious for three to four days before the rash appears and for up to four days while the rash is present.

■ Scope and Distribution

Practically all children developed measles at some stage before vaccination, with the disease being most common in the winter and early spring. Before the introduction of the measles vaccine in 1963, there were 200,000–600,000 cases of measles a year in the United States, and this was probably a gross underestimate of the true scale of the disease. Before vaccination, measles killed more children than polio did. There was a sharp decline in measles cases following mass vaccination, followed by resurgence from 1983. This occurred among those who had not been vaccinated and among previously vaccinated teenagers. By 1989, there were 19,000 reported cases. A revised vaccination strategy, involving two doses instead of one, brought measles under control again. By 1993, cases were down to fewer than 1,000 annually in the United States. Measles has always been a global problem and has a major impact upon child health in developing countries, where vaccination is not readily available. According to the World Health Organization (WHO), there were around 30 million cases of measles around the world in 2004, of which

454,000 proved fatal. Measles can be dangerous to the fetus if a pregnant woman contracts measles in the first three months of pregnancy. Patients with weakened immunity, such as those with HIV/AIDS, are also at risk of complications from measles.

■ Treatment and Prevention

Treatment of measles is often unnecessary, although antibiotics may be given for secondary bacterial infections. Vitamin A may be useful in very severe cases and in countries where this vitamin deficiency is common. The antiviral drug ribavirin may be used in very severe cases also, and in patients with weakened immunity.

The spread of measles can be prevented by good hygiene, including handwashing. People with measles should isolate themselves while they are infectious and not attend school or day care. The best way of preventing measles is by vaccination. A killed vaccine was introduced in 1963, followed by a live vaccine from the late 1960s. It is now usual to give a combined measles, mumps, and rubella (MMR) vaccine—one dose between 12 and 15 months and a second before a child enters school. Most people can take MMR, but it is not usually recommended for people with weakened immunity or for pregnant women. Some parents have concerns over the safety of the MMR vaccine, because it has been linked with autism, and have refused vaccination for their children. In areas where vaccination rates have fallen, for this and other reasons, there have been new and significant measles outbreaks.

■ Impacts and Issues

Measles is the leading cause of vaccine-preventable death among children. The death rate from measles in developed countries is very low but reaches 1–5% in developing countries. The death rate from measles can be as high as 10–30% among malnourished children or those in refugee situations. Around 400,000 children under five years of age die from measles each year. But measles is a disease that could be eradicated from the planet, since humans are the virus' only host. In 2001, the Measles Initiative was established by the American Red Cross, the Centers for Disease Control and Prevention, UNICEF (the United Nations Children's Fund), and the WHO. The Initiative aims to cut deaths from measles by 90% by 2010 compared to figures from the year 2000, using vaccination that can cost less than a dollar per child. In the first five years, the Initiative supported campaigns, with national governments, that led to the vaccination of more than 217 million children, mainly in Africa. This saw measles deaths in Africa drop by 75%—from 506,000 in 1999 to 126,000 in 2005. The Initiative has now expanded its vaccination activities to Asia and is working

WORDS TO KNOW

AEROSOL: Particles of liquid or solid dispersed as a suspension in gas.

KOPLIK'S SPOTS: Koplik's spots, named after American pediatrician Henry Koplik (1858–1927) and also called Koplik's sign, are red spots with a small blue-white speck in the center found on the tongue and the insides of the cheeks during the early stages of measles.

MORTALITY: Mortality is the condition of being susceptible to death. The term "mortality" comes from the Latin word *mors*, which means "death." Mortality can also refer to the rate of deaths caused by an illness or injury, i.e., "Rabies has a high mortality."

in all six WHO regions of the world in an attempt to eradicate measles and its impact on child health.

■ Primary Source Connection

During the late 1970s and early 1980s, the rise of individualism and the popularity of self-help movements in the United States and Western Europe provided a new challenge to public health officials. Individuals began to take control of their own heath care and, in essence, some control and responsibility was wrested away from the physician and other health care workers. This presented a special challenge to public health agencies because a manifestation of the movement toward self directed health care also involved the rejection of traditional vaccinations such as the MMR vaccine.

Over the last decade, many parents further rejected using the MMR vaccine out of fears that the vaccine was linked to autism.

The newspaper article by Mark Porter and commentary below demonstrate different aspects of the scientific and social debate over the MMR vaccine. The article also demonstrates the attempts by scientific community to be both self-correcting and to discipline breeches of ethics. The commentary offers a view that although the original research linking the MMR vaccine to autism appears tainted, the vigorous investigation might lead to future benefits in the way vaccines are developed and tested.

Mark Porter is is a medical doctor who provides regular advice and commentary on medical issues for radio and television programming in the United Kingdom.

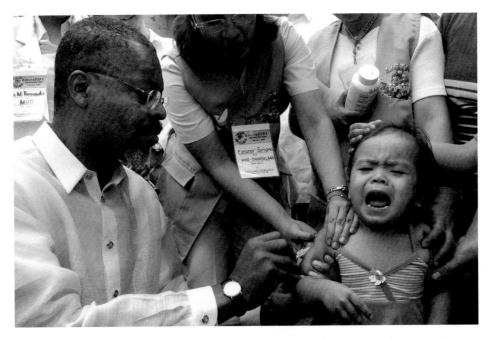

A United Nations Children's Fund (UNICEF) doctor vaccinates a child against measles as part of a national immunization campaign in the Philippines in February 2004. *Jay Directo/AFP/Getty Images.*

Doctor Who Sparked the MMR Debate Faces Misconduct Charge

THE doctor whose research sparked the international scare over the safety of the MMR vaccine is to be charged with serious professional misconduct.

Andrew Wakefield is to be ordered in front of the General Medical Council after publishing a paper in *The Lancet* in 1998 that suggested a link between the jab and autism as well as Crohn's, a bowel disease.

A sheet of preliminary charges accuses him of putting out "inadequately founded" research, of failing to obtain ethical committee approval, obtaining funding "improperly" and of subjecting children to "unnecessary and invasive investigations."

Dr. Wakefield's study is held responsible by many doctors for a dramatic slump in the number of parents allowing their children to have the combined injection against measles, mumps and rubella.

Take-up of the vaccination has fallen to only 12 per cent of children in some areas of London, while city-wide little more than half are having the jab - putting an estimated 100,000 of London children at risk of infection.

In 2004, *The Lancet* withdrew the paper, with the editor declaring it "fatally flawed" after it emerged Dr. Wakefield had been paid [pounds sterling]55,000 (more than $100,000) by lawyers for parents of children who claimed they had been damaged by the MMR vaccine to look for evidence that could be used in legal action. GMC lawyers are working on the list of charges with a hearing expected

next year. If found guilty of serious professional misconduct Dr. Wakefield, 50, faces being struck from the medical register. The GMC decided to bring a case against the doctor contrary to normal procedures. It usually only brings charges when it receives a complaint, but in this case it acted without one, following a two-year investigation.

Why we all owe Wakefield a debt of thanks

COMMENTARY

DR ANDREW WAKEFIELD has had a spectacular fall from grace.

Eight years after sparking worldwide concern about the safety of the MMR vaccine, his research has been rejected by the journal that originally published it, and most of his fellow researchers have distanced themselves from his conclusions.

A promising career in the UK has come to an abrupt end and he has left the country. To cap it all, he is set to be charged with professional misconduct by the General Medical Council. While intrigued by Wakefield's theory that exposure to the measles virus could predispose some children to autism, I have always felt that he was wrong to cast doubts on the safety of MMR without more evidence.

But just because we didn't see eye to eye it doesn't mean that I am comfortable with the public pillorying that he has recently endured. Indeed, I am distinctly uncomfortable with it. We need mavericks like Andrew Wakefield, and his plight can only stifle the sort of independent thinking required to make major breakthroughs in medicine. History has taught us that there is a fine line between being dismissed as an eccentric and being lauded as a genius. Nobel Prize winner Dr. Barry Marshall is a case in point.

At first Dr Marshall's claims that stomach and duodenal ulcers were caused by an infection (*H.pylori*) and could be treated with antibiotics, rather than a lifetime of acid suppressing drugs, were treated with derision.

But he persevered.

Fifteen years later his discovery has transformed the lives of millions of patients and he has become one of medicine's most distinguished academics.

While Dr. Wakefield has achieved notoriety rather than eminence, his enthusiasm left me in little doubt that he really did believe he had stumbled across something that questioned the safety of the MMR vaccine. Time may have proved him wrong, but back in 1998 when he first raised the possibility, we simply didn't have enough data to back the bland reassurances issued by the Department of Health.

Thanks to him sticking his head above the parapet, we now know far more about the MMR vaccine than we ever would have known had he not questioned its safety.

And I suspect the resulting scepticism, both lay and professional, that now surrounds the introduction of new vaccines will benefit us all in the long-term.

Mark Porter

PORTER, MARK. "DOCTOR WHO SPARKED THE MMR DEBATE FACES MISCONDUCT CHARGE." *THE EVENING STANDARD.* JUNE 12, 2006.

SEE ALSO *Childhood Infectious Diseases, Immunization Impacts; Mumps; Rubella.*

BIBLIOGRAPHY

Books

Tan, James S. *Expert Guide to Infectious Diseases.* Philadelphia: American College of Physicians, 2002.

Wilson, Walter R., and Merle A. Sande. *Current Diagnosis & Treatment in Infectious Diseases.* New York: McGraw Hill, 2001.

IN CONTEXT: SCIENTIFIC, POLITICAL, AND ETHICAL ISSUES

With regard to a potential connection between the measles, mumps, and rubella vaccine (MMR vaccine) and autism, scientists at the National Immunization Program (NIP) at Centers for Disease Control and Prevention (CDC) state that "the weight of currently available scientific evidence does not support the hypothesis that MMR vaccine causes autism. CDC recognizes there is considerable public interest in this issue, and therefore supports additional research regarding this hypothesis. CDC is committed to maintaining the safest, most effective vaccine supply in history."

As of May 2007 the CDC further states that, "there is no convincing evidence that vaccines such as MMR cause long term health effects. On the other hand, we do know that people will become ill and some will die from the diseases this vaccine prevents. Measles outbreaks have recently occurred in the UK and Germany following an increase in the number of parents who chose not to have their children vaccinated with the MMR vaccine. Discontinuing a vaccine program based on unproven theories would not be in anyone's best interest. Isolated reports about these vaccines causing long term health problems may sound alarming at first. However, careful review of the science reveals that these reports are isolated and not confirmed by scientifically sound research. Detailed medical reviews of health effects reported after receipt of vaccines have often proven to be unrelated to vaccines, but rather have been related to other health factors. Because these vaccines are recommended widely to protect the health of the public, research on any serious hypotheses about their safety are important to pursue. Several studies are underway to investigate still unproven theories about vaccinations and severe side effects."

SOURCE: *Centers for Disease Control and Prevention, National Immunization Program*

Web Sites

The Measles Initiative. "Home Page." March 16, 2007. <http://www.measlesinitiative.org/index3.asp> (accessed March 20, 2007).

Susan Aldridge

Médecins Sans Frontières (Doctors Without Borders)

■ Introduction

Médecins Sans Frontières (MSF), known in English as Doctors Without Borders, is an international, independent humanitarian organization designed to provide assistance in emergency situations caused by war, drought, famine, epidemics, disasters (either natural or manmade), or lack of available healthcare. It was established in 1971. Among the characteristics that distinguish MSF from other charitable organizations are its independence from government funding (it relies on primarily private donations and is very successful at fundraising) and its ability and willingness to make public opinion statements. Currently, MSF has branches in nearly twenty countries around the world. Roughly 80% of its funding comes from public and private donations; the remaining 20% is received from governmental and international humanitarian agencies.

Médecins Sans Frontières was awarded the Nobel Peace Prize in 1999.

■ History and Scientific Foundations

Because MSF is an independent international organization, it has no political ties or limitations to prevent it from responding to any situation thought likely to benefit from its assistance. It was not designed to become involved in international governmental affairs. For those involved in the local response of MSF, the effort is a humanitarian one. Traveling staff are primarily volunteers (although their personal expenses are paid and they may receive a small stipend) who are willing to make themselves available with very little notice; they are typically deployed in an area for six to twelve months. Assigned locations may be remote and dangerous. MSF hires local staff and provides them with training and materials, and all personnel (MSF core and local staff) work in cooperation with other local and international emergency and relief organizations.

MSF is staffed by physicians, nurses, healthcare providers, logisticians, technicians, technical and non-medical personnel, sanitation and water experts, and administrative workers. There is a small core of paid staff, a large number of volunteer workers, and a significant number of local staffers hired at each major site. MSF participates in an average of nearly 4,000 medically related missions each year.

■ Applications and Research

MSF's primary tasks are the provision of basic and emergency physical and mental health care on-site at hospitals and clinics (either existent or created locally by MSF staff); the performance of surgery; the provision of vaccinations and immunizations; and the operation of feeding centers, primarily for children and mothers of babies. MSF also employs experts who are able to dig and construct wells or bring in potable (safe to drink) water, in order to establish a means of supplying clean drinking water. When necessary, MSF also assists in creating temporary shelters and can supply blankets and plastic sheeting materials.

In addition to their emergency operations, MSF operates longer-term projects to treat infectious and communicable diseases such as HIV/AIDS, tuberculosis, and sleeping sickness, and to provide physical and mental health treatment for marginalized groups and street children. MSF also has an expert epidemiology section, and it has been utilized around the world to diagnose, treat, monitor, and contain epidemics of cholera, meningitis, and measles, among other diseases.

■ Impacts and Issues

By traveling in small teams and enlisting local resources, MSF teams have penetrated war zones and reached

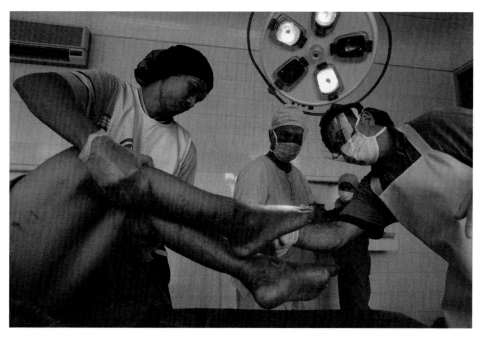

An Australian nurse (right) with Médecins sans Frontières (Doctors Without Borders) examines a patient in Sigli, Indonesia, in January 2005. The patient is about to undergo an operation for an infection in a leg wound acquired during the Indian Ocean Tsunami. *AP Images/James Nachtwey/VII.*

refugee groups and epidemic epicenters. The photograph below shows a makeshift refugee camp in the Democratic Republic of Congo set up by MSF in January 2006 after over 18,000 people fled conflict between the Congolese Army and Mai Mai rebels.

Because of its size, well-trained staff, and ability to hire significant numbers of local people in order to meet personnel needs, MSF is generally able to respond extremely quickly to emergencies. They utilize highly specialized kits and equipment packs that enable them to carry all needed supplies with them when they mobilize, so they are literally able to "hit the ground running," with no delay before they are able to begin emergency operations.

Their field kits are tailored to be an exact match for the type of emergency situation, geographic conditions, terrain, environmental conditions, and estimated patient population size. They can set up portable operating theatres, clinics, and hospitals immediately upon arrival in an affected area. They have created myriad treatment and response protocols that are customized to fit any necessary situation; their kits and protocols have been adopted by emergency and relief organizations worldwide.

One of the unique aspects of MSF, in contrast to nearly all other relief and aid organizations, is its commitment to combining humanitarian medical care with outspoken opinion on the causes of worldwide suffering. It is equally vocal on perceived impediments to the provision of effective medical care. For example, MSF has spoken publicly against pharmaceutical companies that refuse to manufacture pediatric dosages of AIDS-related drugs or to provide affordable and appropriate medications to African countries hardest hit by the AIDS pandemic. MSF has sought (and received) audiences with the United Nations, various international and governmental organizations, and the worldwide media, in an effort to communicate both the needs of their various patient groups and to educate the world on violations of international humanitarian doctrines that they have witnessed or that they argue have been perpetrated across the globe. Researchers, academics, and scientists associated with MSF publish scholarly articles, create media campaigns, engage in public education programs, and offer presentations and exhibits at local and international conferences, in an effort to create public awareness of medical and living conditions in underserved, impoverished, and war-torn areas of the world. MSF has launched a major initiative called the Campaign for Access to Essential Medicines, through which they are trying to help underserved or marginalized populations obtain safe, effective, affordable treatments for such diseases as HIV/AIDS, tuberculosis, and malaria.

■ Primary Source Connection

Médecins Sans Frontières (MSF), or Doctors Without Borders, is an international humanitarian organization that provides emergency medical assistance in over seventy nations. MSF's mission is to provide medical care in

WORDS TO KNOW

EPIDEMIOLOGY: Epidemiology is the study of various factors that influence the occurrence, distribution, prevention, and control of disease, injury, and other health-related events in a defined human population. By the application of various analytical techniques including mathematical analysis of the data, the probable cause of an infectious outbreak can be pinpointed.

NOBEL PEACE PRIZE: An annual prize bequeathed by Swedish inventor Alfred Nobel (1833–1896) and awarded by the Norwegian Nobel Committee to an individual or organization that has "done the most or the best work for fraternity between the nations, for the abolition or reduction of standing armies and for the holding and promotion of peace congresses."

NON-GOVERNMENTAL ORGANIZATIONS (NGOS): A voluntary organization that is not part of any government; often organized to address a specific issue or perform a humanitarian function.

POTABLE: Water that can is clean enough to drink safely is potable water.

to the world's neediest populations, often those touched by war, conflict, epidemic disease, natural disaster, and famine. In the following article, an MSF worker describes the organization's work in Somalia. The story of one patient, Isaac, evidences the significant health threats facing the war-torn region, including tuberculosis, leishmaniasis, and widespread malnourishment.

Isaac

"...WHEN HE FIRST ARRIVED HE WAS TOO WEAK TO STAND AND SO TO SEE HIM WALKING GIVES EVERYONE HOPE."

BY JAKE MCKNIGHT, MARCH 2006

Isaac is seven but he looks much younger. His weak legs barely support the top half of his meagre frame, forcing him to press his hands into his knees to hold himself upright. His movements are further restricted by the horrific damage inflicted by tuberculosis of the spine, which has caused him to effect the hunch of an old man. In his ragged t-shirt and near useless flip-flops, I often see Isaac walking the thirty or so metres from the tuberculosis ward to paediatrics with his head down,

concentrating his efforts against the hot winds that almost carry enough dust to hide his cheerful smile. It would seem that Somalis don't make very good victims.

I have been working for MSF for about a year now, first in Angola and now in Huddur, the small town in central Somalia where I have been for the last six weeks.

On reading a little about Somalia I had felt compelled to come here. For the last century, the country has been at war: firstly with the colonial powers of Italy, France and Britain; secondly with Ethiopia; thirdly with Siad Barre, the dictator who was deposed in 1991. Finally—in the power vacuum that resulted—Somalia has been at war with itself.

Hundreds of clans and sub-clans have split the country into an immensely complex framework of allegiances and ties. All efforts to bring this system under control have failed, earning Somalia the dubious title of being the only country in the world without a government. In addition to this long history of woes, the southern regions—including Huddur—are currently suffering the terrible results of the drought, which is spreading across the horn of Africa.

In such an environment, it would be fair to assume that the Somalis might be quite a bitter people. However, in the late afternoons, when the sun is less fierce and the winds die down, I regularly have the chance to walk around the hospital wards. Despite the cramped conditions and lack of amenities, the patients and their carers sit sometimes in groups, sometimes nursing children and almost always content and peaceful.

Part of the reason for both the lack of space and the happy faces is that MSF is achieving a lot in Somalia. One of the most prevalent serious diseases we treat here is kala azar (leishmaniasis), a condition that mostly affects children. If not treated, kala azar is almost always fatal. When patients arrive in the health centre they are often desperately sick and sometimes malnourished. After careful treatment of the disease and admission into our Therapeutic Feeding Programme for the severely malnourished, it generally takes about five weeks for kala azar patients to be discharged: fat, happy and cured. Word has spread to the surrounding areas and we have noted a month on month increase in patients for over a year.

It will be a while before Isaac leaves the hospital. His condition is serious and unfortunately, although his spine will not become any worse, he will not recover completely. However, when he first arrived he was too weak to stand and so to see him walking gives everyone hope. Doubtless, like the country itself, he has many problems ahead of him. There are no schools, very few hospitals and many of the charities and agencies that would usually be willing to help improve the situation are absent due to the high level of insecurity. Given these factors, the future looks as grim as ever for Somalia but,

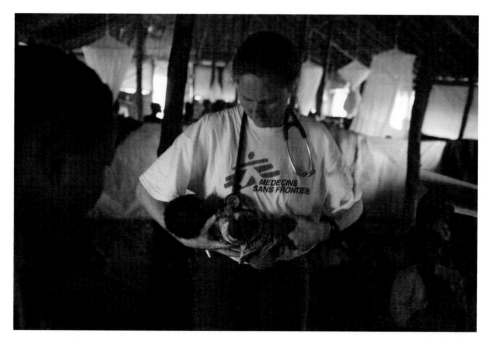

A member of Médecins sans Frontières (Doctors Without Borders) holds an infant at a camp for internally displaced persons in the eastern part of the Ituri province in the Democratic Republic of the Congo in May 2005. Diseases such as cholera and malaria, complicated by malnutrition, have taken millions of lives in the region. *AP Images/Ron Haviv/VII.*

watching Isaac walk, head down against the wind, I feel not pity but hope and admiration for these uniquely brave people.

Jake McKnight

MCKNIGHT, JAKE. *MEDECINS SANS FRONTIERES.* "ISAAC." JUNE 13, 2007. <HTTP://WWW.UK2.MSF.ORG/UKNEWS/LETTERS/ JAKEMCKNIGHTISAAC.HTM> (ACCESSED JUNE 11, 2007).

SEE ALSO *CDC (Centers for Disease Control and Prevention); Developing Nations and Drug Delivery; United Nations Millennium Goals and Infectious Disease; World Health Organization (WHO).*

BIBLIOGRAPHY

Books

Bertolotti, Dan. *Hope in Hell: Inside the World of Doctors Without Borders.* Tonawanda, NY: Firefly Books, 2004.

Médecins Sans Frontières, eds. *In the Shadow of Just Wars: Violence, Politics, and Humanitarian Action.* Translated by Fabrice Weissman and Doctors Without Borders. Ithaca, NY: Cornell University Press, 2004.

Web Sites

Campaign for Access to Essential Medecines. "Companies Not Selling New AIDS Drugs in Africa." <http:// www.accessmed-msf.org/index.asp> (accessed May 15, 2007).

Médecins Sans Frontières/Doctors Without Borders. "About Us." <http://www.doctorswithoutborders.org/ aboutus/index.cfm> (accessed May 15, 2007).

Network for Good. "Doctors Without Borders USA." <http://partners.guidestar.org/controller/search Results.gs?action_gsReport=1&partner=network forgood&ein=13-3433452> (accessed May 20, 2007).

Nobelprize.org. "The Nobel Peace Prize 1999: Médecins Sans Frontières." <http://nobelprize.org/peace/ laureates/1999/index.html> (accessed May 20, 2007).

Paul Davies

Meningitis, Bacterial

■ Introduction

Bacterial meningitis refers to an acute disease caused by several different types of bacteria, in which a membrane called the meninges, which surrounds the brain and the spinal cord, becomes inflamed. Inflammation-related swelling of the membrane can cause serious problems that include septicemia (blood poisoning) brain damage, coma, and death.

A child suffering from bacterial meningitis recovers at a hospital in New Delhi, India, in 2005. The strain of bacterial meningitis killed 14 people in the Indian capital and affected more than 90 others. © Kamal Kishore/Reuters/Corbis.

Bacterial meningitis is the result of a bacterial infection of the blood that spreads to the cerebrospinal fluid, which is the fluid that flows around the meninges. The illness is serious; if not treated, the death rate is high. Those who survive can be left with life-long disabilities that includes impaired hearing due to damage to the hair cells in a portion of the ear that are responsible for converting sound waves to the electrical signals that the brain can interpret. Longer-term problems also include paralysis, mental dysfunction, and paralysis.

■ Disease History, Characteristics, and Transmission

Like other bacterial diseases such as plague and anthrax, bacterial meningitis has likely been occurring for thousands of years. Comparison of the genetic material of the bacteria that cause meningitis with other bacteria—an approach that can indicate whether the bacteria have existed for a long time or have appeared relatively recently—indicates that bacterial meningitis is ancient in its origin. Documented descriptions of the disease date back to 1805, when an outbreak was described in Geneva, Switzerland. In that century, meningitis also decimated the ruling family in Japan.

Bacterial meningitis can be caused by a number of different strains of bacteria. The bacteria that are the most common causes are *Neisseria meningitidis* (also known as meningococcus), *Streptococcus pneumoniae* (also known as pneumococcus), and *Listeria monocytogenes*. Less commonly, *Pseudomonas aeruginosa*, *Staphylococcus aureus*, *Streptococcus agalactiae*, and *Haemophilus influenzae* type b (also known as Hib) can cause meningitis. As well, *Mycobacterium tuberculosis* can be a problem in developing countries.

The less common bacteria are often not a health concern. But, in someone whose immune system is inefficiently functioning due to age, illness, or deliberate immunosuppression (as occurs following organ transplantation to avoid

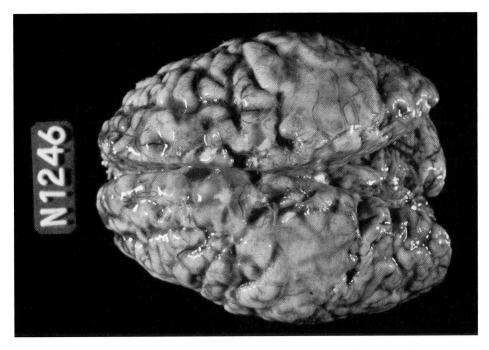

This specimen of a brain shows bacterial meningitis, an infection of the tissues lining the brain.   *CNRI/Photo Researchers, Inc.*

rejection of the transplant) the bacteria are capable of causing meningitis infection.

The source of the infection is sometimes never determined. It is known that bacteria can spread from an ear infection to the meninges. The most common source is the spread of bacteria into the bloodstream from an infection in the heart (endocarditis). In endocarditis, the infecting bacteria can adhere to tissues and produce a colony of bacteria that is enclosed in a slimelike overlay. The organized structure, which is called a biofilm, can then slough off bacteria into the bloodstream.

Infection of the meninges by bacteria usually produces a fever, headache, sensitivity to light, and mental disorientation. As well, when the spinal cord is involved, a person can experience pain in the neck and the legs that becomes progressively worse. These symptoms also occur in the type of meningitis that is caused by viruses. Distinction between the two types of meningitis usually requires obtaining the bacteria from the cerebrospinal fluid. The bacteria are detected when the cerebrospinal fluid is added to a culture, source of nutrients that the bacteria can use. With time, the bacteria grow and divide repeatedly to form a visible mound of cells called a colony.

Bacteria can also be detected by a staining procedure called the Gram stain. Depending on which of two stains the bacteria retain, they can be distinguished as Gram-positive (these bacteria have a single membrane) or Gram-negative (which have two membranes). This distinction is important for determining the most effective antibiotic to use. *Streptococcus pneumoniae* is an example of a Gram-positive bacterium that can cause meningitis. *Neisseria meningitidis* is an example of a Gram-negative bacterium that is a cause of meningitis.

In the meningitis due to *Neisseria meningitidis*, the first symptoms to appear is often a rash that appears as small reddish or purple spots. The rash can spread quickly over the middle part of the body, legs, the conjunctiva in the eyes, and parts of the hands and feet.

■ Scope and Distribution

Bacterial meningitis occurs all over the world. In areas such as Sub-Saharan Africa, the disease is especially prevalent.

The main reason for the global distribution of bacterial meningitis is the equally wide distribution of the bacteria. Some of the bacteria capable of causing meningitis are normally found in the mouth. These can be spread from person to person by coughing or kissing.

In developed countries including the United States, meningitis is rare and occurs as isolated cases. More widespread epidemics still do occur in other parts of the world, in particular northern Africa.

■ Treatment and Prevention

Bacterial meningitis is treated with antibiotics. The choice of the antibiotic depends on the bacterium that is causing the infection. But, when first treating an infection that is suspected of being meningitis, several

WORDS TO KNOW

BIOFILM: Biofilms are populations of microorganisms that form following the adhesion of bacteria, algae, yeast, or fungi to a surface. These surface growths can be found in natural settings such as on rocks in streams, and in infections such as can occur on catheters. Microorganisms can colonize living and inert natural and synthetic surfaces.

MENINGITIS BELT: The Meningitis Belt is an area of Africa south of the Sahara Desert, stretching from the Atlantic to the Pacific coast, where meningococcal meningitis is common.

SEPTICEMIA: Prolonged fever, chills, anorexia, and anemia in conjunction with tissue lesions.

STRAIN: A subclass or a specific genetic variation of an organism.

ASEPTIC AND BACTERIAL MENINGITIS

The meninges are a series of three membranes covering the brain and spinal cord that act to protect and partition the central nervous system (CNS). The membranes comprising the meninges are the dura mater, arachnoid layer, and the pia mater.

Meningitis is an inflammation of the *meninges*—the three layers of protective membranes that line the spinal cord and the brain. Meningitis can occur when there is an infection near the brain or spinal cord, such as a respiratory infection in the sinuses, the mastoids, or the cavities around the ear. Disease organisms can also travel to the meninges through the bloodstream. The first signs may be a severe headache and neck stiffness followed by fever, vomiting, a rash, and, then, convulsions leading to loss of consciousness.

Meningitis generally involves two types: non-bacterial meningitis, which is often called aseptic meningitis, and bacterial meningitis, which is referred to as purulent meningitis.

antibiotics that are effective against the widest variety of bacteria are often used even before the cause of the infection has been identified. This is done because rapid treatment is important to minimizing the danger of the infection. Once the cause of the infection has been determined, the antibiotic therapy can be adjusted to specifically target the particular bacterium.

Antibiotics are usually given intravenously—they are added directly into a vein, where they circulate in the bloodstream. This produces a high level of the antibiotic throughout the body and, because the antibiotic can be continuously supplied, the dose can stay constant during the several weeks of treatment that is usually required.

Vaccines directed towards *Neisseria* and *Haemophilus* have lessened childhood meningitis dramatically. Two *Neisseria meningitidis* vaccines are available in the United States. One has been available since the early 1980s, while the other was approved only in 2005. As well, both newborns and the elderly benefit from vaccines against *Streptococcus pneumoniae*. The American Association of Pediatrics recommends vaccinating newborns against penumococcal meningitis as early as six weeks after birth and the U.S. Centers for Disease Control and Prevention recommends vaccination for everyone over the age of 65.

■ Impacts and Issues

Bacterial meningitis continues to be a great health concern, especially in some under-developed regions of the world. In areas of Sub-Saharan Africa known as the meningitis belt, epidemics of meningitis continue to kill many people. In 1996, more than 250,000 contracted meningitis during one epidemic, and about 25,000 people died of the disease. While outbreaks that large are not common, the occurrence of the disease is a frequent occurrence in some areas of their world.

This continued threat posed by bacterial meningitis is one of the health concerns being addressed by the World Health Organization as part of the Consolidated Appeals Process, which seeks to galvanize support from countries around the globe to assist in aiding under-developed regions.

In both under-developed and developed countries, the disease is a serious health concern for infants less than a year old; the high fever that can be produced can cause seizures. Because bacterial meningitis is contagious, infants in day care facilities are at increased risk for the disease.

Despite the ongoing problem of bacterial meningitis, the introduction of vaccines has greatly reduced the prevalence of the infection. Before a vaccine to *Haemophilus influenzae* type b was introduced in the 1990s, meningitis due to Hib was the leading cause of bacterial meningitis. Now, because of the routine immunization of schoolchildren with a *Haemophilus* vaccine, Hib meningitis is rare.

For survivors of a bacterial meningitis infection, hearing loss can be a consequence. Artificial implants in an area of the ear called the cochlea can sometimes restore hearing to a level that allows normal function. But, the implant must be installed within weeks of the end of an infection to be fully effective. This is because the fluid that has accumulated in the ear changes consistency over time and becomes almost jellylike, making installation of an implant impossible.

SEE ALSO *Bacterial Disease; Childhood Infectious Diseases, Immunization Impacts; Meningitis, Viral.*

BIBLIOGRAPHY

Books

Ferreiros, C. *Emerging Strategies in the Fight Against Meningitis.* Oxford: Garland Science, 2002.

Lax, Alister. *Toxin: The Cunning of Bacterial Poisons.* Oxford: Oxford University Press, 2005.

Periodicals

Wilson-Clark, Samantha D., S. Squires, S. Deeksi "Bacterial Meningitis among Cochlear Implant Recipients—Canada 2002." *Morbidity and Mortality Weekly.* 55: S20-S25 (2006).

Web Sites

Centers for Disease Control and Prevention. "Meningococcal Disease" <http://www.cdc.gov/ncidod/dbmd/diseaseinfo/meningococcal_g.htm> (accessed May 25, 2007).

World health Organization. "Meningitis in Africa: Hundreds of Thousands Vaccinated." <http://www.who.int/mediacentre/news/notes/2007/np12/en/index.html> (accessed May 25, 2007).

Brian Hoyle

Meningitis, Viral

■ Introduction

There are two types of meningitis—an inflammation of the meninges which are the tissues covering the brain and spinal cord. Bacterial meningitis, such as meningiococcal meningitis, is a bacterial infection. Aseptic meningitis is caused by viral, fungal, or other infection. Aseptic meningitis also may have a noninfectious cause such as an underlying illness. Some types of aseptic meningitis respond to antibiotic treatment, but viral meningitis does not. Aseptic meningitis causes between 25,000 and 50,000 hospital admissions per year in the United States alone.

The symptoms of meningitis vary, but severe headache, neck stiffness, and an aversion of light are common. Accurate diagnosis of the cause of meningitis, through examination of the cerebrospinal fluid, is important because treatment for bacterial meningitis needs to begin as soon as possible. Viral meningitis is rarely fatal, but may occasionally cause permanent disability.

■ Disease History, Characteristics, and Transmission

More than 80% of cases of aseptic meningitis are caused by viruses. Many different viruses are implicated, including: enteroviruses, mumps, herpes, HIV, and viruses borne by mosquitoes and ticks, otherwise known as arboviruses. The enteroviruses account for around 90% of cases of viral meningitis. These viruses live in the human intestine. They rarely cause meningitis, but are a common cause of colds, sore throats, stomach upsets, and diarrhea. Until the introduction of the MMR (measles, mumps, and rubella) vaccine, the mumps virus was the most common cause of viral meningitis among children under five years of age.

Although viral meningitis is usually considered to be a mild illness, it often requires physician care or hospitalization for treatment. Some symptoms of viral meningitis are caused by pressure on the brain from inflamed meninges (membranes that envelop the nervous system) and include a severe headache and stiffness of the neck. A high fever and photophobia—an aversion to light—are also common side effects of enterovirus-associated meningitis. Patients may have a strong desire to be in a quiet, dark room.

Many people with viral meningitis experience non-specific symptoms such as vomiting, cough, diarrhea, loss of appetite, and rash. Many such cases are mistaken as influenza (flu). Where symptoms are severe, bacterial meningitis might be suspected and immediate hospital admission is appropriate. Occasionally, the virus affects the brain itself causing encephalitis, an inflammation that can lead to lasting brain damage.

The symptoms of viral meningitis have a rapid onset, usually within three to ten days after exposure. Other causes of aseptic meningitis may produce disease following a slower course. In the early stages, it can be hard to distinguish aseptic and bacterial meningitis. One clue is that the person with aseptic meningitis usually remains alert. Confusion and disorientation may occur with bacterial meningitis, along with neurological abnormalities such as deafness or visual disturbances—such symptoms are uncommon in viral meningitis.

It is more difficult to identify the symptoms of viral meningitis in infants. Fever, fretfulness and irritability, difficulty in waking up, or refusal to eat may be noted.

Anyone with possible meningitis symptoms should seek prompt medical attention. Though viral meningitis is generally less severe, early symptoms of viral and bacterial meningitis may be difficult to distinguish without medical testing. Bacterial meningitis requires antibiotic treatment and can cause permanent disability or death if left to untreated. Diagnosis involves an examination of the cerebrospinal fluid (CSF), the watery fluid that bathes and protects the brain and spinal cord. A sample of CSF is removed from around the spinal cord in a procedure called lumbar puncture. Bacteria can usually be cultured from this in cases of bacterial meningitis.

Most people make a full recovery from viral meningitis, with no lasting effects. Sometimes recovery is slow, with patients experiencing headache, tiredness, fatigue, depression, and loss of concentration for many months.

Transmission of meningitis depends upon the underlying viral cause. Enteroviruses, the most common cause, are spread through direct contact with the saliva, mucus, or nasal mucous of an infected person. Exposure to their coughs and sneezes, shaking hands, or touching something they have handled can cause infection if one then touches their nose or mouth. However, this kind of person-to-person transmission is unusual.

Enteroviruses are also shed into the feces of people who are infected. Children who are not yet toilet-trained may spread the virus in this way. Adults changing the diaper of an infected infant may therefore be at risk. The infectious period lasts from about three days after a person has been infected until ten days after they develop the symptoms of viral meningitis.

■ Scope and Distribution

Viral meningitis is far more common than bacterial meningitis. It is found mainly among babies, children, and adolescents. There are an estimated 300,000 cases per year in the United States, with 25,000–50,000 hospital admissions. Because many mild cases are not reported to the physician, the true number of cases is unknown. Moreover, as the main purpose of hospital investigations is to rule out bacterial meningitis, the specific virus involved in an aseptic case is often not detected.

There are seasonal variations in viral meningitis, depending upon the virus involved. Viruses borne by arthropods, such as mosquitoes and ticks, cause disease most often in late summer and early fall. Enteroviruses follow a similar seasonal pattern. Mumps virus tends to cause meningitis most often in late winter and early spring while herpes meningitis does not have a seasonal pattern.

■ Treatment and Prevention

There is no general anti-viral treatment for viral meningitis, although the anti-viral drug aciclovir might be used if the cause is found to be herpes simplex. Accurate diagnosis is needed to be sure the cause really is viral. Bacterial meningitis and some types of aseptic meningitis respond to antibiotic therapy. Sometimes antibiotics will be started straight away if someone is admitted to hospital with any form of meningitis, but these will be discontinued if the cause is found to be viral. Bed rest, fluids, and medication to relieve pain and fever are the best approach to alleviating the symptoms associated with viral meningitis.

It is difficult to prescribe a specific way of preventing viral meningitis, because there are so many different

WORDS TO KNOW

ARBOVIRUS: An arbovirus is a virus that is typically spread by blood-sucking insects, most commonly mosquitoes. Over 100 types of arboviruses cause disease in humans. Yellow fever and dengue are two examples.

ARTHROPOD: A member of the largest single animal phylum, consisting of organisms with segmented bodies, jointed legs or wings, and exoskeletons.

ENTEROVIRUS: Enteroviruses are a group of viruses that contain ribonucleic acid as their genetic material. They are members of the picornavirus family. The various types of enteroviruses that infect humans are referred to as serotypes, in recognition of their different antigenic patterns. The different immune response is important, as infection with one type of enterovirus does not necessarily confer protection to infection by a different type of enterovirus. There are 64 different enterovirus serotypes. The serotypes include polio viruses, coxsackie A and B viruses, echoviruses and a large number of what are referred to as non-polio enteroviruses.

MENINGITIS: Meningitis is an inflammation of the meninges—the three layers of protective membranes that line the spinal cord and the brain. Meningitis can occur when there is an infection near the brain or spinal cord, such as a respiratory infection in the sinuses, the mastoids, or the cavities around the ear. Disease organisms can also travel to the meninges through the bloodstream. The first signs may be a severe headache and neck stiffness followed by fever, vomiting, a rash, and, then, convulsions leading to loss of consciousness. Meningitis generally involves two types: nonbacterial meningitis, which is often called aseptic meningitis, and bacterial meningitis, which is referred to as purulent meningitis.

causes of the disease. The MMR vaccine will prevent meningitis caused by the measles and mumps virus. Since the majority of cases are caused by enteroviruses, which are spread by infected saliva and other bodily secretions, good personal hygiene stems transmission. Regular and thorough handwashing can stop enteroviruses from spreading. Potentially contaminated surfaces should be cleaned down with soap and water or diluted bleach. These precautions are especially important in institutions such as child care centers, schools, public bathing facilities, and dormitories.

■ Impacts and Issues

Viral meningitis is a serious condition. Though viral meningitis may alleviate without treatment, all people who suspect that they have meningitis should seek medical care. Viral meningitis rarely has serious long-term health consequences in otherwise healthy individuals. Bacterial meningitis, however, can be life-threatening. Since early symptoms of viral and bacterial meningitis are similar, prompt and accurate diagnosis is necessary to distinguish between the two forms of meningitis.

In August 2006, an outbreak of viral meningitis was reported from the region of Khabarovsk, on the Russian Far East border, affecting over 800 children. It is thought they contracted the infection through either swimming in the river Amur or from drinking its waters. There have been ongoing summer outbreaks of viral meningitis in this area for some time, arising usually from fecal contamination of the Amur's waters. Swim-

ming is therefore prohibited in the summer months. During the 2006 outbreaks, public health doctors tried to stem the outbreak by asking parents to keep their children away from social activities, as the meningitis could be spread by infected air droplets.

BIBLIOGRAPHY

Books

Tan, J. *Expert Guide to Infectious Diseases.* Philadelphia: American College of Physicians, 2002.

Wilks, D., M. Farrington, and D. Rubenstein. *The Infectious Diseases Manual* 2nd ed. Malden: Blackwell, 2003.

Web Sites

Centers for Disease Control and Prevention (CDC). "Viral ('Aseptic') Meningitis." Sep 5, 2006 <http://www.cdc.gov/ncidod/dvrd/enterovirus/viral_meningitis.htm> (accessed May 3, 2007).

The Meningitis Trust. "Viral Meningitis The Facts." <http://www.meningitis-trust.org/disease_info/Viral-Meningitis.pdf> (accessed May 3, 2007).

Susan Aldridge

Microbial Evolution

Introduction

Microbial evolution refers to the genetically driven changes that occur in microorganisms and that are retained over time. Some microbial changes can be in response to a selective pressure. The best examples of this are the various changes that can occur in bacteria in response to the presence of antibiotics. These changes can make an individual bacterium less susceptible or completely resistant to the killing action of one or more antibiotics.

Other microbial changes can occur randomly in the absence of any selective pressure. These changes, which often are due to a change in the sequence of the units (nucleotides) that comprise an organism's genetic material, can confer an advantage to the organism, as compared to unaltered organisms. In the classic scenario of evolution, such as advantageous trait will be retained and can be passed on to future generations of the organism.

Gene transfer between bacteria can occur even between species that are not related to one another. This so-called horizontal gene transfer is an important form of microbial evolution that occurs in nature, and it can be important in infectious disease, for example in the acquisition of a gene that determines antibiotic resistance.

In contrast to Darwinian evolution, which takes place over millions of years, microbial evolution can occur within hours. This is because some bacteria are capable of growing and dividing in about 20 minutes under ideal growth conditions. A bacterium containing an altered gene that confers a survival advantage can, over 24 hours, give rise to thousands of progeny that carry the same gene. Each new bacterium can in turn give rise to thousands of progeny by the next day. Thus, a mutation can rapidly spread in a bacterial population and, because the trait is capable of being transferred to unrelated bacteria, to other bacterial populations as well.

Human-imposed selective pressures, such as the overuse or misuse of antibiotics, factory-farm types of agriculture that crowd animals in a small space, and the encroachment of humans on previously undisturbed territory are influencing microbial evolution and the emergence or re-emergence of infectious diseases.

History and Scientific Foundations

Darwinian evolution can be depicted as a tree, with the original organism at the base of the trunk and the myriad evolutionary changes that occur over time generating the branches and even smaller twigs at their tips. Put another way, this route of evolution is vertical, with genetic changes transferred from one generation of a species to succeeding generations.

In contrast, evidence that has been accumulating since the 1970s has firmly established that microbial evolution occurs differently. The tree analogy is inaccurate when describing microbial evolution. Rather, microbial evolution is considered to be more like a web or a net, with the transfer of genetic information occurring between many different species simultaneously, rather than between succeeding generations of one particular type of microbe.

This wider, interspecies transfer is called horizontal transfer. It is one route by which a bacterium can become resistant to one or more antibiotics. A bacterium that carries the genetic determinants for resistance to an antibiotic may be able to transfer the gene to another, unrelated bacterium, which then also becomes resistant to the antibiotic.

The transfer of genes between bacteria can occur in several ways. A gene that resides in the deoxyribonucleic acid (DNA) of a donor bacterium can be transferred to the recipient bacterium through a tube that transiently connects the two cells. Once inside the recipient, the inserted DNA can become part of the recipient's genome (its hereditary information encoded in its DNA) and express its encoded product.

Bacterial genes can also reside on more mobile genetic elements known as plasmids. Plasmids are more

WORDS TO KNOW

ANTIBIOTIC RESISTANCE: The ability of bacteria to resist the actions of antibiotic drugs.

BACTERIOPHAGE: A virus that infects bacteria. When a bacteriophage that carries the diphtheria toxin gene infects diphtheria bacteria, the bacteria produce diphtheria toxin.

HORIZONTAL GENE TRANSFER: Horizontal gene transfer is a major mechanism by which antibiotic resistance genes get passed between bacteria and accounts for many hospital-acquired infections.

MUTATION: A mutation is a change in an organism's DNA that occurs over time and may render it less sensitive to drugs which are used against it.

PLASMID: A circular piece of DNA that exists outside of the bacterial chromosome and copies itself independently. Scientists often use bacterial plasmids in genetic engineering to carry genes into other organisms.

SELECTIVE PRESSURE: Selective pressure refers to the tendency of an organism that has a certain characteristic to be eliminated from an environment or to increase in numbers. An example is the increased prevalence of bacteria that are resistant to multiple kinds of antibiotics.

bacterial host. If the new gene confers an advantage to the second bacterium, it will be retained and passed on to subsequent generations of that bacterium.

The processes described above are directed in the sense that a genetic trait that changes an organism is transferred from one organism to another. In contrast, a final mechanism of microbial evolution—mutation—can occur randomly. A change in the arrangement of nucleotides that makes up a gene can occur by chance during the replication of the DNA. For example, one nucleotide can be substituted for another. Alternatively, additional nucleotides may be accidentally inserted or may be deleted. If the genetic change is not drastic enough to completely disable the gene's action, then the protein produced will be different. Sometimes this difference can be advantageous to the microbe. For example, the altered protein may produce enhanced activity of an enzyme that degrades antibiotics, or it may produce a membrane protein that adopts a different three-dimensional configuration that makes the microbial surface more resistant to antimicrobial compounds. Once again, such an advantageous mutation will be retained and can be passed to subsequent generations.

■ Applications and Research

The ability of bacteria to evolve via horizontal gene transfer has been exploited in genetic engineering that involves the deliberate insertion of a certain gene into a recipient bacterium and the expression of the gene product by the recipient. Indeed, this aspect of biotechnology is essentially a faster version of the natural pace of microbial evolution.

The acquisition of a gene by a microorganism can be tracked. Similar genes can be isolated from various organisms and the sequence of nucleotides that makes up the gene can be deduced. By comparing the gene sequences, researchers can determine how precisely the sequences match. Sequences from different organisms that match exactly provide strong evidence that the gene arose in a single organism and was passed on to another organism. Since changes in a genetic sequence will occur randomly over time, the degree of gene difference can be used as an indication of how recently a gene was acquired by one microbe, relative to another. In this way it is possible to generate a sort of map of the movement of a gene among microbes over a long period of time.

■ Impacts and Issues

The ability of disease-causing microorganisms, particularly bacteria and viruses, to evolve is a fundamentally important factor in infectious diseases. For example, the horizontal acquisition of a gene that encodes for the production of a potent and destructive toxin created *Escherichia coli* O157:H7, which can cause a serious

easily transferable between bacteria. Genes that code for products that render a cell resistant to particular antibiotics can be located on plasmids. If a bacterium that possesses an antibiotic-resistance gene is adjacent to another bacterium (not necessarily the same type of bacterium), a copy of the plasmid can move to the recipient bacterium, which then becomes resistant to the antibiotic(s).

A third genetic mechanism of bacterial evolution involves bacteriophages—viruses that specifically infect a particular type of bacteria (for example, various types of coliphages infect various strains of *Escherichia coli*). When a bacteriophage infects a bacterium, the viral genetic material can insert into the host's genetic material. When the viral material is excised, some of the host's genetic material can be removed as well, to become part of the genome of the bacteriophage. A subsequent infection by the bacteriophage of another bacterium can transfer genes from the first bacterium to the second

and even lethal infection in humans. Without the gene, *E. coli* is a normal and harmless resident of the intestinal tract of warm-blooded creatures, including man. In another example, genetic changes have also spawned a variety of *Mycobacterium tuberculosis* that is resistant to all antibacterial agents currently used to treat tuberculosis. The fact that the bacterium is also easily passed from person-to-person is a cause for concern.

The emergence of avian influenza (caused by an influenza virus designated H5N1) is one example of how human agricultural practices can influence microbial evolution. The tremendous crowding together of poultry that is done to optimize the income generated by a poultry farm made it easier for viral disease to spread in a flock. Then, the ability of many viruses to rapidly mutate allowed the avian influenza virus to spread, first, from bird-to-human and now from human-to-human. While the latter is still rare, the number of cases of human-transmitted H5N1 infection is growing and the geographical range is expanding. The possibility that this serious and sometimes fatal disease will develop into a global epidemic is real and has spurred efforts by agencies, including the World Health Organization (WHO) and the U.S. Centers for Disease Control and Prevention (CDC), to monitor the disease and participate in efforts to develop a vaccine.

The fact that microbial evolution can be manipulated in the laboratory has implications for bioterrorism. In the aftermath of World War II (1939–1945), a number of countries, including the United States, engaged in research aimed at designing more potently infectious bacterial and viral diseases. While this research was discontinued, the advent of molecular biology in the 1970s has created legitimate fears that rogue nations or organizations could design and deploy a deadly version of a contagious microorganism.

■ Primary Source Connection

Harvey B. Simon is a physician and an associate professor of medicine at Harvard Medical School. He also serves as a consultant in infectious disease at Massachusetts General Hospital in Boston, Massachusetts. In this article appearing in *Newsweek* magazine in December 2006, Simon discusses the evolution of some increasingly troublesome microorganisms.

Old Bugs Learn Some Noew Tricks; As more drugs are created to fight infection, bacteria mutate and strike in another form

When antibiotics arrived 60 years ago, many experts thought it was the beginning of the end for infectious diseases. Sadly, they were wrong. Infections caused by viruses, fungi and other assorted critters never respond

to antibiotics. As special drugs are developed for some of them, new foes such as bird flu crop up. And even bacteria, the true targets of antibiotics, have found ways to beat the rap. In most cases they change their genes to thwart antibiotics. Smart scientists fight back by creating new drugs—but, more often than not, the bugs find a way to give them the slip.

To see how it works—and what we can do about it—consider three important bugs that have recently found new ways to make us sick. The first is staph aureus, which has been part of the human condition since the beginning of recorded history. The bacterium's natural habitat is the human nose; at any one time, at least 25 percent of us harbor the germ. In most, it's a harmless fellow traveler, but it often travels from nose to hand to skin, where it causes pesky boils and infects "ingrown" hairs and nails. In an unlucky few, staph causes devastating infections of the blood and organs. These were highly lethal until penicillin came along. The drug was dramatically effective, but the bug rapidly changed its genes to produce penicillinase, an enzyme that chews up the antibiotic. Penicillin-resistant strains appeared first in hospitals, then spread to the community. By now, 95 percent of staph shrug off penicillin.

In response to the growing problem, researchers developed penicillinase-proof antibiotics. The first, in 1959, was methicillin, and a family of related drugs soon followed. But by 1960, methicillin-resistant staph aureus (MRSA) began to crop up in hospitals; by now it constitutes the majority of strains in some hospitals and has also exploded in the community.

Hospitals try to contain the spread of MRSA by handling infected patients with latex gloves and other precautions. At home, we should stress handwashing with soap and water as well as alcohol-based rubs. So far, community strains of MRSA are reassuringly susceptible to certain older oral antibiotics, but major infections should be treated with the same injected drugs used for hospital patients.

Compared with staph, *Clostridium difficile* (C. diff) is a newcomer. It was first diagnosed in 1978, when it appeared as an occasional cause of diarrhea in patients who were taking a particular antibiotic (clindamycin). By now, though, it is clear that virtually any antibiotic can trigger the problem. *C. diff* strikes at least 300,000 people in the United States each year, even some who haven't taken antibiotics. Many healthy people harbor a few *C. diff* among the millions of bacteria in the colon. When *C. diff* hangs out in the form of inert spores, it's harmless. But if antibiotic therapy knocks off the normal bacteria, *C. diff* springs to life, producing two toxins that attack the colon. Doctors can treat most cases by stopping the offending drug and prescribing metronidazole or vancomycin, oral antibiotics that target *C. diff*. But spore forms of the bug defy even these drugs, and diarrhea often recurs when treatment stops.

The next threat is a novel, highly virulent strain of *C. diff* that produces 16 to 23 times more toxin than its predecessors. Because the bug is so new, doctors have not yet determined if revised treatment guidelines are warranted. This new and dangerous form of *C. diff* makes it even more urgent that people with diarrhea, or people caring for people with diarrhea, scrupulously wash their hands with soap and water after any possible contact with the infected material to avoid spreading the germ or becoming infected themselves.

Finally, there's tuberculosis—a historic scourge of humankind. Even now, it is the leading infectious cause of death in the world, accounting for more than 2 million deaths a year. We've been much luckier in this country. As a result of improved social and economic conditions, the incidence of TB began to decline around 1900 and nearly disappeared with the discovery of anti-TB drugs in mid-century. But in 1984, an alarming upturn developed. It was fueled by HIV and homelessness, and it featured a rise in multidrug-resistant (MDR) TB. Ordinary TB can be cured by six months of combination therapy. But MDR strains defy the standard drugs.

In this country, TB plateaued in 1992 and has declined steadily since because of aggressive diagnosis and strict isolation of cases. Still, there's no room for complacency. In 2006, doctors in South Africa identified a new, extensively drug-resistant (XDR) strain of TB. So far it has been confined to AIDS patients in South Africa, but it's a small world, and infections respect no borders. We need new drugs for TB. But we also need to use the resources that we already have to deliver medical care to the developing world. If we fight the war against TB on that turf, we may not have to fight it on our own turf.

Harvey B. Simon

SIMON, HARVEY B. "OLD BUGS LEARN SOME NEW TRICKS; AS MORE DRUGS ARE CREATED TO FIGHT INFECTION, BACTERIA MUTATE AND STRIKE IN ANOTHER FORM." *NEWSWEEK* (DEC 11, 2006): 74.

SEE ALSO *Antibiotic Resistance; Emerging Infectious Diseases.*

BIBLIOGRAPHY

Books

Ewald, Paul. *Plague Time: The New Germ Theory of Disease.* New York: Anchor, 2002.

Schopf, J. William. *Life's Origin: The Beginnings of Biological Evolution.* Berkeley: University of California Press, 2002.

Seifert, H. Steven, and Victor J. Dirta, eds. *Evolution of Microbial Pathogens.* Washington, DC: ASM Press, 2006.

Brian Hoyle

Microorganisms

■ Introduction

Microorganisms are life forms that are too small to be seen with the naked eye, but that play an important role in human health and disease. The main types of microorganisms are bacteria, fungi, protozoa, and viruses. The first three are single-celled organisms, of which only bacteria have a nucleus. Viruses, however, need to be inside a host cell in order to survive.

Microbes occupy a wide range of ecological niches. Some live inside the human intestine or on the skin, others are found in soil, on the ocean floor, or even in the Arctic ice cap. Microbes have potential for both benefit and harm. They help keep the digestive system healthy and play an important role in decomposing dead plants and animals. However, microbes also cause a wide range of diseases, from colds and flu, to tuberculosis, AIDS, and cholera.

■ History and Scientific Foundations

The first microbes were observed by the Dutch biologist Anton van Leeuwenhoek (1632–1723) in 1674 using a primitive microscope he had invented. He observed what he called "animalcules" of all shapes and sizes in samples from many sources. The origin and function of these life forms was widely discussed over the next two centuries, but it was not until the nineteenth century that the scientific foundations of microbiology were laid down by Louis Pasteur (1822–1895) and Robert Koch (1843–1910).

Pasteur's work in the 1870s and 1880s showed that putrefaction depended upon the action of microbes. He went on to develop pasteurization, a technique of gentle heating that stops food and drink from spoiling by decreasing their levels of microbial contamination. Meanwhile, Koch isolated the anthrax bacillus in 1876 and the tuberculosis bacillus in 1882. By the end of the century, the microbes responsible for plague, meningitis, gonorrhea, typhoid, tetanus, diphtheria, dysentery, and pneumonia had been discovered and characterized.

Koch pushed forward the germ theory of disease, which rested on his four postulates. First, the responsible microorganism had to be isolated from infected animals, and then cultivated and identified in the laboratory. Finally, on re-injection to other lab animals, the disease had to be reproduced.

Microbes are classified according to the hierarchical system adopted for plants and animals, with related species being grouped together in the same genus. For example, *Staphylococcus aureus* and *Staphylococcus epidermidis* are two species belonging to the *Staphylococcus* genus. This name comes from the Greek word "staphyl," meaning bunch of grapes and "coccus," which means grain or berry, and refers to the appearance of the bacteria under the microscope.

Bacteria are single-celled organisms of average length two micrometers and average diameter of 0.5 micrometers. They occur in a range of characteristic shapes from which their names are sometimes derived—for instance, rods (bacilli), spheres or ovals (cocci), and spirals (spirochaetes). Bacteria do not have a nucleus and their genetic material (DNA) lies free in the cell or on tiny circular structures called plasmids. They cause a range of infections, including sore throats, pneumonia, and food poisoning.

Fungi and protozoa have a cell structure that is more like that of a human cell, with a nucleus carrying their DNA. Protozoa are single-celled microbes, including algae and trypanosomes, which often have complex lifecycles and interactions with their human hosts. They cause some serious tropical diseases, including malaria. The fungi group includes yeasts, molds and mushrooms. They play an important part in decomposing biological material, such as dead plants, and in the food and drink industry. Some fungi cause diseases of the skin and hair, such as athelete's foot. Fungal infections can also cause health problems in people with reduced immunity, such as those with HIV/AIDS.

Viruses were first discovered in the late 1880s when it was realized that some disease agents could pass through filters that would usually hold back the smallest bacteria. These filtrates were implicated in diseases such as yellow fever and foot and mouth disease (a disease of

COLONIZATION: Colonization is the process of occupation and increase in number of microorganisms at a specific site.

ERADICATION: The process of destroying or eliminating a microorganism or disease.

PATHOGEN: A disease causing agent, such as a bacteria, virus, fungus, etc.

RESISTANT ORGANISM: Resistant organisms are bacteria, viruses, parasites, or other disease-causing agents that have stopped responding to drugs that once killed them.

animals). Unlike other microbes, viruses need a living cell in which to replicate themselves. Without a host, they die. Viruses are responsible for a range of human diseases, including hepatitis, AIDS, colds, influenza and some forms of pneumonia and meningitis.

Applications and Research

Understanding microbiology leads to a better appreciation of many diseases, which can allow for more accurate diagnosis and effective treatment. Sometimes one microorganism can cause many different diseases, such as *S. aureus* which causes strep throat, scarlet fever, and toxic shock syndrome. On the other hand, one disease can often be caused by many different microorganism. For instance, pneumonia can be caused by adenovirus, respiratory syncytial virus, influenza virus, parainfluenza virus, and cytomegalovirus. Among the bacteria that can cause pneumonia are *Streptococcus pneumoniae*, *Chlamydia pneumoniae*, *Haemophilus influenzae*, *Klebsiella pneumoniae* and *Pseudomonas aeruginosa*. The disease can also be caused by mycoplasma, which are organisms that have some of the characteristics of both bacteria and viruses.

Most microorganisms are actually harmless to human health. Pathogens—microbes that cause disease—are of two kinds, strict pathogens and opportunistic pathogens. A strict pathogen is always associated with disease; these include *Mycobacterium tuberculosis*, which causes tuberculosis (TB), and rabies virus. However, most human infections are caused by opportunistic pathogens, which colonize, or normally live on the skin or in the nose or mouth, or in the surroundings without causing any problems. However, if they enter unprotected sites like the blood, they may cause disease. Among the most common of the opportunistic pathogens are *Pneumocystis carinii*,

Candida albicans, and cytomegalovirus, which often cause complications among those with HIV/AIDS.

Impacts and Issues

Infectious diseases including HIV/AIDS, malaria, and tuberculosis, continue to claim millions of lives each year. There are also emerging infections such as SARS and bird flu, which have the potential to cause pandemics. However, science has shown that infections can be defeated—smallpox has been eradicated and polio and measles could be eradicated in the near future.

Antibiotics—which are active against bacteria, fungi, but not viruses—have been the major weapon against infection. Starting with the introduction of penicillin in the 1940s, doctors now have a wide range of drugs against infections like TB. Anti-viral drugs are also making AIDS a chronic disease rather than a death sentence. However, microorganisms are developing resistance against these chemical weapons so it is vital that scientists continue to extend their understanding of microbial physiology so that new drugs against infection can be developed.

Vaccines are the other major tool against microbial disease. They generally contain either a killed or weakened version of the microbe or a part of the organism, such as a protein borne on its surface, which can elicit an immune response. There is an urgent need for the development of vaccines against malaria, AIDS, and hepatitis C.

A new and more detailed level of understanding of microbiology may come from genetics. The genomes of several medically significant microbes have now been solved. Their genes have been recorded and will now, hopefully, be identified. These include *Hemophilus influenzae*, which can cause meningitis or pneumonia, *Nesseria meningitidis*, another meningitis organism, and *Streptococcus pneumoniae* which causes meningitis and pneumonia. The genomics approach means a better understanding of how microorganisms cause human illnesses and new opportunities for developing more effective antibiotics, antivirals, and vaccines.

SEE ALSO *Antibiotic Resistance; Germ Theory of Disease; Koch's Postulates; Microbial Evolution; Microscope and Microscopy.*

BIBLIOGRAPHY

Books

Lock, Stephen, Stephen Last, and George Dunea. *The Oxford Illustrated Companion to Medicine.* Oxford: Oxford University Press, 2001.

Murray, Patrick, Ken Rosenthal, and Michael Pfaller. *Medical Microbiology.* 5th ed. Philadelphia: Elsevier, 2005.

Susan Aldridge

Microscope and Microscopy

■ Introduction

The microscope is a powerful tool for investigating the complexity of biological life. This includes looking at the identity and structure of microorganisms, which is essential in the diagnosis of many infectious diseases. Microorganisms are not visible to the human eye, owing to their small size. The light microscope focuses visible light upon a clinical specimen and allow the microbe to be magnified through a series of lenses.

Staining a specimen that may contain microorganisms is an additional aid to identification. Some microbes will absorb a certain stain while others will not, which provides a way of identifying them. Modern microscopic technologies allow for quick and accurate identification of microorganisms involved in human disease. However, microscopic identification alone is only part of the investigations underlying a diagnosis of an infectious disease. The patient's medical history and biochemical tests upon clinical specimens are equally important.

■ History and Scientific Foundations

The magnifying power of lenses—curved pieces of glass that can bend light—was first mentioned in the writings of the Roman philosophers Seneca and Pliny the Elder during the first century AD. But they were not put to practical use until the development of spectacles towards the end of the thirteenth century. The Dutch spectacle makers Zaccharias Janssen and his son Hans began to experiment with the magnifying properties of combinations of lenses in the late sixteenth century. News of their work spread to Galileo who produced a primitive microscope in 1609. But it was Anthony van Leewenhoek (1632–1723), the Dutch biologist, who first realized the potential of the microscope for the study of the world of microorganisms.

Looking at specimens from many different sources, he described the appearance of what he called animalcules—namely, yeast, bacteria, and protozoa. During his life, he wrote over 100 papers on his discoveries for both the Royal Society of England and the French academy. The English scientist Robert Hooke went on to confirm van Leewenhoek's work and improved on the design of his light microscope. Towards the end of the nineteenth century, there were some major advances in microscope manufacture. The American pioneer Charles A. Spencer founded an industry based upon instruments with fine optical systems, which are similar to today's basic light microscopes.

Magnifications of 1,250 are achievable with ordinary white light and up to 5,000 if blue light is used. The microscope is a compound optical system. A condensing lens focuses a bright beam of light upon the clinical specimen, which is placed on a platform called a stage and covered with a thin sheet of glass called a cover slip. The objective lens, near the specimen, forms an intermediate magnified image, which is magnified again by the eyepiece, which is close to the eye.

The magnification of a light microscope is limited by the wavelength of the light used to illuminate the specimen. It cannot distinguish objects that are smaller than half the wavelength of the light. Thus, white light has an average wavelength of around 0.55 micrometers, so any two lines that are closer together than half of this—0.275 micrometers—will shown up as a single line and an object that is smaller than this in diameter will show up as a blur, or not at all. Smaller objects, such as viruses, can only be seen with the aid of the electron microscope, in which the beam of illuminating light is replaced by a beam of electrons. Electron microscopes were invented in the late 1940s and are much more expensive than light microscopes. However, they have allowed not only the study of viruses but also of so called biological ultrastructure, which is the fine details of cells, tissues, and their activities in health and disease.

WORDS TO KNOW

ELECTRON: A fundamental particle of matter carrying a single unit of negative electrical charge.

LENS: An almost clear, biconvex structure in the eye that, along with the cornea, helps to focus light onto the retina. It can become infected with inflammation, for instance, when contact lenses are improperly used.

MICROORGANISM: Microorganisms are minute organisms. With the single yet-known exception of a bacterium that is large enough to be seen unaided, individual microorganisms are microscopic in size. To be seen, they must be magnified by an optical or electron microscope. The most common types of microorganisms are viruses, bacteria, blue-green bacteria, some algae, some fungi, yeasts, and protozoans.

STAINING: Staining refers to the use of chemicals to identify target components of microorganisms.

WAVELENGTH: A distance of one cycle of a wave; for instance, the distance between the peaks on adjoining waves that have the same phase.

ANTONI VAN LEEUWENHOEK

Antoni van Leeuwenhoek (1632–1723) who, using just a single lens microscope, was able to describe organisms and tissues, such as bacteria and red blood cells, which were previously not known to exist. In his lifetime, Leeuwenhoek built over 400 microscopes, each one specifically designed for one specimen only. The highest resolution he was able to achieve was about 2 micrometers.

■ Applications and Research

The chemical and dyestuffs industry that began in Germany in the nineteenth century provided microscopists with a range of stains that made the identification of specific microorganisms much easier. Many of these are still used in modern microbiology laboratories. For instance, Gram's stain distinguishes between bacteria on the basis of the thickness and composition of their cell wall. Gram-positive bacteria, such as *Corynebacterium, listeria* and *Bacillus* species, which have a more complex cell wall, do absorb the stain, trapping it between the layers of this wall. Gram-negative bacteria, such as *Salmonella* and *Shigella* species, do not retain the stain because their walls lack one of the layers.

Ziehl-Nielsen stain is useful for identifying the mycobacteria that cause tuberculosis (TB), and silver methenamine stains chitin, a carbohydrate that is found in the walls of fungi and of *Pneumocystis carinii*, the microorganism that causes an otherwise rare form of pneumonia among HIV/AIDS patients. Giemsa stain is found useful in identifying malaria and other parasites, such as *Leishmania*.

Immunofluorescence is a modern microscopy technique that uses antibodies labeled with a fluorescent marker to bind to specific parts of a microbial pathogen. When the specimen is examined under ultraviolet light, the antibody will glow with a green fluorescence, if the pathogen is present.

Microsocopy aids diagnosis by examining the clinical specimens that are likely to be infected with the causative organism. Therefore, sputum is examined for TB, blood for malaria, stool samples for parasites, and urine to detect bacteria causing urinary tract infections. Viruses are detected, although not routinely, with an electron microscope. There are many other laboratory methods for the detection of microorganisms that complement microscopy.

The optics of a light microscope are adjustable depending on the type of result desired. In light field microscopy, the specimen is visualized by light passing from the condenser through the specimen, while dark field microscopy uses oblique illumination that gives higher resolution of detail, if this is needed. Phase contrast microscopy involves modification to the condenser and objective to give an optical interference pattern in the viewed image. This is very valuable for transparent specimens because it makes details appear darker against a light background.

■ Impacts and Issues

A microscope must be operated by a skilled scientist, if findings are to be of clinical value. Some microorganisms are easy to identify under the microscope, especially if the specimen is given the correct preparation, including staining. However, it is not always possible to distinguish between a pathogen and a harmless organism present within the same specimen.

But sometimes inadequate preparation will give faulty results and an important diagnosis may be missed. Use of the microscope is also relatively insensitive as a diagnostic tool in that many organisms must be present for a positive result to be given. Infections caused by relatively few bacteria may be missed.

It also takes time and experience to come to a correct conclusion based upon microscope findings. If lab technicians are handling a large number of specimens—from a cervical cancer screening program, for example—they may miss positive findings. Cancer cells have different features under the microscope compared to healthy cells. Sometimes these differences may be missed, leading to a false negative. The microscope is just one of many diagnostic tools at the disposal of the pathology laboratory for the diagnosis of infectious and other diseases.

SEE ALSO *Microorganisms; Rapid Diagnostic Tests for Infectious Diseases.*

BIBLIOGRAPHY

Books

Gillespie, Stephen, and Kathleen Bamford. *Medical Microbiology and Infection at a Glance.* Oxford: Blackwell, 2000.

Web Sites

Molecular Expressions(tm). "Optical Microscopy Primer." March 6, 2005. <http://micro.magnet.fsu.edu/ primer/index.html> (accessed May 8, 2007).

Susan Aldridge

ELECTRON MICROSCOPES

There are two types of electron microscope, the transmission electron microscope (TEM) and the scanning electron microscope (SEM). The TEM transmits electrons through an extremely thin sample. The electrons scatter as they collide with the atoms in the sample and form an image on a photographic film below the sample. This process is similar to a medical x ray, where x rays (very short wavelength light) are transmitted through the body and form an image on photographic film behind the body. By contrast, the SEM reflects a narrow beam of electrons off the surface of a sample and detects the reflected electrons. To image a certain area of the sample, the electron beam is scanned in a back and forth motion parallel to the sample surface, similar to the process of mowing a square section of lawn. The chief differences between the two microscopes are that the TEM gives a two-dimensional picture of the interior of the sample while the SEM gives a three-dimensional picture of the surface of the sample. Images produced by SEM are familiar to the public, as in television commercials showing pollen grains or dust mites.

Monkeypox

■ Introduction

Monkeypox is an infectious viral disease that is very similar to smallpox but milder. There is very low prevalence of this disease, with almost all cases occurring in west and central Africa. The first outbreak in the United States occurred in 2003. This disease causes smallpox-like symptoms, including fever, headache, muscle aches, backache, exhaustion, and discomfort in addition to a papular rash over the body. One symptom common in monkeypox but not smallpox is the swelling of the lymph nodes.

Monkeypox is a zoonosis, a disease humans can contract from an infected animal. It is usually contracted via an animal bite, or by coming into contact with the bodily fluids of infected animals. There is no treatment for monkeypox, but fatality rates are low, with most patients recovering in 2–4 weeks. Monkeypox can be prevented by controlling the transmission of the disease from animals to humans. This involves reporting diseased animals, and taking appropriate action to prevent transfer of the virus to humans.

■ Disease History, Characteristics, and Transmission

Monkeypox is a rare disease caused by the monkeypox virus. This virus belongs to the orthopoxvirus group of viruses, which also includes smallpox and cowpox. Monkeypox was first discovered in 1958. It was first identified in laboratory monkeys and later in rodents. The first human case of monkeypox was reported in 1970.

Monkeypox is found in many animals including monkeys, mice, rats, rabbits, and squirrels. All mammals are thought to be susceptible to this virus. Humans become infected with monkeypox when they come into direct contact with an infected animal's bodily fluids— either through an animal bite or by touching its lesions. This virus can also be transmitted by airborne droplets from the respiratory tract. Therefore, face to face contact

between an infected animal and a human also can spread this virus. Contact with contaminated items, such as bed sheets, can also spread the disease.

Monkeypox is a milder version of smallpox, presenting similar, although less severe, symptoms. Approximately 12 days after infection with the monkeypox virus, a person will develop an illness characterized by fever, headache, muscle aches, backache, exhaustion, and discomfort. Unlike smallpox, monkeypox also causes the lymph nodes to swell. A few days after these initial symptoms, a papular rash (raised bumps on the skin) begins to form. This rash usually develops first on the face before spreading across the body. The bumps develop, crust

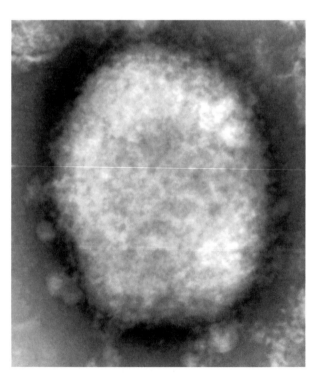

The monkeypox virus. *CDC/Science Source.*

556

over, and finally fall off. The infection usually lasts 2–4 weeks. Between 1% and 10% of the people in Africa who contract monkeypox will die of the disease. No monkeypox fatalities have been reported outside of Africa.

■ Scope and Distribution

Monkeypox was first found in Africa. Most cases of monkeypox occur in central and western Africa, particularly in Zaire, and the countries in which it occurs are characterized by tropical rainforest. There is a low prevalence of the disease. Between 1970 and 1986, only 400 cases worldwide were reported by the World Health Organization.

In 2003, the first ever cases of monkeypox occurred in the United States. Of at least 79 reports of monkeypox, 29 were confirmed as true cases of monkeypox. It is argued that the virus was transmitted to humans by tame prairie dogs that were earlier in contact with infected Gambian rats from Africa. The tame prairie dogs probably contracted the virus from the Gambian rats.

Although the virus is similar to smallpox, which devastated populations prior to its eradication, monkeypox is not as transmissible as smallpox. While smallpox spread rapidly from person to person, only one-third of monkeypox cases arise in this way.

The people most at risk of developing monkeypox are those exposed to infected animals or infected patients. This includes investigators of current monkeypox outbreaks, veterinarians, health care workers, laboratory workers, and friends or family of monkeypox patients.

■ Treatment and Prevention

There is no safe, specific treatment for monkeypox. However, a good health care system, including adequate supportive care for symptoms, as well as good nutrition, aids recovery. The illness normally lasts 2–4 weeks and a person is no longer infectious when the rash lesions are crusted. No fatalities have been reported outside of Africa. However, within rural African regions, where health care is generally poor, monkeypox fatalities may reach 10% of reported cases.

There is no vaccination against monkeypox, although the smallpox vaccination has been found to be effective against monkeypox. However, the CDC does not recommend widespread smallpox vaccination. Instead, use of the vaccine is recommended only for high risk individuals, such as those caring for monkeypox patients, or people who have been in contact with infected animals and are at risk of becoming infected. Vaccination after exposure to the virus has been found to help prevent or reduce the severity of infection. However, vaccination should be avoided in patients with weakened immune systems or patients with life-threatening allergies to the smallpox vaccine and its

> # WORDS TO KNOW
>
> **CHAIN OF TRANSMISSION:** Chain of transmission refers to the route by which an infection is spread from its source to susceptible host. An example of a chain of transmission is the spread of malaria from an infected animal to humans via mosquitoes.
>
> **FOMITE:** A fomite is an object or a surface to which an infectious microorganism such as bacteria or viruses can adhere and be transmitted. Transmission is often by touch.
>
> **ENDEMIC:** Present in a particular area or among a particular group of people.
>
> **PAPULAR:** A papule is a small, solid bump on the skin; papular means pertaining to or resembling a papule.
>
> **ZOONOSES:** Zoonoses are diseases of microbiological origin that can be transmitted from animals to people. The causes of the diseases can be bacteria, viruses, parasites, and fungi.

ingredients, since the smallpox vaccine could be more harmful than the monkeypox virus in these cases.

In order to prevent spread of this disease, infected animals are separated from human populations as soon as possible. These animals are reported to the health department, and appropriate action is taken to keep the animal from transmitting the disease. As contact with fomites (contaminated surfaces such as clothing) and bedding can also result in transmission of the disease, these items must be washed with hot water and detergent to remove the virus.

■ Impacts and Issues

Monkeypox is not a widespread disease. While low mortality outbreaks occur in Africa, few outbreaks have been reported outside of African countries. Prior to 2003, monkeypox had not appeared in the United States and was not considered a threat. Since 2003, there has been one outbreak of monkeypox in the United States and, although the disease was contained, it is now considered a possible threat for United States citizens.

The outbreak in the United States included at least 29 confirmed cases of monkeypox. However, no deaths occurred due to this disease. The effect of this disease on victims in the United States was noticeably milder than its effect on African populations. A better national health care network is thought to have resulted in a more efficient and

IN CONTEXT: REAL-WORLD RISKS

The Centers for Disease Control and Prevention (CDC) states that "past data from Africa suggests that the smallpox vaccine is at least 85% effective in preventing monkeypox." CDC states that: "for most persons who have been exposed to monkeypox, the risks from monkeypox disease are greater than the risks from the smallpox vaccine."

"Studies of monkeypox in West Africa—where people live in remote areas and are medically underserved—showed that the disease killed 1% to 10% of people infected. In contrast, most people who get the smallpox vaccine have only expected minor reactions, like mild fever, tiredness, swollen glands, and redness and itching at the place where the vaccine is given. However the smallpox vaccine does have more serious risks too. Based on past experience, it is estimated that between 1 and 2 people out of every 1 million people vaccinated will die as a result of life-threatening reactions to the vaccine."

SOURCE: *Centers for Disease Control and Prevention*

thus more effective containment of the disease. This health care network includes better nutrition, access to good supportive care, and availability of a vaccine.

Future outbreaks in the United States and in other countries outside of Africa are still possible. However, not only are the chances of transmission throughout a population low, but it is unlikely that a chain of transmission would be sustained within a human community.

There has been some debate within the United States over the potential for monkeypox to be used by terrorists as a biological weapon. However, the efficient containment of this disease during the 2003 outbreak, coupled with the low likelihood that this disease would spread rapidly through the population, significantly reduces its risk as a bioweapon.

SEE ALSO *Bioterrorism; Smallpox; Smallpox Eradication and Storage; Viral Disease; Zoonoses.*

BIBLIOGRAPHY

Periodicals

Huhn, G.D., et al. "Monkeypox in the Western Hemisphere." *New England Journal of Medicine* 350 (April 22, 2004): 1790–1791.

Web Sites

Centers for Disease Control and Prevention. "Questions and Answers about Monkeypox." November 4, 2003. <http://www.cdc.gov/ncidod/monkeypox/qa.htm> (accessed March 6, 2007).

Illinois Department of Public Health. "Monkeypox." <http://www.idph.state.il.us/health/infect/monkeypox.htm> (accessed March 6, 2007).

Stanford University. "Monkeypox." Winter 2000. <http://www.stanford.edu/group/virus/pox/2000/monkeypox_virus.html> (accessed March 6, 2007).

University of Alabama. "History of Monkeypox." May 25, 2005. <http://www.bioterrorism.uab.edu/EI/monkeypox/history.html> (accessed March 6, 2007).

Mononucleosis

■ Introduction

Mononucleosis is a self-limiting viral disease caused by the Epstein-Barr virus (EBV). EBV is considered to be one of the most common viruses among humans and most people become infected with the virus at some point during their lives. When infection with EBV occurs during adolescence or young adulthood, the infection develops into mononucleosis 35–50% of the time. The disease occurs worldwide.

EBV infection during early childhood is usually asymptomatic. When an adolescent or young adult develops mononucleosis the symptoms include fever, sore throat, swollen glands, swollen lymph nodes, and general fatigue. In severe cases, patients may display symptoms for months, but usually they will resolve within four weeks of initial infection. There is no vaccine to prevent mononucleosis and treatment of symptoms relies largely on rest and rehydration.

No areas have been identified as having an increased risk of infection and most cases occur sporadically with no reports of outbreaks. The long incubation period of infection coupled with the universal presence of the viral agent makes epidemiological control impractical.

■ Disease History, Characteristics, and Transmission

Mononucleosis is also known as Pfeiffer's disease, Filatov's disease, the kissing disease, glandular fever, or, simply, mono. The disease was first termed glandular fever by a group of German physicians in the 1880s due to the obvious swelling of the lymph nodes and glands. In 1920, scientists discovered that the infection was associated with white blood cells called mononuclear leukocytes, and thus it was also called infectious mononucleosis. The causative agent wasn't identified as EBV until 1968, when Michael Epstein (1921–) and Yvonne Barr (1932–) discovered the virus.

EBV is a member of the family of human herpes viruses. It is one of the most common human viruses and is responsible for 90% of mononucleosis cases. Cytomegalovirus is another member of this family of viruses and may cause mononucleosis in a small number of cases. EBV causes mononucleosis by infecting lymphocytes, or white blood cells, which subsequently reduces host immunity for the period of infection. EBV has also been implicated in more severe diseases, such as post-transplant lymphoproliferative disease, Hodgkin's disease, nasopharyngeal carcinoma, and Burkitt's lymphoma.

Mononucleosis has an incubation period of 4–7 weeks, during which symptoms may not be present. Most children are exposed to EBV at a young age, which generally results in a mild, asymptomatic infection. If initial infection occurs during adolescence or young adulthood, symptoms may present as a persistent cold or flu and may include fever, enlarged lymph nodes on the neck, sore throat, muscle aches, fatigue, and white patches on the tonsils. Enlargement of the spleen occurs in 25–75% of cases and poses threat of further complications due to the possibility of rupture. Other symptoms may include abdominal pain, headache, jaundice, depression, weakness, skin rash, and swollen liver. The broad spectrum of possible symptoms means that almost all cases of mononucleosis are unique to each patient.

Generally the infection is self-limiting within 2–4 weeks, but in some cases the course of disease is considered chronic and patients may suffer from symptoms for months, or even years. In most cases, hospitalization is seldom required unless complications, such as ruptured spleen or liver problems, arise. There have been no indicating factors to suggest why some people develop more serious symptoms than others, however it is postulated that external stressors in a patient's life could potentially play a key role. The EBV infection does not necessarily affect only people with compromised immunity and quite often, those that contract mononucleosis appear fit and healthy.

Mononucleosis is considered relatively contagious and is transmitted through contact with saliva or mucus,

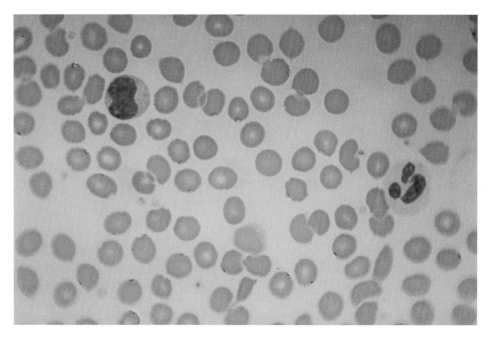

Infectious mononucleosis is caused by the Epstein-Barr virus. The patient's blood contains large, atypical mononuclear cells, which are activated lymphocytes. © *Lester V. Bergman/Corbis.*

which can occur by kissing or by the sharing of drinks and utensils. In some instances, transmission has been linked to blood and may occur through transfusion. Infected people may be contagious while symptomatic but even asymptomatic persons can carry and spread the virus for life, and, as such, remain a primary reservoir for transmission.

◼ Scope and Distribution

EBV is found worldwide. Mononucleosis most frequently occurs in young adults between 15 and 17 years of age, but it potentially affects people of all ages. One to three percent of college students are affected annually.

Generally, most people will contract EBV at some stage of their life and in the United States, 95% of 35 to 40 year-olds have previously been infected. In most cases, previous infection will have occurred without recognition or diagnosis. This is due to the fact that during early childhood, infection is mild, usually producing no symptoms, or only mild symptoms similar to the common cold.

The statistics are much the same for developing nations, where 90% of children contract asymptomatic EBV when under five years old. These individuals are then not susceptible to mononucleosis caused by EBV. It is interesting to note that mononucleosis is a disease that more commonly affects people in developed countries than those in developing countries. Variations in social etiquette and acceptable social behaviors may account for such differences, since mononucleosis is a disease that requires direct contact with saliva for transmission, such as through intimate kissing. Another theory accounting

for this difference is that in developing countries, individuals are likely to be exposed to EBV while young, and so would develop a mild form of the infection. In developed countries, individuals may be protected from the virus until adolescence. Without the immunity conferred by prior infection, mononucleosis would develop.

There does not appear to be a strong link between the health status of a person and the extent to which they will develop mononucleosis, but potentially people who have a compromised immune systems may be at higher risk of developing mononucleosis when infected with EBV.

The global scope of EBV almost certainly ensures the continued transmission of the disease. Most cases of mononucleosis occur sporadically and outbreaks are rare. In most cases, people presenting symptoms of the disease have no recollection of possible exposure to the virus, and it is uncommon that infection would be transmitted to a group from a single source. In any large adult group environment, over 90% of the people will probably have been exposed to the EBV previously and, in such situations, an outbreak is unlikely.

There are no known ethnic, racial, or sexual factors that predispose a person to develop mononucleosis. However, it is interesting to note that, in developed countries, infection more often occurs in persons belonging to a higher socioeconomic class. This may be attributed to differences in lifestyle and increased opportunities for the social interactions associated with this disease. In addition, the fact that these individuals receive a higher level of protection from childhood

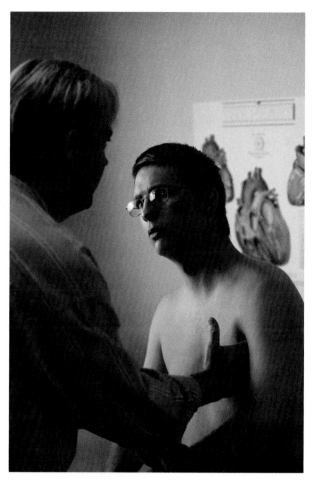

A doctor examines the lymph nodes of a person who has contracted mononucleosis. © *Steve Raymer/Corbis.*

infections may also play a role. The only gender-related factor associated with mononucleosis is that 90% of cases of ruptured spleens occur in males.

■ Treatment and Prevention

Diagnosis of mononucleosis may be confirmed through serological testing to determine the presence of abnormal white blood cells. The "mono spot" test is a specific test designed to detect the presence of antibodies that have developed as a result of the viral infection. These are known as heterophile antibodies and usually develop about one week after onset of the disease. They peak during the first month of illness, but may persist in the blood for several months and up to one year. Some people infected with mononucleosis may never develop these antibodies and so the test may return a false negative result. Generally, the testing is accurate with false positive results occurring in only a small number of patients.

There is no vaccine or preventative medicine available for mononucleosis, largely due to the fact that it

results from a viral infection. However, the severity of other infections related to EBV, in addition to a further understanding of the virus, has prompted scientists to investigate avenues for creating a potential vaccine. It is likely that the vaccine would be targeted towards minimizing the clinical manifestations of primary infection with EBV, rather than towards malignancies associated with the disease.

The fact that EBV infection in early childhood seldom results in development of mononucleosis, while primary infection occurring after adolescence develops into the disease in 35–50% of cases has encouraged researchers. This observation suggests that a vaccine generating a minimized immune response may potentially limit the clinical symptoms of mononucleosis. The limiting factor in this area of research is that such a vaccine requires the use of an attenuated (weakened) virus, which has been deemed unsafe for administration to healthy adolescents. For this reason, it is unlikely that the vaccine would meet strict licensing laws.

In most cases, mononucleosis resolves within four weeks after symptoms first arise, during which time treatments are targeted at the symptoms of the infection. Rest is one of the key elements to recuperation and maintenance of fluid intake is essential. Patients are also advised to avoid heavy activity for at least one month following initial infection to reduce the risk of spleen rupture. Nonsteroidal anti-inflammatory (NSAID) medication may be used to treat pain and reduce fever and swelling, and dietary supplements may help boost the immune system. Antibiotics may be useful in treating throat infections often accompanying mononucleosis, but will not be effective against EBV. It is not recommended that patients use aspirin due to the possibility of developing Reye's syndrome, a potentially fatal disease.

The typically benign and self-limiting course of mononucleosis, in addition to the ubiquitous nature of the virus, makes prevention virtually impossible. With over 90% of the western adult population returning positive tests for previous infection, person-to-person infection remains highly likely in societies worldwide.

Prevention of the disease may not be beneficial. As noted, childhood infection with EBV typically results in few or no symptoms. In contrast, infection during adolescence tends to result in a more serious disease. This suggests that intentional early primary exposure could potentially be used as a method of preventing the later onset of mononucleosis.

■ Impacts and Issues

The statistics show that inevitably, at some stage of their life, almost the entire world population will be exposed to, contract, and harbor the Epstein-Barr virus. However, the majority of people who encounter infection during early childhood will not even develop

WORDS TO KNOW

ANTIBODY: Antibodies, or Y-shaped immunoglobulins, are proteins found in the blood that help to fight against foreign substances called antigens. Antigens, which are usually proteins or polysaccharides, stimulate the immune system to produce antibodies. The antibodies inactivate the antigen and help to remove it from the body. While antigens can be the source of infections from pathogenic bacteria and viruses, organic molecules detrimental to the body from internal or environmental sources also act as antigens. Genetic engineering and the use of various mutational mechanisms allow the construction of a vast array of antibodies (each with a unique genetic sequence).

CHRONIC FATIGUE SYNDROME: Chronic fatigue syndrome (CFS) is a condition that causes extreme tiredness. People with CFS have debilitating fatigue that lasts for six months or longer. They also have many other symptoms. Some of these symptoms are pain in the joints and muscles, headache, and sore throat. CFS appears to result from a combination of factors.

EPSTEIN BARR VIRUS (EBV): Epstein-Barr virus (EBV) is part of the family of human herpes viruses. Infectious mononucleosis (IM) is the most common disease manifestation of this virus, which once established in the host, can never be completely eradicated. Very little can be done to treat EBV; most methods can only alleviate resultant symptoms.

MONO SPOT TEST: The mononucleosis (mono) spot test is a blood test used to check for infection with the Epstein-Barr virus, which causes mononucleosis.

MONONUCLEAR LEUKOCYTE: A mononuclear leukocyte is a type of white blood cell active in the immune system.

they may miss classes during this time. In addition, being removed from social groups for extended periods may generate emotional issues among adolescents. This is especially significant considering that the disease commonly occurs at an important time in social development.

In addition, social pressures can occur when adults contract mononucleosis. Adults may lose income due to an inability to work, which may put economic pressures on families and further strain family relationships. Such concerns may lead individuals to shorten their recovery period and return to their regular activities earlier than recommended. In these cases, symptoms of fatigue may persist for longer than usual and result in lower productivity.

In some chronic cases of the disease, patients suffer symptoms for more than six months and sometimes for years. In many chronic cases, it is considered that the mononucleosis contributed to the development of chronic fatigue syndrome (CFS). Although the exact causes of CFS have not been identified, approximately 10% of mononucleosis patients will go on to suffer from it and so CFS is considered a possible side effect of the disease. In these situations, people are unable to work, study, or socialize for long periods of time and, sometimes, permanently.

Cases of mononucleosis are generally much more severe in people with compromised immunity, and the complications that develop from such infections may prove fatal. Immunocompromised individuals include those who have undergone organ or marrow transplants, individuals receiving chemotherapy, and those with autoimmune diseases. The development of an immune disorder later in life may also result in a severe relapse of mononucleosis infection among people who previously only carried the virus in a latent form. While fatalities resulting from mononucleosis were previously a rare occurrence, the growing numbers of people suffering from immune disorders makes this a potentially significant threat in the future.

Bone marrow has been identified as one site of latent EBV persistence within the body. It has also been observed that an EBV-positive individual who receives a bone marrow transplant from an EBV-negative donor is found to be EBV-negative following transplantation. This means that this recipient is again susceptible to infection and most likely, if the transplant occurs during adulthood, will develop mononucleosis. This raises a new concern—the loss of immunity to certain diseases following transplantation. This could become a more serious problem as organ transplantation becomes a more common procedure.

■ Primary Source Connection

A diagnosis of mononucleosis can mean a period of convalescence for about two months, and that is usually a difficult order for an otherwise healthy teenager or

mononucleosis. It is the omnipresence of EBV that prevents the eradication of the infection.

The impact of mononucleosis may be seen on a personal level. Severe cases may keep patients in bed and away from their normal activities for many weeks or even months. This is a particular problem for students, since

young adult, who are the prime ages for infection with the viruses that cause mono. In the following article from the *FDA Consumer*, author Judith Levine Willis discusses mono and it's implications for physical and social limitations for young people. At the time the article was published in 1998, Judith Levine Willis was on the public affairs staff of the Food and Drug Administration. She has since authored, as Judith Levine, books about gender, health, and consumer issues.

Mono: Tough for Teens and Twenty-Somethings

Missed parties. Postponed exams. Sitting out a season of team sports. And loneliness. These are a few of the ways that scourge of high school and college students known as "mono" can affect your life.

The disease whose medical name is infectious mononucleosis is most common in people 10 to 35 years old, with its peak incidence in those 15 to 17 years old. Only 50 people out of 100,000 in the general population get mono, but it strikes as many as 2 out of 1,000 teens and twenty-somethings, especially those in high school, college, and the military. While mono is not usually considered a serious illness, it may have serious complications. Without a doubt your lifestyle will change for a few months.

You've probably heard people call mono the "kissing disease." But if your social life is in a slump, you may wonder, "How did I get this 'kissing disease' when I haven't kissed anyone romantically recently?"

Here's how. Mono is usually transmitted though saliva and mucus—which is where the "kissing disease" nickname comes from. But the kissing or close contact that transmits the disease doesn't happen right before you get sick. The virus that causes mono has a long incubation period: 30 to 50 days from the time you're exposed to it to the time you get sick. In addition, the virus can be transmitted in other ways, such as sipping from the same straw or glass as an infected person—or even being close when the person coughs or sneezes. Also, some people can have the virus in their systems without ever having symptoms and you can still catch it from them.

Two viruses can cause mono: Epstein-Barr virus (EBV) and cytomegalovirus (CMV). Both viruses are in the herpes family, whose other members include viruses responsible for cold sores and chickenpox.

EBV causes 85 percent of mono cases. About half of all children are infected with EBV before they're 5, but at that young age, it usually doesn't cause any symptoms. If you don't become infected with EBV until you're a teen or older, you're more likely to develop mono symptoms. After you're infected, the virus stays with you for life, but usually doesn't cause any additional symptoms. Still, every now and then you may produce viral particles in your saliva that can transmit the virus to other people, even though you feel perfectly fine. By age 40, 85 to 90 percent of Americans have EBV antibodies, indicating they have the virus in their systems and are immune to further EBV infection.

CMV is also a very common virus. About 85 percent of the U.S. population is infected with it by the time they reach adulthood. As with EBV, CMV is frequently symptomless, and mono most often results when infection occurs in the teens and 20s. Sore throat is less common in people who have CMV mono than in those infected with EBV.

As another one of its nicknames—glandular fever—implies, perhaps the most distinguishing mono symptom is enlarged glands or lymph nodes, especially in the neck, but also in the armpit and groin.

Another common mono symptom is fever. A temperature as high as 39.5 degrees Celsius (103 degrees Fahrenheit) is not uncommon. Other symptoms include a tired achy feeling, appetite loss, white patches on the back of the throat, and tonsillitis.

"My tonsils got so swollen they were touching each other in back," says Heidi Palombo of Annandale, Va., who had mono when she was a senior in college. She recalls her throat being "so hot and swollen that the only thing that felt good was ice water."

Cold drinks and frozen desserts are both ways to relieve sore throat symptoms. Doctors also recommend gargling with saltwater (about half a teaspoon salt to 8 ounces of warm water) and sucking on throat lozenges available over the counter in pharmacies and other stores. If throat or tonsils are infected, a throat culture should be taken so the doctor can prescribe an appropriate antibiotic. Ampicillin is usually not recommended because it sometimes causes a rash that can be confused with the pink, measleslike rash that 1 out of 5 mono patients develops.

For fever and achiness, you can take acetaminophen (marketed as Tylenol, Datril and others) or ibuprofen (marketed as Advil, Motrin, Nuprin, and others). If you're under 20, don't take aspirin unless your doctor approves it. In children and teens, aspirin taken for viral illnesses has been associated with the potentially fatal disease Reye syndrome. Sometimes a person with mono may have trouble breathing because of swelling in the throat, and doctors have to use other medications and treatment. A person who has mono—or those caring for the person—should contact a doctor immediately if the person starts having breathing problems.

Some people with mono become overly sensitive to light and about half develop enlargement of the spleen, usually two to three weeks after they first become sick. Mild enlargement of the liver may also occur.

Whether or not the spleen is enlarged, people who have mono should not lift heavy objects or exercise vigorously—including participating in contact sports—for two months after they get sick, because these activities increase the risk of rupturing the spleen, which can be life-threatening. If you have mono and get a severe sharp, sudden pain on the left side of your upper abdomen, go to an emergency room or call 911 immediately.

Because its symptoms can be very similar to those of other illnesses, doctors often recommend tests to find out exactly what the problem is.

"I was misdiagnosed at first and told I was bit by a spider," writes John L. Gipson, of Kansas City, Mo., in a note he posted to a Website. "That's what I thought because I had killed a spider in my room. I figured I'd been bitten by a spider in my sleep. A few days after. I had no energy, a fever. and those pea-sized bumps on the back of my neck." Gipson returned to his doctor, who did blood tests and diagnosed mononucleosis.

Other diagnostic problems can result because enlarged lymphocytes, a type of white cell, are common with mono, but can also be a symptom of leukemia. Blood tests can distinguish between the type of white cell seen in leukemia and that with mono.

If your throat is sore, having a throat culture is usually a good idea for several reasons. First, the symptoms of mono and strep infection (including that caused by Strep-A, a particularly serious form of strep) are very similar. Second, strep throat or other throat infections can develop anytime during or shortly after in the disease. In any case, it's important that throat infections be diagnosed as soon as possible and treated with antibiotics that can kill the organism responsible for the infection.

The test most commonly used to tell whether you have mono or some other ailment is the mononucleosis spot test. This blood test detects the antibodies (proteins) that the body makes to fight EBV or CMV. Because it takes a while for antibodies to develop after infection, your doctor may need to order or repeat the test one to two weeks after you develop symptoms. At that time the test is about 85 percent accurate.

Other tests your doctor might order include a complete blood count (CBC) to see if your blood platelet count is lower than normal and if lymphocytes are abnormal, and a chemistry panel to see if liver enzymes are abnormal.

Bed rest is the most important treatment for uncomplicated mono. It's also important to drink plenty of fluids. Mono is not usually a reason to quarantine students. Many people are already immune to the viruses that

cause it. But if you have mono you'll want to stay in bed and out of classes for several days, until the fever goes down and other symptoms abate. Even when you've started to get better, you can expect to have to curtail your activities for several weeks, and it can take two to three months or more until you feel your old self again.

The author of this article had mono herself when she was 16. Though she didn't mind getting out of all that homework (or at least putting it off), having to delay finals only added to her anxiety about college applications that many high school juniors experience. And then there was that guy who never called again.

When you add the time spent recuperating to the fact that most people are not exactly anxious to get close to a person with mono, you can understand why some students find themselves combating loneliness on top of their other troubles.

Getting through mono may be both challenging and depressing—and seem to take forever. But if you rest when your body tells you to, you can lessen the chances of complications and get back your life.

Judith Levine Willis

WILLIS, JUDITH LEVINE. "MONO: TOUGH FOR TEENS AND TWENTY-SOMETHINGS." *FDA CONSUMER* (MAY, JUNE 1998): 32,3.

SEE ALSO *Blood Supply and Infectious Disease; Cancer and Infectious Disease; Childhood Infectious Diseases, Immunization Impacts; Demographics and Infectious Disease; Viral Disease.*

BIBLIOGRAPHY

Books

Collier, L., and J. Oxford. *Human Virology.* New York: Oxford University Press, 2006.

Mandell, G.L., J.E. Bennett, and R. Dolin. *Principles and Practice of Infectious Diseases.* 6th ed. Philadelphia: Elsevier, 2004.

Tselis, A., and H.B. Jenson. *Epstein-Barr Virus.* New York: Taylor & Francis, 2006.

Umar, C.S. *New Developments in Epstein-Barr Virus Research.* New York: Nova Science Publishers, 2006.

Web Sites

Centers for Disease Control and Prevention. "Epstein-Barr Virus and Infectious Mononucleosis." 2007. <http://www.cdc.gov/ncidod/diseases/ebv.htm> (accessed March 7, 2007).

Mosquito-borne Diseases

Introduction

Mosquitoes have harmed more humans than any other group of insects. The scientific names conveyed upon mosquitoes reflect the torment that they can cause: *Psorophora horrida*, *Culex perfidiosus*, *Mansonia perturbans*, *Aedes vexans*, and *Aedes tormentor*. However, the annoyance caused by mosquitoes pales in comparison to the widespread suffering and millions of deaths that these insects cause. These flies from the order Diptera transmit some of the most devastating diseases.

There are over 2,500 different species of mosquitoes throughout the world. The vast majority of mosquitoes are harmless to humans, feeding only on nectar or other plant juices. Only females of some species consume blood. These mosquitoes transmit such diseases as malaria, yellow fever, dengue, filariasis and encephalitis (St. Louis encephalitis [SLE], Western Equine encephalitis [WEE], LaCrosse encephalitis [LAC], Japanese encephalitis [JE], Eastern Equine encephalitis [EEE] and West Nile virus [WNV]) to humans and to animals.

Disease History, Characteristics, and Transmission

A vector-borne disease results from an infection transmitted to humans and other animals by blood-feeding

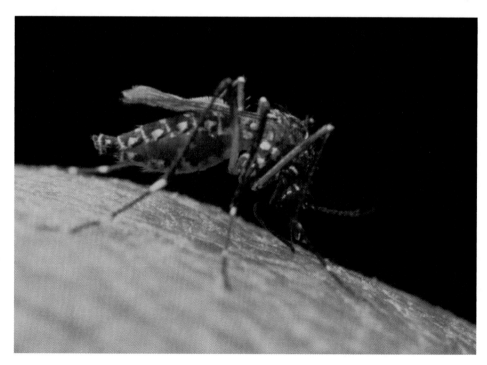

The female *Aedes aegypti* mosquito is primarily responsible for the spread of dengue fever. *Aedes aegypti* is a domestic, day-biting mosquito that prefers to feed on humans. *Martin Dohrn/Photo Researchers, Inc.*

IN CONTEXT: SCIENTIFIC, POLITICAL, AND ETHICAL ISSUES

Developed during the 1940s, the pesticide dichloro-diphenyl-trichloroethane (DDT) was used to fight malaria and other insect-borne diseases—and was considered by many to be a so-called miracle pesticide. During three decades of use, approximately 675,000 tons of DDT were applied in the United States.

Although DDT can greatly reduce the burden of mosquito-borne disease in the 1960s, DDT use remains controversial. DDT is an environmentally persistent chlorinated hydrocarbon that accumulates in the food chain and has significant environmental consequences that offset its benefits in the control of disease. The pesticide was banned in many developed nations, including the United States since 1972, because of its potential to damage ecosystems and wildlife. It is, however, still used for disease control in some countries. Proponents of DDT use assert that its environmental impact has been overstated, and that prohibitions on DDT use and

manufacturing may have contributed to worldwide deaths from mosquito-borne diseases over the past several decades. It is again recommended for limited use in targeted areas because of its effectiveness in removing this severe public health hazard. Others assert that safer insecticides than DDT should be used in all locations.

American biologist and author Rachel Louise Carson (1907–1964), was a seminal figure in the environmental movement during the 1950s and early 1960s. Carson's book *Silent Spring* was an indictment of overzealous pesticide use and its effects on the environment, was published in 1962 and quickly became a controversial and enduring contribution to the environmental literature. Carson argued against indiscriminate pesticide use without consideration of its ecological consequences. Largely as a result of *Silent Spring*, DDT was banned by the United States in 1972 and is currently illegal in many other countries.

anthropods, such as mosquitoes. Female mosquitoes take a blood meal by bending back a troughlike protective scabbard to permit other mouthparts to penetrate the skin. The piercing "needle" is a long tube composed of six long, separate, stilettolike stylets wet with saliva that adhere to each other. The tube is traversed by two channels, a wide one through which the blood is sucked into the digestive system and a narrow one through which saliva containing an anticoagulant can be injected into the vertebrate host. Pathogens are transmitted from the mosquito to the host at this point.

In 1878, English parasitologist Patrick Manson discovered the link between bloodsucking insects and disease. European and American infectious disease experts subsequently focused on the most common mosquito-borne diseases in these regions: malaria and yellow. The rapid worldwide movement of goods and people has also helped mosquitoes to cross the globe. By the end of the twentieth century, scientists battled mosquito-borne diseases that were worldwide plagues.

West Nile fever, caused by a mosquito-borne virus related to yellow fever, made its first appearance in the Western Hemisphere in New York City in 1999. First isolated and identified in Uganda in 1937, West Nile came to the United States via an infected mosquito, a sick person, or an infected bird. A human source is improbable because human blood generally contains too little virus to contaminate a mosquito. It may have come to New York in mosquitoes that stowed away on an airplane. However, the most likely scenario is that it arrived in illegally imported birds that had been not been quarantined before entering the country. It has subsequently spread by migrating birds, and is now present in all 48 contiguous states in the U.S.

■ Scope and Distribution

Malaria occurs in tropical areas of Central and South America, Africa, Asia, and the East Indies. Until the mid-twentieth century, it was far more widespread. Malaria was established in virtually all subtropical and tropical areas as well as some temperate areas. Malaria receded because breeding sites for mosquitoes were drained for agricultural and industrial purposes. Meanwhile, people moved into in better housing that was less open to mosquitoes. While the disease has been all but obliterated from most of the developed world, it continues to kill elsewhere. More than one million people, mostly in Africa, die annually from malaria with a child succumbing every 30 seconds.

Several different species of the *Aedes* and *Haemogogus* (South America only) mosquitoes transmit the yellow fever virus. While control programs successfully eradicated mosquito habitats in the past, particularly in South America, these programs have lapsed. As a result, mosquito populations have jumped and there is an accompanying rise in the risk of yellow fever epidemics. There are 200,000 estimated cases of yellow fever with 30,000 per year. However, the World Health Organization (WHO) suspects that yellow fever may be underreported.

Dengue is also spread by the Aedes mosquito. Dengue haemorrhagic fever (DHF) is a potentially lethal complication. WHO estimated in 2007 that there were 50 million cases of dengue annually, but the disease is rapidly spreading worldwide. DHF, mostly found in Asia, is a leading cause of hospitalization among children with over 500,000 requiring such care annually.

Treatment and Prevention

The best method of preventing mosquito-borne diseases is to kill mosquitoes. To eradicate mosquitoes, public health experts advise emptying containers of standing water that attract egg-laying females. Some governments kill mosquitoes through insecticide spraying programs or swamp-draining efforts. Exposure to mosquito-borne diseases can be minimized by limiting outdoor movement. Screens are effective at keeping mosquitoes from entering homes.

Infection with the parasite that causes malaria is treated with chloroquine, unless the parasite is resistant to this medication, in which case quinine sulfate and antibiotic combinations are used. As many other mosquito-borne diseases are viral in nature, treatment is mostly supportive or in some cases, involves antiviral medications.

Vaccines are available to protect against Japanese encephalitis and yellow fever. However, vaccine development for dengue and DHF is difficult because any of four different viruses may cause disease. Protection against only one or two dengue viruses could actually increase the risk of more serious illness. Other vaccines are in development. As of 2005, at least one potential vaccine for malaria was ready for clinical trial in humans.

Impacts and Issues

In some regions, mosquitoes have shown the ability to become resistant to pesticides. *Anopheles* mosquitoes in some areas are no longer killed by applications of DDT. Pesticide can also be prohibitively expensive. In 2007, Uganda announced that it could not spray DDT to fight malaria because it had failed to raise the 400 million United States dollars necessary to purchase the pesticide. An estimated 320 Ugandans die of malaria daily.

Several international organizations and charities have been instrumental in the fight against mosquito-borne diseases. The Bill and Melinda Gates Foundation supports mosquito-borne disease research and prevention efforts worldwide, including the development of effective and affordable drugs, improvement of existing preventative measures, and vaccine development. RAPIDS (Reaching HIV-Affected People with Integrated Development and Support), a consortium of several organizations, targets its efforts against mosquito-borne diseases in HIV/AIDS affected communities in Zambia. RAPIDS distributes protective netting and provides in-home follow-up care, ensuring that mosquito netting is properly used.

Promotion of specific sanitation measures is underway in areas where mosquito-borne diseases pose public health threats. Biological control methods, such as wasps that kill mosquitoes, are also being investigated. Researchers are also

---

WORDS TO KNOW

BEDNETS: A type of netting that provides protection from diseases caused by insects such as flies and mosquitoes. It is often used while sleeping to prevent insects from biting while still allowing air to flow through its mesh structure.

GENETIC ENGINEERING: Genetic engineering is the altering of the genetic material of living cells in order to make them capable of producing new substances or performing new functions. When the genetic material within the living cells (i.e., genes) is working properly, the human body can develop and function smoothly. However, should a single gene—even a tiny segment of a gene go awry—the effect can be dramatic: deformities, disease, and even death.

INSECTICIDE: A chemical substance used to kill insects.

MOSQUITO COILS: Mosquito coils are spirals of inflammable paste that, when burned, steadily release insect repellent into the air. They often used in Asia, where many coils release octachlorodipropyl ether, which can cause lung cancer.

MOSQUITO NETTING: Fine meshes or nets hung around occupied spaces, especially beds, to keep out disease-carrying mosquitoes are called mosquito netting. Mosquito netting is a cost-effective way of preventing malaria.

PESTICIDE: Substances used to reduce the abundance of pests, any living thing that causes injury or disease to crops.

---

developing and investigating the use of genetically engineered mosquitoes to fight malaria. The modified mosquitoes are resistant to malaria, and breed at a faster rate than unmodified, non-resistant mosquitoes. Researchers hope that such mosquitoes can be introduced into malaria-prone regions and overtake wild disease-carrying mosquito populations. However, little is known about the impact genetically engineered mosquitoes could have on the transmission or development of other diseases.

Outdoor time-released insecticide misting systems are increasing in popularity, particularly in the United States, as means of controlling mosquitoes. These systems utilize various synergized formulations of natural pyrethrins or synthetic pyrethroids that are dispensed into the environment at intervals determined by the user. Some systems

IN CONTEXT: LIVING WITH DISEASE

It was once argued that malaria could be eradicated. The draining of marshlands and the use of the pesticide DDT dramatically reduced the six million cases a year that the U.S. experienced in the first decades of the twentieth century. By 1960, the World Health Organization (WHO) had established antimalarial policies in 100 nations and was confident that the disease could be eradicated.

A number of sociopolitical factors, however, combined to slow the advance of medicine. People became complacent about malaria and public health programs were allowed to falter and lapse. Without outside aid, poor nations did not have the money for malarial control methods. Additionally, countries torn by war focused resources on fighting, not on medical care. Meanwhile, malarial microbes evolved in response to drugs, while the ready availability of air travel brought new strains into areas that lacked immunity to them. Global warming is expected to bring malaria back to northern Europe, and it never completely left southern Europe or the United States. WHO now forecasts a 16 percent growth rate in the disease per year.

also utilize minimum risk pesticides to control or repel mosquitoes. The American Mosquito Control Association (AMCA) opposes this method of dispensing pesticides as inconsistent with the Integrated Mosquito Management practices approved by the Environmental Protection Agency as part of the Pesticide Environmental Stewardship Program. The AMCA specifically fears unnecessary insecticide use, indiscriminate killing of beneficial insects, pesticide exposure to humans, and promotion of insecticide resistance.

The regular use of insecticide-impregnated curtains and bednets can reduce the rate of such diseases, particularly among children. The success of using bednets for sustained mosquito control is dependent upon regular treatment of the nets with pyrethroid insecticide once or twice a year. Dip-it-yourself kits have been distributed for this purpose in some countries, and researchers are developing better, longer-lasting insecticide-impregnated fabrics for netting, drapery, and clothing.

Travelers visiting areas known for major outbreaks of mosquito-borne diseases are advised to use mosquito repellent insecticide. The use of mosquito coils, and protective clothing and bedding is also often recommended, along with available vaccinations.

IN CONTEXT: PERSONAL RESPONSIBILITY AND PROTECTION

In October 2006 the Division of Global Migration and Quarantine at Centers for Disease Control and Prevention (CDC) issued an updated list of measures to prevent bites from mosquitoes, ticks, fleas and other insects and arthropods. The preventative measures were designed to "reduce the possibility of being bitten by insects or arthropods that can transmit diseases (vector-borne), such as malaria, dengue, and tickborne encephalitis (TBE)." CDV recommendation include:

- Use an insect repellent on exposed skin to repel mosquitoes, ticks, fleas and other arthropods. EPA-registered repellents include products containing DEET (N,N-diethylmetatoluamide) and picaridin (KBR 3023). DEET concentrations of 30% to 50% are effective for several hours. Picaridin, available at 7% and 15 % concentrations, needs more frequent application. DEET formulations as high as 50% are recommended for both adults and children over 2 months of age.
- Protect infants less than 2 months of age by using a carrier draped with mosquito netting with an elastic edge for a tight fit.
- When using sunscreen, apply sunscreen first and then repellent. Repellent should be washed off at the end of the day before going to bed.

- Wear long-sleeved shirts which should be tucked in, long pants, and hats to cover exposed skin. When you visit areas with ticks and fleas, wear boots, not sandals, and tuck pants into socks.
- Inspect your body and clothing for ticks during outdoor activity and at the end of the day. Wear light-colored or white clothing so ticks can be more easily seen. Removing ticks right away can prevent some infections.
- Apply permethrin-containing (e.g., Permanone) or other insect repellents to clothing, shoes, tents, mosquito nets, and other gear for greater protection. Permethrin is not labeled for use directly on skin. Most repellent is generally removed from clothing and gear by a single washing, but permethrin-treated clothing is effective for up to 5 washings.
- Be aware that mosquitoes that transmit malaria are most active during twilight periods (dawn and in the evening).
- Stay in air-conditioned or well-screened housing, and/or sleep under an insecticide treated bed net. Bed nets should be tucked under mattresses and can be sprayed with a repellent if not already treated with an insecticide. Daytime biters include mosquitoes that transmit dengue and chikungunya viruses and sand flies that transmit leishmaniasis.

SOURCE: *Centers for Disease Control and Prevention, National Center for Infectious Diseases, Division of Global Migration and Quarantine.*

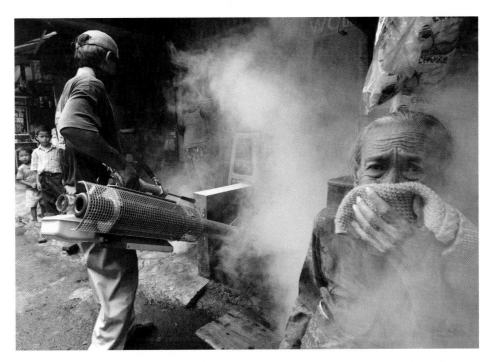

An elderly Indonesian woman covers her nose as a health department worker sprays pesticide in a slum area of Jakarta during an outbreak of the dengue fever in 2004. © *Dadang Tri/Reuters/Corbis.*

BIBLIOGRAPHY

Speilman, Andrew, and Michael D'Antonio. *Mosquito: A Natural History of Our Most Persistent and Deadly Foe.* New York: Hyperion, 2001.

Web Sites

Centers for Disease Control Division of Vector-Borne Infectious Diseases. "Division of Vector-Borne Infectious Diseases." February 23, 2007 <http://www.cdc.gov/ncidod/dvbid/> (accessed April 25, 2007).

Caryn E. Neumann

MRSa

Introduction

MRSa is an acronym for methicillin-resistant *Staphylococcus aureus*, which is a particular type (strain) of *S. aureus*. The bacterium is important because of its antibiotic resistance and because it can cause a number of severe diseases. One such disease is necrotizing fasciitis, more popularily known as "flesh-eating disease." MRSa is also known as oxacillin-resistant *S. aureus* (oxacillin is another antibiotic) and multiple-resistant *S. aureus*.

Until the beginning of this century, MRSa was almost exclusively found in hospitals, because the tremendous antibiotic use in hospitals provided a powerful selection pressure, that is, an environment where only the most resilient bacteria could survive. In 2007, the prevalence of MRSa in environments outside of the hospital is increasing. This form of the bacterium (whether it is different from the hospital form of MRSa is not known) has been designated as community associated-MRSa or CA-MRSa.

Disease History, Characteristics, and Transmission

MRSa is resistant to methicillin, a synthetic penicillin antibiotic. It is also resistant to all of the penicillin class of antibiotics. This wide range of resistance makes the bacterium hard to treat, since commonly used antibiotics are will not kill it.

MRSa has been evident almost as long as methicillin has been in use. Methicillin was introduced in 1959 to treat strains of *S. aureus* that had developed resistance to penicillin. By chemically altering the structure of penicillin, scientists were able to produce methicillin, and the penicillin-resistant *S. aureus* were killed by the newly synthesized antibiotic. But this beneficial effect did not last long. By 1961, MRSa were making a comeback, despite the use of methicillin in the United Kingdom (UK). Soon, reports of MRSa came from other countries in Europe, Japan, Australia, and North America. By 2005, thousands of hospital deaths in the UK were caused by MRSa, and the organism accounted for almost 50% of all hospital-acquired infections.

Methicillin resistance is caused by the presence of a gene (a section of genetic material that codes for the production of a protein or other compound) that codes for a protein that binds to the antibiotic and prevents the antibiotic from entering the bacteria. The *S. aureus* that is susceptible to methicillin does not have this gene. It is the transfer of this gene from one bacterium to another that has spread the resistance through populations of *Staphylococcus* around the globe.

The spread of MRSa has been aided by the fact that *S. aureus* is normally found in the environment. The

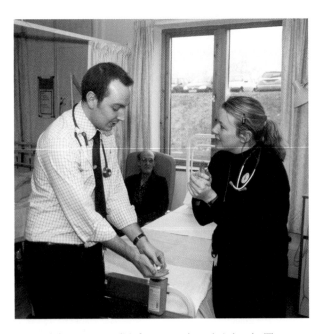

Hospital doctors use a disinfectant to clean their hands. The disinfectant will reduce the amount of bacteria on their hands and is more convenient to use than a sink.   *John Cole/Photo Researchers, Inc.*

bacterium is present in soil and in our bodies. Studies of the bacteria present in certain areas of the body have revealed that approximately 30% of healthy adults harbor *S. aureus*, including MRSa, on the surface of their skin or in other places, like their noses. In these environments, the bacterium is harmless. But, if MRSa gets into a wound and/or if a person's immune system is not functioning efficiently, illness can result.

MRSa is sometimes capable of causing necrotizing fasciitis, an extremely invasive disease that progresses rapidly. Sometimes amputation of the infected limb is the only way to save the patient's life. MRSa can also carry genes that code for the production of potent toxins. If these toxins get into the bloodstream, the resulting effects can be devastating to the body.

■ Scope and Distribution

Since *S. aureus* has a worldwide distribution, it is not surprising that MRSa has a similar distribution. In the past, MRSa was usually found in hospitals and athletic facilities, since both are places where abrasions, cuts, and scrapes occur. In 2007, however, MRSa is becoming increasingly prevalent in the community, which raises the possibility that certain illnesses, such as necrotizing fasciitis, may become more common.

It is estimated that over 50 million people around the globe carry MRSa in their bodies. In the United States, about 32% of people are colonized with *S. aureus* in their noses. Colonization refers to bacteria (or other pathogens) that establish a presence on a tissue. Fewer than one percent of otherwise healthy individuals colonized with MRSa will develop a MRSa-related disease.

Having another infection can increase the likelihood of developing a MRSa infection. For example, individuals with cystic fibrosis often have recurring lung infections that require treatment with a number of different antibiotics. This situation increases the risk that MRSa will be able to gain a foothold in these patients.

Ominously, in February of 2007, an article appeared in *Clinical & Infectious Disease* detailing the person-to-person spread of CA-MRSa via sexual contact. This is the first time this route of transmission has been reported for MRSa.

■ Treatment and Prevention

Treating MRSa is challenging. Only a few antibiotics remain effective against the bacterium. One of these is vancomycin. It has the disadvantage of not being absorbed easily into the body; it cannot be given by mouth because there will be little active compound left by the time the antibiotic circulates through the bloodstream to the site of the infection. Rather, vancomycin must be given intravenously—via a needle inserted into a

WORDS TO KNOW

COLONIZATION: Colonization is the process of occupation and increase in number of microorganisms at a specific site.

PATHOGEN: A disease causing agent, such as a bacteria, virus, fungus, etc.

RESISTANCE: Immunity developed within a species (especially bacteria) via evolution to an antibiotic or other drug. For example, in bacteria, the acquisition of genetic mutations that render the bacteria invulnerable to the action of antibiotics.

SELECTION PRESSURE: Selection pressure refers to factors that influence the evolution of an organism. An example is the overuse of antibiotics, which provides a selection pressure for the development of antibiotic resistance in bacteria.

vein. This usually means that a person being treated must be hospitalized.

The search continues for new antibiotics that will be effective against MRSa. This research is literally a race against time. The development of new antibiotics must at least keep pace with the evolution of resistance by MRSa.

Another potential treatment option is called phage therapy. Phage is short for bacteriophage, which is a virus that specifically infects and forms new phage particles inside of a bacterium. The phage-bacterium association is specific—a certain type of phage infects a certain type of bacterium. In doing so, the phage ultimately destroys the bacterial cell. Scientists are experimenting with a phage that targets MRSa. If this technique proves successful, it would be a powerful treatment, since resistance to a phage does not typically develop.

Contact precautions, including handwashing, are critical in preventing MRSa infection. In a hospital, washing hands before and after caring for a patient is the most important method of preventing the spread of MRSa from patient to patient. Many hospitals now have alcohol-based hand cleansers in each room, sometimes right by each patient's bed. Washing with an alcohol-based wash takes only a few seconds, and, thus, is easier for busy health care providers to do. Moreover, MRSa is usually sensitive to alcohol. Compliance with handwashing precautions is surprisingly low. Surveys in the United States and Europe have confirmed that health care providers only wash their hands about half as much as is optimum for reducing the spread of infection. The Centers for Disease Control and Prevention has estimated that properly performed handwashing could save 30,000 lives a year that are currently lost due to hospital-acquired infections, including MRSa infections.

◾ Impacts and Issues

Studies have indicated that a hospitalized patient who acquires MRSa is about five times more likely to die than a patient in the same hospital that does not carry the bacterium.

Variants of MRSa are appearing that are resistant even to vancomycin. These new forms of the bacterium, which are called vancomycin intermediate-resistant *Staphylococcus aureus*, are especially troublesome, as they can be treated with only a very few compounds. With time, further resistance could develop, and, if newer and more powerful (and likely more expensive) antibacterial agents have not been discovered and tested, there could be no means of combating the infections.

In 2006, researchers published a paper in *Nature* describing the development of a new antibiotic produced by a fungus. This antibiotic, called platensimycin, successfully treats MRSa infections, but further preclinical studies and human clinical trials are necessary before the drug can be approved for human use.

Community-acquired MRSa is a great concern. The organism tends to more aggressively invade tissues and produces a more severe infection than that produced by hospital-acquired MRSa, for reasons that are not yet clear. In addition, it has been discovered that MRSa can grow and divide inside another microscopic organism called *Acanthamoeba*. *Acanthamoeba* can become airborne and drift for a considerable distance on air currents. This may mean that MRSa is acquiring the ability to spread great distances, which would make treatment even harder.

SEE ALSO *Antibiotic Resistance; Contact Precautions; Resistant Organisms.*

BIBLIOGRAPHY

Books

Brunelle, Lynn, and Barbara Ravage. *Bacteria.* Milwaukee, WI: Gareth Stevens Publishing, 2003.

DiClaudio, Dennis. *The Hypochondriac's Pocket Guide to Horrible Diseases You Probably Already Have.* New York: Bloomsbury, 2005.

Roemmele, Jacqueline A., and Donna Batdorff. *Surviving the Flesh-eating Bacteria: Understanding, Preventing, Treating, and Living with Necrotizing Fascitis.* New York: Avery, 2003.

Periodicals

Cook, H., et al. "Heterosexual Transmission of Community-associated Methicillin-resistant Staphylococcus aureus." *Clinical & Infectious Disease* (2007) 44: 410–413.

Wang, J., et al. "Platensimycin Is a Selective FabF Inhibitor with Potent Antibiotic Properties." *Nature* (2006) 441: 358–363.

Brian Hoyle

Mumps

■ Introduction

Mumps is an acute viral illness whose main symptom is parotitis, an inflammation of the salivary glands in the neck. It was first described by the great Greek physician,

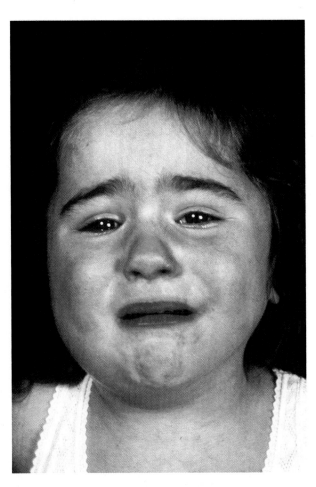

A child's face shows the telltale signs of mumps—swollen cheeks. *Biophoto Associates/Photo Researchers, Inc.*

Hippocrates, in the fifth century BC. Before an effective vaccination program was introduced in 1968, mumps was one of the most significant childhood diseases.

Mumps is as infectious as influenza and rubella (German measles), but somewhat less so than measles and chickenpox. Many of those infected with the virus have no symptoms at all. Mumps usually clears up within a week or so, and those infected then have lifelong immunity. However, the virus can spread through the lymph glands to cause a number of complications, including permanent deafness, so protecting children from mumps through vaccination is important. The introduction of vaccination for mumps has cut the rate of infections in the United States by 98%. However, local epidemics still sometimes occur.

■ Disease History, Characteristics, and Transmission

Mumps, also known as infectious parotitis, is caused by a paramyxovirus, which consists of single-stranded RNA (its genetic material [ribonucleic acid], as opposed to DNA [deoxyribonucleic acid]) surrounded by a protein envelope. The incubation period of the virus is 12–25 days, during which time it infects the upper respiratory tract and may pass to the glandular tissue of the ovaries, testes, or pancreas through the lymphatic system.

The most common symptom of mumps is parotitis, an inflammation of the salivary glands. The patient will experience pain, tenderness, and swelling in the jaw area, which may be accompanied by an earache. Approximately half of mumps infections are accompanied by parotitis. However, bacterial infection by *Staphylococcus* species can also cause parotitis, and that may be confused with mumps on diagnosis. Headache is another common symptom of mumps, and malaise, fever, and loss of appetite may also occur, especially in the early stages. Parotitis peaks about two days after its onset and the infection begins to clear within a week, with the vast

573

WORDS TO KNOW

MALAISE: Malaise is a general or nonspecific feeling of unease or discomfort, often the first sign of disease infection.

OOPHORITIS: Oophoritis is an inflammation of the ovary, which happens in certain sexually transmitted diseases.

ORCHITIS: Orchitis is inflammation of one or both testicles. Swelling and pain are typical symptoms. Orchitis may be caused by various sexually transmitted diseases or escape of sperm cells into the tissues of the testicle.

PANCREATITIS: Pancreatitis is an inflammation of the pancreas, an organ that is important in digestion. Pancreatitis can be acute (beginning suddenly, usually with the patient recovering fully) or chronic (progressing slowly with continued, permanent injury to the pancreas).

PARAMYXOVIRUS: Paramyxovirus is a type of virus that contains ribonucleic acid as the genetic material and has proteins on its surface that clump red blood cells and assist in the release of newly made viruses from the infected cells. Measles virus and mumps virus are two types of paramyxoviruses.

PAROTITIS: Parotitis is inflammation of the parotid gland. There are two parotid glands, one on each side of the jaw, at the back. Their function is to secret saliva into the mouth.

REPORTABLE DISEASE: By law, occurrences of some diseases must be reported to government authorities when observed by health-care professionals. Such diseases are called reportable diseases or notifiable diseases Cholera and yellow fever are examples of reportable diseases.

RIBONUCLEIC ACID (RNA): Any of a group of nucleic acids that carry out several important tasks in the synthesis of proteins. Unlike DNA (deoxyribonucleic acid), it has only a single strand. Nucleic acids are complex molecules that contain a cell's genetic information and the instructions for carrying out cellular processes. In eukaryotic cells, the two nucleic acids, ribonucleic acid (RNA) and deoxyribonucleic acid (DNA), work together to direct protein synthesis. Although it is DNA (deoxyribonucleic acid) that contains the instructions for directing the synthesis of specific structural and enzymatic proteins, several types of RNA actually carry out the processes required to produce these proteins. These include messenger RNA (mRNA), ribosomal RNA (rRNA), and transfer RNA (tRNA). Further processing of the various RNAs is carried out by another type of RNA called small nuclear RNA (snRNA). The structure of RNA is very similar to that of DNA, however, instead of the base thymine, RNA co

---

majority of patients making a full recovery. One attack of mumps confers lifelong immunity, therefore it does not recur.

However, mumps does sometimes cause complications and, indeed, is responsible for one death a year, on average, in the United States. When the virus spreads to the glands, it can cause orchitis (inflammation of the testicles), oophoritis (inflammation of the ovaries), pancreatitis, arthritis, and encephalitis. Central nervous system involvement in the form of asymptomatic meningitis is common, while symptomatic meningitis with headache and stiff neck occurs in up to 15% of patients, although this usually resolves itself within several days. Around one in 10,000–20,000 cases of mumps will lead to permanent deafness, with sudden onset. In 80% of these cases, the deafness is confined to one ear.

The mumps virus is spread by airborne transmission and through the droplets created by coughs and sneezes. Those infected will spread the virus about a week before they develop symptoms—if any occur—and will remain infectious for up to ten days after the symptoms begin. People without symptoms may still be infectious.

■ Scope and Distribution

The mumps virus affects both children and adults around the world, with the peak of infection occurring in late winter and early spring, although cases occur throughout the year as well. However, mass vaccination has had a dramatic impact on the number of cases of mumps where it is used. In World War I (1939-1945), only gonorrhea and influenza caused more hospitalizations than mumps among the military.

When it comes to the complications of mumps, adults appear to be more susceptible than children. Men in the 15–29 age group are the most susceptible to orchitis, which affects 20–50% of those developing mumps. In

30% of these cases, both testicles are affected, which raises the threat of infertility. However, although shrinkage of the testicles does occur in some cases of orchitis, infertility rarely results. Around 5% of young women with mumps will develop oophoritis, which may cause severe pelvic pain, but this complication is not linked to infertility. Pregnant women who develop mumps run an increased risk of spontaneous abortion. Mumps has been a reportable disease in the United States for several years.

■ Treatment and Prevention

Treatment of mumps infection includes hydration and painkillers. If headache is severe, then lumbar puncture may bring relief. Strong painkillers may be needed in cases of orchitis, because the pain can be quite severe. Children and adults with mumps should be excluded from school or work during the infectious period.

Mumps can be prevented by immunization with a live mumps vaccine. This is part of the measles, mumps and rubella (MMR) vaccine, which is given as childhood immunization—once at 12–15 months and again between four and six years of age. Although the mumps vaccine is generally safe, it should not be given to pregnant women, those with a fever, or patients with weakened immunity. There have been occasional side effects of mumps vaccine on the central nervous system, some of which have led to deafness. As with all airborne diseases, good personal hygiene helps prevent transmission. Therefore, people should always cover their nose and mouth when they cough or sneeze, and wash their hands regularly.

■ Impacts and Issues

Mumps was once a major childhood disease with occasional serious complications, such as deafness and infertility. Vaccination has changed that. Mumps became a reportable disease in the United States in 1968, when vaccination was introduced. Before that, there were an estimated 212,000 cases per year. However, between 1983 and 1985, there were only around 3,000 cases reported annually, demonstrating the value of mass vaccination.

In 1986 and 1987, there was a relative resurgence of mumps, with around 13,000 cases being reported in the United States. Most occurred in the 10–19 age group, who were born before vaccination was introduced. Since mumps can affect adults too, this was not unexpected. There were several outbreaks among highly vaccinated school populations, which suggested that a single dose might not be sufficient to protect children.

Since 1989, there has been a marked decline in the number of reported cases of mumps, from 5,712 cases to a total of 258 cases in 2004. But childhood infections like mumps can still come back unexpectedly. In 2006, there were outbreaks in several states, mostly among young adults, which led to a total of more than 6,000

IN CONTEXT: SCIENTIFIC, POLITICAL, AND ETHICAL ISSUES

With regard to a potential connection between the measles, mumps, and rubella vaccine (MMR vaccine) and autism, scientists at the National Immunization Program (NIP) at Centers for Disease Control and Prevention (CDC) state that "the weight of currently available scientific evidence does not support the hypothesis that MMR vaccine causes autism. CDC recognizes there is considerable public interest in this issue, and therefore supports additional research regarding this hypothesis. CDC is committed to maintaining the safest, most effective vaccine supply in history."

As of May 2007 the CDC further states that, "there is no convincing evidence that vaccines such as MMR cause long term health effects. On the other hand, we do know that people will become ill and some will die from the diseases this vaccine prevents. Measles outbreaks have recently occurred in the UK and Germany following an increase in the number of parents who chose not to have their children vaccinated with the MMR vaccine. Discontinuing a vaccine program based on unproven theories would not be in anyone's best interest. Isolated reports about these vaccines causing long term health problems may sound alarming at first. However, careful review of the science reveals that these reports are isolated and not confirmed by scientifically sound research. Detailed medical reviews of health effects reported after receipt of vaccines have often proven to be unrelated to vaccines, but rather have been related to other health factors. Because these vaccines are recommended widely to protect the health of the public, research on any serious hypotheses about their safety are important to pursue. Several studies are underway to investigate still unproven theories about vaccinations and severe side effects."

SOURCE: *Centers for Disease Control and Prevention, National Immunization Program*

---

reported cases. Most of these cases had received either one or two shots of MMR, but possibly had not developed a full immune response for some reason.

Introduction of mumps vaccine has been associated with a shift in the age at which people get the disease. Previously, 90% of cases occurred among children aged 15 or younger. But since 1990, those aged 15 or older have accounted for 30–40% of cases each year, with males and females being affected equally. These trends may reflect the effect of vaccine coverage in the population, and also the tendency of mumps to affect both children and young adults. Mumps is a disease that should not be taken lightly. Any lapse in vaccination coverage could lead to more outbreaks, with the attendant—albeit rare—complications.

SEE ALSO *Childhood Infectious Diseases, Immunization Impacts; Measles (Rubeola); Rubella.*

IN CONTEXT: SOCIAL AND PERSONAL RESPONSIBILITY

Social issues can still arise out of even the most effective and seemingly well-intended of medical advances. For example, although childhood diseases such as measles, mumps, whooping cough, and diphtheria have been effectively controlled by childhood vaccinations, some parents resist or reject vaccinating their own children because they feel that the small personal risk is not mitigated by the larger social benefit of disease control. By opting out of the system (by relying on the immunizations of others to reduce the risk of disease) they rely upon the acts their social group to offer their open children personal protection.

BIBLIOGRAPHY

Books

Wilks, David, Mark Farrington, and David Rubenstein. *The Infectious Disease*. 2nd ed. Malden: Blackwell, 2003.

Wilson, Walter R., and Merle A. *Current Diagnosis & Treatment in Infectious Diseases*. New York: McGraw Hill, 2001.

Web Sites

Centers for Disease Control and Prevention. "Pink Book—Mumps." <http://www.cdc.gov/nip/publications/pink/mumps.pdf> (accessed March 25, 2007).

Susan Aldridge

Mycotic Disease

■ Introduction

Mycotic diseases are caused by fungi, which are present in many forms in the environment. Many fungi are found in soil and are transmitted to humans either via cuts in the skin or by inhalation of the spores or cells of the fungi. Fungi can also inhabit moist environments, such as damp clothing, shoes, and showers. Transmission occurs when a person's skin comes in contact with the fungi. Other fungi may already be present in the human body at a certain population level (this is termed colonization) and cause infection only when the fungal population grows. An example of this is the common fungal infection of the mouth known as thrush.

Symptoms of a fungal disease can range from skin irritations to organ damage, such as lung disease. Fungi are characterized by the area of the body that they affect. Some fungi affect the outer layer of the skin, while others affect the cutaneous and subcutaneous layers of the skin. Furthermore, some fungi develop first in the lungs before spreading to other regions, while other fungi are opportunistic and develop wherever they can. Fungal infections are generally treated with antifungal drugs taken internally or applied externally. However, many of these drugs are toxic and cause side effects. In addition, some fungi are beginning to develop resistance to treatment making it difficult to eradicate an infection.

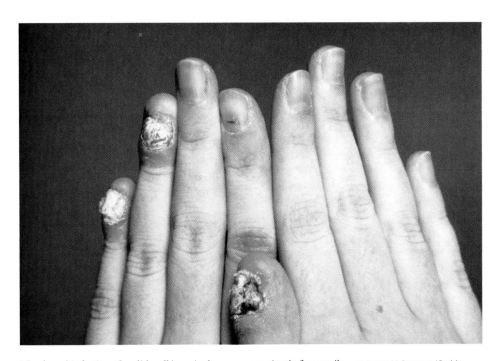

The fungal infection *Candida albicans* is shown on a patient's fingernails. © *Lester V. Bergman/Corbis.*

WORDS TO KNOW

COLONIZATION: Colonization is the process of occupation and increase in number of micro-organisms at a specific site.

CUTANEOUS: Pertaining to the skin.

IMMUNOCOMPROMISED: A reduction of the ability of the immune system to recognize and respond to the presence of foreign material.

OPPORTUNISTIC INFECTION: An opportunistic infection is so named because it occurs in people whose immune systems are diminished or are not functioning normally; such infections are opportunistic insofar as the infectious agents take advantage of their hosts' compromised immune systems and invade to cause disease.

SPORE: A dormant form assumed by some bacteria, such as anthrax, that enable the bacterium to survive high temperatures, dryness, and lack of nourishment for long periods of time. Under proper conditions, the spore may revert to the actively multiplying form of the bacteria.

Disease History, Characteristics, and Transmission

Different types of fungi affect different regions of the body and mycotic diseases are characterized according to the region being affected. Superficial infections involve the outer layers of the skin and hair; cutaneous infections involve the epidermis, hair and nails; and subcutaneous infections involve the dermis, subcutaneous tissues, and muscle. There are also systemic infections that are caused by either primary fungi or opportunistic fungi. Primary fungi originate in the lungs before spreading infection to other organ systems. Opportunistic fungi infect anywhere in the body. Opportunistic fungal infections tend to occur most commonly in people with a suppressed or weakened immune system, when their health is already compromised.

Fungal infections cause a range of symptoms depending on the body region they infect. Cutaneous (skin) infections such as tinea, which is a disease of the skin, tend to result in itchy, peeling skin, sometimes with pus or inflamed areas. These symptoms are usually not life threatening, but can cause discomfort and irritation. Subcutaneous infections tend to occur when fungi enter under the skin and forms lesions as they grow. Systemic fungi originate in the lungs and eventually spread to other organs, potentially causing tissue damage, ulcers, and pulmonary symptoms. Opportunistic fungi can potentially cause disease in any region of the body.

Humans develop fungal infections when they come in contact with a fungus. Some fungi are present in the soil. Therefore, when soil is disturbed, for example, during an earthquake or while gardening, fungal spores can become airborne and be inhaled. The fungi can then cause infection. Other fungi thrive in moist, dark conditions. Therefore, moist clothing, shoes, or certain rooms, such as bathrooms, can harbor fungi. When humans come in contact with these fungi, infection can occur. One example is athlete's foot, a type of tinea. Often the fungi responsible for this disease will develop in shoes or in showers and can be spread from these sources. One common fungi from the genus *Candida* gives rise to thrush, a common infection that causes an itchy rash. This infection can occur in the genital area, in the mouth, or in the bloodstream. The fungus is already present in humans in small amounts, and infection occurs when the fungus grows out of control, often in response to a hormonal imbalance.

Scope and Distribution

There are a range of mycotic diseases worldwide. A common fungal infection is tinea, which refers to cutaneous infection of various parts of the body. This infection is common on the feet where it is known as athlete's foot, and in the crotch where it is known as jock itch. Both of these infections can be present in males and females and spread of this disease is facilitated by shared locker rooms or showers where people tend to walk around barefoot.

Some infections occur more commonly in certain people, or people with certain conditions. Genital thrush, which is caused by the fungus *Candida*, is very common in women, and is also more common during pregnancy, in women with diabetes mellitus, or in women using broad-spectrum antibiotics or corticosteroid medications.

Immunocompromised people appear to be at a significantly greater risk of developing fungal infections. Even fungi that normally do not cause infections in healthy people have been found to cause illness in people with compromised immune systems, such as are caused by certain conditions including cancer, diabetes, or AIDS. In addition, some fungal infections can cause more severe symptoms when they develop in these people. For example, HIV-infected people may develop severe pulmonary disease leading to death following infection by the fungus *Coccidioides immitis*. Other factors such as stress can also increase the likelihood of a fungal infection.

Fungal infections occur worldwide, although specific infections may be found only in some locations. Cryptococcosis, a fungal infection that causes potentially fatal meningitis, can be found in soils worldwide. Coccodioidomycosis on the other hand is endemic to areas in the United States, Mexico, and South America. The potential to pick up a fungal infection depends on whether it is present within the country, and whether living or working conditions promote the growth and transmission of the fungus. Sporotrichosis occurs in hay and is transferred via cuts in the skin. Therefore, individuals, such as farmers, who handle hay on a regular basis are more susceptible to this fungal infection.

■ Treatment and Prevention

Fungal infections are generally treated using antifungal drugs. These drugs can be taken orally, via the genital tract, or applied externally. Some common antifungal treatments contain azole derivatives and actively prevent the fungus from producing ergosterol. Ergosterol is used by fungal cells to produce a cell membrane, and lack of ergosterol results in cell death and death of the fungus. However, many treatments for fungal infections are extremely toxic and can cause serious side effects, if used incorrectly.

As no vaccines are available for mycotic diseases, avoidance or removal of fungi is the best method of prevention. Maintaining high sanitary standards can help avoid coming into contact with potentially dangerous fungi. For example, wearing bath shoes in communal showers, avoiding wearing moist clothes, or drying damp shoes can all help prevent contracting the fungus responsible for athlete's foot. Thorough cleaning of contaminated items, such as clothing and bedclothes, using hot water and detergent may remove the fungi from these items, and prevent infection.

For fungi that can be transmitted via airborne spores or cells, avoiding areas in which soil has been disturbed will help minimize contact with fungal spores. For example, in an area where soil fungi are a potential problem, wearing a facemask following an earthquake may help prevent infection. Wearing gloves can also provide protection against soil fungi that are transmitted via cuts in the skin. This is one way to avoid sporotrichosis, which is caused by fungi present in bales of hay or other plant materials that are often harvested and used by humans.

■ Impacts and Issues

The U.S. Centers for Disease Control and Prevention, Division of Bacterial and Mycotic Diseases reports that mycotic infections are becoming an increasing risk to the

---

IN CONTEXT: FUNGI

Fungi play an essential role in breaking down organic matter and thereby allowing nutrients to be recycled in nature. As such, they are important decomposers and without them living communities would become buried in their own waste. Some fungi, the saprobes, get their nutrients from nonliving organic matter, such as dead plants and animal wastes, clothing, paper, leather, and other materials. Others, the parasites, obtain nutrients from the tissues of living organisms. Both types of fungi obtain nutrients by secreting enzymes from their cells that break down large organic molecules into smaller components. The fungi cells can then absorb the nutrients.

Although the term fungus invokes unpleasant images and can be a source of disease, fungi are also a source of antibiotics, vitamins, and industrial chemicals. Yeast, a form of fungi, is used to ferment bread and alcoholic beverages.

In addition to human diseases fungi also cause food spoilage, wheat and corn diseases, and, perhaps most well known, the Irish potato famine of 1843–1847 (caused by the fungus *Phytophthora infestans*), which contributed to the deaths of 250,000 people in Ireland.

---

public health. Immunocompromised people, such as cancer patients, HIV-infected individuals, and people with diseases such as diabetes, are at a high risk of developing fungal infections due to opportunistic fungi, such as aspergillosis, candidiasis, and cryptococcosis. Furthermore, new forms of old fungal infections, such as coccidioidomycosis, are occurring in these patients. In addition, previously harmless fungi, which normally grow in rotting food, soil, or plants, are now causing potentially fatal or debilitating infections in immunocompromised individuals.

Another issue of significant concern is the development of resistance to antifungal drugs by certain strains of fungi. This has occurred in response to the use of antifungal treatments for fungal infections. For example, in some people, *Candida* fungi, which cause thrush, have developed resistance to the antifungal treatments used to eradicate this infection. Therefore, fewer treatment options are available as the fungi become resistant to the certain drugs.

The rise in the number of mycotic infections has led to a increased research into the control and prevention of fungal diseases. Mycotic disease research involves determining the cause of outbreaks, risk of outbreaks, outbreak trends, and methods of control.

SEE ALSO *Antibiotic Resistance; Aspergillosis; Blastomycosis; Candidiasis; Coccidioidomycosis;*

Cryptococcus neoformans Infection; Histoplasmosis; Opportunistic Infection; Ringworm; Sporotrichosis.

BIBLIOGRAPHY

Books

Dismukes, W. E., P.G. Pappas, and J.D. Sobel. *Clinical Mycology.* New York: Oxford University Press, 2003.

Howard, D.H. *Pathogenic Fungi in Humans and Animals.* New York: Marcel Dekker, 2003.

Web Sites

Centers for Disease Control and Prevention. "WHO Collaborating Center for the Mycoses." February 5, 2007. <http://www.cdc.gov/ncidod/dbmd/mdb/index.htm> (accessed March 6, 2007).

Southern Illinois University. "Mycotic Infections." <http://www.cehs.siu.edu/fix/medmicro/mycotic.htm> (accessed March 6, 2007).

National Institute of Allergy and Infectious Diseases

■ Introduction

The National Institute of Allergy and Infectious Diseases (NIAID) is part of the National Institutes of Health (NIH). The NIH, in turn, is an arm of the United States Department of Health and Human Services of the U.S. federal government. NIAID's mission is to conduct and support research into the causes of allergic, immunologic, and infectious diseases and to develop better ways to prevent, diagnose, and treat such illnesses. It does so both by funding its own researchers and by granting billions of dollars annually to researchers in universities and industry to pay for research. Scientists wishing to receive grants must apply to NIAID for them competitively. Some of

NIAID's many areas of investigation are acquired immunodeficiency syndrome (AIDS, also cited as acquired immune deficiency syndrome), allergic diseases, defense of the public against possible terrorism using bacteria or viruses, radiation exposure, emerging infectious diseases, genetics and transplantation, immune-mediated diseases such as asthma and organ rejection, vaccine development, sexually transmitted infections, and malaria.

■ History of Organization

In 1948, two government-funded biology laboratories, the Rocky Mountain Laboratory and Biologics Control

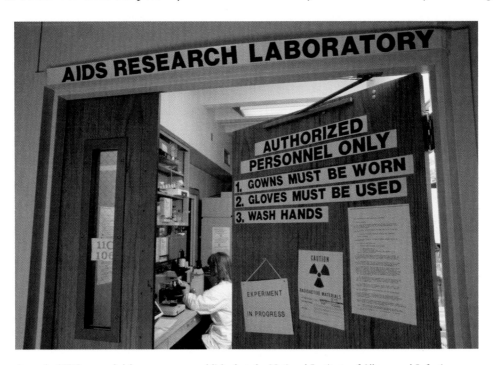

An early AIDS research laboratory was established at the National Institute of Allergy and Infectious Diseases. © Nathan Benn/Corbis.

WORDS TO KNOW

EMERGING INFECTIOUS DISEASE: New infectious diseases such as SARS and West Nile virus, as well as previously known diseases such as malaria, tuberculosis, and bacterial pneumonias that are appearing in forms that are resistant to drug treatments, are termed emerging infectious diseases.

GENOME: All of the genetic information for a cell or organism. The complete sequence of genes within a cell or virus.

PANDEMIC: Pandemic, which means all the people, describes an epidemic that occurs in more than one country or population simultaneously.

STRAIN: A subclass or a specific genetic variation of an organism.

T-CELL VACCINE: A T-cell vaccine is one that relies on eliciting cellular immunity, rather than humoral antibody-based immunity, against infection. T cell vaccines are being developed against the human immunodeficiency virus (HIV) and hepatitis C.

Intramural Research, and (7) Division of Microbiology and Infectious Diseases.

Several of these divisions are devoted specifically to supporting medical research:

- The Division of AIDS was founded in 1986. Its mission is to increase basic scientific knowledge of the disease in order to end the AIDS epidemic (as of early 2007, almost 40 million people were infected with AIDS worldwide and over 25 million had already been killed by the disease).

- The Division of Allergy, Immunology, and Transplantation supports research to unravel the mechanisms underlying disease of the immune system, with the goal of more effective treatment and prevention.

- The Division of Intramural Research oversees research by the 17 laboratories owned and operated by NIAID, all located in Maryland and Montana.

- The Division of Microbiology and Infectious Diseases supports research to control and prevent diseases caused by infectious agents other than human immunodeficiency virus (HIV), the cause of AIDS. For example, this division funds projects to sequence the genomes of infectious agents. NIAID-funded researchers have sequenced the genomes (the complete genetic content of an organism) of the bacterium that causes Lyme disease (*Borrelia burgdorferi*) and a number of others.

■ **Impacts and Issues**

Due to the scope of NIAID's efforts, basic scientific knowledge of many diseases has been greatly increased. Further, a number of vaccines have been developed using NIAID funds. In 2005, NIAID made its first cash research grants under Project Bioshield, the Federal program to defend the public against possible bioterrorism. Its attempt to fund private-sector development of a vaccine for anthrax, one of the candidate organisms for use as a terror weapon, has not yet proved successful, as the vaccine was not successfully developed by its original target date.

Other vaccine challenges for the NIAID include the pursuit of a vaccine to protect against HIV/AIDS. The current NIAID-sponsored candidates for an HIV vaccine are not formulated to prevent infection as do most vaccines, but instead could delay the onset of AIDS by keeping the levels of HIV in the blood in check. Called T-cell vaccines, these types of vaccines could also reduce the ability of an infected individual to transmit the HIV virus to others. Several T-cell vaccines will soon begin expanded clinical trials, and although they have potential benefits in the battle against HIV/AIDS, the NIAID continues to pursue a traditional type vaccine that would prevent the establishment altogether of HIV infection.

Influenza, in both its seasonal and potential pandemic forms, is also major focus of NIAID research and

Laboratory (both founded in 1902), were combined with two divisions of the National Institute of Health into a single organization, the National Microbiological Institute. This was the organization that eventually became NIAID. In 1951, the National Microbiological Institute began distributing cash grants to support research by scientists, and in 1955 was renamed NIAID. In the following decades, the types of research supported by NIAID multiplied and its organizational structure was repeatedly reorganized to deal with this widening range of concerns. For example, in 1986, the organization established an Acquired Immunodeficiency Syndrome Program to coordinate the institute's support of research into AIDS, then a recently-discovered disease.

A number of research laboratories have been established by NIAID over the years. For example, the Laboratory of Immunoregulation was established in 1980, the Laboratory of Molecular Microbiology in 1981, the Laboratory of Immunopathology in 1985, the Laboratory of Allergic Diseases in 1994, and so forth. In 2002, as part of the national response to the terrorist attacks of 2001, an Office of Biodefense Research Affairs was established within the Division of Microbiology and Infectious Diseases.

Today, NIAID is organized into seven divisions: (1) Office of the Director, (2) Vaccine Research Center, (3) Division of Acquired Immunodeficiency Syndrome, (4) Division of Allergy, Immunology, and Transplantation, (5) Division of Extramural Activities, (6) Division of resources. In April 2007, the NIAID announced that its researchers, along with an international team, used antibodies taken from humans who survived the H5N1 avian influenza (bird flu) to successfully treat mice infected with H5N1, and also to successfully prevent uninfected mice from acquiring the disease. NIAID researchers plan to move ahead with this research by further testing in animals, and if successful, then in human volunteers. Ultimately, this line of research could yield both a vaccine and an effective treatment for H5N1, a strain (type) of influenza virus often cited by scientists as a likely candidate to begin a new influenza pandemic.

SEE ALSO *CDC (Centers for Disease Control and Prevention); Epidemiology; Public Health and Infectious Disease.*

BIBLIOGRAPHY

Books

Brower, Jennifer, and Peter Chalk. *The Global Threat of New and Reemerging Infectious Diseases: Reconciling U.S. National Security and Public Health Policy.* Santa Monica, CA: Rand Corporation, 2003.

Periodicals

Kaiser, Jocelyn. "Quick Save for Infectious-Disease Grants at NIAID." *Science.* 303(2004):941.

Web Sites

National Institute of Allergy and Infectious Diseases. <http://www3.niaid.nih.gov/> (accessed February 9, 2007).

Necrotizing Fasciitis

■ Introduction

Necrotizing fasciitis is a rare, and often fatal, infection by the bacterium *Streptococcus pyogenes*, also known as group-A streptococcus or GAS. Varieties of this bacterium also cause a wide range of other diseases, including strep throat, impetigo, cellulitis, erysipelas, scarlet fever, rheumatic fever, and more. To necrotize tissue is to kill it, and the word fasciitis signifies inflammation of the fascia, which are the thin sheaths of fibrous connective tissue that cover the muscles and other organs. In necrotizing fasciitis,

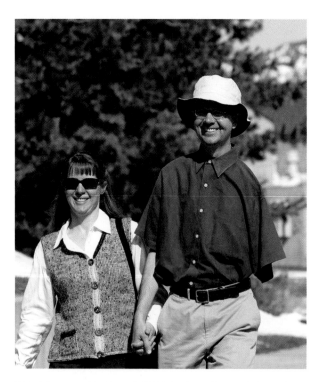

Nobel laureate Eric Cornell (1961–), shown here with his wife, Celeste Landry, had to have his left arm and shoulder amputated to stop necrotizing fasciitis. *AP Images.*

group-A streptococci infect the deeper layers of the skin and the fascia in the tissue underneath the skin. Although this disease has often been referred to in the press as being caused by "flesh-eating bacteria," GAS is not flesh-eating; that is, it does not actually eat away the flesh of victims of necrotizing fasciitis. Rather, GAS releases toxins that cause the body's own immune system to dissolve certain tissues. Necrotizing fasciitis first became popularly known in the 1990s. There was fear that it would become widespread, but it has remained rare. Necrotizing fasciitis is only one form of invasive group-A streptococcus infection. Other closely related forms include streptococcal toxic-shock syndrome (multi-organ infection) and bacteremia (infection of the blood).

■ Disease History, Characteristics, and Transmission

The German-Austrian surgeon Christian Theodor Billroth (1829–1894) first described the streptococci bacterium. Billroth discovered *Streptococcus pyogenes* growing in infected wounds. The streptococci are gram-positive bacteria that tend to clump in pairs or chains and are classed into two basic types based on their ability to cause partial or complete hemolysis (breakdown of blood cells). Group A streptococci, which cause complete hemolysis, are further subdivided into a series of alphabetically labeled groups called Lancefield groups. In the 1930s, Rebecca Lancefield (1895–1981) defined the Lancefield groups using standard laboratory tests. She also showed that a protein in the GAS cell wall, M protein, is important to this bacterium's disease-causing power. Varying types of M protein can be used to distinguish over 120 different varieties of *S. pyogenes*, including those that cause necrotizing fasciitis.

Shifts in the M proteins and other substances produced by various strains of *S. pyogenes* are caused by genetic mutations and by genetic alterations caused by viruses (which can change the DNA of bacteria and other cells).

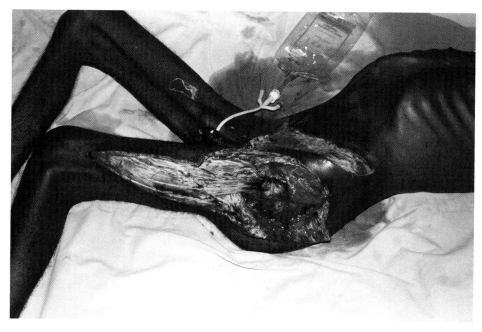

The leg of a 15-year-old African AIDS patient shows extensive tissue loss due to necrotizing fasciitis, a bacterial infection of connective tissue.   *Dr. M.A. Ansary/Photo Researchers, Inc.*

Because of these changes, the virulence (tendency to cause disease) of various *S. pyogenes* strains waxes and wanes over time. During World War II (1939–1945), for example, there were reports of GAS bacteria causing toxic shock and destruction of tissue. These reports then abated until the late 1980s, when clusters of such infections began appearing in Australia, New Zealand, Scandinavia, and the central United States. A survey of four American states by the U.S. Centers for Disease Control and Prevention (CDC) conducted from 1989 to 1991 estimated that 10,000–15,000 invasive group A streptococcus infections were occurring in the U.S. each year. British tabloid writers coined the phrase "flesh-eating bacteria" to describe the new type of GAS infection. Necrotizing fasciitis has continued to occur at a more or less steady rate in the years since, neither disappearing nor becoming epidemic.

There are several types of life-threatening, invasive streptococcus A infections. Necrotizing fasciitis is a deep-seated infection of the tissues beneath the outer skin that destroys fascia and fat but may or may not destroy muscle and skin. It can be caused not only by *S. pyogenes* but, less commonly, by *Clostridium perfringens* or *C. septicum*. Necrotizing fasciitis may be caused by a blend of organisms in patients with diabetes or open wounds contaminated with fecal matter. An early term for the condition was "streptococcal gangrene." Infections can begin at the site of a major or even invisible breakage of the skin. Typically, within 24 hours a lesion or sore spot appears at the wound site that is red, hot, and painful to the touch. There may also be fever. In the next 24–48 hours, the lesion becomes purple, violet, or

blue, and blisters appear. Influenzalike symptoms occur in about 20% of cases, with symptoms including nausea, diarrhea, confusion, weakness, and tiredness. In three to four days gangrene may appear, with the entire limb, in some cases, appearing necrotic. The disease can cause death through shock, kidney failure, and respiratory arrest.

S. pyogenes is transmitted by direct contact or via airborne saliva droplets released by sneezing or coughing. Necrotizing fasciitis occurs when an appropriate strain of *S. pyogenes* enters a break in the skin. The break may be a large wound or a pinprick; in half of all cases, the break through which the pathogen entered cannot be identified.

■ Scope and Distribution

Severe invasive group-A streptococcal disease, including necrotizing fasciitis, is primarily found in Europe and North America. In 2004, 3,833 cases of severe group A streptococcal disease were reported to the CDC.

■ Treatment and Prevention

Necrotizing fasciitis is treated with antibiotics, including penicillin, erythromycin, and clindamycin. In some cases, treatment may require amputation or other surgery to remove damaged tissue. Prompt care is essential. Without antibiotics, the death rate for invasive group-A streptococcus infection, including necrotizing fasciitis, is

WORDS TO KNOW

CLINICAL TRIALS: According to the National Institutes of Health, a clinical trial is "a research study to answer specific questions about vaccines or new therapies or new ways of using known treatments." These studies allow researchers to determine whether new drugs or treatments are safe and effective. When conducted carefully, clinical trials can provide fast and safe answers to these questions.

FASCIA: Fascia is a type of connective tissue made up of a network of fibers. It is best thought of as being the packing material of the body. Fascia surrounds muscles, bones, and joints and lies between the layers of skin. It functions to hold these structures together, protecting these structures and defining the shape of the body. When surrounding a muscle, fascia helps prevent a contracting muscle from catching or causing excessive friction on neighboring muscles.

GANGRENE: Gangrene is the destruction of body tissue by a bacteria called *Clostridium perfringens*, or a combination of streptococci and staphylococci bacteria. C. perfringens is found widespread in soil and the intestinal tracts of humans and animals. It becomes dangerous only when its spores germinate, producing toxins and destructive enzymes, and germination occurs only in an anaerobic environment (one almost totally devoid of oxygen). While gangrene can develop in any part of the body,

it is most common in fingers, toes, hands, feet, arms, and legs, the parts of the body most susceptible to restricted blood flow. Even a slight injury in such an area is at high risk of causing gangrene. Early treatment with antibiotics, such as penicillin, and surgery to remove the dead tissue will often reduce the need for amputation. If left untreated, gangrene results in amputation or death.

HEMOLYSIS: The destruction of blood cells, an abnormal rate of which may lead to lowered levels of these cells. For example, Hemolytic anemia is caused by destruction of red blood cells at a rate faster than which they can be produced.

M PROTEIN: M protein is an antibody found in unusually large amounts in the blood or urine of patients with multiple myeloma, a form of cancer that arises in the white blood cells that produce antibodies.

MUTATION: A mutation is a change in an organism's DNA that occurs over time and may render it less sensitive to drugs which are used against it.

NECROTIC: Necrotic tissue is dead tissue in an otherwise living body. Tissue death is called necrosis.

STREPTOCOCCUS: A genus of bacteria that includes species such as *Streptococci pyogenes* a species of bacteria that causes strep throat.

IN CONTEXT: TRENDS AND STATISTICS

The Division of Bacterial and Mycotic Diseases at Centers for Disease Control and Prevention (CDC) states that About 9,400 cases of invasive GAS disease occurred in the United States in 1999. Of these, about 300 were streptococcal toxic shock syndrome (STSS) and 600 were necrotizing fasciitis. In contrast, there are several million cases of strep throat and impetigo each year.

SOURCE: *Centers for Disease Control and Prevention (CDC), Coordinating Center for Infectious Diseases, Division of Bacterial and Mycotic Diseases*

nearly 100%. Even with treatment the death rate is estimated by various experts at 25% to as much as 70%. In the 1990s, when public concern over this disease was at

its height, Dr. Vincent Fischetti of Rockefeller University in New York advised the public that "If you see a rapidly progressing reddening area that is hot and quite sore to the touch and if you are running a fever, I would go to the doctor very quickly."

■ Impacts and Issues

Public consciousness of invasive group A streptococcal disease, including necrotizing fasciitis, has been out of proportion to the number of deaths it causes as compared to many other diseases and behaviors. Undoubtedly, one reason for this is the dramatic nature of the disease. A bacterial infection that "eats flesh" and has a 25–70% fatality rate even with the best medical care is certainly attention-getting. In addition, there have been a number of well-publicized deaths from the disease, including leading British economist David Walton (1963–2006), who died within 24 hours of diagnosis.

A vaccine for group-A streptococcus is being investigated, but remains elusive. According to the World Health Organization (WHO), clinical trials—experiments in human volunteers designed to test the vaccine's effectiveness and safety—are under way, but will probably take years to complete.

SEE ALSO *Impetigo; Puerperal Fever; Scarlet Fever; Streptococcal Infections, Group A; Streptococcal Infections, Group B.*

BIBLIOGRAPHY

Books

ICON Health Publications. *Necrotizing Fasciitis.* San Diego, CA: ICON Health Publications, 2004.

Periodicals

Factor, Stephanie H., et al. "Invasive Group A Streptococcal Disease: Risk Factors for Adults." *Emerging Infectious Diseases* 9 (2003): 970–977.

Factor, Stephanie H., et al. "Risk Factors for Pediatric Invasive Group A Streptococcal Disease." *Emerging Infectious Diseases* 11 (2005): 1062–1066.

Kolata, Gina. "A Dangerous Form of Strep Stirs Concern in Resurgence." *New York Times* (June 8, 1994).

Musher, Daniel M., et al. "Trends in Bacteremic Infection Due to *Streptococcus pyogenes* (Group A Streptococcus), 1986–1995." *Emerging Infectious Diseases* 2 (1996): 54–56.

Stevens, Dennis L. "Streptococcal Toxic-Shock Syndrome: Spectrum of Disease, Pathogenesis, and New Concepts in Treatment." *Emerging Infectious Diseases* 1 (1995): 69–76.

IN CONTEXT: REAL-WORLD RISKS

The Division of Bacterial and Mycotic Diseases at Centers for Disease Control and Prevention (CDC) states that "two of the most severe, but least common, forms of invasive GAS disease are necrotizing fasciitis and streptococcal toxic shock syndrome. Necrotizing fasciitis (occasionally described by the media as 'the flesh-eating bacteria') destroys muscles, fat, and skin tissue. Streptococcal toxic shock syndrome (STSS) causes blood pressure to drop rapidly and organs (e.g., kidney, liver, lungs) to fail. STSS is not the same as the 'toxic shock syndrome' frequently associated with tampon usage. About 20% of patients with necrotizing fasciitis, and more than half with STSS, die. About 10%–15% of patients with other forms of invasive group A streptococcal disease die."

SOURCE: *Centers for Disease Control and Prevention (CDC), Coordinating Center for Infectious Diseases, Division of Bacterial and Mycotic Diseases.*

Web Sites

National Institute of Allergy and Infectious Diseases. "Group A Streptococcal Infections." November 2005. <http://www.niaid.nih.gov/factsheets/strep.htm> (accessed February 14, 2007).

National Necrotizing Fasciitis Foundation. "Home Page." January 28, 2007. <http://www.nnff.org/> (accessed February 14, 2007).

Nipah Virus Encephalitis

Introduction

Nipah virus is best known as the causative agent of a large outbreak of disease among pigs in Malaysia in 1999. It is a member of the Paramyxoviridae family of viruses and is naturally harbored in fruit bats of the *Pteropus* genus in Malaysia.

The virus may be transmitted to pigs in contact with bat urine or feces and subsequently spread to humans through contact with the pig's bodily fluids on pig farms and in abattoirs (slaughterhouses). In humans, Nipah virus infection presents as encephalitis and respiratory disease and carries a significant mortality rate. Treatment is limited to reducing symptoms, but appropriate preventative measures may be implemented to limit spread.

Nipah virus is considered an emerging infectious disease and is argued to pose a significant potential threat to human health. The impact of this viral infection is evident both economically and socially and the recent evidence of person-to-person transmission raises significant cause for public concern.

Disease History, Characteristics, and Transmission

Nipah virus was first isolated in 1999 during an outbreak of encephalitis and respiratory illness among a group of men in Malaysia. The outbreak resulted in 265 cases of encephalitis, 105 of which were fatal. The virus was named after the location in which it was first detected, Sungai Nipah New Village. Affecting pigs and humans, Nipah virus is a member of the *Henipavirus* genus of the Paramyxoviridae family. The natural reservoir of the virus is argued to be *Pteropus* fruit bats.

Transmission from bats to pigs is thought to occur when pigs are exposed to the urine and feces of the bats. Humans may contract the disease following exposure to contaminated tissue and bodily fluids of infected pigs.

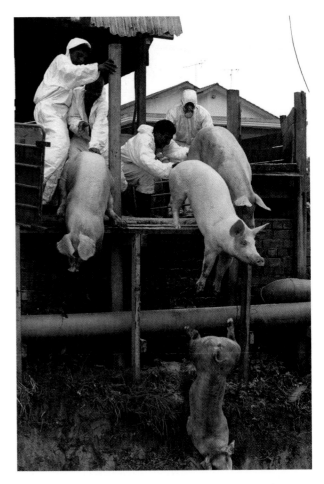

Farm workers hurl pigs into a large grave in Malaysia during a 1999 outbreak of a disease caused by a newly emergent pathogen called the Nipah virus. In an effort to halt the transmission of the epidemic, health authorities killed more than 300,000 pigs that were suspected of carrying the virus. The epidemic killed more than 100 people in Malaysia. *AP Images.*

Person-to-person transmission has been suspected in more recent cases.

In humans, infections are primarily encephalitic after an incubation period of 4–18 days. Symptoms initially include fever and headache, followed by drowsiness and disorientation, nausea, weakness, and in some cases, respiratory illness. In 60% of patients, these signs and symptoms may progress to coma within 24–48 hours. In pigs, the virus generally produced only mild illness, characterized by respiratory distress.

■ Scope and Distribution

It has been observed that the *Pteropus* genus of fruit bats are susceptible to Nipah virus infection, but do not develop illness. Populations of these bats are distributed across a wide area, including the northern, eastern and southeastern regions of Australia, Indonesia, Malaysia, the Philippines, and other Pacific islands.

This disease has a wide host range, which accounts for the emergence of Nipah virus as a zootic pathogen. Those people most at risk of contracting the disease are those working in close association with infected pigs in areas of where the virus is endemic (naturally present).

Nipah virus was first implicated in encephalitis in the outbreak of neurological and respiratory disease that occurred on Malaysian pig farms in 1999. Cases also occurred in Singapore in 1999 and were attributed to pigs that had been imported from the infected Malaysian pig farms. Between 2001 and 2005, six outbreaks occurred in India and Bangladesh. These were all in areas where *Pteropus* fruit bats live, suggesting that the spread of the virus is limited to those areas where these fruit bats are found.

■ Treatment and Prevention

During the initial outbreaks of Nipah virus infection, the antiviral drug ribavirin was used and was deemed helpful in reducing the duration of feverish illness and the severity of the disease. However, the precise clinical usefulness of the drug remains uncertain. The usual treatment for infected persons is intensive supportive care. Researchers have made progress in identifying the way in which the virus enters cells and replicates, and this knowledge could potentially lead to an effective treatment for the virus.

Nipah virus infection may be prevented by avoiding contact with animals known to harbor the infection and by using appropriate personal protective equipment when handling infected tissue. Transmission of the virus from bats to pigs may be avoided by minimizing the overlap of the habitats of these animals, thus reducing the likelihood that pigs will come into contract with bat urine, feces, or partially eaten fruits.

WORDS TO KNOW

EMERGING INFECTIOUS DISEASE: New infectious diseases such as SARS and West Nile virus, as well as previously known diseases such as malaria, tuberculosis, and bacterial pneumonias that are appearing in forms that are resistant to drug treatments, are termed emerging infectious diseases.

ENDEMIC: Present in a particular area or among a particular group of people.

HOST: Organism that serves as the habitat for a parasite, or possibly for a symbiont. A host may provide nutrition to the parasite or symbiont, or simply a place in which to live.

STRAIN: A subclass or a specific genetic variation of an organism.

■ Impacts and Issues

Nipah virus is classified as an emerging infectious disease by the United States Centers for Disease Control and Prevention (CDC). It is considered a cause for public concern due to the significant mortality rates observed following infection, as well as the social impacts of the infection.

Later human outbreaks of the disease in Bangladesh were characterized by a high rate of respiratory disease, which potentially increases the chances of person-to-person transmission and may indicate the emergence of more dangerous strains (types) of the virus. It is assumed that the virus did not emerge suddenly, but has been slowly adapting to humans as a host and therefore poses an greater threat.

Nipah virus infection among pigs carries a significant economic impact. The 1999 outbreak in Malaysia caused about one million pigs to be slaughtered. This loss of potential income exacts an economic toll on both individual farmers and the community as a whole.

SEE ALSO *Antiviral Drugs; Emerging Infectious Diseases; Viral Disease; Zoonoses.*

BIBLIOGRAPHY

Books

Mandell, G.L., J.E. Bennett, and R. Dolin. *Principles and Practice of Infectious Diseases.* 6th ed. Philadelphia: Elsevier, 2004.

Periodicals

Butler, D. "Fatal Fruit Bat Virus Sparks Epidemics in Southern Asia." *Nature* 429 (May 6, 2004): 7.

Pulliam, J.R., H.E. Field, and K.J. Olival. "Nipah Virus Strain Variation." *Emerging Infectious Diseases* 11 (December 2005): 1978–1979.

Web Sites

Centers for Disease Control and Prevention. "Hendra Virus Disease and Nipah Virus Encephalitis." August 23, 2004. <http://www.cdc.gov/ncidod/dvrd/spb/mnpages/dispages/nipah.htm> (accessed March 28, 2007).

Commonwealth Scientific and Industrial Research Organisation (CSIRO). "Fighting Nipah Virus." May 23, 2006. <http://www.csiro.au/science/ps1so.html> (accessed March 28, 2007).

World Health Organization. "Nipah Virus." September 2001. <http://www.who.int/mediacentre/factsheets/fs262/en/> (accessed March 28, 2007).

Nocardiosis

Introduction

Nocardiosis is a serious infectious disease with a high mortality (death) rate. It is caused by funguslike bacteria that affect the lungs (pulmonary nocardiosis), skin (nocardiosis), or the entire body (disseminated or systemic nocardiosis), especially the brain and meninges. According to the U.S. Centers for Disease Control and Prevention (CDC), the majority of cases—about 80%—involves lung infections, brain abscesses, or disseminated (widespread) diseases. The other 20% of cases involve

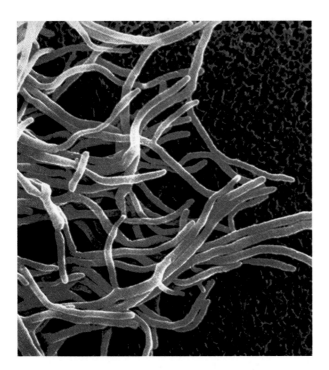

This colored scanning electron micrograph (SEM) shows the *Nocardia* bacteria. One species of this gram-positive bacteria causes nocardiosis, a rare pulmonary infection that affects people with weakened immune systems. *BSIP/Photo Researchers, Inc.*

the skin. With respect to cures, when the skin and soft tissues are involved, cure rates are about 100%; when the lungs are involved, the cure rate is about 90% of the cases; disseminated cases are cured about 63% of the time; and when the brain is involved, the cure rate drops to 50% These cure rates are only achieved when proper therapy is given in a timely manner.

The infection itself is caused by bacteria of the genus *Nocardia*. At least 15 species have so far been identified, with new species still being found. The bacteria that cause infection the most frequently are: *Nocardia astreoides* and *Nocardia brasiliensis*. However, *N. farcinica*, *N. nova*, *N. transvalensis*, and *N. pseudobrasiliensis* also cause infection. *N. astreoides* is responsible for about 50% of all invasive cases, and is the species responsible for the most cases of nocardiosis in the United States.

Disease History, Characteristics, and Transmission

Nocardia are often found in soil and dust particles. They cause occasional disease in humans and animals around the world. Transmission of pulmonary nocardiosis is usually accomplished by inhalation of the organisms when they are within airborne dust particles. Transmission of systemic nocardiosis usually occurs by direct contact with soil through puncture wounds. Abrasions (scrapes) can also be a route for transmission, but less frequently than the other two means. There are no known cases of human-to-human transmission of *Nocardia*. The incubation period is not known, however, it is suspected to be several weeks.

Symptoms of the pulmonary form are usually chills, fever, cough (similar to pneumonia or tuberculosis), thick (often bloody) sputum, night sweats, and chest pain. When the bacteria affect the brain, symptoms usually include severe headaches, lethargy, disorientation, confusion, dizziness, nausea and seizures, problems with

WORDS TO KNOW

CUTANEOUS: Pertaining to the skin.

IMMUNOCOMPROMISED: A reduction of the ability of the immune system to recognize and respond to the presence of foreign material.

MORTALITY: Mortality is the condition of being susceptible to death. The term "mortality" comes from the Latin word *mors*, which means "death." Mortality can also refer to the rate of deaths caused by an illness or injury, i.e., "Rabies has a high mortality."

SYSTEMIC: Any medical condition that affects the whole body (i.e., the whole system) is systemic.

walking, and sudden neurological problems. These symptoms are often more severe in patients with compromised immune systems. If a brain abscess (localized area of infection) ruptures, the infection can often lead to meningitis (infection of the outer covering of the brain, or meninges). When the skin is affected, rashes, lumps, and sores are usually present, along with swollen lymph nodes. They are often located in the skin or directly underneath the skin. Lesions may also form in the kidneys, liver, and bones.

■ Scope and Distribution

Nocardiosis is found throughout the world. People of all ages can contract the infection, although it occurs more frequently in people 40–49 years of age. Nocardiosis is more common in males than females by a three to one ratio. It is especially common in people with impaired immune systems and people who have chronic lung problems, such as emphysema.

About 0.4 cases occur in 100,000 people in the United States. According to the CDC, about 500–1,000 new cases are reported annually. No accurate statistics are available internationally. People with lowered immune systems are especially vulnerable; however, people with no history of serious diseases can also get the disease. It cannot be transmitted from person to person.

Immunocompromised persons are at increased risk from *Nocardia*. This risk includes such groups as people with cancer, connective tissue disorders, bone marrow transplants, solid organ transplants, high-dose cortico-

steroid use, and HIV/AIDS (human immunodeficiency virus/acquired immunodeficiency syndrome).

■ Treatment and Prevention

The diagnosis is sometimes difficult because *Nocardia* grow more slowly than most bacteria, and so cultures are often not analyzed for a sufficient amount of time in the clinical laboratory. In addition, the infection inside cultures of sputum or discharge is not easily identifiable. It is most often identified from respiratory secretions, abscess aspirates, and skin biopsies. Physicians also use special staining techniques. In addition, they take a complete medical history to help evaluate the patient. Lung biopsies and chest x rays are also sometimes taken. For brain infections, computer tomography (CT) or magnetic resonance imaging (MRI) scans are usually used.

A treatment usually lasts at least six months, but sometimes 12–18 months or longer is needed to cure the infection. Bed rest is recommended during antibiotic drug treatment. Short-term antibiotic treatment does not work. Sometimes, co-trimoxazole or sulfonamide drugs (in high doses) are used. Sulfadiazine is often used. The combination of trimethoprim-sulfamethoxazole (TMP-SMX) is generally the drug treatment preferred by the medical community. If patients do not respond to these medicines, ampicillin, erythromycin, or minocycline may be added to them.

Recently, according to the CDC Division of Bacterial and Mycotic Diseases, the drug combination of sulfonamide, ceftriaxone, and amikacin has shown promising results, especially when TMP-SMX is difficult to administer. Treatment sometimes also includes surgery to excise dead tissue and drain abscesses. Bed rest is recommended while the patient recovers, however, activity may slowly resume. Sometimes with chronic cases, a therapy called chronic suppressive therapy is used that includes prolonged, low-dose antibiotic therapy. The prognosis is best for the patient when nocardiosis is diagnosed early and before it reaches the brain.

Diagnosis has been difficult in the past. However, new diagnostic tools, including molecular diagnostic and subtyping methods, are helping to better identify the infection.

■ Impacts and Issues

Nocardia infections are difficult for physicians because they cause a wide variety of diseases, especially in immunocompromised patients, that require extra expertise. The number of cases has been increasing. However, this increase in numbers is generally attributed to improvements in diagnostic techniques and to the overall increase in the number of severely immunocompromised persons throughout the world.

Recovery may be slow. Treatments are usually able to control the infection. Sometimes, allergies to the antibiotics prescribed to treat the infection occur, and alternatives may need to be provided. The prognosis is generally good when the diagnosis and treatment are prompt and on target. However, the outcome is generally poor after the infection has spread widely in the body, and treatment has not been prompt. Three of the major complications are rib lesions, brain abscesses, and skin infections.

SEE ALSO *Antibacterial Drugs; Bacterial Disease; CDC (Centers for Disease Control and Prevention).*

BIBLIOGRAPHY

Books

Handbook of Diseases. 3rd ed. Philadelphia: Lippincott Williams & Wilkins, 2004.

IN CONTEXT: TRENDS AND STATISTICS

The Division of Bacterial and Mycotic Diseases at Centers for Disease Control and Prevention (CDC) estimates that "500 to 1,000 new cases of Nocardia infection occur annually. An estimated 10% to 15% of these patients also have HIV infection."

SOURCE: *Centers for Disease Control and Prevention (CDC), Coordinating Center for Infectious Diseases, Division of Bacterial and Mycotic Diseases.*

Web Sites

Centers for Disease Control and Prevention. "Nocardiosis." October 13, 2005. <http://www.cdc.gov/ncidod/dbmd/diseaseinfo/nocardiosis_t.htm> (accessed March 15, 2007).

Norovirus Infection

■ Introduction

A Norovirus infection is a type of stomach ailment known as viral gastroenteritis. The infection is also commonly (and incorrectly) known as the stomach flu, and is not related to the respiratory symptoms caused by the influenza virus.

The infection is caused by Noroviruses, which have also been termed Norwalk-like viruses and caliciviruses.

■ Disease History, Characteristics, and Transmission

Noroviruses are named after the "Norwalk virus," which was the cause of a gastroenteritis outbreak in a school in Norwalk, Ohio, in 1968. Once called Norwalk-like viruses, they have since been officially designated as Noroviruses.

An infection caused by a Norovirus is usually not life threatening, but can certainly cause a person to feel miserable. Typically, a person develops the symptoms of infection suddenly and becomes ill for several days. Vomiting and diarrhea occur many times during the illness; the loss of fluids can cause dehydration. Dehydration can be serious in infants, elderly people, and people whose immune systems are not functioning efficiently.

Recovery is usually complete, with no lingering symptoms or infection. However, as different strains (types) of the Norovirus exist, repeated gastrointestinal infections throughout a person's life are possible.

Norovirus are found in the intestinal tract. A Norovirus infection can occur when fecal material is transferred to food, liquid, or an object; most often this occurs when food has been handled or an object like a doorknob is handled by someone who has not properly washed their hands after having had a bowel movement. The virus is ingested by eating the contaminated food or handling the object and then touching that hand to the mouth—this is called the fecal-oral route. A person becomes contagious from the moment they display symptoms to as long as two weeks after the symptoms have ended.

There is no evidence that the virus can by transferred by inhaling virus-laden air, even though it has been shown that vomiting does release virus particles into the air.

■ Scope and Distribution

Norovirus infection is common. The United States Centers for Disease Control and Prevention (CDC) estimates that about 23 million cases of Norovirus infection occur in the United States each year, with over 50% of all foodborne disease outbreaks being due to Noroviruses. Most of the foodborne outbreaks are due to the handling of food by someone whose hands are contaminated with virus-laden fecal material.

A wide variety of foods can be contaminated including salad dressing, deli-style meats, bakery items, cake icing, fruits, and vegetables. Seafoods such as oysters can become contaminated and can concentrate the virus in high numbers when they filter Norovirus-laden water and then eating the raw oysters can transmit the virus to people. Drinking water can also be contaminated with Norovirus.

Norovirus infections occur anywhere in the world. Indeed, because the virus is easily spread among persons,

---

WORDS TO KNOW

GASTROENTERITIS: Gastroenteritis is an inflammation of the stomach and the intestines. More commonly, gastroenteritis is called the stomach flu.

difficult to kill, and contagious, the probability exists of repeated, large-scale outbreaks.

Treatment and Prevention

Treatment for a Norovirus infection consists of keeping a person hydrated and as comfortable as possible while waiting for the infection to subside.

Good personal hygiene is the best prevention strategy. Proper handwashing is crucial in preventing transfer of the virus. Similar to the viruses that cause the common cold and influenza, having an infection does not produce an immunity to future infections since there are many, slightly different version of Norovirus. An immune response to one version is not protective against other versions of the virus.

Washing fruits and vegetables before eating them, especially those labeled organically grown, is wise, as some organic produce is fertilized with manure. Because virus particles require a host cell before they can replicate, Norovirus particles that adhere to produce can remain capable of causing an infection for a long time.

Impacts and Issues

The intensity of the symptoms of a Norovirus infection is of most concern when the infection occurs in settings such as a day care, cruise ship, school, or a hospital. This is because the rapid loss of fluid that occurs with repeated bouts of diarrhea and vomiting can be quickly dehydrating. In an infant or an infirmed person, the combination of the infection and dehydration can be dangerous.

The consequences of the immune catch-up response that occurs when a new version of Norovirus appears can be enormous. An example involves the high number of Norovirus infections that occurred in the United States and Europe in 2002 with the appearance of a new Norovirus variant. The majority of cases occurred in hospitals, cruise ships, and nursing homes. In some cases, patient and surgical wards and the emergency room were temporarily shut down, crippling hospital services and escalating medical costs. Cruise lines cancelled cruises, quarantined ill crewmembers, and kept ships out of service for cleaning and sanitizing. Outbreaks of Norovirus occurred in 25 cruise ships bound for U.S. ports in 2002, affecting almost 3,000 passengers. Cruise ships sailing into U.S. ports are required to notify the CDC of each case of gastroenteritis diagnosed aboard ship 24 hours prior to arrival. If the number of affected passengers or crew reaches 2%, the ship must file an alert informing U.S. health authorities of the outbreak. The CDC monitors reports of outbreaks of gastroenteritis aboard cruise ships on a daily basis, and helps to identify the causative agent.

IN CONTEXT: PERSONAL RESPONSIBILITY AND PROTECTION

With regard to preventing norovirus gastroenteritis, the Centers for Disease Control and Prevention (CDC), National Center for Infectious Diseases states:

- "Many local and state health departments require that food handlers and preparers with gastroenteritis not work until 2 or 3 days after they feel better. In addition, because the virus continues to be present in the stool for as long as 2 to 3 weeks after the person feels better, strict handwashing after using the bathroom and before handling food items is important in preventing the spread of this virus. Food handlers who were recently sick can be given different duties in the restaurant so that they do not have to handle food (for example, working the cash register or hostessing)."

- "People who are sick with Norovirus illness can often vomit violently, without warning, and the vomit is infectious; therefore, any surfaces near the vomit should be promptly cleaned and disinfected with bleach solution and then rinsed. Furthermore, food items that may have become contaminated with Norovirus should be thrown out. Linens (including clothes, towels, tablecloths, napkins) soiled to any extent with vomit or stool should be promptly washed at high temperature. Oysters should be obtained from reputable sources and appropriate documentation kept. Washing raw vegetables thoroughly before eating and appropriate disposal of sewage and soiled diapers also help to reduce the spread of norovirus and prevent illness. In small home-based catering businesses or family owned or operated restaurants, sick children and infants in diapers should be excluded from food preparation areas."

SOURCE: *Centers for Disease Control and Prevention, National Center for Infectious Diseases*

Another outbreak of Norovirus among people in close quarters occurred in the Reliant Astrodome in Houston, Texas, during September 2005, when it was used to house evacuees from hurricane Katrina. Approximately 1,500 evacuees and relief workers received treatment for gastroenteritis at the Astrodome complex between September 2–12, 2005. The causative agent was later identified as a Norovirus, and despite the rapidly changing population of evacuees, the outbreak was contained within one week by isolating persons with symptoms within one area of the complex, distributing hand sanitizer, conducting handwashing awareness campaigns, and installing additional portable sinks in the facility.

Protection against Noroviruses in the form of a vaccine is not available, although at least one pharmaceutical

IN CONTEXT: TRENDS AND STATISTICS

With regard to the disease burden of norovirus gastroenteritis, in August 2006 the Centers for Disease Control and Prevention (CDC) estimated that:

- 23 million cases of acute gastroenteritis are due to Norovirus infection, and it is now thought that at least 50% of all foodborne outbreaks of gastroenteritis can be attributed to noroviruses.
- Among the 232 outbreaks of norovirus illness reported to CDC from July 1997 to June 2000, 57% were foodborne, 16% were due to person-to-person spread, and 3% were waterborne; in 23% of outbreaks, the cause of transmission was not determined. In this study, common settings for outbreaks include restaurants and catered meals (36%), nursing homes (23%), schools (13%), and vacation settings or cruise ships (10%).
- Most foodborne outbreaks of Norovirus illness are likely to arise though direct contamination of food by a food handler immediately before its consumption. Outbreaks have frequently been associated with consumption of cold foods, including various salads, sandwiches, and bakery products. Liquid items (e.g., salad dressing or cake icing) that allow virus to mix evenly are often implicated as a cause of outbreaks. Food can also be contaminated at its source, and oysters from contaminated waters have been associated with widespread outbreaks of gastroenteritis. Other foods, including raspberries and salads, have been contaminated before widespread distribution and subsequently caused extensive outbreaks.
- Waterborne outbreaks of Norovirus disease in community settings have often been caused by sewage contamination of wells and recreational water.

SOURCE: *Centers for Disease Control and Prevention, National Center for Infectious Diseases*

company is attempting to develop an inhalable vaccine. Norovirus infection also has consequences for the military. The debilitating and contagious natures of the infection can lessen the combat readiness of troops. Recognizing this, the vaccine development effort is being largely funded by U.S. defense agencies.

SEE ALSO *Gastroenteritis (common causes); Handwashing; Viral Disease.*

BIBLIOGRAPHY

Books

Janse, Allison. *The Germ Freak's Guide to Outwitting Colds and Flu: Guerilla Tactics to Keep Yourself Healthy at Home, at Work and in the World.* Deerfield Beach: HCI, 2005.

Periodicals

Maunula, Leena. "Norovirus Outbreaks from Drinking Water." *Emerging Infectious Diseases.* 11: 1716–1722 (2005).

Palacio, H., et al. "Norovirus Outbreak among Evacuees from Hurricane Katrina - Houston, Texas, September 2005." *Morbidity and Mortality Weekly.* 54: 1016–1019 (2005).

Splete, Heidi. "Raspberries Implicated in Norovirus Outbreaks." *Family Practice News.* 36: 23–24 (2006).

Brian Hoyle

Nosocomial (Healthcare-Associated) Infections

■ Introduction

Nosocomial infections—also called healthcare-associated infections—are infections contracted in health-care settings, usually hospitals. Such infections have occurred for as long as doctors have handled patients, but their source only began to be widely understood in the mid- to late nineteenth century. Nosocomial infections occur primarily at sites where objects such as catheters, scalpels, needles, breathing tubes, and similar devices are introduced into the body, providing a place for bacteria to grow. Infections caused in this way are an increasing problem, partly due to the ongoing evolution of resistance to many antibiotics by bacteria. Approximately 1.4 million people worldwide acquire healthcare-associated infections at any given time. These infections claim many tens of thousands of lives every year and occur in both developed and developing nations. Countermeasures include handwashing, glove-wearing, increasing blood-supply safety, improvement of injection practices, immunization of health-care workers and others, and improvement of water supply quality and waste management.

■ Disease History, Characteristics, and Transmission

The word "nosocomial" comes from the Greek word *noso-komos*, meaning "person who tends the sick." The idea that physicians might themselves be a major cause of disease did not occur until the 1790s, when a few doctors began to notice that puerperal fever, a disease caused by the group-A streptococcus bacterium *Streptococcus pyogenes*, was afflicting women after childbirth and seemed to be transmitted to patients by doctors. These observations received little attention from the medical world as a whole, however, until the mid-nineteenth century. At that time, puerperal fever was common in hospitals, where *S. pyogenes* was transmitted by physicians' unwashed hands as they went from patient to patient. During childbirth, women were often infected with

the *S. pyogenes* that contaminated their doctors' hands as they moved between patients, or from the autopsy room directly to the delivery room. This commonly resulted in death rates in maternity wards of 10–25%, with occasional epidemics wiping out entire wards.

In 1843, writer and physician Oliver Wendell Holmes (1809–1904) published a seminal essay titled "The Contagiousness of Puerperal Fever." In it, he argued forcefully against the widespread medical opinion that puerperal fever was not a contagious disease. "The

---

WORDS TO KNOW

PUERPERAL FEVER: Puerperal fever is a bacterial infection present in the blood (septicemia) that follows childbirth. The Latin word *puer*, meaning boy or child, is the root of this term. Puerperal fever was much more common before the advent of modern aseptic practices, but infections still occur. Louis Pasteur showed that puerperal fever is most often caused by *Streptococcus* bacteria, which is now treated with antibiotics.

RESISTANT ORGANISM: An organism that has developed the ability to counter something trying to harm it. Within infectious diseases, the organism, such as a bacterium, has developed a resistance to drugs, such as antibiotics.

STANDARD PRECAUTIONS: Standard precautions are the safety measures taken to prevent the transmission of disease-causing bacteria. These include proper hand washing, wearing gloves, goggles, and other protective clothing, proper handling of needles, and sterilization of equipment.

disease known as Puerperal Fever," he wrote, "is so far contagious as to be frequently carried from patient to patient by physicians and nurses." He noted that in case after case, a string of maternal deaths could be traced to a series of visits by a single doctor or midwife. In one instance, he documented a string of deaths 40 cases long—all caused by a single doctor.

Also in the 1840s, Hungarian-German physician Ignaz Semmelweis (1818–1865) documented similar facts in the Vienna General Hospital. The death rate in the section of the hospital in which women in childbirth were attended by doctors was three times higher than that in which they were attended by midwives. Semmelweis concluded that doctors were infecting patients by visiting them with unwashed hands after performing autopsies (dissecting corpses). He managed to institute a program of handwashing using a chlorine solution, greatly reducing the death rate. In the 1860s and 1870s, French scientist Louis Pasteur (1822–1895) established that infectious disease was caused by germs, that is, living organisms too small to be seen by the naked eye. With this discovery, Pasteur finally explained the mechanism by which unwashed hands can transmit disease. By the end of the century, medical opinion had shifted towards a nosocomial origin for puerperal fever. However, there were still many doctors who washed their hands after delivering babies, but not before.

In the twentieth century, nosocomial puerperal fever rapidly became a thing of the past, at least in industrialized countries. However, other forms of nosocomial infection eventually became more common for two reasons. The first is the proliferation of various devices—hypodermic needles, catheters, intravenous lines, breathing tubes, and the like—for delivering air or fluid to or from the body. The second is the rise, especially in health-care settings, of antibiotic-resistant bacteria. Intrusive medical devices and antibacterial drugs have saved many lives that would otherwise been lost, but not as many as they could have saved without the nosocomial infections that accompanied their use.

Nosocomial infections of the respiratory tract, associated with breathing tubes, are the most common; in particular, ventilator-assisted pneumonia is common in intensive-care units. The next most common sources of nosocomial infection, in order of decreasing frequency, are central lines (also called central venous catheters, tubes inserted into large veins and left in place for days or weeks), urinary drainage catheters, and surgical wounds. Two factors combine to cause a typical nosocomial infection. The first is decreased immune-system function in a patient who is already ill, and the second is the introduction of bacteria into the patient, usually by some type of invasive device. The National Nosocomial Infection Surveillance system of the United States Centers for Disease Control and Prevention has found that about 83% of nosocomial pneumonia cases are associated

with breathing machines (ventilators), 97% of urinary-tract infections are associated with catheters, and 87% of cases of bacteremia (infection of the bloodstream) are associated with central lines.

The most common cause of nosocomial infection is the *Staphylococcus aureus* bacterium. Some strains of this bacterium have evolved resistance to all penicillin-type antibiotics and others. For example, the USA300 strain of *S. aureus*, first identified in 2000, has evolved resistance to cefalexin, erythromycin, doxycycline, beta lactams, dindamycin, tetracycline, ciprofloxacin, and mupirocin. When a patient is infected with the bacteria, physicians may need to search by trial-and-error for an antibiotic that will work. During this time, an infection may progress and even kill a patient.

■ Treatment and Prevention

Nosocomial bacterial infections are treated with antibiotics, although antibiotic-resistant strains of bacteria are making this increasingly difficult. Prevention is accomplished through infection control and standard precautions by health-care workers, including handwashing, flushing of catheters and intravenous lines using saline (salt water) solution or other chemicals, wearing disposable gloves, using disposable needles, and properly sterilizing surgical instruments. In 2005, the World Health Organization announced an initiative called the Global Patient Safety Challenge 2005–2006, with the motto "Clean Care is Safer Care." This was an effort to reduce nosocomial infection risks throughout the world by improving practices related to the purity of blood products, injection practices, water and sanitation, emergency care, and hand hygiene.

■ Scope and Distribution

Of all patients admitted to hospitals in the industrialized world, between 5% and 10% acquire a nosocomial infection—sometimes more than one. For patients admitted to intensive care (also called critical care, often requiring the use of breathing machines and other high-tech support devices), the rate is between 15% and 40% because these patients are subject to more invasive devices. In poor countries, the nosocomial infection rate for hospital patients is 2–20 times higher (i.e., can approach 100% in some locations). More than half the babies in neonatal care units in developing countries acquire a nosocomial infection, with death rates ranging from 5% to 56%.

Health-care workers may not only transmit nosocomial infections but acquire them. During the SARS (severe acute respiratory syndrome) epidemic of 2002–2003, health-care workers accounted for 20–60% of cases around with the world, depending on location.

■ Impacts and Issues

In the United States, as of 2005, 1 out of 136 patients admitted to a hospital became seriously ill from a nosocomial infection. This entailed a caseload of 2 million nosocomially infected patients yearly with an annual monetary cost probably over $5 billion and some 80,000 deaths per year. For comparison, a little over 40,000 people die each year in the U.S. from car accidents. In Mexico, the per capita nosocomial infection rate is somewhat higher: Mexico sees about half the number of deaths from this cause in a population about a third the size of the U.S. population.

According to the medical journal *The Lancet*, "perhaps the most important topic in infection control is handwashing; yet health-care workers are notoriously bad at washing their hands each time that they should." Thus, ironically, the same behavioral problem that caused thousands of women's deaths from puerperal fever in the nineteenth century—dirty hands—remains a problem in twenty-first century medicine.

Nosocomial infection is a growing problem worldwide, partly because more patients are suffering serious underlying illnesses, such as AIDS (acquired immunodeficiency syndrome). In many health-care settings in industrialized countries, rushed health care workers often comply poorly with rules for hand-cleansing. In poorer countries, dirty instruments, crowding, lack of safe water sources, and dirty overall conditions also help spread nosocomial infections.

SEE ALSO *Antibiotic Resistance; Blood Supply and Infectious Disease; Infection Control and Asepsis; Streptococcal Infections, Group A.*

BIBLIOGRAPHY

Books

Wenzel, Richard P. *Prevention and Control of Nosocomial Infections.* Philadelphia: Lippincott Williams & Wilkins, 2003.

Periodicals

Diep, Binh An, et al. "Complete Genome Sequence of USA300, An Epidemic Clone of Community-Acquired Meticillin-Resistant *Staphylococcus aureus.*" *The Lancet* 367 (March 4, 2006): 731–740.

Pittet, Didier, et al. "Effectiveness of a Hospital-Wide Programme to Improve Compliance with Hand Hygiene." *The Lancet* 356 (October 14, 2000): 1307–1312.

Vincent, Jean-Louis. "Nosocomial Infections in Adult Intensive-care Units." *The Lancet* 361 (June 14, 2003): 2068–2077.

Web Sites

Centers for Disease Control and Prevention. "National Nosocomial Infections Surveillance System." February 16, 2005. <http://www.cdc.gov/ncidod/dhqp/nnis.html> (accessed February 20, 2007).

World Health Organization. "Global Patient Safety Challenge 2005–2006: Clean Care is Safer Care." 2005. <http://www.who.int/entity/patientsafety/events/05/GPSC_Launch_ENGLISH_FINAL.pdf> (accessed February 20, 2007).

Larry Gilman

Notifiable Diseases

■ Introduction

Notifiable diseases are infectious diseases whose occurrence must be reported by physicians and laboratories to a public health agency. This monitoring is necessary to prevent or contain outbreaks of disease, and to maintain surveillance about current disease patterns. Reporting notifiable diseases is mandatory at the state level, and diseases that are required to be reported vary slightly by state. Reporting is voluntary at the federal level, although all fifty states and districts cooperate to report information about cases of notifiable infectious diseases to the Centers for Disease Control and Prevention (CDC).

Examples of some notifiable diseases in the United States include acquired immunodeficiency syndrome (AIDS, also cited as acquired immune deficiency syndrome), anthrax, cholera, diphtheria, giardiasis, influenza (both bacterial and viral), Lyme disease, malaria, measles, mumps, plague, severe acute respiratory syndrome (SARS), tuberculosis, and yellow fever. The list of notifiable diseases changes with time as emerging infectious diseases present new public health concerns, or as an older disease becomes more prevalent. An example of a newly emerging notifiable disease is SARS, which was added to the list following the outbreak in Asia, Canada, and elsewhere in 2003. An example of a disease that has assumed a greater prominence due to its resurgence and development of heightened antibiotic resistance is tuberculosis.

■ History and Scientific Foundations

In the United States, the history of notifiable diseases dates back to 1878, when Congress authorized the predecessor of the present-day public health service to collect reports of overseas deaths due to infectious diseases that were prevalent at the time such as smallpox, cholera, and yellow fever. The intention was to use the knowledge to institute quarantine for people coming into the United States from the affected regions to prevent domestic outbreaks of these diseases.

The following year, the authority for collection of notifiable disease information was extended to state and local public health officials. By 1928, every U.S. state and territory was contributing information to a national report of 29 designated infectious diseases. CDC assumed

IN CONTEXT: REAL-WORLD REPORTING

Below is the Centers for Disease Control and Prevention (CDC) list of nationally notifiable infectious diseases, revised in mid-2007 to include novel, or unusual type-A influenza. By encouraging states to report a newly observed type-A influenza, scientists aim to recognize a candidate for a pandemic flu virus and respond in its early stages. Physicians, laboratories, and other health providers are mandated to report notifiable diseases to state health authorities, and reporting at the federal level is voluntary.

- Acquired immunodeficiency syndrome (AIDS)
- Anthrax
- Arboviral neuroinvasive and non-neuroinvasive diseases (California serogroup, Eastern equine encephalitis, Powassan, St. Louis encephalitis, West Nile, and Western equine encephalitis viruses)
- Botulism (food-borne, infant, other [wound and unspecified])
- Brucellosis
- Chancroid
- *Chlamydia trachomatis*, genital infections
- Cholera
- Coccidioidomycosis
- Cryptosporidiosis
- Cyclosporiasis
- Diphtheria
- Ehrlichiosis (human granulocytic, human monocytic and human, other or unspecified agent)
- Giardiasis
- Gonorrhea
- *Haemophilus influenzae*, invasive disease
- Hansen disease (leprosy)
- Hantavirus pulmonary syndrome
- Hemolytic uremic syndrome, post-diarrheal
- Hepatitis, viral, acute (A, B, B virus, perinatal infection, C)
- Hepatitis, viral, chronic (B, C virus [past or present]
- HIV infection (adult [13 years], pediatric [13 years])
- Influenza-associated pediatric mortality
- Legionellosis
- Listeriosis
- Lyme disease
- Malaria
- Measles

- Meningococcal disease
- Mumps
- Novel influenza A virus infections
- Pertussis
- Plague
- Poliomyelitis, paralytic
- Poliovirus infection, nonparalytic
- Psittacosis
- Q fever
- Rabies (animal, human)
- Rocky Mountain spotted fever
- Rubella
- Rubella, congenital syndrome
- Salmonellosis
- Severe acute respiratory syndrome-associated Coronavirus (SARS-CoV) disease
- Shiga toxin-producing *Escherichia coli* (STEC)
- Shigellosis
- Smallpox
- Streptococcal disease, invasive, Group A
- Streptococcal toxic-shock syndrome
- *Streptococcus pneumoniae*, drug resistant, invasive disease
- *Streptococcus pneumoniae*, invasive in children 5 years
- Syphilis (primary, secondary, latent, early latent, late latent, latent/unknown duration, Neurosyphilis, late, non-neurological, syphilitic Stillbirth, congenital
- Tetanus
- Toxic shock syndrome (other than Streptococcal)
- Trichinellosis (Trichinosis)
- Tuberculosis
- Tularemia
- Typhoid fever
- Vancomycin - intermediate *Staphylococcus aureus* (VISA)
- Vancomycin - resistant *Staphylococcus aureus* (VRSA)
- Varicella (morbidity)
- Varicella (deaths only)
- Vibriosis
- Yellow fever

SOURCE: *Centers for Disease Control and Prevention (CDC)*

responsibility for the collection and reporting of the information in 1961. As of 2007, 58 diseases comprise the list of nationally notifiable diseases. Information on some of these diseases is issued weekly in a CDC publication called the *Mortality and Morbidity Weekly Report*, and annually in the *Summary of Notifiable Diseases*.

■ Applications and Research

A key part of CDC's National Notifiable Diseases Surveillance System is a computerized and Internet-linked communications network called the National Electronic Telecommunications System for Surveillance (NETSS). The network was established in 1985 (it was then called the Epidemiologic Surveillance Project) and was linked to all states by 1989. It is via NETSS that the weekly data is conveyed to CDC by U.S. states and territories. While participation is voluntary, all states, territories and the District of Columbia participate.

The criteria for reporting of notifiable diseases was published in 1990 by CDC in collaboration with the Council of State and Territorial Epidemiologists. The disease-by-disease criteria ensure that the information for a given notifiable disease is sufficient. For example, some diseases require the inclusion of laboratory data while other diseases, particularly those like salmonellosis that can arise due to eating contaminated food, require epidemiological information such as the food eaten at the gathering and the number of cases.

Data gathered on notifiable diseases also typically includes information such as the detected date of the illness, geographical information (state, county), and aspects of those affected including their age, gender, and race/ethnicity. Information is also gathered on the disease itself including its type, severity, diagnosis, treatment history, and health care facilities and public health response capabilities in the affected region. Personal information such as the name and address of those who become ill are recorded with some diseases that require tracing and notifying close contacts who could have been exposed to the disease.

■ Impacts and Issues

The nationwide network established in the United States, Canada, England, and other countries around the world for the prompt and regular reporting of infectious diseases deemed to have a significant potential for spread and whose effects can be debilitating and even fatal has likely saved countless lives, as it has allowed public health officials to detect and respond to infectious illnesses faster and in a more coordinated fashion.

The disease surveillance networks have also become useful in monitoring illnesses that might result from a deliberate release of an infectious agent. By monitoring the pattern of an illnesses' spread, experts can gauge whether the infection has appeared and progressed naturally (cases appear geographically as a sort of bull's-eye, with concentration in one region and subsequent spread out from this region) or unnaturally (cases suddenly appear in similar numbers in different areas of a region).

The storage of the information in electronic databases is of some concern to those who argue that the databases can be tampered with or information extracted and used for malicious purposes. Countering this, security surrounding the databases is very robust. State and the federal health authorities must take steps to safeguard as much as possible the privacy of someone's personal information gained via the report of a notifiable disease. Typically, names and other personal information are indexed by numbers or other blind identifiers in databases, which allows access to data, but not specific personal information.

As new diseases emerge, they may be added to the list of notifiable diseases. For example, in mid-2007 the list was revised to include reporting of influenza A virus subtypes that are different from the typical influenza A viruses common in circulation at a given time. With the reporting of novel influenza type A viruses, scientists aim to quickly spot influenza viruses with pandemic potential.

The United States also abides by the International Health Regulations (IHR), which guide the World Health Organization (WHO) and member states in responding to and reporting international health emergencies. The IHR also added novel influenza virus subtypes to the list of diseases that should be immediately reported to the WHO.

SEE ALSO *Epidemiology; Public Health and Infectious Disease.*

BIBLIOGRAPHY

Books

Schneider, Mary Jane. *Introduction to Public Health.* 2nd ed. Boston: Jones & Bartlett Publishers, 2005.

Szklo, M., and F. Javier Nieto. *Epidemiology: Beyond the Basics.* Boston: Jones & Bartlett Publishers, 2006.

Turnock, Bernard J. *Public Health, Third Edition: What It Is and How It Works.* Boston: Jones & Bartlett Publishers, 2004.

Web Sites

Centers for Disease Control and Prevention (CDC). "National Notifiable Diseases Surveillance System." <http://www.cdc.gov/epo/dphsi/nndsshis.htm> (accessed May 26, 2007).

Brian Hoyle

Opportunistic Infection

■ Introduction

An opportunistic infection is one that is caused by a bacterium, fungus, or virus that would normally be kept in check by the immune system. The advent of AIDS (acquired immunodeficiency syndrome) focused attention upon the problem of opportunistic infections. As the name suggests, AIDS results in weakened immunity, giving normally harmless microbes the opportunity to invade the body and cause infection.

Besides AIDS, other medical conditions associated with opportunistic infections include cancer, severe burns, malnutrition, and diabetes. Medical treatments such as cancer chemotherapy and the long-term immunosuppressant drug therapy needed after organ transplantation also undermine immunity. Among the most common of the opportunistic pathogens (disease-causing organisms) are *Pneumocystis carinii* (recently renamed *P. jiroveci*), *Candida albicans*, and cytomegalovirus. None of these pathogens would normally cause disease in a healthy person. Treatment of an opportunistic infection is therefore two-fold. The infection is treated with antibiotics or other drug therapy, and then the underlying immune problem should also be addressed.

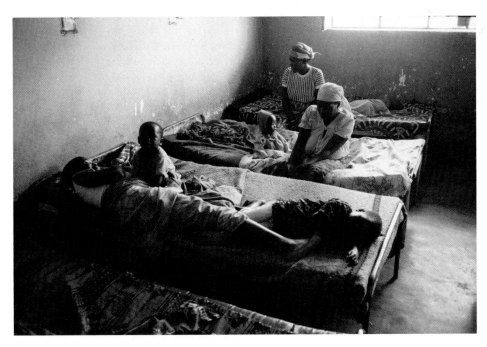

HIV-positive patients are shown at a clinic for tuberculosis (TB) treatment in Rwanda. TB progresses more rapidly and causes more severe disease in people infected with HIV.   *Chris Sattlberger/Photo Researchers, Inc.*

WORDS TO KNOW

COLONIZATION: Colonization is the process of occupation and increase in number of microorganisms at a specific site.

GRAM-NEGATIVE BACTERIA: All types of bacteria identified and classified as a group that does not retain crystal-violet dye during Gram's method of staining.

GRAM-POSITIVE BACTERIA: All types of bacteria identified and classified as a group that retains crystal-violet dye during Gram's method of staining.

HOST: Organism that serves as the habitat for a parasite, or possibly for a symbiont. A host may provide nutrition to the parasite or symbiont, or simply a place in which to live.

IMMUNOCOMPROMISED: A reduction of the ability of the immune system to recognize and respond to the presence of foreign material.

MORTALITY: Mortality is the condition of being susceptible to death. The term "mortality" comes from the Latin word *mors*, which means "death." Mortality can also refer to the rate of deaths caused by an illness or injury, i.e., "Rabies has a high mortality."

PROPHYLAXIS: Treatment to prevent the onset or recurrence of disease.

Disease History, Characteristics, and Transmission

The fungus *Pneumocystis carinii* infects nearly everyone at some point during their lives, but is normally completely harmless. The reporting of cases of *P. carinii*-associated pneumonia among previously healthy young men in the early 1980s was one of the early warning signs of the emergence of AIDS, as *P. carinii* pneumonia is normally a very rare occurrence.

The symptoms of an opportunistic infection depend upon the nature of the associated organism. Nearly all microbes—bacteria, fungi, viruses, and protozoa—can become pathogenic, given the right opportunity. However, certain organisms have a strong association with specific types of impaired immunity.

Gram-positive bacteria, such as *Staphylococcus aureus*, tend to invade the skin and implanted devices such as catheters. Gram-negative bacteria, including *Pseudomonas aeruginosa* are associated with a form of immune deficiency known as granulocytopenia. This refers to depletion of a type of white blood cell called a granulocyte, a condition that is found in leukemia and during chemotherapy for cancer. The terms Gram-positive and Gram-negative refer to a classification of bacteria according to how they react with Gram's stain, which is used in preparation of samples for microscopy.

Tuberculosis infection from *Mycobacterium tuberculosis* may be reactivated among those whose immune systems are impaired because of age or AIDS. The fungus *C. albicans* can infect blood or solid organs in cases of granulocytopenia. Finally, *Toxoplasma gondii* is another protozoan that commonly causes opportunistic infection among AIDS patients.

Transmission of an opportunistic infection depends upon the organism involved. Many of these organisms will normally be present on the skin or in the body in amounts less than necessary to cause infection. This is known as colonization. It is only because the defenses of the immune system are breached that they can take hold and cause infection.

Scope and Distribution

Many different groups are at especial risk of opportunistic infections. The common factor is an abnormality or defect in the immune system or any related host defense system, such as the skin, which acts as a natural barrier.

Rarely, an immune deficiency can be present from birth. More commonly, immune deficiency is acquired, as in AIDS, where the human immunodeficiency virus attacks and destroys the immune system. Certain underlying diseases, including cancer, diabetes, cystic fibrosis, sickle cell anemia, and severe burns undermine immunity, making a person prone to opportunistic infection.

Various drug treatments impair immunity, such as steroids, immunosuppressants, cancer chemotherapy, and prolonged antibiotic therapy. Medical devices, including indwelling catheters and prosthetic heart valves also attract opportunistic infection. Finally, the very young and the very old tend to have weaker immunity, which puts them at higher risk of opportunistic infection.

Treatment and Prevention

Diagnosis of an opportunistic infection can be difficult, as most of the causative agents are normally benign (not harmful). Once the microbe has been identified, the treatment will generally consist of the appropriate antibiotic or antifungal drug, if the opportunistic infection is caused by a bacterium or fungus. Cytomegalovirus infection is generally treated with antiviral drugs like ganciclovir.

Prevention of opportunistic infections depends upon the organism involved and the medical condition of the patient. Sometimes, antibiotic and antiviral prophylaxis (preventative treatment) may be used. Scrupulous personal hygiene around patients with compromised immunity is always essential; for instance, hospital visitors and medical staff should wash their hands thoroughly and regularly before and after touching patients.

■ Impacts and Issues

Opportunistic infections can be a challenge because they usually involve organisms that are normally not harmful. The incidence of opportunistic infections is likely to increase as the population ages, persons with HIV/AIDS live longer, more organ transplants are performed, and other populations of immunocompromised persons (those with weakened immune systems) increase.

In developing countries, malnutrition leaves millions of children with weakened immune systems and in turn, more vulnerable to infections. Acute infections such as diarrheal diseases, respiratory infections, measles, and malaria account for more than half of childhood mortality (deaths) in developing countries, and malnutrition is associated with over fifty percent of these deaths, according to the World Health Organization (WHO). When malnutrition is present, some health authorities broaden the definition of the term opportunistic infection to include a synergistic relationship between malnutrition and communicable disease: malnutrition weakens natural immunity, leading to increased susceptibility to infection, and more frequent, severe, and prolonged episodes of infection. The cycle is perpetuated when infection aggravates malnutrition by decreasing intake and increasing the body's metabolic needs. For example during a 2005 outbreak of measles in Somali refugees in Kenya, measles was considered an opportunistic infection due to malnutrition brought on by Somali crop failures after drought and conflict.

SEE ALSO *AIDS (Acquired Immunodeficiency Syndrome); Candidiasis; Pneumocystis carinii Pneumonia; Toxoplasmosis (Toxoplasma Infection).*

BIBLIOGRAPHY

Books

Tan, James S. *Expert Guide to Infectious Diseases.* Philadelphia: American College of Physicians, 2002.

Periodicals

Rice, Amy L., et al. "Malnutrition as an Underlying Cause of Childhood Deaths Associated with Infectious Diseases in Developing Countries." *Bulletin of the World Health Organization* 78 (2000): 1207-1218.

Web Sites

Centers for Disease Control. "Guidelines for Preventing Opportunistic Infections Among HIV-Infected Persons." June 14, 2002. <http://www.cdc.gov/mmwr/preview/mmwrhtml/rr5108a1.htm> (accessed May 28, 2007).

Susan Aldridge

Outbreaks: Field Level Response

◼ Introduction

Outbreaks of infectious disease range in size and severity. A prompt response at local—or field—level can limit the spread of an outbreak and help to prevent future episodes. Response is an important component of epidemiology, which is the study of the occurrence of disease among the population. Epidemiology involves surveillance and case reporting, so that outbreaks can be identified. Emergency response can include treatment and isolation measures, but needs to be coupled with a thorough investigation so that the causes of the outbreak can be recognized and halted.

Health authorities need to put in place advance plans for dealing with outbreaks covering the three components of surveillance, response, and investigation. The World Health Organization (WHO) and the Centers for Disease Prevention and Control (CDC) in the United

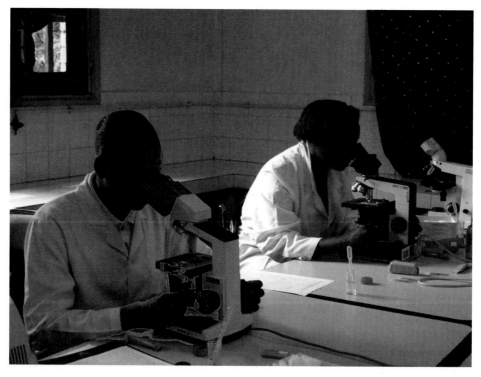

The Pasteur Institute of Madagascar hosted a week of talks and practical training for fellow scientists from nine other African countries hit by the plague in 2004. According to the World Health Organization (WHO), about 20,000 cases of the disease have emerged in Africa since 1980—95 percent of bubonic plague and 5 percent of pneumonic and septicaemic plague. The African continent accounts for three-quarters of the cases of plague in the world. *AFP/Getty Images.*

States have developed structures, guidelines, and networks which allow responses to be mounted to infectious disease outbreaks, including deliberate outbreaks of disease due to a bioterrorist attack.

History and Scientific Foundations

The English physician John Snow (1813–1858) demonstrated one of the earliest recorded responses to a disease outbreak. In 1854, he began to investigate an outbreak of cholera in his local area of London. He constructed a detailed street map showing the location of cases and deduced that the source of the infection was the local water pump.

He either removed the pump handle himself, or ordered it to be removed, and shortly afterwards, the number of cholera cases began to decline. It is not possible to prove that Snow's action, in itself, limited the outbreak—it may have been on the decline naturally—but the principle of removing the cause of the infection was correct. It is this same principle which guides effective field response to outbreaks today.

A field response to an outbreak occurs at a local level and often involves the facilities of the nearest hospital, particularly its emergency department. The hospital needs to have sufficient capacity to deal with an outbreak in terms of medical supplies, such as vaccines and antibiotics, trained medical staff, and beds to care for seriously ill patients. Naturally, many hospitals may not have this capacity on site, but they must be able to access it if necessary.

Adequate and prompt communication between the hospital, primary care, the emergency services or public health organization, and the media is essential while responding to an outbreak. The local health authorities have detailed plans for responding to an outbreak at the field level, and this is tested in simulation exercises to identify gaps and weaknesses. As infectious agents know no boundaries, states and countries work together to respond to an outbreak.

Applications and Research

Countries, especially developing countries, cannot be expected to deal with outbreaks of infectious disease on their own. In 2000, the World Health Organization set up the Global Outbreak Alert and Response Network (GOARN), which is a collaboration of over a hundred technical institutions, non-governmental organizations and networks, creating a pooled resource for alert and response operations.

Investigative teams from GOARN will arrive at the site of an outbreak within 24 hours. They will offer on-the-spot investigation, confirmation of diagnosis, handling of

---

WORDS TO KNOW

EPIDEMIC: From the Greek *epidemic*, meaning "prevalent among the people," is most commonly used to describe an outbreak of an illness or disease in which the number of individual cases significantly exceeds the usual or expected number of cases in any given population.

GLOBAL OUTBREAK ALERT AND RESPONSE NETWORK (GOARN): A collaboration of resources for the rapid identification, confirmation, and response to outbreaks of international importance.

ISOLATION: Isolation, within the health community, refers to the precautions that are taken in the hospital to prevent the spread of an infectious agent from an infected or colonized patient to susceptible persons. Isolation practices are designed to minimize the transmission of infection.

NON-GOVERNMENTAL ORGANIZATION (NGO): A voluntary organization that is not part of any government; often organized to address a specific issue or perform a humanitarian function.

PATHOGEN: A disease causing agent, such as a bacteria, virus, fungus, etc.

SURVEILLANCE: The systematic analysis, collection, evaluation, interpretation, and dissemination of data. In public health, it assists in the identification of health threats and the planning, implementation, and evaluation of responses to those threats.

---

dangerous pathogens (disease-causing organisms), case detection, patient management, containment, and provision of staff and supplies. All of these elements are needed to safely contain an outbreak, but many may not be available on site.

Since early 2000, WHO and GOARN have launched international responses to disease outbreaks in countries around the world including Afghanistan, Bangladesh, India, Pakistan, Sudan, Tanzania, and Uganda. Recently, WHO has strengthened GOARN's outbreak response logistics with specialized transport and communication facilities, which are particularly valuable in areas with weak local infrastructures. Many other non-governmental organizations (NGO), such as the humanitarian group Médicins sans Frontières, and national health authorities, like the

Centers for Disease Control and Prevention (CDC), also get involved responding to situations in developing countries.

In a recent report, WHO describes its involvement in dealing with an outbreak of meningococcal meningitis in Burkina Faso. In the early months of 2007, the Ministry of Health in Burkina Faso reported 22,255 suspected cases including 1,490 deaths, meaning that 34 districts were over the threshold considered to be an epidemic. Cerebrospinal fluid samples from all affected areas tested positive for the bacteria *Neisseria meningitides*. This lab work was essential for describing the extent of the outbreak, implying what needed to be done to contain it.

A vaccination campaign was completed in 15 districts, reaching 100% of those at risk, and was ongoing at the time of the last report. The vaccine came from an international stockpile, which was able to supplement those held by the Ministry of Health of Burkina Faso. Financial support for the vaccination campaign was forthcoming from the international community via many non-governmental organizations, such as the United nations Central Emergency Response Fund and the United States Agency for International Development.

Response to outbreaks in countries with well-developed health infrastructures is usually coordinated by a national body, such as the CDC's Emergency Preparedness and Response Department, or the Health Protection Agency in the United Kingdom. Typical incidents might include food poisoning or measles outbreaks, and response would be part of the surveillance, case reporting, and investigation strategy. The response might involve actions such as closing schools, child care centers, or restaurants to eliminate the cause of the infection or limit its spread.

Public information dissemination is an important part of response to an outbreak at field level, including warning people of symptoms and advising them on how to avoid infection. Medical treatments include vaccination, drug administration, and hospitalization, but the specifics depend upon the illness involved in the outbreak.

The most testing situation for an outbreak response team is when a new or unusual infection is involved. Thus, the manner in which outbreaks of severe acute respiratory syndrome (SARS) and H5N1 avian influenza have been dealt with in recent years has come under scrutiny. The WHO commented on some aspects of the way the Ministry of Health of China handled an outbreak of SARS among laboratory workers in 2004. The response was judged, overall, to have been prompt with isolation of cases and tracing of possible contacts, although there was delay in identifying the early cases and initially, there was secrecy towards fellow citizens and the international scientific community. The Chinese Ministry of Health later stated it would learn from this outbreak and further strengthen its response system for the future.

Current research includes developing vaccines for use before and during outbreaks of disease (such as two vaccines approved in 2006 that protect against rotaviruses, a common cause of diarrhea outbreaks), developing effective and inexpensive personal protective equipment for responders and community members, and especially, developing rapid diagnostic tests to identify particular pathogens and diseases in the field during the initial stages of an outbreak.

■ Impacts and Issues

When it comes to outbreaks of well-known diseases, such as *Salmonella* food poisoning and meningitis, public health authorities are well-practiced in mounting a response. However, there are new threats, from emerging diseases such as H5N1 avian influenza to the possibility of bioterrorist attacks. A major issue is whether there is the capacity and preparedness within the health system to deal effectively with these.

In 2003, the United States General Accounting Office (GAO) conducted a survey of major hospitals to find out more about their public health response capacity. This showed that bioterrorism preparedness efforts mounted since the terror attacks of September 11, 2001, had indeed improved overall response capacity, but gaps remained. These included workforce shortages and shortfalls in laboratory capacity to deal with an emergency situation. There was also a lack of planning between states.

The GAO did find that states had plans for receiving and distributing medical supplies (even if these were not on site) and plans for mass vaccinations. Staff had participated in basic planning for large infectious disease outbreaks, but some hospitals lacked sufficient isolation facilities and staff to treat a large increase in the number of patients that might result from an emergency outbreak of influenza or a bioterrorist attack.

■ Primary Source Connection

In 2003, as a serious new infectious disease threat (SARS) emerged in China, the Chinese government initially took measures to keep the outbreak a secret. Only after the disease spread beyond the borders of China and a few journalists and physicians found a way to communicate the urgency of the disease to the international scientific community did fully coordinated field-level response to the SARS epidemic begin. By this time, there were multiple outbreak sites requiring response. In this excerpt from the magazine *Foreign Policy*, Karl Taro Greenfeld unravels the story of how the mystery disease was communicated to the world. At that time, Greenfeld was the editor of *Time Asia in Hong Kong*, and has since published a book about the emergence of SARS in China entitled *China Syndrome: The True Story of the 21st Century's First Great Epidemic*. China has now adopted a policy of international cooperation and participation in networks that report, track, and respond to outbreaks of infectious disease.

The Virus Hunters: When the Deadly SARS Virus Struck China Three Years Ago, Beijing Responded with a Massive Coverup. If It Weren't for the Persistence of Two Young Reporters and One Doctor Who Had Seen Enough, SARS Might Have Killed Thousands More. There's No Guarantee the World Will Be So Lucky Next Time.

In April 2003, as thousands of Chinese were infected and the dying were quarantined in squalid hospital wards, the Chinese government covered up the SARS outbreak, allowing the killer virus to spread around the world. That was hardly surprising. The first response to an epidemic is usually denial. From the perspective of a head of state, a mayor, a governor, or any ruling body, infectious disease remains among the hardest issues to manage. There is almost no calamity, save starvation or siege, that can so quickly reduce a city to panic and despair. Why should China's mandarins behave any differently? When confronted with a new infectious disease caused by the SARS virus, they initially downplayed the danger and assumed a tacit policy of wishing the microbe back into whatever species from which it had jumped. What did they really have to go on at first? A few hundred cases? In a nation of more than a billion? Indeed, with infectious disease outbreaks a far more common occurrence in China than in, say, the United States, it is on one level understandable how China's minister of health, Zhang Wenkang, could have initially downplayed the threat posed by a respiratory infection thousands of miles from the capital. If it hadn't jumped international borders, then the outbreak might have remained a minor medical curiosity.

Yet the SARS epidemic of 2003 now appears a useful blueprint of how the next pandemic might begin. As the planet struggles to deflect another imminent viral emergence, the lessons learned from SARS are more relevant than ever. Although the work of virologists, physicians, nurses, and public health officials was instrumental in beating back the virus, it is frightening to consider that if it weren't for the courage of one iconoclastic Chinese physician who came forward to tell the truth at enormous personal risk, the SARS epidemic would have been even more devastating.…

A BITTER DISCOVERY

He had watched this before, 71-year-old Dr. Jiang Yanyong recalled. He hd seen the best and the brightest brought down because of a lie, for the government's prevarications, recalcitrance, and duplicity. Jiang had been on duty the evening of June 3, 1989, when the People' Liberation Army (PLA) massacred the students in Tiananmen Square.…

Today, Jiang holds a military rank equivalent to general because of his title as chief of surgery at the hospital. For a moment, when you first see him, you think he must be in his 50s—his hair is an unnatural crow black—but there is an age droop to his eyes, as if the ocular muscles themselves have worn out from squinting into so many surgical incisions.

Throughout March 2003, Jiang had been spending more time indoors, like many people around the world, watching television for news of the war in Iraq. The SARS virus was only a crawl on China Central Television (CCTV), a glowing proclamation that "SARS is under control and there has never been a better time to visit Guangdong Province." The SARS outbreak has so far been reported as primarily a Hong Kong problem; the disease, if it were in China at all, had probably been brought in by foreigners, the official Chinese media were reporting.

Among international public health officials, of course, there was increasing consensus that the outbreak in China was far worse than the Chinese government was admitting. The State Council Information Office was reporting 12 SARS cases and 3 fatalities in Beijing. It seemed impossible: There were thousands of cases in Guangdong and Hong Kong, and hundreds in the provinces throughout China. How could Beijing have just 12 cases? Jiang found that discrepancy curious but gave it little thought.

But near the end of that month, a good friend of Jiang's fell ill with lung cancer and, naturally, Jiang was brought in to consult on the case. The patient, a medical professor, was brought to 301 Hospital. Surprisingly, he developed a high fever and a spot was found on his lung. After another specialist was brought in, Jiang's friend was diagnosed with SARS and transferred to the intensive care unit before he was removed and sent to 309 Hospital, deemed the official SARS Control and Prevention Center for the People's Liberation Army. Jiang, checking on the treatment his friend might receive, phoned respiratory specialists at 309 who were former students of his from Beijing University Medical College. "They sounded very upset," Jiang recalls. "I didn't understand why. There were just a few cases and that was such a big hospital."

There were 60 cases, Jiang was told, dozens of them medical staff themselves. Seven patients had already died of the disease. He called other colleagues and found that there were similar outbreaks occurring at 302 Hospital, which had 40 cases, and even at his own 301 Hospital, which had 46 SARS cases. "This is a terrible disease," one of his colleagues told him. "It acts so quickly. I've never seen any disease progress this fast. You go from breathing normally to intubation in three days. You die in a week."

Why, then, did the health minister, Zhang Wenkang, appear on television on April 3 to reassure the public that there were only 12 cases in all of Beijing, when there were 60 in just one hospital?...

A DUTY TO SPEAK

...Jiang decided to pen a note, explaining who he was and the facts about the number of SARS cases in the No. 301, No. 302, and No. 309 hospitals. "As a doctor who cares about people's lives and health, I have a responsibility to aid international and local efforts to prevent the spread of SARS." He faxed it to the government-controlled CCTV-4 and Hong Kong's Phoenix-TV, two of China's biggest networks, using the fax number for viewer comments and suggestions. He assumed they would quickly get in touch with him to check his credentials before airing it. They never called.

THE OFFICIAL NUMBES WERE LIES

Our Beijing correspondent, Susan Jakes, was asked to prepare a file about the general state of the Chinese healthcare system. She had no contacts in the Ministry of Health. Trying to think of a way into the subject, she decided to call a political source. Susie's connections in the dissident community had been useful in the past, but it was unlikely those connections would extend into the Chinese medical community. Still, desperate, Susie called one of her political contacts, Harold, who had ties to party officials.

She asked him if he knew anything about SARS in Beiing.

There was silence on the line. "Call me back from a safe phone."

Often, in China, we suspected our land lines and even our cell phones were bugged. When we needed to talk specifics about sensitive subjects, Matt or Susie would switch the SIM cards in their phones from a local Beijing number to an international exchange that was billed through a foreign phone company we believed far less likely to be tapped. Or, even safer, the reporter would find a pay phone—which are still common in China—and call from there.

Susie threw on her denim jacket, walked out of the bureau, and hurried to a nearby pay phone.

"I'm going to send you an email," Harold said when she called him back. "In that e-mail, there will be a URL to a secure Web site. At that Web site, you'll need a password. Type in your old Hong Kong phone number and you will be able to download a Word file. Read that and call me back."

Susie ran back to the office to check her e-mail. Harold's message had already arrived. Following his instructions, she downloaded the Word document. At the top, it read

Jiang Yanyong, Doctor, and said that he was a longtime Chinese Communist Party member. It also gave his phone number. She read the note. The letter indicated that the number of patients infected with SARS was significantly higher than the official statistics from China's Ministry of Health. It went on to describe at least 60 patients at one Beijing hospital. Most amazing, this letter was signed by this doctor.

She went back to the pay phone and called Harold.

"Who is this guy?"

"He is who he says he is. A doctor. A party member."

Susie was nervous this letter would be difficult to verify. "Can I call this guy? Will he talk to me?"

"Call him," Harold assured her. "He's at home."

Susie knew what she had now had. A big story about a big lie.

Still using the pay phone, Susie called the number on the letter. Dr. Jiang Yaonyong answered.

When she identified herself, Jiang told her, "Everything I want to say is in the letter."

"But I need to ask you some more questions," Susie pleaded, "to flesh this out a little bit."

He paused for a moment, and then, speaking in a lower voice, said, "Okay, let's meet at the teahouse at 4 o'clock in the Ruicheng Hotel, in the western part of Beijing, near the 301 Military Hospital."

But, when Susie returned to the bureau, she received another call, this one from a labor lawyer she had called the day before asking if he knew anyone who knew anything about SARS.

"Why don't you come to my office right now," he suggested. "I think I might have something you want to hear."

When Susie returned from the bureau, she took a taxi to his offices, on the fourth floor of a modern office building, and when she walked in, after he closed the door, he told her that he had a cousin who is a doctor at the Military Academy of Sciences.

"Will she talk to me?" Susie asked.

"No," the lawyer explained, "But I can call her and you can listen while we speak."

Susie would later realize that this had been prearranged by the lawyer ad his cousin to screen them from any possible accusations of talking to a foreign reporter and violating a gag order that was handed down on March 7 forbidding doctors and public health officials from talking to the media about SARS. As for the veracity of the source, we had worked with this lawyer before on several stories, and found him to be reliable.

The lawyer dialed his cousin's cell phone.

"Tell me again what you told me before," he said, handing the phone to Susie.

Susie listened as the doctor spoke of a situation even more terrifying than that described in Jiang's letter. She described the first case to come to Beijing—a woman who had driven from Shanxi and seeded the Beijing outbreak. To Susie's surprise, that had been in early March, during the National People's Congress. The hospital director at the Military Academy of Sciences had told his staff that there was SARS in Beijing, but that no one was to mention a word of it outside the hospital, so as not to interfere with the National People's Congress and leadership transition.

Since then, the woman continued, there were numerous cases at several hospitals. No. 1 and No. 2 hospitals each had dozens of cases. "They are practically filled," the woman said. And 309 Hospital, specifically mentioned in Jiang's letter, had 40 new cases in just the last week. 301 and 302 hospitals were also being overwhelmed.

The official numbers were lies.

Susie arrived at the Ruicheng Hotel in Western Beijing at 2:45 that afternoon. With each Chinese businessman entering, Susie would glance up, wondering if he were Jiang. When he finally walked in, he paused a moment and then, seeing Susie, the only foreigner, he gestured her with a quick wave to follow him. She took off after him as he headed for a corner of the lobby. He led her through a service entrance, up an elevator, and down a hall, where he asked a hotel employee for directions. Susie realized he didn't know where he was going as he walked into a cafeteria, which, besides clandestine business meetings, was the primary purpose for these little teahouse rooms. Susie's first impression was that he was nervous. But once they ordered and began to chat, he calmed down. He talked about his work as a surgeon, spoke in very clear Chinese, and gave the names of medical procedures in very good English. He was, Susie quickly deduced, exactly who he said he was in the letter.

Finally, Susie asked, "Why did you write this?"

He paused. "As a doctor, I cannot stand by while there is a terrible disease threatening the people and they are not hearing the truth about it."...

'WE ARE ASHAMED'

Huang had already tapped out his most obvious contacts. He began calling friends and asking if they knew anyone who worked in Beijing's hospitals or public health sectors, not really expecting to come up with a source. Yet a friend of his suggested a doctor from the China-Japan Friendship Hospital whom he vaguely knew and gave Huang his mobile phone number.

Huang called and quickly explained who he was and that they shared a mutual friend, and what we had learned about the coverup.

The doctor was silent.

Fearing he would hang up, Huang added that what they knew was going to be published anyway, and this was merely an attempt to make sure they had the facts correct.

Huang listened as the doctor took a deep breath and sighed, "It's true."

The doctor then recounted to Huang the story of the WHO's April visit to the China-Japan Friendship Hospital. The hospital had 56 SARS patients, 31 of whom were doctors, nurses, and other medical workers. A few minutes before the WHO team arrived, a fleet of ambulances pulled into the horseshoe driveway in front of the hospital. The hospital director ordered the stricken healthcare workers loaded onto gurneys, and staff scrambled to move these patients into the waiting ambulances. As the team of WHO experts inspected the hospital, the fleet of white vans took a leisurely tour around Beijing, keeping its deadly cargo of 31 coughing health care workers a secret from the world.

The doctor was now confirming with Huang that this was more than a "hole"; it was a pattern of deception the scope and scale of which were hard to imagine.

Huang asked him, "How could you do this?"

The doctor said, softly, "We are ashamed."...

Karl Taro Greenfeld

GREENFELD, KARL TARO. "THE VIRUS HUNTERS: WHEN THE DEADLY SARS VIRUS STRUCK CHINA THREE YEARS AGO, BEIJING RESPONDED WITH A MASSIVE COVERUP. IF IT WEREN'T FOR THE PERSISTENCE OF TWO YOUNG REPORTERS AND ONE DOCTOR WHO HAD SEEN ENOUGH, SARS MIGHT HAVE KILLED THOUSANDS MORE. THERE'S NO GUARANTEE THE WORLD WILL BE SO LUCKY NEXT TIME." *FOREIGN POLICY* (MARCH, APRIL 2006): 153, 42.

SEE ALSO *Epidemiology; Public Health and Infectious Disease.*

BIBLIOGRAPHY

Web Sites

Centers for Disease Control and Prevention (CDC). "Emergency Preparedness & Response." <http://www.bt.cdc.gov/> (accessed May 12, 2007).

United States General Accounting Office. "Infectious Disease Outbreaks." Apr 9, 2003 <http://www.gao.gov/new.items/d03654t.pdf> (accessed May 12, 2007).

World Health Organization Epidemic and Pandemic Alert and Response. "Global Outbreak Alert & Response Network." <http://www.who.int/csr/outbreaknetwork/en> (accessed May 12, 2007).

World Health Organization Western Pacific Region. "Investigation into China's recent SARS Outbreak Yields Important Lessons for Global Public Health." July 2, 2004 <http://www.wpro.who.int/sars/docs/update/update_07022004.asp> (accessed May 12, 2007).

Susan Aldridge

Pandemic Preparedness

Introduction

Pandemic influenza is one of the greatest infectious disease threats facing the world. A pandemic is a disease epidemic that affects a large proportion of the population over a wide geographic area. In the worldwide pandemic influenza attacks of 1918, 1958, and 1968, about 30% of the U.S. population developed some degree of illness. It is likely that another pandemic will strike the same percentage of the population. With about 301,717,000 people in the United States in 2007, a pandemic could sicken over 90 million people in America alone.

There is little doubt in the medical community that a pandemic will strike—only its timing, severity, and exact microbial strain (type) remain unknown. If a pandemic is severe, the effects of it will be far-ranging. Damage to critical infrastructure will have both economic and social consequences. Accordingly, a number of governments, mostly in developed nations, along with the World Health Organization (WHO), have developed plans to tackle an influenza pandemic.

Disease History, Characteristics, and Transmission

Influenza is a respiratory disease that historically has killed more people than the Black Death (plague). The dead are usually those with weakened immune systems, typically the already-ill, the very young, or the very old. However, the average age of death during the Spanish Influenza pandemic of 1918 was 33. Otherwise healthy adults in that deadly year may have produced an intense localized inflammation that overwhelmed their bodies. Transmission of the next pandemic may be from human to human or, in the possible case of avian flu, initially from bird to human.

Scope and Distribution

Public health experts anticipate a gap between the supply of vaccine and the demand for vaccine during an

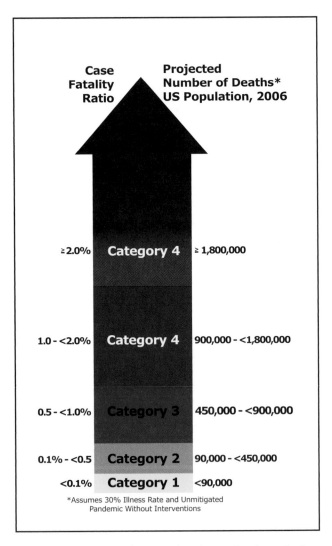

The Pandemic Severity Index categorizes the severity of a pandemic using case fatality ratios. The index helps government officials forecast the impact of influenza on a population and make recommendations for measures, such as school closings, that could reduce the spread of the disease.   *Courtesy, PandemicFlu.gov*

influenza pandemic. To reduce the impact of an influenza pandemic, the WHO recommends a non-pharmaceutical approach, such as infection control, as well as a pharmaceutical approach, such as the use of vaccines and antiviral medications for treatment and prophylaxis. Unfortunately, the availability of a pandemic vaccine will be delayed for several months after influenza first appears because of the requirements for vaccine formulation and production. The widespread nature of a pandemic means that there will be insufficient production capacity to supply everyone seeking vaccine with medication, at least in the initial months of an outbreak.

For these reasons, pandemic planning must include the assumption that a range of individuals will be struck down by disease. The U.S. government estimates that 40% or more of workers may be out sick or afraid to go to work for fear of exposure. Community outbreaks may last for six to eight weeks, with multiple waves of disease outbreaks in a calendar year. Further complicating the situation, today's highly mobile population may result in simultaneous disease outbreaks throughout the nation.

A pandemic will likely dramatically reduce the number of workers available to provide goods and services. As a result, the critical infrastructure (food, banking, water, energy, telecommunications, transportation, postal and shipping, emergency services, healthcare) and key resources (government facilities, dams, nuclear power plants, commercial facilities) will lack the staff to function without interruption.

■ Treatment and Prevention

In 2005, U.S. President George W. Bush announced a comprehensive plan to prepare for and combat pandemic influenza. The plan emphasizes the need for all levels of government and the private sector to cooperate in developing a response. In 2006, the U.S. Homeland Security Council distributed *The National Strategy for Pandemic Influenza Implementation Plan*. It requires federal government departments and agencies to develop operational plans addressing the protection of employees, the maintenance of essential functions and services, support for federal responses, and communication about pandemic planning and response. State, local, and tribal governments bear the responsibility for limiting an outbreak within and beyond the community's borders, establishing plans, educating key spokespersons in risk communication, providing public education on pandemic influenza, and establishing stockpiles of essential goods. The plan also includes a pandemic severity index that uses case fatality ratios (the proportion of deaths among persons with a particular illness) to make specific recommendations for action based upon the impact of the pandemic.

WORDS TO KNOW

CASE FATALITY RATIO: A ratio indicating the amount of persons who die as a result of a particular disease, usually expressed as a percentage or as the number of deaths per 1,000 cases.

PANDEMIC: Pandemic, which means all the people, describes an epidemic that occurs in more than one country or population simultaneously.

QUARANTINE: Quarantine is the practice of separating people who have been exposed to an infectious agent but have not yet developed symptoms from the general population. This can be done voluntarily or involuntarily by the authority of states and the federal Centers for Disease Control and Prevention.

STRAIN: A subclass or a specific genetic variation of an organism.

IN CONTEXT: TERRORISM AND BIOLOGICAL WARFARE

Pandemic preparedness programs may also help safeguard against potential bitoterrorism. One example is the National Pharmaceutical Stockpile Program (NPS). The stockpile of antibiotics, vaccines, and other medical treatment countermeasures can be rapidly deployed to the site of a domestic attack. For example, in the aftermath of the deliberate release of *Bacillus anthracis* (the bacteria that causes anthrax) in 2001, the U.S. government and some state agencies were able to quickly provide an antibiotic called ciprofloxacin (Cipro) to those potentially exposed to the bacterium.

Following these bioterrorist attacks, increased funding for the NPS was authorized. The additional funds were designated to help train medical personnel in the early identification and treatment of disease caused by the most likely pathogens.

Advocates of increased research capabilities argue that laboratory and hospital facilities must be increased and modernized to provide maximum scientific flexibility in the identification and response to biogenic threats. The CDC has already established a bioterrorism response program that includes increased testing and treatment capacity along with an enhanced ability to recognize and respond to the illness patterns that are characteristic of the deliberate release of an infectious agent.

■ Impacts and Issues

With 83% of critical infrastructure in the United States in the hands of the private sector, developing individual and system-wide business continuity plans are a priority for planning for a possible pandemic. Businesses should assess the regulations and issues that could affect their supply chain, transportation, priority for municipal services, and workplace safety. Companies, such as restaurants, that rely on unavoidable public contact and those with shared workplaces, such as plants, will be especially hard-hit by limitations on face-to-face encounters.

It is possible that a pandemic response might involve closing places of assembly, isolating those with the disease, quarantining people who have been exposed to the disease, and furloughing non-essential workers. Meanwhile, the WHO has developed a Global Vaccine Action Plan to increase the supply of a vaccine during an influenza pandemic and thereby reduce the expected gap between supply and demand.

■ Primary Source Connection

During a pandemic, governmental agencies such as the Centers for Disease Control and Prevention will play a key role in tracking the disease, assisting state health agencies, and distributing key personnel and medical supplies. Planning at the community level is also important to maintain vital services during a pandemic, while limiting the spread of the disease. In the following excerpt from a guidebook for communities planning for a pandemic, the CDC recommends measures that promote limiting social contact during a pandemic, such as closing schools and voluntary quarantine for those who are ill with the disease.

Community Strategy for Pandemic Influenza Mitigation in the United States

The pandemic mitigation framework that is proposed is based upon an early, targeted, layered application of multiple partially effective nonpharmaceutical measures. It is recommended that the measures be initiated early before explosive growth of the epidemic and, in the case of severe pandemics, that they be maintained consistently during an epidemic wave in a community. The pandemic mitigation interventions described in this document include:

1. Isolation and treatment (as appropriate) with influenza antiviral medications of all persons with confirmed or probable pandemic influenza. Isolation may occur in the home or healthcare setting, depending on the severity of an individual's illness and/or the current capacity of the healthcare infrastructure.

2. Voluntary home quarantine of members of households with confirmed or probable influenza case(s) and consideration of combining this intervention

with the prophylactic use of antiviral medications, providing sufficient quantities of effective medications exist and that a feasible means of distributing them is in place.

3. Dismissal of students from school (including public and private schools as well as colleges and universities) and school-based activities and closure of childcare programs, coupled with protecting children and teenagers through social distancing in the community to achieve reductions of out-of-school social contacts and community mixing.

4. Use of social distancing measures to reduce contact between adults in the community and workplace, including, for example, cancellation of large public gatherings and alteration of workplace environments and schedules to decrease social density and preserve a healthy workplace to the greatest extent possible without disrupting essential services. Enable institution of workplace leave policies that align incentives and facilitate adherence with the nonpharmaceutical interventions (NPIs) outlined above.

All such community-based strategies should be used in combination with individual infection control measures, such as handwashing and cough etiquette. Implementing these interventions in a timely and coordinated fashion will require advance planning. Communities must be prepared for the cascading second- and third-order consequences of the interventions, such as increased workplace absenteeism related to child-minding responsibilities if schools dismiss students and childcare programs close.

Centers for Disease Control and Prevention

CENTERS FOR DISEASE CONTROL AND PREVENTION. "INTERIM PRE-PANDEMIC PLANNING GUIDANCE: COMMUNITY STRATEGY FOR PANDEMIC INFLUENZA MITIGATION IN THE UNITED STATES." WASHINGTON, DC: U.S. DEPARTMENT OF HEALTH AND HUMAN SERVICES, FEBRUARY 2007, PAGE 8. ALSO AVAILABLE ONLINE AT <HTTP://WWW2A.CDC.GOV/PHLP/DOCS/COMMUNITY_MITIGATION.PDF>

BIBLIOGRAPHY

Web Sites

U.S. Department of Health and Human Services. "Pandemic Flu.gov." April 26, 2007. <http://www.pandemicflu.gov/index.html> (accessed April 28, 2007).

World Health Organization. "Epidemic and Pandemic Alert Response." 2007. <http://www.who.int/csr/disease/influenza/nationalpandemic/en/index.html> (accessed April 28, 2007).

World Health Organization. "Global Pandemic Influenza Action Plan to Increase Vaccine Supply." 2006. <http://www.who.int/vaccines-documents/DocsPDF06/863.pdf> (accessed April 28, 2007).

Caryn E. Neumann

Parasitic Diseases

Introduction

A parasite is an organism that lives on or in a host organism. It is dependent upon the host for food and protection. For millions of years, parasites and humans have co-existed. Many parasites do no damage, particularly protozoa in low numbers, but some can cause significant harm. Parasitic infections, such as toxoplasmosis, malaria, and Guinea worm, strike millions of people annually in every region of the world. These infections are often painful, debilitating, or deadly.

There are three main classes of parasites that can cause disease in humans: protozoa, helminths, and ectoparasites. Protozoa are microscopic, one-celled organisms. A serious infection can develop from just a single organism that then multiplies. Helminths are flatworms, thorny-headed worms, and roundworms. Ectoparasites are ticks, fleas, mites, and lice that burrow into the skin. Arthropods, including mosquitos, serve as the vectors of many different pathogens (disease-causing organisms).

Disease History, Characteristics, and Transmission

Transmission of protozoa typically occurs by a fecal-oral route through contaminated food or water or by person-to-person contact. Arthropod vectors, such as ticks, transmit protozoa that thrive in human blood or tissue. Helminths are spread by ingestion, usually through contaminated meat or water.

Scope and Distribution

Parasitic diseases occur most often in the topics and subtropics, but can also occur in more moderate climates, or anywhere the parasite and its host or vector resides. Worldwide, parasitic diseases, of which malaria is the

leader, kill more than two million people annually. The World Health Organization estimates that over one person in four harbors some sort of parasitic helminth

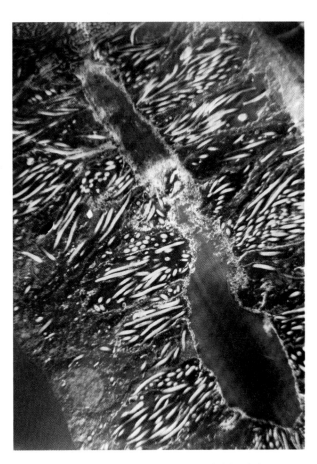

This colored transmission electron micrograph (TEM) shows malaria sporozoites in mosquito salivary glands. The sporozoites (*Plasmodium* [yellow]) develop after the mosquito feeds on an infected human. They migrate to the salivary glands (red), move into the central salivary duct (dark blue area), and are injected into a human as the mosquito feeds. *LSHTM/Photo Researchers, Inc.*

WORDS TO KNOW

ARTHROPOD: A member of the largest single animal phylum, consisting of organisms with segmented bodies, jointed legs or wings, and exoskeletons.

ECTOPARASITES: Parasites that cling to the outside of their host, rather than their host's intestines. Common points of attachment are the gills, fins, or skin of fish.

HELMINTH: A representative of various phyla of worm-like animals.

HOST: Organism that serves as the habitat for a parasite, or possibly for a symbiont. A host may provide nutrition to the parasite or symbiont, or simply a place in which to live.

PATHOGEN: A disease causing agent, such as a bacteria, virus, fungus, etc.

PROTOZOA: Single-celled animal-like microscopic organisms that live by taking in food rather than making it by photosynthesis and must live in the presence of water. (Singular: protozoan.) Protozoa are a diverse group of single-celled organisms, with more than 50,000 different types represented. The vast majority are microscopic, many measuring less than or 5 one-thousandths of an inch (0.005 millimeters), but some, such as the freshwater Spirostomun, may reach 0.17 inches (3 millimeters) in length, large enough to enable it to be seen with the naked eye.

VECTOR: Any agent, living or otherwise, that carries and transmits parasites and diseases. Also, an organism or chemical used to transport a gene into a new host cell.

(worm). In the United States, trichomoniasis is the most common parasitic infection, with over seven million cases diagnosed per year.

The increased movement of people from region to region has also spread parasites. Chagas, an insect-borne parasitic disease, once rarely appeared in the United States. Immigration from Central and Latin America is a contributing factor in an increased incidence of Chagas parasite, *Trypanosoma cruzi*, in the United States. The American Red Cross now screens blood donors for the parasite to prevent transmission. In the Los Angeles area, the parasite was found in one in 3,800 donors by 2006.

Another disease, cysticercosis, caused by tapeworm larvae, is also on the rise in the United States. However, the disease disproportionately affects foreign-born residents, especially Hispanics who immigrated from Mexico and Central America, most of whom contracted the disease in their home countries.

■ Treatment and Prevention

The first step in treating a parasitic disease is to identify it but this is complicated by the number of diseases with similar symptoms that exist in the world. In 2006, a device known as GreeneChip became generally available to detect parasites. It is a microscope slide covered with bits and pieces of genetic information from nearly 30,000 different viruses, bacteria, fungi, and parasites. First used by the World Health Organization (WHO), the $125 slide has subsequently been delivered to the Centers for Disease Control and Prevention (CDC).

If a parasite is detected in a host early enough, strong anti-protozoal drugs such as nifurtimox can bring the parasite to undetectable levels or eliminate it entirely. In other cases, such as the common Latin American and Middle Eastern blight leishmaniasis, medication derived from the chemical element antimony and anti-fungal drugs have stopped the parasite.

Patients with severe infections must also undergo weekly blood tests and electrocardiograms to make sure that their kidneys, liver, and heart remain healthy throughout treatment. Some parasites, such as the one that causes Chagas, may have multiplied over years and decades. In these cases, infected individuals may require treatment with heart-regulating drugs or regulation via an implanted pacemaker.

As of May 2007, there were no vaccines licensed to prevent parasitic diseases. Research and development of potential vaccines focus on three distinct ways to stop the spread of parasitic diseases. Anti-disease vaccines target blood forms and parasite-produced toxins. Transmission-blocking vaccines prevent the development of the parasite within a host. Anti-infection vaccines target parasites in stages where they are most likely to infect.

Several ongoing animal studies are testing possible vaccines against helminth and arthropod-borne parasitic diseases. As of 2005, at least one potential malaria vaccine was ready for clinical testing in humans. However, researchers have already noticed that some forms of vaccination may have unintended consequences. In some studies, parasites that survived in immunized animals displayed increased virulence. Such virulent strains of parasitic diseases such as malaria could be resistant to existing anti-malarial drugs or thwart emerging vaccines. Thus, many health officials assert that more must be done to identify and combat sources of parasites.

■ Impacts and Issues

Many parasitic diseases no longer have geographic borders. Physicians must consider that parasites which are common in distant regions may be seen in immigrants or travelers.

Regular access to potable water for drinking, cooking, and washing can virtually eliminate water-borne parasitic diseases. However, the WHO estimates that one billion people worldwide live without access to clean water. Improved access to uncontaminated water, personal hygiene and food safety education, and construction of sewer-sanitation systems—even as basic as proper latrines—dramatically reduce incidence of parasite related illnesses.

Parasitic disease prevention can have environmental consequences. Pesticides are often spread over large areas to reduce parasite-transmitting insect populations. Pesticides are powerful chemicals that can contaminate drinking water and soil. People who work around pesticides must take precautions to avoid exposure.

Use of some pesticides, such as dichloro-diphenyl-trichloroethane (DDT) remains controversial, but pesticides are an important part of parasitic disease control that save thousands of lives each year. To minimize environmental damage, researchers are working to develop better pesticides, many directed at killing parasite-transmitting insects, or the parasites themselves, while reducing toxicity to humans and animals. Health workers also promote responsible use of pesticides. For example, in the fight against mosquito-borne diseases, health workers advocate the use of insecticide-treated nets to minimize the need for topical insecticides applied directly to the skin.

Research indicates that global climate change may impact the incidence of parasitic infections in humans. Recent studies in Kenya indicate a strong correlation between rising temperatures, more variable rainfall, and a greater incidence of mosquitoes spreading malaria into highland areas previously protected from the parasite. A 2007 report by the Intergovernmental Panel on Climate Change (IPCC) advised that millions of people may be affected by similar shifts in the spread of parasitic diseases. Other studies dispute these findings, asserting that increased migration of people and animals has a more significant impact on parasite distribution.

Malaria remains the top parasitic killer in the world, causing from one to two million deaths around the world each year, mostly among children. On June 30, 2005, U.S. president George W. Bush announced the President's Malaria Initiative (PMI), a cooperative program with the goal of cutting malaria deaths in half by 2008 in target African nations. The PMI funds research, anti-malarial drugs, and treatment as well as distributes insecticide-treated mosquito nets. Many other nations, international agencies, and nongovernment organizations have similar anti-malaria campaigns. Among nongovernment charitable entities, the Bill and Melinda Gates Foundation is one of the world's leading sponsors of anti-malaria programs and malaria vaccine research, thus far granting over $400 million.

BIBLIOGRAPHY

Web Sites

Bill & Melinda Gates Foundation. <http://www.gatesfoundation.org/default.htm> (accessed May 31, 2007).

Department of Health and Human Services, Centers for Disease Control and Prevention. "Parasitic Diseases." February 16, 2007 <http://www.cdc.gov/ncidod/dpd/index.htm> (accessed April 30, 2007).

Caryn E. Neumann

Personal Protective Equipment

Introduction

Personal protective equipment is equipment used in a healthcare setting to prevent direct contact with infectious microorganisms or contact with body fluids that might contain a disease-causing (pathogenic) microorganism.

Gloves, gowns or aprons, masks and respirators, goggles, and face shields are all examples of personal protective equipment. The degree of protection offered by such equipment varies depending on the infectious disease being dealt with. Treating someone who has a common cold may only require the use of medical gloves, for example, while a public health response to the dispersal of *Bacillus anthracis* (the cause of anthrax) requires personnel to wear full body suits, including sealed gloves and respirators that block the inhalation of the tiny bacterial spores.

History and Scientific Foundations

The use of personal protective equipment is centuries old. Records from England dating back to the seventeenth century describe the protective headgear, gowns, and masks worn by physicians treating plague victims. At the time, some physicians assumed that plague could be transmitted through the air. Although scientists later discovered that plague is caused by a bacterium called *Yersinia pestis* that is transmitted by the bite of an infected flea, the use of protective clothing was a wise precaution.

Through the early decades of the nineteenth century, surgeons did not wear any special clothing when they performed operations. Surgeries were done by physicians who literally walked in off the street into an open-air operating theater. The realization that dedicated surgical clothing prevented the transmission of infections from patient to patient revolutionized medicine and made post-surgical infections less common. In this sense, the clothing was protective to the patient. However, with time the protective value of clothing to healthcare providers also was recognized.

Then as now, the premise of personal protective equipment is simple—protective clothing and other gear presents a barrier to the transmission of infectious microorganisms.

Applications and Research

The types of personal protective equipment used depend on a number of factors. One factor is the setting. For example, a researcher at a biosafety level 4 facility, which is designed to deal with dangerously contagious microorganisms, must be completely enclosed in a protective suit that is connected to an air supply. On the other hand, a general practitioner who is examining a person who has a cold may only elect to wear a face mask as a barrier to virus-laden droplets that could be expelled by a cough.

Another factor is the anticipated type of exposure. More extensive face and body coverage is required if there is the potential for splashing or spraying of body fluids, for example. Related to this is the appropriateness of the protective equipment for the task. For example, when confronting a dangerous respiratory infection, a respirator can be more appropriate than a mask, since the respirator is designed to exclude small droplets that can pass through the mask fabric. As a second example, an apron that does not absorb liquids is a safer choice when dealing with a victim of Ebola (where a great deal of bleeding usually occurs) than a surgical gown made of absorbent cotton.

A third factor is the fit of the protective equipment. One size does not fit all. Trying to care for a patient or respond to a medical emergency while wearing protective equipment that is too small or too large is certainly inconvenient and can be dangerous. Ill-fitting protective gear may restrict movement and, in the case of a respirator that is too large and fits sloppily on the face, may render the equipment useless.

Gloves are the most common personal protective equipment in hospitals and other healthcare settings. The choice of glove depends on the task. Gloves are available in a variety of materials, may be sterile (free of microorganisms) or non-sterile, and may be intended for single use or repeated use. However, gloves are only as effective as the person wearing them. For example, if a healthcare provider fails to change gloves after leaving one patient and moving on to treat another patient, infections may be spread. Even when treating a single patient, a healthcare worker should change gloves after examining a body site that is infected and before examining other non-infected sites on the same patient.

The use of approved respirators are required when dealing with certain infections. One example is tuberculosis. The bacterium that is responsible for the respiratory infection (*Mycobacterium tuberculosis*) can be expelled inside small droplets, which can be inhaled by someone close by the patient. N95, N99, and N100 respirators are designed to exclude droplets that are less than 5 microns (a micron is one-millioneth of a meter) in diameter. Avian influenza—a potentially lethal infection caused by the H5N1 virus that has evolved to include the capability of person-to-person transmission—is another infection that requires a healthcare provider to use a respirator.

■ Impacts and Issues

When properly used and worn, personal protective equipment is an efficient means of minimizing the

IN CONTEXT: TERRORISM AND BIOLOGICAL WARFARE

Fear of bioterrorism, periodically heightened by news events, sometimes causes panic buying of equipment that may be ill-designed to meet real threats. For example, military surplus gas masks generally provide only the illusion of protection. They offer no real protection against biological agents and should not be bought for that purpose. Personnel stockpiling of antibiotics is also unwise. The potency of antibiotics such as Cipro declines with time. Moreover, the inappropriate use of antibiotics can actually lead to the development of bacterial resistance and a consequential lowering of antibiotic effectiveness.

General preparedness is always prudent. A few days supply of food and water and the identification of rooms in homes and offices that can be temporarily sealed with duct tape to reduce outside air infiltration is a wise precaution. More specific response plans and protective measures, however, must be based upon the specific dangers posed by organisms that produce disease. For example, Anthrax (*Bacillus anthracis*), Botulism (*Clostridium botulinum* toxin), Plague (*Yersinia pestis*), Smallpox (*Variola major*), Tularemia (*Francisella tularensis*), viral hemorrhagic fevers (e.g., Ebola, Marburg), and arenaviruses (e.g., Lassa) are considered high-risk potential bioterrorism agents. These agents share a common trait of being easily spread from person to person. And they all can kill many of those who are infected. However, the natures of the diseases they cause are very different. A response that is effective against one microorganism may well be useless against another.

spread of infectious disease from those who are infected to their healthcare providers, and, via the healthcare provider, to other patients. For example, before surgeons began to wear surgical garments, operations were a last resort due to the high post-surgical death rate. When surgeons began to wear special clothing that was changed between operations, the rate of post-surgical infection decreased dramatically. Today, the Occupational Safety and Health Administration enforces the Bloodborne Pathogens Standard, last updated in 2001, which specifies the personal protective practices and equipment that must be available for healthcare workers and patients in the United States.

But there are difficulties involved in the use of protective equipment. For example, in an emergency, there may not be time to properly clean protective clothing or to maintain the supply of disposable protective equipment, such as gloves or disposable needles. As a result, protective equipment may be re-used when it should not be, and the contaminated equipment can continue the spread of infection. During the first documented outbreak of Ebola hemorrhagic fever in Zaire in 1976, the virus quickly spread to hospital workers when non-disposable needles were reused and protective barriers, such as non-permeable gowns and face shields, were not available.

As shown in the months following the September 11, 2001, terrorist attacks on the United States, the deliberate airborne release of an infectious organism, such as *B. anthracis*, can easily occur. A large scale release of such a pathogen could affect a wide geographical area, requiring the rapid deployment of many personnel. It is unlikely that their need for protective equipment could be met from a central source, since even facilities dedicated to the study of highly infectious microbes usually have only a limited number of full-body protective suits on hand. This is an issue that those responsible for emergency planning need to address.

SEE ALSO *Bioterrorism; Contact Precautions; Infection Control and Asepsis; Isolation and Quarantine; Standard Precautions.*

BIBLIOGRAPHY

Books

Lawrence, Jean, and Dee May. *Infection Control in the Community.* New York: Churchill Livingstone, 2003.

Tierno, Philip M. *The Secret Life of Germs: What They Are, Why We Need Them, and How We Can Protect Ourselves Against Them.* New York: Atria, 2004.

Brian Hoyle

Pink Eye (Conjunctivitis)

■ Introduction

Pink eye refers to a chemical- or allergy-related inflammation, or a viral or bacterial infection, of the transparent covering of the eyelid and a portion of the eyeball. The transparent covering is called the conjunctiva, and so the inflammation or infection is known as conjunctivitis.

The designation pink eye indicates the appearance of the inflamed or infected conjunctiva, due to the increased prominence of blood vessels, which changes the color of the white portion of the eye to red or pink.

■ Disease History, Characteristics, and Transmission

Infection-related conjunctivitis can be caused by viruses or bacteria. The microbes that are responsible are those that cause colds, ear infections, sore throats, and sexually transmitted diseases. Bacteria include *Staphylococcus*, *Streptococcus*, *Chlamydia*, *Gonorrhea*, and *Hemophilus*. Viruses include adenoviruses, rhinoviruses, coronaviruses, echoviruses, paramyxoviruses, and coxsackieviruses. Viral conjunctivitis is more common than the bacterial infections.

Infants can be infected during birth by bacteria in the mother's birth canal. While harmless in the mother, the bacteria are capable of causing an infection in the infant, whose immune system is not yet operating at full efficiency. The bacteria are described as being opportunitistic pathogens—they normally cause no harm, but can cause disease given the appropriate circumstances. Screening of the mother prior to the birth can detect and treat the infection. Newborn conjunctivitis is treated by the application of an antibiotic ointment to the eyes soon after birth.

The redness of the affected eye(s) is a hallmark of pink eye. Another common symptom is the feeling that something foreign is in the eye. Many people also complain of a gritty or itchy sensation in the infected eye(s). Other symptoms include blurred vision, increased sensitivity to light, increased formation of tears, and a dis-

charge from the infected eye(s) that can become crusty during sleep.

Conjunctivitis can also be caused by an allergic reaction to pollen or some other substance. A part of the allergic response is the production of an antibody called immunoglobulin E, which in turn triggers cells in the

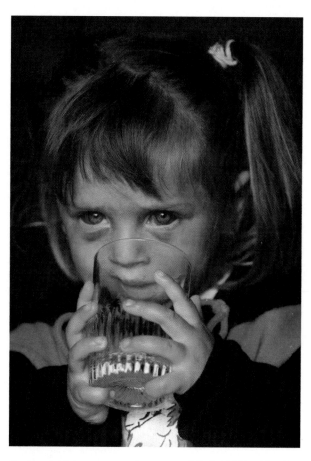

Conjunctivitis is a common disease, especially in children, that is usually caused by bacteria or viruses and is limited to the clear membrane that covers the white part of the eye.   *AP Images.*

eyes and airway to release various compounds. One of these compounds, histamine, produces a variety of allergic responses including allergic conjunctivitis.

While the allergic response cannot be passed from person to person, viral and bacterial conjunctivitis are highly contagious.

Scope and Distribution

Pink eye is global in occurrence and can affect anyone. Pink eye, like most minor contagious infections, spreads easily among groups of children. Viral and bacterial pink eye often affect children who live in group settings or attend school or day care.

Treatment and Prevention

People who develop bacterial or viral pink eye should avoid close contact with others. This is especially important for infants in day care and school-age children.

The cause of pink eye can be determined. If caused by a bacterial infection, pink eye is easily treated using antibiotics. Typically, the antibiotic is applied as an eye-drop solution, although an ointment can be used for infants and younger children. The infection usually clears up within several days. Even so, the antibiotic needs to be used for as long as has been prescribed to make sure all the infecting bacteria are killed. If treatment is stopped too early, some bacteria may survive and develop resistance to the antibiotic, making treatment of the recurring infection more difficult.

Allergic pink eye can be treated by use of eyedrops containing compounds that lessen symptoms. Rubbing

the eye should be avoided, as it can introduce allergens and trigger more symptoms.

Good personal hygiene, especially handwashing and minimizing rubbing of the eyes, reduces the risk of developing pink eye. Frequently washing of bathroom and bedroom linens and avoiding sharing pillows and cosmetic applicators further lessen the risk of conjunctivitis.

Impacts and Issues

While conjunctivitis is usually an inconvenience rather than a health concern, there is a risk that it can lead to problems with the cornea of the eye. As well, the infection in newborns can led to more serious health issues, including loss of vision. Prompt treatment can eliminate this concern.

In the United Kingdom, researchers and public health officials are currently studying the costs and benefits of changing common medical approaches to the treatment of viral and bacterial conjunctivitis. Since many cases of pink eye can disappear without medical intervention, researchers are developing new protocols for when parents should seek medical attention for children with conjunctivitis and how physicians should treat conjunctivitis. Public health officials have noted that antibiotic eyedrops are frequently prescribed, even before a clinical diagnosis of bacterial pink eye can be made. Use of antibiotics does not treat viral pink eye and only negligibly reduces recovery time for most cases of bacterial pink eye. Researchers worry that overzealous prescription of antibiotics could lead to bacterial resistance. Health officials note that patients' costs associated with treating many mild forms of pink eye—including eyedrops, antibiotics, missed work, missed school, and doctors' visits—may be unnecessarily high.

SEE ALSO *Childhood Infectious Diseases, Immunization Impacts; Contact Lenses and* Fusarium *Keratitis.*

BIBLIOGRAPHY

Books

Douglas, Ann. *The Mother of All Toddler Books.* New York: John Wiley & Sons, 2004.

Ernest, Paul H. *How to Have Healthy Eyes for Life.* New York: Hudson Mills Press, 2003.

Weizer, Jennifer S., and Sharon Fekrat. *All about Your Eyes.* Raleigh: Duke University Press, 2006.

Brian Hoyle

CONJUNCTIVA AND TEARS

A fine mucus membrane, the conjunctiva, covers the cornea and also lines the eyelid. Blinking lubricates the cornea with tears, providing the moisture necessary for its health. The cornea's outside surface is protected by a thin film of tears produced in the lacrimal glands located in the lateral part of the orbit below the eyebrow. Tears flow through ducts from this gland to the eyelid and eye, and they drain from the inner corner of the eye into the nasal cavity. A clear watery liquid, the aqueous humor, separates the cornea from the iris and lens. The cornea contains no blood vessels or pigment and gets its nutrients from the aqueous humor.

Pinworm (*Enterobius vermicularis*) Infection

■ Introduction

Pinworm infection, or enterobiasis, is a common helminth infection that arises when humans drink water or eat food contaminated by eggs of parasitic pinworms. Enterobiasis is considered the most common roundworm infection in the United States. Although it can affect any human, it is more common in children.

Pinworms live in the general area of the body known as the rectum (lower part of intestine). The small, thin (threadlike), white pinworm is about 0.4 in (1 cm) in length, with the adult male ranging from 0.04–0.16 in (0.1–0.4 cm) in length and the adult female having a length of 0.32–0.50 in (0.8–1.3 cm). A pinworm possesses a long, pin-shaped posterior, which gives the worm its common name. Pinworms are nematodes in the family Oxyuridae, genus *Enterobius*. Pinworm infection is most commonly caused by the species *Enterobius vermicularis*, the threadworm. A second species, *Enterobius gregorii*, recently has been found to cause the infection in Africa, Asia, and Europe.

■ Disease History, Characteristics, and Transmission

The pinworm is a roundworm, which is the common name of any non-segmented worm located in freshwater, marine, or terrestrial environments. Roundworms are

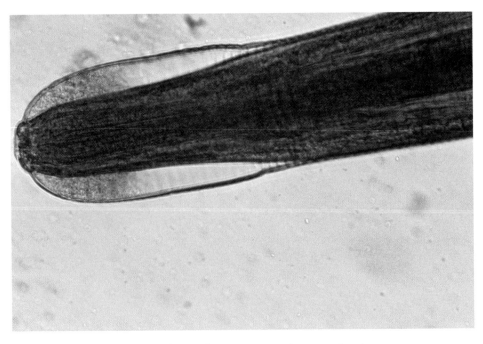

Adult pinworm, *Enterobius vermicularis*, is shown. *Pr. Bouree/Photo Researchers, Inc.*

found almost anywhere around the world, living frequently in the surface layers of soils.

Pinworms develop to adulthood within the host's intestines, specifically in the lower small intestine and the upper colon. On rare occasions they are found in the abdominal lining, fallopian tubes, liver, uterus, and vagina. Generally, they are not found in the bloodstream or in other organs besides the intestines.

The male pinworm dies after mating. The female moves from the intestine to the anal area where she lays 10,000–20,000 eggs. Within four to six hours, the eggs become mature and, thus, infectious. The female soon expels a sticky substance that causes itching in the host. Intense itching causes the human to transfer eggs to the fingers, which then transfer the eggs to other objects. The eggs can live outside of a host for up to two weeks—in some cases, three weeks. The eggs are often accidentally ingested. The larvae then hatch and move to the intestine. They mature within 30–45 days. Their overall lifespan is about 60 days. The larvae can also hatch outside the host and then move through the anus and into the intestines. In some cases, the eggs become airborne and are inhaled by the host.

Symptoms are usually mild, and sometimes there are no symptoms at all. When present, symptoms include itching, intestinal problems, vomiting, nervousness and irritability, restless sleep, and sometimes skin reddening and infection around the anus. Other than these mild symptoms, the infection usually does not cause permanent damage.

■ Scope and Distribution

Pinworm infection is found worldwide, although it is found more commonly in temperate regions of Western Europe and North America. It is only occasionally found in tropical areas. The infection is frequently found when humans live in crowded environments. It is estimated that between 200 million and 500 million people worldwide are infected annually. The Division of Parasitic Diseases (DPD) of the National Center for Infectious Diseases (U.S. Centers for Disease Control and Prevention) estimates that approximately 40 million people are infected each year in the United States. About 50% of all children become infected at some time during their childhoods.

In the United States, according to the DPD, pinworm infection is most common in school-age children, followed by preschool-age children and people in institutional care facilities and children at day care facilities. Mothers are also frequently infected.

■ Treatment and Prevention

Diagnosis of pinworm infection is made by an examination of the patient's anal region. A tape test is usually used, which involves placing the sticky side of a trans-

> ## WORDS TO KNOW
>
> **HELMINTH:** A representative of various phyla of worm-like animals.
>
> **HOST:** Organism that serves as the habitat for a parasite, or possibly for a symbiont. A host may provide nutrition to the parasite or symbiont, or simply a place in which to live.
>
> **LARVAE:** Immature forms (wormlike in insects; fishlike in amphibians) of an organism capable of surviving on its own. Larvae do not resemble the parent and must go through metamorphosis, or change, to reach the adult stage.
>
> **NEMATODES:** Also known as roundworms; a type of helminth characterized by long, cylindrical bodies.

> ## *IN CONTEXT*: TRENDS AND STATISTICS
>
> The Division of Parasitic Diseases at the Centers for Disease Control and Prevention (CDC) states that "pinworm is the most common worm infection in the United States. School-age children, followed by preschoolers, have the highest rates of infection. In some groups nearly 50% of children are infected. Infection often occurs in more than one family member. Adults are less likely to have pinworm infection, except mothers of infected children. Child care centers, and other institutional settings often have cases of pinworm infection."
>
> SOURCE: *Centers for Disease Control and Prevention, National Center for Infectious Diseases, Division of Parasitic Diseases.*

parent adhesive or cellophane tape against the skin around the anus. The procedure should be performed immediately after waking up, before bathing and using the toilet, so that any eggs in the anal area will be picked up. The materials that stick to the tape are then examined under a microscope for the presence of pinworms. The infected person may also see worms crawling on bed sheets or clothing.

Treatment includes various antiparasitic drugs that have been found effective in treating the infection. These drugs include albendazole, mebendazole, piperazine, and pyrantel pamoate. If one person in a household has the infection, all family members are often advised to take the drug treatment.

These medicines kill the worms about 95% of the time. However, they do not kill the eggs. To kill the eggs, a second round of medicine is recommended two weeks after the completion of the first round. If this treatment does not eliminate the infection, then additional treatments should be administered. In addition, a thorough search should be made for the source of the infection, including other children, household members, and anyone or anything else that has come in contact with the infected person. Four to six treatments spaced two weeks apart are sometimes recommended for difficult cases.

To avoid becoming re-infected, an array of hygiene practices are advised, including disinfecting eating utensils and bed linens; cleaning the toilet daily; keeping fingers away from the nostrils and mouth; bathing when first waking; changing and washing underwear daily; changing bed clothing frequently and after each treatment; providing plenty of sunlight or artificial light (pinworms are light sensitive); trimming fingernails (scratching of anal area may place pinworms underneath nails); and not scratching bare anal areas.

■ Impacts and Issues

When treated properly, pinworm infection is fully curable. Even though the prognosis for pinworm infection is very good, complications can set in. Among the most common complications are salpingitis (pelvic inflammatory disease, an infection of the lining of the uterus, fallopian tubes, or ovaries), vaginitis (any infection or inflammation of the vagina), and reinfestation (further reoccurrence of the infection).

Children who are being treated for pinworm infection need not be kept home from school, and it is not appropriate to conclude that a child with pinworms has an unclean environment. Pinworm infections are extremely common among children, with half of all children eventually becoming infected due to the large amount of time spent outdoors playing in dirt and sand. Parents can minimize the chances of their children getting the infection by promoting handwashing and sanitation within and outside the home. Prompt medical care, medication, and preventive hygiene practices will eliminate pinworms from children and adults in a quick and safe manner.

SEE ALSO *CDC (Centers for Disease Control and Prevention); Public Health and Infectious Disease; Roundworm (Ascariasis) infection.*

BIBLIOGRAPHY

Books

Cheng, Liang, and David G. Bostwick, eds. *Essentials of Anatomic Pathology.* Totowa, NJ: Humana Press, 2006.

Rudolph, Collin D., et al., eds. *Rudolph's Pediatrics.* New York: McGraw-Hill, 2003.

Web Sites

Centers for Disease Control and Prevention. "Enterobiasis (*Enerobius vermicularis*)." May 5, 2004. <http://www.dpd.cdc.gov/dpdx/HTML/Enterobiasis.htm> (accessed March 16, 2007).

KidsHealth for Parents. "Infections: Pinworm." April 2005. <http://www.kidshealth.org/parent/infections/parasitic/pinworm.html> (accessed March 16, 2007).

U.S. Department of Health and Human Services. National Institute of Allergy and Infectious Diseases. "Parasitic Roundworm Diseases." February 2005. <http://www.niaid.nih.gov/factsheets/roundwor.htm> (accessed March 16, 2007).

Plague, Early History

■ Introduction

Plague has shaped the development of all civilizations. In the recorded histories of Chinese civilization, epidemic disease thrice wiped out one-quarter to over one-third of its population. The Black Death transformed the social, political, and economic landscape of medieval Europe.

Most scientists and historians link bubonic plague in antiquity to rats. *Yersina pestis*, the bacterium that causes bubonic plague, lives inside the guts of a flea. When inside the flea, *Yersina pestis* can multiply and blocks the flea's throat area, making the flea quite hungry and in search of new hosts, whether rats or humans. When

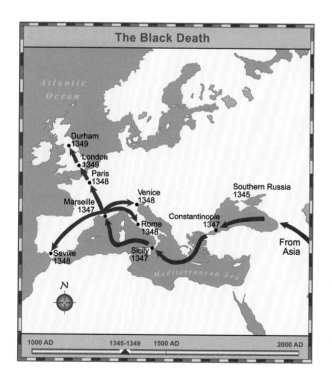

The Black Death

This map shows the migration of the bubonic plague during the 14th century from Asia and Europe. © *MAPS.com/Corbis.*

the flea bites, some of the bacteria is spit out into the bite wound, transmitting the disease.

However, pestilence or plague as recorded in the annals of history does not refer to only one disease. "Plague" did not always describe bubonic plague or the Black Death. Measles, smallpox, flu, dysentery, or typhoid all could have produced a sudden rise in mortality and were referred to in antiquity as plague.

Epidemic disease has likely always been part of human history, but the first written account of its devastating effects originates in the ancient Middle East. The development of horticulture permitted the development of towns, concentrating populations in relatively small areas and facilitating the spread of some diseases. Many historians assert that infectious disease agents spread and thrived because there was a large supply of non-immune, disease-susceptible people that diseases could attack. People often shared their living quarters with farm animals. Diseases such as cowpox could affect humans or become genetically modified to create epidemics, such as smallpox.

■ History

Plague in Ancient Egypt, the Middle East, and China

Ancient literature often provides a historical account of ancient epidemics. The Babylonian *Epic of Gilgamesh* from the seventh-century BC claimed that a visit from the god of pestilence was more preferable than a flooding disaster, and an Egyptian text from 2000 BC compared "fear of Pharaoh with fear of the god of disease in the year of pestilence." Biblical texts such as the Book of Exodus also report the plagues in Egypt in the form of skin pustules, and the Plague of the Philistines in I Samuel supposedly killed 70,000 in Israel.

In ancient China, references to plague in the Yangtze River Valley were likely endemic malaria or Dengue Fever, a disease common in low-lying areas borne by mosquitoes. The Chinese also were beset by smallpox,

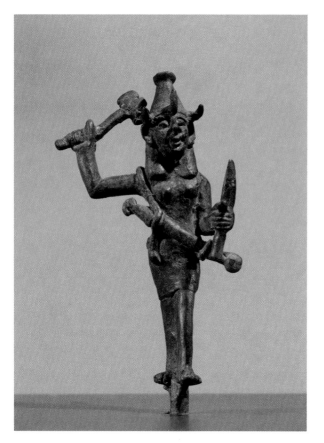

Bronze figurine of the Canaanite god Reshef, god of the nether world and of plagues. *Erich Lessing/Art Resource, NY.*

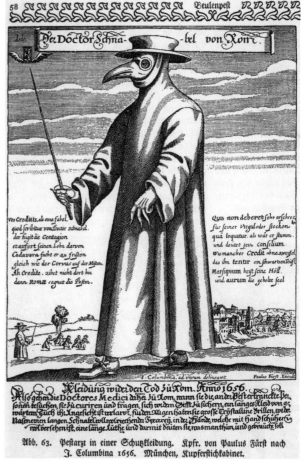

A 17th-century illustration shows a physician wearing protective clothing, including a mask, to shield him against the plague. *© Bettmann/Corbis.*

and they invented the first techniques of effective prevention in 590 BC called "pock-sowing." They would grind dried skin scabs from smallpox victims along with musk and apply the mixture to the noses of the healthy. The Chinese also placed matter from the smallpox pustules that arose on the skin into a scratch in the arm of a recipient, in a process called variolation. Exposure to the pathogen usually produced a mild case and gave the recipient immunity, but sometimes a full-blown case would develop. (Effective and safe vaccination for smallpox did not occur until the eighteenth century).

However, another Egyptian text, called the Ebers Papyrus, from 1500 BC does describe an epidemic disease with symptoms similar to the bubonic plague, a bacterial infection that causes buboes, or swelling of the lymph glands. The Ebers Papyrus mentions an illness that "has produced a bubo, and the pus has petrified, the disease has hit."

Plague in Ancient Greece and Rome

In contrast with Egypt or China where rivers brought irrigation as well as disease-borne vectors, ancient Greece was relatively free of disease. The Greek agriculture did not alter the environment nearly as much as

Chinese rice paddies. As a result, the agricultural revolution in Greece did not bring exposure to new diseases.

Threat of epidemics came from the expansion of cities in Greece, increased population density, and exposure to new pathogens from travelers and trade. Ancient Greece was made up of a number of small independent city-states and economics was driven by trade—contact with other peoples brought contact with new diseases. In the fifth century BC, Athens was the most prominent Greek city-state, and it initiated a protracted war with rival city-state Sparta. Expecting to win with its powerful navy, Athens was instead brought to its knees with the appearance of a mysterious epidemic in 430-429 BC that wiped out one-quarter of the Athenian land forces. The ancient Greek historian Thucydides (460–399 BC) in his *History of the Peloponnesian War* argues the epidemic was the main reason for Athens military defeat—a defining event in subsequent Mediterranean political history.

The identity of this epidemic has been a matter of debate, ranging from scarlet fever to smallpox to

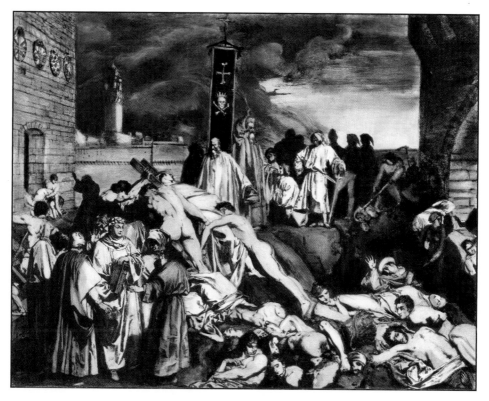

A 14th-century engraving by Giovanni Boccaccio (1313–1375) depicts an outbreak of the plague in Florence, Italy. © *Bettmann/Corbis.*

bubonic plague to the effects of ergot or a mold on the grain supply. Regardless of the source or causative agent of disease, Athenians had little immunity to it. Because the disease entered the Athenian population with sudden ferocity and then disappeared, several scientists and historians theorize that the pathogen came by sea and soon died out after provoking an accelerated immune response in the local population. The Spartans, more geographically isolated on the Peloponnesian peninsula, were untouched, giving them a decisive military advantage.

Ancient Rome was highly prone to plagues. During the reign of emperor Marcus Aurelius (121–180), the Roman Empire was struck by a destructive epidemic that began in 166 AD and occurred with intermittent frequency until 189 AD. The accounts of the Greek physician Galen (c.130–c.200) about the plague, particularly the incidence of skin rash and gastrointestinal bleeding, have led some scholars to conclude it was probably smallpox. The mortality rate was 7 to 10 percent among the local population, and 10 to 15 percent in the army for a total of five million deaths over the 23-year period. Unlike in China, treatment in the Western World was relatively ineffectual, though it was common knowledge that smallpox survivors were immune to the disease. As early as 430 BC, those who had survived the disease were encouraged to nurse others through the illness, and the Romans also advocated this practice.

The Late Roman Empire and the First Pandemic of the Bubonic Plague

The first pandemic of bubonic plague occurred during the reign of Roman emperor Justinian (483–565). The pandemic probably originated in lower Egypt in 542 and spread via trade routes to Alexandria and then to Constantinople, which served as the capital of the eastern part of the Roman Empire (known as Byzantium) at the time. Forty percent of the population in Constantinople perished. The medical writer Procopius of Caesarea (c.500–c.565) clearly identified the disease as bubonic plague, remarking, "The fever made its attack suddenly. Generally on the first or second day, but in a few instances later, buboes appeared, not only in the groin, but also in the armpits and below the ears." The plague then continued to Italy, Spain, Britain, Denmark, and ended up in China in 610 AD, and it has been estimated it killed 100 million people, approximately 50% of the human population. As Procopius relates in his *History of the Wars*, doctors had little recourse or understanding how to treat the disease. They did observe in some patients however that their buboes grew to a large size and ruptured. The patient usually recovered, but tended to have muscle tremors; doctors therefore would lance the buboes in an attempt to increase chances of survival.

WORDS TO KNOW

ENDEMIC: Present in a particular area or among a particular group of people.

ETIOLOGY: The study of the cause or origin of a disease or disorder.

PLAGUE: A contagious disease that spreads rapidly through a population and results in a high rate of death.

QUARANTINE: Quarantine is the practice of separating people who have been exposed to an infectious agent but have not yet developed symptoms from the general population. This can be done voluntarily or involuntarily by the authority of states and the federal Centers for Disease Control and Prevention.

VACCINATION: Vaccination is the inoculation, or use of vaccines, to prevent specific diseases within humans and animals by producing immunity to such diseases. The introduction of weakened or dead viruses or microorganisms into the body to create immunity by the production of specific antibodies.

VARIOLATION: Variolation was the pre-modern practice of deliberately infecting people with smallpox in order to make them immune to a more serious form of the disease. It was dangerous, but did confer immunity on survivors.

Land went uncultivated leading to food shortages, entire villages in rural areas were abandoned, the army shrunk in size, and monastic houses with their close-knit populations were decimated. As the tax base severely declined, civic building projects ceased and public services, including the burial of the dead, virtually disappeared.

Along with these severe cultural effects, the plague in Justinian's reign also greatly affected the history and survival of the Roman Empire. In the West, the Roman Empire had been vulnerable to attacks from Germanic tribes such as the Vandals, Goths, and Ostrogoths, and the western part of the empire had been captured in the fifth century AD. Previous to the outbreak of the disease, Justinian had however made significant inroads in re-taking much of Italy from the Ostrogoths and Northern Africa from the Vandals. The eastern part of the Roman Empire was prospering, silk manufacture in Syria adding to its wealth. Population increased in Greece, Asia Minor, and the Balkans. Justinian had also used

his increased revenues to engage in a building program in Constantinople constructing great churches like Hagia Sophia. As Josiah C. Russell remarked in his article "That Earlier Plague," Justinian's "building program was part of a kind of Golden Age in which literature enjoyed a fine period: Rome still seemed eternal." In 540, the prospect that the Empire might be restored without straining its resources seemed entirely probable.

However, the devastation of the plague weakened the eastern Roman Empire at a critical juncture. Justinian's army shrunk from 350,000 men to 150,000 on his death in 565. As the plague tended to be especially fatal to young people over ten years of age and pregnant women, the devastation to the population meant that fresh military recruits were increasingly scarce. The offensive in the West was thus abandoned after 565. The resulting power vacuum, along with the birth of Islam, promoted the rise of the Arabic empires in the seventh century.

The Bubonic Plague in Medieval Europe

After the plague epidemics in the sixth and seventh centuries, the disease reappeared sporadically, but did not re-emerge with ferocity until the mid-fourteenth century, erupting in the Gobi Desert in the late 1320s. It is not well understood why the bubonic plague reappeared, but the climate of earth had begun to cool at this time, producing a phenomenon known as the "Little Ice Age," and this change in environment may have had an effect. We do know that the cooler temperatures resulted in poor harvests and there were famines in Western Europe from 1315–17, which weakened the population and made it vulnerable to epidemic disease. Ultimately, one-third of the population of Western Europe perished, and populations did not return to their previous levels until the sixteenth century. Urban areas like Florence lost between half and three-quarters of their population.

As in the sixth century, the plague followed trade routes in its spread westward, reaching Sicily by 1347, and in late 1347, the Italian mainland, arriving in Germany via Rhine trade routes, and then France and England in 1348 when the plague was at its peak. From reading primary sources, it seems the plague took two forms in the fourteenth century: a septicaemic plague, which attacks the blood, and pneumonic plague, which infects the lungs and is an especially virulent airborne disease.

Medical treatment ranged from the sophisticated to the folkloric. Some theologians opined that it was the result of vengeance of God and nothing could be done, but many of the Italian city-states such as Milan and Venice, took more practical measures and attempted to quarantine sufferers, walling up houses found to have inhabitants with plague. The quarantine, the pest house, and health boards often just crowded the susceptible poor together causing higher mortality, while the urban wealthy fled the city, segregating themselves in the country away from plague sufferers.

Many correctly thought the disease was thought to be transmitted by air, but in an era with no knowledge of microorganisms, it was thought bad smells or *miasmas* caused infections. Incense and aromatic oils were hawked as cures, as were posies of flowers to be held to the face.

Pope Clement VI (1291–1352) consulted the Parisian medical faculty in 1348 to get their opinion, and they theorized that the disaster was due to astrological events, an unfortunate conjunction of Saturn, Jupiter and Mars that caused hot, moist conditions, which in turn caused the earth to exhale poisonous vapors. Astrology and medicine were intricately intertwined at this time, with the macrocosm of the universe thought to affect the "little world" or microcosm of the body, so their explanation was taken quite seriously. The physicians advised not to eat any food thought to be hot or moist that would add to the effect of the vapors and particularly thought fish were dangerous to include in the diet.

Some expressed their despair at events via religious fanaticism. Groups of flagellants whipped themselves in public to do penance for sins, some believing the end of the world was approaching. Others blamed religious and ethnic minorities such as Jews, Moors, or Roma, accusing them of poisoning town wells and causing the disease. There were pogroms, or mass-killings, of Jews and Roma in the fourteenth and fifteenth centuries. In Strasbourg in 1349, nearly 200 Jews were burned to death. In response to this persecution, some of the Jewish population moved into Eastern Europe into areas of Poland and Lithuania.

The massive population loss also had great economic effects. Labor shortages meant that wages rose, and landlords attempted, often forcefully, to hold on to the serfs they had and to enforce more labor duties. It is little surprise that in the 1380s there were a number of peasant revolts (the Jacquerie in 1358, the Peasants' Revolt in England in 1381, and the Catalonian Rebellion in 1395) as laborers asserted their rights in a market that should have been favorable to them.

Landlords shifted production on the land from foodstuffs, the demand for which was declining with a smaller population, to pastoral agriculture (sheep and cattle raising). Grazing cattle or sheep required less farm labor. Women also found their labor in demand. The two centuries after the plague have been described as an "early golden age for women" as several female guild masters and business owners appeared. Marriage rates also decreased after the bubonic plague. The disease seemed to disproportionately kill young men, so many women married late or not at all, and thus turned to convents or cottage businesses to earn their livings.

These disruptions and changes to the social and economic fabric of medieval society have caused many

IN CONTEXT: CULTURAL IMPACTS

In 1687, English physicist Sir Isaac Newton (1642–1727) published a law of universal gravitation in his important and profoundly influential work *Philosophiae Naturalis Principia Mathematica* (*Mathematical Principles of Natural Philosophy*). Newton articulated a law of universal gravitation that states that bodies with mass attract each other with a force that varies directly as the product of their masses and inversely as the square of the distance between them. This mathematically elegant law, along with Newton's laws of motion, became the guiding models for the future development of physical law.

Born in Woolsthorpe, Lincolnshire, England, Newton did not initially distinguish himself in school, and he was removed by his mother in the late 1650s to work on the family farm, but Newton proved a worse farmer than scholar. His uncle, however, encouraged the boy to go to Cambridge in 1660. Five years later Newton graduated, even though he had failed a scholarship exam in 1663 due to his lack of knowledge concerning geometry.

Newton returned to the farm in 1665 to escape the bubonic plague, which at the time was decimating London. In his year of enforced isolation, his *annus mirabilis* or miracle year, he invented the calculus, discovered the color spectrum of light, and derived his law of universal gravitation.

historians to claim that the plague was the dividing line between the Middle Ages and the Renaissance. Certainly it seems that more secular values that became more important in the Renaissance, as opposed to the spiritual values of the medieval era, began to dominate society. For a variety of political reasons, the popes during the plague also did not live in the spiritual home of Rome and the Vatican, but in southern France in Avignon to the scandal of many. The Crusades in the 1290s had also been resolute failures and the Holy Lands were lost.

Accompanied by the disaster of the plague, the loss of faith in the church may have set the stage for Renaissance secularism. The Catholic Church seemed unable to offer the degree of spiritual comfort required in an era of great loss, and many adopted the "live for today" attitude, enjoying life while they could in uncertain times. For instance, the Italian author Giovanni Boccaccio's (1313–1375) *Decameron*, written shortly after the plague, is a literary masterpiece which has as it premise a group of lords and ladies who escaped Florence to the country town of Fiesole during the epidemic. While in exile they told stories to amuse themselves and pass the time, often displaying themes of lust, love, and a decidedly commercial, urban, and secular ethic.

The bubonic plague, though it never reoccurred in as virulent a manner as in 1348, did return several times in the fifteenth century, and there were local epidemics until the mid-seventeenth century. The last occurrence of the bubonic plague in Western Europe was in 1665 in London just before the Great Fire burned the medieval wooden houses and seemingly cleansed the capital of fleas and rats responsible for the disease.

In 1665, a young man called Isaac Newton (1642–1727) fled the plague raging in Cambridge to his parent's home in Woolsthorpe, Lincolnshire. In his year of enforced isolation, his *annus mirabilis* or miracle year, he invented the calculus, discovered the color spectrum of light, and derived his law of universal gravitation.

■ Current Issues

Another great pandemic of plague spread through China, southeast Asia, and India beginning in 1855. The advent of the railway and increased migration helped the disease spread rapidly in Asia, India, and parts of Russia. Over the following 50 years, plague (predominantly pneumonic) spread to every inhabited continent. The so-called Third Pandemic killed 12 million people, primarily in Manchuria and Mongolia.

Several scientists have theorized that the Second Pandemic, the Black Death, may not have involved bubonic plague, but another form of plague that is not present today. Others assert that the Black Death was too virulent to have been bubonic plague, suggesting that a highly contagious hemorrhagic fever—akin to modern Ebola or Marburg—was the epidemic disease of the medieval plague. The theories are controversial and *Yersina pestis* remains the predominantly accepted culprit of the Black Death.

While researchers have been scouring written sources for years for clues about ancient plagues, they had been limited to matching described symptoms to known disease behaviors. Archaeological and forensic research may aid the identification of past epidemics. Eva Panagiotakopulu, an archaeologist from the University of Sheffield, theorizes that Egypt was the very source of the deadly bubonic plague, which has been commonly thought by historians to have its origins from the Near East. Panagiotakopulu found fossilized fleas in ancient Egyptian's habitations, as well as remains of Nile rats that could have carried the disease. She speculates that the Nile River Valley was a natural habitat for flea-carrying rats and that endemic flooding drove large rat populations into urban areas.

■ Primary Source Connection

Often, key components of research published in scientific journals are written in accessible language. Journal articles usually follow a structured form, with an abstract or overview followed by supporting data and arguments, and end with a summary. The abstract, at the top of the article, introduces the reader to the key components of the research using as broad and easily understandable terms as possible. The methods and body of the research and evidence follow, and in the conclusions, much of the abstract is restated as it relates to the evidence presented. By reading the abstract and conclusions of scientific literature, the reader can often gain a basic picture of the research. Although the body of the article can contain arguments and data that are designed for scientists, the abstract and summary or conclusion sections often contain valuable and readable information for non-scientists.

In this extract from the journal *Emerging Infectious Diseases*, the author Michel Drancourt presents his evidence that *Yersinia pestis* was the cause of at least two historical pandemic plagues using the classic form for reporting in scientific journals. Michel Drancourt is professor of medical microbiology in Unité des Rickettsies, Marseille Medical School, Marseille, France. His research interests are paleomicrobiology of plague and bartonelloses.

Yersinia pestis Orientalis in Remains of Ancient Plague Patients

Abstract

Yersinia pestis DNA was recently detected in human remains from 2 ancient plague pandemics in France and Germany. We have now sequenced *Y. pestis* glpD gene in such remains, showing a 93-bp deletion specific for biotype Orientalis. These data show that only Orientalis type caused the 3 plague pandemics.

Three historical pandemics have been attributed to plague. The causative agent, *Yersinia pestis*, was discovered at the beginning of the ongoing third pandemic. The etiology [origin or cause] of the 5th–7th-century first pandemic and the 14th–18th-century second pandemic, however, remained putative until recently....

THE STUDY

We had historical evidence that 3 mass graves excavated in France were used to bury bubonic plague victims. In Vienne, 12 skeletons, including 5 children, buried within the ruins of a Roman temple have been dated from the 7th–9th centuries both by a 5th-century coin and ^{14}C dating. In Martigues, 205 skeletons buried in 5 trenches were dated from 1720 to 1721 on the basis of coins and detailed parish bills that listed the victims. In Marseille, 216 skeletons buried in a huge pit dated from a May 1722 epidemic relapse. We previously confirmed the diagnosis of plague at this site. Eighteen teeth from 5 skeletons in Vienne, 13 teeth from 5 skeletons in Martigues, and 5 teeth from 3 skeletons in Marseille were processed for the search for *Y. pestis* DNA in the dental pulp. The teeth were processed according to

IN CONTEXT: CULTURAL CONNECTIONS

Plague created panic and desperation in the pre-modern world and those fears lingered in the social psyche—often manifesting themselves in bizarre form.

Mistakes in pronouncement of death—and premature burial—are now highly unlikely in the industrialized world, but until the twentieth century there were less definitive means of determining death. As a result, it was not unheard of for a person ill with plague to fall into a coma or a stupor and to appear to observers to be dead when, in fact, the patient was still alive. Plague often led to fears of premature burial.

Bodies were often quickly buried, particularly in times of plague or cholera. There have been numerous tales, dating back to very early history, of the apparently dead spontaneously reviving and living on for extended periods of time. One such story is that of Marjorie Halcrow Erskine of Chirnside, Scotland. She was reported to have died in 1674 and was buried in a rather shallow grave by the village sexton, who planned to rob her grave and steal her jewelry. As the sexton attempted to cut off the woman's finger in order to obtain one of her rings, she suddenly revived. Ms. Erskine was able to return home, and she lived a full life, giving birth to and raising two sons.

In the seventeenth through nineteenth centuries, in times of plague, cholera, and smallpox epidemics, a substantial number of premature burials were reported. A nineteenth century researcher named William Tebb published a book in 1896 titled *Premature Burial and How It May Be Prevented*. In it, he detailed 219 instances of near premature burial, 149 cases of genuine premature burial, ten cases of dissection before actual death, and two cases in which embalming began before death had occurred.

During the eighteenth and nineteenth centuries, various methods were employed to ensure that an individual was, in fact, dead. In one method, a hot poker was applied to the deceased patient, while another involved pouring liquid into the patient's mouth. Yet another creative strategy required the attending physician to stick the finger of the apparently deceased into his (the

physician's) ear in an effort to feel the *buzz* or *hum* of life. In 1846, a French physician named Eugene Bouchut suggested that the stethoscope be used to determine when the heart stopped beating in order to determine that death had occurred.

The most extreme measures for preventing premature burial occurred in Germany between 1790 and 1860. There, roughly fifty centers called *Leichenhäuser*, or waiting mortuaries, were built. In these buildings, corpses were kept in warm rooms. Each corpse had strings wrapped around fingers and toes, with the other ends of the strings attached to bells. The bells were meant to be rung by the awakening person, but there is no report of a bell ever ringing. The bodies were maintained until evidence of putrefaction was unequivocally present (complete with requisite stench). Some of the waiting mortuaries had luxury and common rooms—some were even open for public observation. A later Leichenhaus in Vienna utilized an electronic bell system.

Individuals went to elaborate lengths to prevent premature burial. Some requested that their heads be severed. Others wanted their arteries slashed (Danish writer Hans Christian Anderson, 1805–1875), their bodies dissected (Polish composer Frédéric Chopin, 1810–1849), or their bodies embalmed. All these measures were designed to ensure with absolute certainty that the individual was dead before he or she was buried.

In 1896, Count Karnice-Kamicki, a chamberlain to the Russian tsar, invented a device to be affixed to a coffin in order to avoid premature burial—or, rather, to provide a means of correcting that unfortunate situation. His mechanism was comprised of a tube running from the inside of the coffin to an airtight box several feet above the ground. A spring, which ran the length of the tube, was attached to a glass sphere sitting on the chest of the body. The slightest movement of the body would trigger the spring, causing the lid of the airtight box to pop open, thus allowing light and air into the interior of the coffin via the connecting tube. The box above the grave also contained a flag, a bell or a buzzer, and a light that could be seen and heard from a considerable distance.

---

published criteria for authenticating molecular data in paleomicrobiology: 1) there should be no positive control; 2) negative controls, as similar as possible to the ancient specimens, should test negative; 3) a new primer sequence targeting a genome region not previously amplified in the laboratory should be used (suicide PCR); 4) any amplicon should be sequenced; 5) a second amplified and sequenced target should confirm any positive result; and 6) an original sequence that differs from modern homologs should be obtained to exclude contamination.

Accordingly, DNA samples were submitted for suicide-nested PCR conducted by using 1 negative control (18th-century teeth from skeletons of persons without anthropologic and macroscopic evidence of infection) for every 3 specimens.... The sequences were compared in the GenBank database (www.ncbi.nlm.nih.gov/GenBank)

using the multisequence alignment Clustal within the BISANCE environment.

CONCLUSIONS

In this study, contamination of the ancient specimens is unlikely because of the extensive precautions we took, including use of the suicide PCR protocol excluding positive controls. Accordingly, glpD gene had never been investigated in our laboratory before this study, and negative controls remained negative. The specificity of the amplicons was ensured by complete similarity of experimental sequences with that of the Υ. *pestis Orientalis* glpD gene. One site (Marseille, 1722) was previously positive for Υ. *pestis* after sequencing of 2 different targets (chromosome-borne rpob and plasmid-borne pla genes) in other specimens collected in other persons's remains.

These results therefore confirm the detection of *Y. pestis*-specific DNA in plague patients' remains from the first and second epidemics. We observed a 93-bp in-frame deletion within the glpD gene sequences obtained from ancient dental pulp specimens. This deletion has been found only in Orientalis biotype isolates in 2 independent studies comprising a total of 77 and 260 *Y. pestis* isolates, respectively, of the 4 biotypes.

After previous demonstration of *Y. pestis* Orientalis-type multiple spacer type sequences in Justinian and medieval specimens, we now have cumulative evidence using 2 different molecular approaches that *Y. pestis* closely related to the Orientalis biotype was responsible for the 3 historical plague pandemics.

Michel Drancourt

DRANCOURT, M, ET AL. "*YERSINIA PESTIS ORIENTALIS* IN REMAINS OF ANCIENT PLAGUE PATIENTS." *EMERGING INFECTIOUS DISEASES*. (FEBRUARY 2007): AVAILABLE AT <HTTP://WWW.CDC.GOV/EID/CONTENT/13/2/332.HTM> (ACCESSED MAY 28, 2007).

BIBLIOGRAPHY

Books

Boccaccio, Giovanni. *The Decameron*. Mark Musa, trans. New York: Signet, 1992.

Bollet, Alfred J. *Plagues and Poxes: The Impact of Human History on Epidemic Disease*. New York: Demos Medical Publishing, 2004.

Carmichael, Anne G. *Plague and the Poor in Renaissance Florence*. Cambridge: Cambridge University Press, 1986.

McNeill, William Hardy. *Plagues and Peoples*. New York: Doubleday, 1998.

Procopius, *History of the Wars*. H. B. Dewing, trans. Cambridge, Mass.: Harvard University Press, 1914, Vol. I, pp. 451–473.

Wrigley, E.A., and R.S. Scofield. *The Population History of England, 1541–1871: A Reconstruction*. Cambridge, Mass: Harvard University Press, 1984.

Periodicals

Gross, C.P., and K.A. Sepkowitz. "The myth of the medical breakthrough: smallpox, vaccination, and Jenner reconsidered." *International Journal of Infectious Disease* 3 (1998), pp.54–60.

Littman, R.J., and M.L. Littman. "Galen and the Antonine Plague." *The American Journal of Philology* 94, 3 (Autumn 1973), pp. 243–255.

Morgan, Thomas E. "Plague or Poetry? Thucydides on the Epidemic at Athens." *Transactions of the American Philological Association* 124 (1994), pp. 197–209.

Russell, Josiah C. "That Earlier Plague." *Demography* 5, 1 (1968), pp. 174–184.

Web Sites

Walker, Cameron. "Bubonic Plague Traced to Ancient Egypt." *National Geographic News*. March 10, 2004. <http://news.nationalgeographic.com/news/2004/03/0310_040310_blackdeath.html> (accessed May 17, 2007).

Anna Marie E. Roos

Plague, Modern History

■ Introduction

Plague is a greatly feared disease that has killed millions of people since medieval times. It is caused by the bacterium *Yersinia pestis*, which is carried by flea-infested rodents, and mortality rates are more than 50% if the disease is left untreated. The third pandemic of plague extended into the twentieth century and stimulated research into the cause and transmission of the disease.

There have been no major epidemics of plague in the United States for many years, although occasional cases still occur in the southwestern states. Globally, from 1,000 to 3,000 cases annually are reported to the World Health Organization (WHO), most of which occur in Africa, Southeast Asia, and Latin America. It may not be possible to eradicate plague, but outbreaks can be prevented by reducing rodent populations. Constant vigilance regarding plague is also necessary because it has some potential as an agent of a bioterrorist attack.

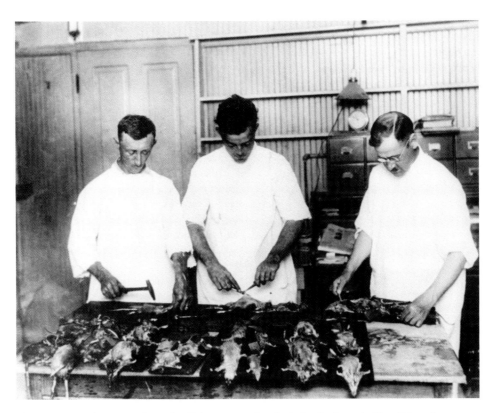

Three men examine rats to determine if they are carrying the bubonic plague in New Orleans in 1914. © *Corbis*.

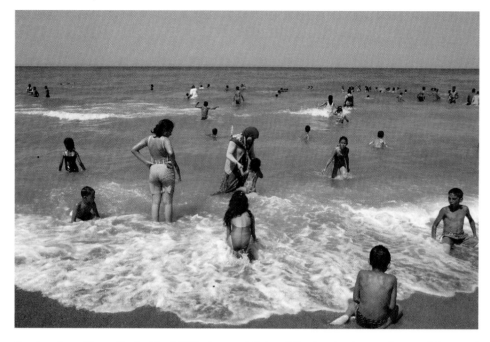

People swim at Tipaza Beach, 40 mi (70 km) west of Algiers, following the closure of some of the capital city's more popular beaches in July 2003. The closures were made as a precaution against the spread of a rare outbreak of both the plague and meningitis. At least ten people had contracted the bubonic plague during the previous month. *Hocine Zaourar/AFP/Getty Images.*

■ Disease History, Characteristics, and Transmission

Yersinia pestis is a Gram-negative bacillus—rod-shaped—bacterium, which was discovered as the cause of plague by the Swiss researcher Alexander Yersin in 1894. The term Gram-negative refers to the way in which the bacterium absorbs the Gram stain used to prepare bacterial cultures for microscopy. The incubation period of *Y. pestis* is between two and eight days, and the microbe produces three types of plague: bubonic, pneumonic, and septicemic.

Bubonic plague accounts for 90–95% of all cases and is marked by sudden onset of fever, chills, weakness, and headache. Initially, these could be mistaken for flu symptoms. Shortly after, multiplication of the bacteria within the lymph glands of the armpits and groin cause characteristic swellings, called buboes, which are extremely tender, typically 0.8–4 in (2–10 cm) in diameter, and hot to the touch.

The disease often progresses to bleeding from the gastrointestinal, respiratory or genitourinary tract—leading to the name "Red Death." Gangrene—death of tissue from lack of oxygen—may occur on the nose or penis, leading to the name "Black Death." This name also was given to some of the plague epidemics in history. These complications are caused by the spread of the bacterium throughout the bloodstream and the effects

of associated toxins. Untreated bubonic plague has a death rate of more than 50%.

Pneumonic plague may occur as a complication of bubonic plague, and also accounts for 5% of primary cases. Symptoms include bloody sputum, chest pain, coughing, and breathlessness. The disease is highly infectious and 100% fatal if left untreated. Septicemic plague has similar symptoms to bubonic plague—apart from the buboes—and accounts for around 5% of cases, with extensive bloodstream infection being the most significant feature.

Plague is a zoonosis—a disease of animals that can infect humans. Rodents act as the animal reservoir for the disease. When fleas bite an animal infected with *Y. pestis*, they can carry the disease to other rodents. The animals become sick, and when they start to die, the fleas will seek out human hosts as an alternative source of blood meals. The main flea vector is the oriental rat flea, *Xenopsylla cheopsis*.

Humans generally become infected with plague through the bite of an infected flea or from handling an infected animal and coming into contact with its tissues or body fluids. In the United States, wild rodents are the most common animal reservoirs for plague, with the rock squirrel being implicated in the majority of cases in the Southwest. In the Pacific States, the California ground squirrel is the most important source of plague. Prairie dogs, wood rats, chipmunks, and other burrowing rodents have also been involved in U.S. cases of plague. Other, less frequent, sources include wild rabbits, wild carnivores, and domestic cats and dogs, who pick up infected fleas from wild rodents. In addition, pneumonic plague can be spread from person-to-person through inhalation of infected secretions.

The *Y. pestis* bacteria quickly enter the bloodstream and enter white blood cells, where they multiply and produce toxins. They spread throughout the blood and may cause disseminated intravascular coagulation—multiple tiny blood clots—which lead to the complications of plague.

■ Scope and Distribution

Plaque has been responsible for three known pandemics during the course of human history. The first began in the middle of the sixth century and is known as the Justinian plague. It was followed in the middle of the fourteenth century by the pandemic popularly known as the Black Death. The Third or Modern pandemic of plague began in the mid-1800s in China and spread throughout the world to cause nearly 30 million cases and over 12 million deaths between 1896 and 1930.

By the time of the Third pandemic, scientists had developed methods for investigating microbial causes of disease that could be applied to this serious public health problem. Alexander Yersin discovered *Y. pestis* in 1894 and the transmission of plague via fleas was reported by Paul-Louis Simond in 1890. This new understanding, together with the later introduction of antibiotics, meant that plague began to exact less of a toll on human life in many countries. Modern techniques of analyzing DNA have led to new insights into ancient cases of plague from previous pandemics, using samples from the dental pulp of victims' remains.

Today plague causes both sporadic cases and epidemics involving hundreds of people, the numbers involved depending upon geographical location. The disease is found in Africa, Southeast Asia, Latin America, and in the southwestern United States. In Africa, there have been severe outbreaks in recent years in Kenya, Tanzania, Zaire, Botswana, and Mozambique. Smaller outbreaks have occurred in other East African countries. Sporadic cases have been reported from North and West Africa. The disease also occurs regularly in Madagascar, where multi-drug resistance has been reported. In Asia, countries that are particularly affected by plague include Burma (Myanmar), Vietnam, and Indonesia. In Latin America, plague is found in the Andean mountain region and in Brazil. However, there is no plague today in Australia or Europe.

In North America, most human cases of plague occur in two specific regions. One is in northern New Mexico, northern Arizona, and southern Colorado. The other is in California, southern Oregon, and far western Nevada. The highest rates are in Native Americans, par-

WORDS TO KNOW

BIOWEAPON: A weapon that uses bacteria, viruses, or poisonous substances made by bacteria or viruses.

BUBO: A swollen lymph gland, usually in the groin or armpit, characteristic of infection with bubonic plague.

EPIDEMIC: From the Greek *epidemic*, meaning "prevalent among the people," is most commonly used to describe an outbreak of an illness or disease in which the number of individual cases significantly exceeds the usual or expected number of cases in any given population.

FLEA: A flea is any parasitic insect of the order *Siphonaptera*. Fleas can infest many mammals, including humans, and can act as carriers (vectors) of disease.

GRAM-NEGATIVE BACTERIA: All types of bacteria identified and classified as a group that does not retain crystal-violet dye during Gram's method of staining.

MULTI-DRUG RESISTANCE: Multi-drug resistance is a phenomenon that occurs when an infective agent loses its sensitivity against two or more of the drugs that are used against it.

NOTIFIABLE DISEASE: A disease that the law requires must be reported to health officials when diagnosed; also called a reportable disease.

PANDEMIC: Pandemic, which means all the people, describes an epidemic that occurs in more than one country or population simultaneously.

RESERVOIR: The animal or organism in which the virus or parasite normally resides.

ZOONOSES: Zoonoses are diseases of microbiological origin that can be transmitted from animals to people. The causes of the diseases can be bacteria, viruses, parasites, and fungi.

ticularly Navajos, hunters, veterinarians and pet owners handling infected animals, and among campers or hikers entering areas with outbreaks of animal plague. The last urban epidemic of plague in the United States occurred in Los Angles in 1924–1925.

Worldwide, between 1,000 and 3,000 cases of plague are reported to the WHO each year. In 2003, there were

2,118 cases reported from nine countries, including 182 deaths. Nearly all of these came from Africa. In the United States, there is an average of around 15 cases of plague each year, of which one in seven proves fatal. In Africa, Asia, and Latin America there were major outbreaks each year in the 1980s. These cases tend to be associated with domestic rats and were more common among those living in small towns, villages, and agricultural areas than among the population in urban areas.

The major risk factor for epidemic plague is poor living conditions with rodent and flea infestation, coupled with human overcrowding. Lab workers handling plague bacteria are also at high risk wherever they are located.

The WHO received reports of outbreaks of pneumonic plague in the Democratic Republic of Congo (DRC) in 2005 and 2006. The disease has long been endemic in the Ituri region, and, indeed, this region is the most active natural focus of plague in the world today. There was an outbreak near the town of Zobia, in mid–2005 in a forest area that had attracted several thousand people responding to reports of the discovery of diamonds there. The outbreak involved 124 cases of pneumonic plague and 56 deaths. Investigators from the WHO found suspect rodents and poor sanitary conditions at the affected site. The situation was made worse by panic, with many people fleeing the outbreak and dying along forest trails, spreading this highly infectious disease. It was no surprise, therefore, when there were further outbreaks in the DRC in the months following.

In October 2006, there were apparently 626 more suspected cases of pneumonic plague, including 42 deaths, in the DRC. But this would be an unusually low death rate for pneumonic plague, so the WHO thought there might have been an over-estimation of the number of cases. A team from the humanitarian group Médicins sans Frontières (Doctors without Borders) worked with the WHO and the local health authority in Congo doing lab tests, case management, and contact tracing to bring the outbreak under control. However, further outbreaks are almost inevitable and, if they occur in a city, many deaths will result.

Plague is notifiable to the Centers for Disease Control and Prevention (CDC) whose center in Fort Collins, Colorado, is a WHO Collaborating Center for Reference and Research on Plague Control, reporting all human plague cases in the United States to the WHO. Also, the National Notifiable Disease Surveillance System carries out surveillance on animal plague, reports human cases, and carries out lab testing on fleas, animal tissues, and blood samples.

■ Treatment and Prevention

Antibiotic treatment reduces the mortality rate of plague from over 50% to around 10%. Streptomycin is the preferred drug, but tetracycline or chloramphenicol can be used as alternatives. Anyone with plague must be isolated and hospitalized. However, given prompt diagnosis and treatment, nearly everyone with plague can expect to recover.

The contacts of plague cases must be traced and treated with antibiotics to help stop the infection from developing. They should also be disinfested of any fleas they may be carrying. Passengers traveling back from plague endemic areas are generally subject to quarantine regulations in case they are incubating the disease.

Preventive antibiotics can be taken if someone has been exposed to the bites of wild rodent fleas during an outbreak, or to the tissues or fluids of a plague-infected animal. The same treatment is appropriate for those who have been exposed to a person or pet with suspected plague, especially if it is pneumonic plague. Tetracycline, chloramphenicol, or sulfonamide antibiotics are preferred for this kind of prophylactic treatment. However, since multi-drug resistance has begun to emerge in Madagascar, it has to be assumed that it could also happen elsewhere.

Although vaccines against plague have been used in the past, these are not available in the United States currently. Research has shown that the vaccine does not help reduce the number of cases or the spread of infection during an outbreak. However, it may have a role to play in protecting those who are repeatedly exposed through lab or healthcare work.

Prevention of plague among the population currently depends upon controlling fleas and rodents. People living in those regions of the United States where plague infection is active need to take care to avoid exposure. Sick or dead rodents, which may be infected with plague, should be reported to local health authorities and should never be handled.

Keeping homes, workplaces, and recreation areas clear of food and nesting places for rodents is extremely important. Junk, firewood, and rock piles should be removed to make these places rodent-proof. Insect repellents applied to clothing and skin can reduce the risk of exposure to potentially infected fleas. Cats and dogs need to be regularly treated with flea control agents and should not be allowed to roam freely, in case they come into contact with infected rodents. Investigation of outbreaks and sporadic cases of plague often lead to the identification of a clustered area of animal die-offs that is the exposure source and needs to be disposed of.

■ Impacts and Issues

Plague has been a public health problem for several centuries and, unlike polio and smallpox, it is unlikely that it can ever be eradicated. Between outbreaks, *Y. pestis* lives on in certain rodent populations without actually wiping them out, thereby constituting a silent, long-term reservoir of infection. The best that can be hoped for is to employ control and precautionary measures in those places where humans and flea-infested rodents are likely to interact.

Although sporadic cases of plague do occur in the southwestern United States, these can be avoided as far as possible with common sense precautions regarding contact with potentially infected rodents. Efforts to control plague probably need to be focused where conditions create a risk of disease outbreak or even epidemics. This means managing unsanitary rat-infested environments to make places where people live, work, or play safer.

Control of rat populations in rural and urban areas of many less developed countries has not yet been achieved to the extent that it has in most developed countries. Close surveillance of both rodents and humans for plague is the first step in tightening controls. Insecticides can be used to control rodent fleas in danger areas and efforts made to reduce the local population of rodents in human-inhabited areas by removing potential food sources and nesting sites.

In the future, however, plague may become even more unpredictable. Changing climate, due to global warming, and population movements may create new environments where flea-infested rodents can flourish and put people at risk of plague.

A further threat of the spread of plague comes from its potential use as a bioweapon. The concern centers around pneumonic plague, which is highly infectious and can spread rapidly from person to person. An aerosol-based biological weapon could introduce Υ. *pestis* into the population without warning, causing a severe epidemic within just a few days. Containment would depend upon rapid detection of cases and treatment of these people, and their contacts, with antibiotics within 24 hours. Public health authorities in the United States—probably a potential major target for such an attack—do hold large stocks of the appropriate antibiotics, and the CDC says these could be made available anywhere to any location where they are needed within 12 hours.

People may, however, feel more reassured if they were already vaccinated against plague, rather than hoping that the response to an attack will be prompt and sufficiently effective. However, there is currently no plague vaccine available in the United States. Research into such a vaccine by academics and the U.S. Army is ongoing, but the CDC says it will be several years before one becomes widely available.

The threat of bioterrorism has re-focused attention on plague as a disease problem that has been largely absent from developed countries, including the United States, for many years except in sporadic form. In many African countries and in parts of Southeast Asia, plague is still an endemic public health issue that leads to hundreds of deaths each year. The U.S. bioterrorism effort can learn from what is known of the natural history of plague in other countries and use molecular technologies to better understand the disease. A bioterrorist attack with Υ. *pestis* may never happen, but the knowledge gained in preparing for a potential attack may help better diagnosis, treatment, and prevention efforts in those places where the disease occurs naturally.

SEE ALSO *Plague, Early History.*

BIBLIOGRAPHY

Books

Wilson, Walter R., and Merle A. Sande. *Current Diagnosis & Treatment in Infectious Diseases.* New York: McGraw Hill, 2001.

Periodicals

Drancourt, M., and D. Raoult. "Molecular Insights into the History of Plague." *Microbes and Infection* 4 (January 2002): 105–109.

Web Sites

Centers for Disease Control and Prevention. "CDC Plague Home Page." <http://www.cdc.gov/ncidod/dvbid/plague/index.htm> (accessed May 13, 2007).

Centers for Infectious Diseases Research and Policy. "Plague Outbreak Highlighted Ongoing Problem in Africa." May 27, 2005. <http://www.cidrap.umn.edu/cidrap/content/bt/plague/news/may2705plag.html> (accessed May 13, 2007).

Susan Aldridge

Pneumocystis carinii Pneumonia

■ Introduction

Pneumocystis carinii pneumonia (PCP) is the most common opportunistic infection occurring among people with AIDS (acquired immunodeficiency syndrome). Although rates of the infection have fallen with the advent of drugs against HIV, PCP is still a leading cause of mortality in this patient group in the United States.

P. carinii is a fungus that is found in the respiratory tract of humans and other mammals. Its distribution is widespread and most children will have been exposed to it by the age of three or four. However, *P. carinii* only causes disease among those with impaired immunity. Its appearance among previously healthy homosexual men in the early 1980s was an early warning sign of the emergence of HIV/AIDS. Other groups at risk include those who have cancer or are receiving immunosuppressive drugs following an organ transplant.

Fortunately, PCP is treatable with antibiotics and survival rates have improved in recent years. People at risk can also be given preventive drugs to stop PCP infection taking hold.

■ Disease History, Characteristics, and Transmission

P. carinii was first thought to be a trypanosome, then a protozoan. More detailed biochemical studies have now established that the organism is a fungus. The organism that actually causes PCP was recently re-named *Pneumocystis jiroveci* after Otto Jirovec, the researcher who first isolated it from human subjects (although the new name is not yet in common use).

P. carinii is harmless in a healthy person, but if immunity is weakened for any reason, it can invade the lungs, causing pneumonia. The symptoms of PCP may be of gradual onset and include breathlessness, fever, chills, weight loss, a non-productive cough, and weight loss. PCP

proves fatal in 10–20% of cases. Survival rates have improved in recent years for those with HIV (human immunodeficiency virus), but not for non-HIV patients.

P. carinii is spread by airborne transmission. Most people have been infected by *P. carinii* in early childhood. Research suggests that PCP occurs through new

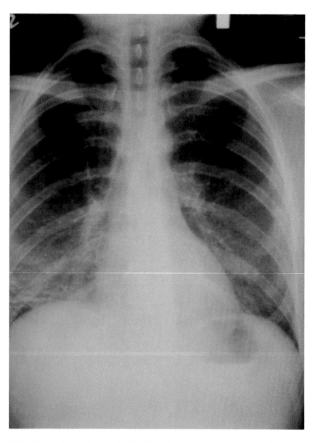

This X-ray shows interstitial infiltration of pneumonia-causing *Pneumocystis carinii* protozoans. Pneumocystis pneumonia is among the most common causes of death in patients with acquired immunodeficiency syndrome (AIDS). © *Lester Bergman/Corbis.*

infection, by inhalation, rather than by re-activating an old infection.

Scope and Distribution

PCP was first noted during World War II among malnourished and premature infants in Central and Eastern Europe. Prior to the 1980s, PCP was rare in the United States, with fewer than 100 cases a year occurring—mainly during cancer chemotherapy and after solid organ transplantation. In 1981, the U.S. Centers for Disease Control and Prevention reported an unusual finding—five cases of PCP in previously healthy homosexual men. It was the first warning of the advent of AIDS. Since the causative agent, HIV, attacks and destroys the immune system, *P. carinii* is able to cause PCP, an opportunistic infection.

However, PCP is less of a problem than it was in the past. Before the introduction of highly active antiretroviral therapy (HAART), 70–80% of those with HIV/AIDS would develop PCP, but these rates have been much reduced. Similarly, 88% of lung transplant recipients developed PCP, but the disease is now rare in this patient group.

It used to be assumed that PCP was less common in the developing world, but this may not be so. Apparently lower rates could merely reflect lack of access to diagnostic facilities. It now appears that PCP could be on the increase in Africa, with the infection affecting around 80% of HIV-positive children who present with pneumonia.

Treatment and Prevention

Although it is a fungus, *P. carinii* does not actually respond to anti-fungal drugs. However, there are a number of antibiotics that can be used to treat PCP. These include trimethoprim-sulfamethoxazole and pentamidine. Steroids may also be used in severe cases. Prophylactic treatment with these drugs, and with other drugs, can help those at risk avoid developing PCP. Giving up smoking is also essential in helping prevent PCP.

Impacts and Issues

PCP is an ongoing threat to people with HIV/AIDS. It mainly seems to affect those whose CD4+ t-cell count is less than 200 per microliter. CD4+ t-cells are a type of white blood cell that is targeted by the HIV virus. CD4+ t-cell counts are an essential monitor of the condition of someone with HIV and a drop in the count indicates a

---

WORDS TO KNOW

AIRBORNE TRANSMISSION: Airborne transmission refers to the ability of a disease-causing (pathogenic) microorganism to be spread through the air by droplets expelled during sneezing or coughing.

CD4+ T CELLS: CD4 cells are a type of T cell found in the immune system, which are characterized by the presence of a CD4 antigen protein on their surface. These are the cells most often destroyed as a result of HIV infection.

MORTALITY: Mortality is the condition of being susceptible to death. The term "mortality" comes from the Latin word *mors*, which means "death." Mortality can also refer to the rate of deaths caused by an illness or injury, i.e., "Rabies has a high mortality."

OPPORTUNISTIC INFECTION: An opportunistic infection is so named because it occurs in people whose immune systems are diminished or are not functioning normally; such infections are opportunistic insofar as the infectious agents take advantage of their hosts' compromised immune systems and invade to cause disease.

---

vulnerability to PCP that should be addressed. Although treatment, both to prevent and cure the infection, is available, PCP is still a significant cause of mortality (death) among those with HIV/AIDS.

SEE ALSO *AIDS (Acquired Immunodeficiency Syndrome); Opportunistic Infection; Pneumonia.*

BIBLIOGRAPHY

Books

Wilks, Robert, Mark Farrington, and David Rubenstein. *The Infectious Diseases Manual.* 2nd ed. Malden, UK: Blackwell Publishing, 2003.

Web Sites

McLean, Joseph. "Pneumocystis carinii Pneumonia." *eMedicine*, September 11, 2006. <http://www.emedicine.com/MED/topic1850.htm> (accessed April 18, 2007).

Pneumonia

■ Introduction

Pneumonia is an inflammatory response of the lungs to the entry of an infective organism or other foreign material. It is an important disease, as it is the sixth leading cause of death in the United States, and the major cause of death from infection.

Pneumonia is a complex disease with many different causes and risk factors. It can affect people of any age, anywhere, although the very young and the very old are most vulnerable to an attack. Pneumonia is classified in two ways—according to its cause and according to its setting.

The cause of pneumonia can be viral, bacterial, mycobacterial, fungal, or even non-infective irritants.

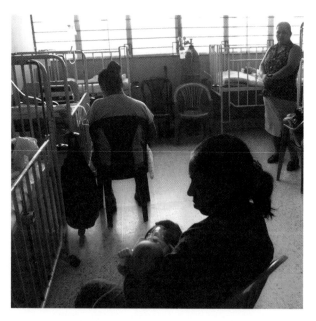

A one-month-old baby is held by his aunt at the Benjamin Bloom Children's Hospital in San Salvador, El Salvador, during a 2003 pneumonia outbreak that caused several hundred deaths in the country. *AP Images.*

The setting may be either within the community or in the hospital. These distinctions are important because they influence the choice of treatment. Before the advent of antibiotics, pneumonia was a greatly feared disease because it could kill so easily. Today, with effective treatment, most people can expect to make a full recovery from pneumonia.

■ Disease History, Characteristics, and Transmission

Pneumonia is unlike many other infectious diseases in that it cannot be attributed to infection by one, or just a few, specific microbes. The respiratory tract, consisting of the nose, pharynx (back of the throat), trachea (windpipe), and lungs, has various mechanisms to protect itself from microbes as well as foreign bodies, such as particulate pollution, food, liquid, or gas. The nose and trachea are lined with mucous membranes, which bear tiny beating hairs called cilia. The thick mucous traps any microbes or foreign particles as they enter through the nose and mouth and the cilia propel them back to the nose and mouth where they are expelled, by nose blowing, or are swallowed. This mechanism protects the bronchi, which are the tiny tubes fanning out to connect the trachea with the alveoli, the tiny air sacs making up the lung tissue.

The cough reflex is another of the lungs' defenses against infection, expelling foreign material before it enters the lungs. Added to this is the immune system, which will trigger cells or antibodies to destroy any threatening microbes or other material. Therefore, microorganisms may colonize the upper part of the respiratory tract, without causing disease, or they may cause an infection such as a cold or influenza. With the usual defenses in place, they do not invade the lungs.

If these defenses break down for any reason—for instance, because of the use of a mechanical ventilator in the intensive care unit, or because of weakened

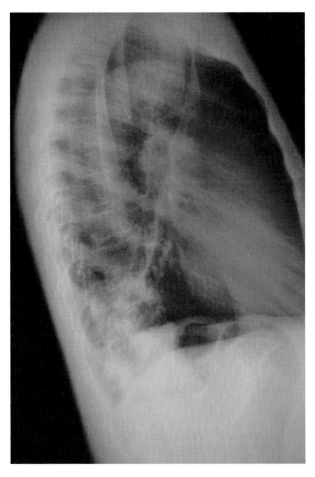

A chest X-ray shows pneumonia in the lower lobe of a patient's right lung. © *Visuals Unlimited/Corbis.*

Among AIDS patients, *Pneumocystis carinii* is a major cause of pneumonia as an opportunistic infection. Before the advent of AIDS, *P. carinii* pneumonia was rare and its sudden appearance alerted researchers to the emergence of a new disease. *P. carinii* is a fungus-like organism. Other fungi that cause pneumonia include *Histoplasma capsulatum* and *Cryptococcus neoformans.*

Pneumonia may follow an attack of influenza or even a cold, but it can also arise on its own. Anyone who suddenly starts to feel worse after flu or a cold needs to get medical advice immediately. The symptoms of pneumonia vary from mild to very severe, and they may be either gradual or sudden in onset. The nature of the symptoms also varies depending upon the infecting microbe and patient characteristics. A cough, which may be either dry or productive of green or rust-colored phlegm (a discharge from the lungs), is probably the most common symptom of pneumonia. Sometimes the patient will even cough up blood. Fever, chills, and breathlessness may also occur and there may be chest pain. However, older people may have few symptoms other than mental confusion.

Bacterial pneumonia tends to come on suddenly with fever, shaking chills, sweating, and chest pain. The cough usually produces thick greenish or yellow phlegm. The symptoms are usually more dramatic among those previously in good health.

In viral pneumonia, which is more common in the winter months, there is a dry cough, headache, fever, muscle pain, and fatigue. Breathlessness tends to develop as the disease goes on and the cough starts to produce white phlegm. Viral pneumonia is a particular threat to those with pre-existing heart or lung disease. If it does not clear up, a secondary bacterial pneumonia may take hold.

Mycoplasma pneumonia is sometimes called "walking pneumonia" because the symptoms are gradual and mild—indeed, patients are not always aware that they are ill. This form of pneumonia often strikes schoolchildren and young adults. It may account for up to one-third of all childhood cases.

The examining doctor will look for signs of pneumonia, such as an increase in respiration and pulse rate. Pneumonia also is associated with characteristic chest sounds—bubbling, cracking sounds called rales, and rumblings called ronchi—that indicate the presence of fluid within the alveoli. These can be heard when the doctor puts a stethoscope to the chest. Chest x-ray, and possibly computed tomography (CAT) scanning, are an important part of the diagnosis of pneumonia, since they will reveal characteristic opacities or shadows on the affected lung. (Pneumonia may affect one or both lungs.)

The complications of pneumonia include blood poisoning, pleural effusion, and lung abscess. The alveoli are in close contact with the bloodstream and so the infection may enter the bloodstream, causing what is commonly known as blood poisoning or septicemia. When bacteria

immunity—infection may spread down to the lungs. The alveoli mediate gas exchange between the lungs and the blood—oxygen in, carbon dioxide out. They deal with anything that threatens this function, such as invading microbes or particulate matter, with a strong inflammatory response, which is the underlying mechanism of pneumonia. One of the main features of this inflammation is the production of a thick secretion or exudate by the lung tissue.

Over 100 different organisms can cause pneumonia, and the most significant of these depends on patient characteristics and the setting—whether in the community or in the hospital. Some of the most important viral causes of pneumonia include adenovirus, respiratory syncytial virus, influenza virus, parainfluenza virus, and cytomegalovirus. Among the bacteria that can cause pneumonia are *Streptococcus pneumoniae, Chlamydia pneumoniae, Haemophilus influenzae, Klebsiella pneumoniae,* and *Pseudomonas aeruginosa.* Mycoplasma, which are organisms that have some of the characteristics of both bacteria and viruses, can also cause pneumonia.

WORDS TO KNOW

ANTIBIOTIC RESISTANCE: The ability of bacteria to resist the actions of antibiotic drugs.

ASPIRATION: Aspiration is the drawing out of fluid from a part of the body; it can cause pneumonia when stomach contents are transferred to the lungs through vomiting

CILIA: Cilia, which are specialized arrangements of microtubules, have two general functions. They propel certain unicellular organisms, such as paramecium, through the water. In multicellular organisms, if cilia extend from stationary cells that are part of a tissue layer, they move fluid over the surface of the tissue.

NOSOCOMIAL: A nosocomial infection is an infection that is acquired in a hospital. More precisely, the Centers for Disease Control and Prevention in Atlanta, Georgia, defines a nosocomial infection as a localized infection or one that is widely spread throughout the body that results from an adverse reaction to an infectious microorganism or toxin that was not present at the time of admission to the hospital.

OPPORTUNISTIC INFECTION: An opportunistic infection is so named because it occurs in people whose immune systems are diminished or are not functioning normally; such infections are opportunistic insofar as the infectious agents take advantage of their hosts' compromised immune systems and invade to cause disease.

enter the bloodstream, they can reach the other organs of the body in a short time, possibly resulting in multi-organ failure and death. In pleural effusion, fluid leaks from the lungs into the space between the pleura, which are the membranes covering the lungs and the inner surface of the chest wall. This fluid could become infected—a condition known as empyema—and may have to be drained or removed surgically. Finally, an abscess, which is a cavity containing pus-infected material, may form within the lungs as a result of pneumonia. Although treatable with antibiotics, a lung abscess occasionally must be removed surgically.

The complications of pneumonia are more common among the elderly, the frail, and those with weakened immunity, such as HIV/AIDS patients. The prognosis of pneumonia depends upon the setting and the patient. In those over 65, mortality ranges from 5% to 65%. The overall death rate for community-acquired pneumonia (CAP) is less than 1%. This rises to around 14% for nosocomial or hospital-acquired pneumonia (HAP) and to around 40% for patients in the intensive care unit.

Pneumonia is not transmitted from one person to another. Instead, it involves aspiration of microbes into the lungs from a previously colonized airway, implying that the normal defense mechanisms of the respiratory tract have broken down for some reason. It can also develop through aspiration of stomach contents, gas, or particulate pollution, all of which may inflame lung tissue.

■ Scope and Distribution

The public health burden of pneumonia in the United States is considerable. There are three million cases of pneumonia each year, accounting for ten million physician visits, 600,000 hospital admissions, and more than 60,000 deaths. It is the sixth most common cause of death and the leading cause of death from infection. Pneumonia accounts for half of all deaths from infection in the United States. Worldwide, pneumonia is the leading cause of death among infants less than one year old.

Pneumonia can strike at any age, but infants and children under four years of age and those over 65 years old are most at risk. The elderly account for almost 90% of all deaths from pneumonia and influenza. In adults, strong risk factors for pneumonia include existing illnesses such as congestive heart failure, kidney disease, diabetes, chronic obstructive pulmonary disease, removal of the spleen, malnutrition, alcoholism, institutionalization, and dementia. Children and young adults with cystic fibrosis are especially at risk of pneumonia. For infants, low birth weight and low maternal age have been found to be risk factors for pneumonia.

Community-acquired pneumonia (CAP) refers to pneumonia contracted outside a hospital setting—that is, either at home in the community or in a nursing home, day care setting, school, or other place where people congregate. The cause of CAP is often viral, but bacteria are also important causes of CAP. Different species of bacteria are involved in causing CAP in different age groups. *Streptococcus* and pneumococcus are the most common causes of pneumonia, accounting for up to 35% of all cases. *Streptococcus* and *Staphylococcus* species of bacteria are found to be especially important in cases of pneumonia in newborns, while *S. pneumoniae* and *H. influenzae* infections are common in older children. *S. pneumoniae* infection is also found often in elderly people with pneumonia.

Hospital-acquired pneumonia (HAP) is one of the most significant nosocomial infections. It refers to pneumonia that develops 48 hours after hospital admission. HAP occurs at a rate of 5–10 per 1,000 hospital admissions in the United States. Most cases occur in the intensive care unit or in post-surgical recovery. The risk of HAP is 6–20 times greater among those on mechanical ventilation. This is because ventilation involves inserting a tube into the trachea, which disrupts the natural defenses of the respiratory tract. The microbiology of HAP has been found to differ from that of CAP with *Klebsiella pneumoniae*, *Pseudomonas aeruginosa*, *Serratia*, and *Enterobacter* species, all of which are gram-negative bacilli, being most often involved. The term gram-negative (or positive) refers to the way a bacterial species reacts with a common stain used in microscopic studies.

■ Treatment and Prevention

Some cases of pneumonia need to be treated in the hospital and prompt assessment by a physician is needed, because the condition can progress rapidly. An increased respiratory rate, decreased blood pressure, increased temperature, and confusion are all potential indicators for hospital admission. Microbiological tests are often needed to confirm the infective organism.

However, the physician often needs to start empiric antibiotic treatment before the microbiology results are available. There is no effective treatment for viral pneumonia, which usually clears up on its own. In particular, antibiotics will not work against viruses. For those recovering from pneumonia at home, bed rest is important, along with plenty of fluids to help loosen mucus in the lungs. These patients should also be sure to stay away from those with weakened immunity, which may mean not visiting anyone in the hospital.

Many different antibiotics can be used to treat pneumonia. The American Thoracic Society has established guidelines to help physicians make a good choice of antibiotic for pneumonia, based upon the patient and the setting. For out-patients, amoxicillin, azithromycin, and levofloxacin are often used. The latter is one of a relatively new group of drugs called the respiratory fluoroquinolones, which are valuable because they can treat drug-resistant bacteria. In-patients not in intensive care may be given cefotaxime, while intensive care patients may be treated with a combination of drugs, such as cefotaxime with a fluoroquinolone. Sometimes treatment is given by injection, to get to the infection as quickly as possible. Patients with cystic fibrosis often need high doses of antibiotics and in combination.

Immunization against *H. influenzae* and pneumococcus is valuable in the prevention of CAP in the over-65s and in those otherwise at risk, such as patients with cystic fibrosis. The latter protects against 23 different types of pneumococcus. HAP is preventable by good hospital hygiene, especially relating to mechanical ventilation. Elevation of the bed has been found useful in protecting the lower respiratory tract from infection. Prevention of pneumonia is important, because the com-

> ### *IN CONTEXT:* DISEASE IN DEVELOPING NATIONS
>
> Pneumonia is an infection of the lung that can be caused by nearly any class of organism known to cause human infections, including bacteria, viruses, fungi, and parasites. In the United States, pneumonia is one of the most common diseases leading to death, and the most common fatal infection acquired by already hospitalized patients. In developing countries, pneumonia and diarrhea are the most common causes of death.

plications of the condition can be so serious. And with the growth of drug-resistant strains of bacteria that can cause pneumonia, effective treatment can no longer be relied upon.

■ Impacts and Issues

William Oster, the great nineteenth century Canadian physician, called pneumonia "the old man's friend" because it often releases an elderly, frail, terminal patient from a catalog of severe medical complaints. However, not all patients with pneumonia fall in this category. HAP is the second most common nosocomial infection in the United States and the most serious in terms of morbidity and mortality, with 300,000 new cases a year, accounting for 1.2 billion U.S. dollars in healthcare costs.

The causes of HAP need addressing when they are preventable, such as violations in infection control, including insufficient handwashing, and the use of equipment that could be contaminated. However, the risk of HAP is inextricably linked to the nature of modern medicine, especially when it comes to intensive care. Mechanical ventilation may save the lives of the desperately ill, but it is also the leading cause of HAP because of the way in which it breaches the natural defenses of the respiratory tract against infection. Other invasive devices that are linked with a high risk of HAP include nasogastric intubation (a tube leading from the nasal passages to the stomach) for feeding an unconscious patient, and chest, abdominal, and head and neck surgery. Again, these can be life saving treatments, and health care workers and researchers are attempting to develop technologies and practices within the intensive care and surgical setting that can minimize the risk of pneumonia.

Another major concern arising from HAP is that the cause is often a multi-drug resistant organism. This means that the patient's upper respiratory tract has been colonized with such a resistant organism and it may be difficult to find an antibiotic within the armory available to the physician that can treat the pneumonia successfully.

Antibiotic resistance is also a concern in CAP, as penicillin-resistant *S. pneumoniae* is increasingly common. The fight against antibiotic resistance is two-fold. Researchers must develop new classes of antibiotic, which act by mechanisms not previously known. And both existing and new antibiotics must be used sparingly. Overuse or misuse of antibiotics promotes the emergence of resistant strains. On exposure, the weaker strains die, leaving the more resistant ones to flourish. This is especially likely to happen when a patient does not finish a prescribed course because symptoms of the infection clear up. This is as true of pneumonia as of any other infection. Patients must be responsible and take their medication exactly as prescribed. Only then are the chances of killing resistant bacteria maximized.

■ Primary Source Connection

In the following journal article, author Carol Potera discusses a type of aspiration (inhalation) pneumonia seen after the 2004 Asian tsunami that was termed "tsunami lung." Potera is a contributor to *Environmental Health Perspectives*, a journal devoted to the interaction between environmental factors and human and animal health.

In Disaster's Wake: Tsunami Lung

When the Asian tsunami struck on 26 December 2004, health authorities braced for an onslaught of waterborne illnesses including malaria and cholera, which often follow such disasters. But saltwater flooded the freshwater breeding grounds of the mosquitoes that spread malaria, and relief agencies quickly distributed bottled water, thwarting a cholera epidemic. Instead, a type of aspiration pneumonia named "tsunami lung" emerged and afflicted some survivors.

Tsunami lung occurs when people being swept by tsunami waves inhale saltwater contaminated with mud and bacteria. The resulting pneumonia-like infections normally are treated with antibiotics. However, the 2004 tsunami "wiped out the medical infrastructure, and antibiotics were not available to treat infections in the early stages," says David Systrom, a pulmonologist at Massachusetts General Hospital in Boston. Consequently, victims' lung infections festered, entered the bloodstream, and spread to the brain, producing abscesses and neurological problems such as paralysis.

Systrom and colleagues volunteered to work on a medical disaster team with Project HOPE (Health Opportunities for People Everywhere) aboard the hospital ship U.S. Naval Ship *Mercy* off the coast of Banda Aceh, Sumatra. When they arrived three weeks after the tsunami hit, "we saw infections not seen in the United States since before the development of antibiotics," says Systrom. Among them were about 25 cases of tsunami lung. "No one expected the number of tsunami lung cases we saw," says Systrom. "It was not on the radar screen."

The diagnosis of tsunami lung requires a chest radiograph and computed tomography scan of the brain to confirm abscesses. This sophisticated equipment was available on the hospital ship. "Only the most severe cases with central nervous system involvement made it to the ship," says Systrom. The team suspects that hundreds of milder cases went unreported.

In the 23 June 2005 issue of the *New England Journal of Medicine*, the team describes the case of a 17-year-old girl who aspirated water and mud while engulfed by a wave and carried about half a mile. She developed pneumonia two weeks later and was treated at a local clinic with unknown medicines. A week later, the right side of her face drooped, her right arm and leg became paralyzed, and she stopped talking.

A chest radiograph revealed air and pus outside the lining of the lung (a condition known as hydropneumothorax), and a brain scan showed four abscesses. After the doctors treated her with a combination of intravenous antibiotics (imipenem until the stock of that drug ran out, then vancomycin, ceftazadime, and metronidazole), her speech and facial movement recovered first. When she moved her right leg and arm for the first time, she "burst into peals of laughter," according to the report. She was transferred to an International Committee of the Red Cross-Crescent field hospital. "I suspect she'll fully recover," says Sydney Cash, a neurologist at Massachusetts General Hospital and member of the team, who has since received pictures of her walking.

A combination of microbes likely contributes to tsunami lung, but no lab facility was available to culture and identify those found in the Indonesian patients before the Mercy arrived. However, in a letter published in the 4 April 2005 issue of the *Medical Journal of Australia*, Anthony Allworth, director of infectious diseases at Royal Brisbane and Women's Hospital, describes culturing *Burkholderia pseudomallei* from two tsunami lung patients in a land-based hospital and *Nocardia* species from a third.

B. pseudomallei lives in the Asian soil and water. Mark Pasternack, an infectious disease specialist at Massachusetts General Hospital who also served on the Mercy, says, "You do not have to directly aspirate *Burkholderia* to produce pneumonia .... After the tsunami, people had soft tissue injuries from being forced into objects, so they could have gotten *Burkholderia* from wounds or aspiration."

Cash echoes this thought: "Natural disasters produce odd combinations of pathogens and unexpected ways for the body to be damaged that lead to unexpected clinical circumstances. [Medical disaster physicians need to] keep an open mind and expect the unexpected."

Could an infection like tsunami lung emerge in victims of Hurricane Katrina? Probably not, speculates Pasternack.

Although the water sweeping the Gulf Coast area may have been contaminated, "it was not forced down peoples' lungs by high-speed waves," he says. Therefore, aspiration pneumonia and its complications are unlikely to appear commonly during the Gulf Coast relief efforts.

Carol Potera

POTERA, CAROL. "IN DISASTER'S WAKE: TSUNAMI LUNG." *ENVIRONMENTAL HEALTH PERSPECTIVES* 113 (2005): 11, 734.

SEE ALSO Chlamydia pneumoniae; Haemophilus influenzae; *MRSA; Nosocomial (Healthcare-Associated) Infections;* Pneumocystis carinii *Pneumonia.*

BIBLIOGRAPHY

Books

Gates, Robert H. *Infectious Disease Secrets.* 2nd ed. Philadelphia: Hanley and Beltus, 2003.

Tan, James S. *Expert Guide to Infectious Diseases.* Philadelphia: American College of Physicians, 2001.

Wilson, Walter R., and Merle A. Sande. *Current Diagnosis & Treatment in Infectious Diseases.* New York: McGraw Hill, 2001.

Web Sites

American Lung Association. "Pneumonia Fact Sheet." April 2006. <http://www.lungusa.org/site/apps/nl/content3.asp?c=dvLUK9O0E&b=2060321&content_id={08C669B0-E845-4C9C-8B1E-285348BC83BD}&notoc=1> (accessed March 25, 2007).

Mayo Clinic. "Pneumonia." May 12, 2005. <http://www.mayoclinic.com/health/pneumonia/DS00135> (accessed March 25, 2007).

Susan Aldridge

Polio (Poliomyelitis)

■ Introduction

Polio, short for poliomyelitis, is a highly infectious viral disease that can cause rapid paralysis of the limbs and the muscles used in breathing. Also known as infantile paralysis, polio mainly affects children under the age of five, although it can also affect adults.

First described at the end of the eighteenth century, there have been many epidemics of polio both in the United States and in other countries around the world. Once an effective vaccine was introduced in 1955, however, the number of cases of polio began to fall dramatically. In 1988, the World Health Organization (WHO), along with other charities and organizations, launched the Global Polio Eradication Initiative. This relies on ensuring that all children are vaccinated against polio. The initiative has led to a dramatic drop in the number of cases of polio around the world—from around 350,000 in 1988 to fewer than 2,000 in the year 2005.

■ Disease History, Characteristics, and Transmission

The word poliomyelitis comes from *polio*, the Greek word for gray, and *myelon*, the Greek word for marrow (indicating the spinal cord). It is the effect of the poliovirus on the spinal cord that causes the paralysis associated with this disease. There are three types of poliovirus—1, 2, and 3—all of which cause very similar infections. Polioviruses belong to the enterovirus group and are part of the picornavirus family of RNA viruses (that is, their genetic material is composed of RNA rather than DNA). John F. Enders (1897–1985), Thomas Weller (1915–), and Frederick Robbins (1916–2003) of Harvard School for Public Health, first grew poliovirus in tissue culture in 1948, and were awarded the Nobel Prize for this work in 1954.

Polio occurs mainly in the summer and fall seasons in temperate climates, but has no seasonal pattern in tropical climates. The incubation time of poliovirus is 7–14 days, during which time it multiplies in the cells lining the intestines and the respiratory tract. In 90% of

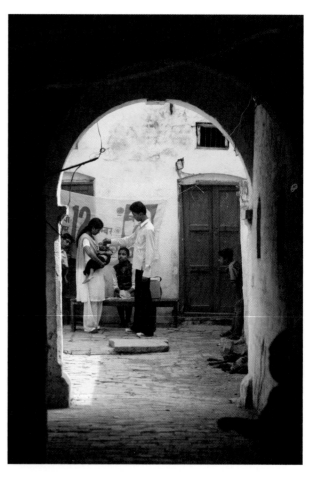

A health worker gives polio drops to a child in the Indian state of Uttar Pradesh in late 2006. At that time, authorities had detected 25 new polio cases over the past week in India's most populous state, stoking fears of a resurgence of the disease that was once nearly eradicated in the country. *AP Images.*

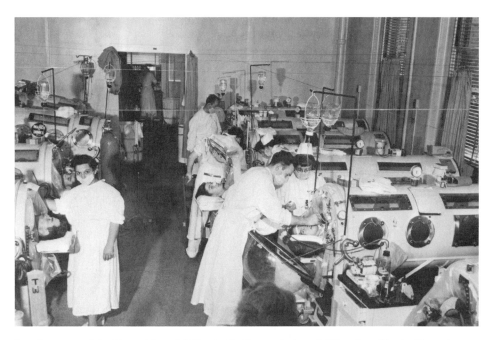

Iron lungs crowd the Hynes Memorial Hospital in Boston during a 1955 polio epidemic. The early ventilators used negative pressure to enable patients with weakened respiratory muscles to breathe.
© *Bettmann/Corbis.*

cases, the infection causes no symptoms at all. Another 5% will have relatively mild symptoms including headache, fever, fatigue, and vomiting. These symptoms are indistinguishable from those of many other viral illnesses and usually clear up within a week.

One to two percent of polio infections result in nonparalytic aseptic meningitis, which causes stiffness of the neck, back, and/or legs. This condition tends to clear up within a week or so and complete recovery is usual. In one percent of cases, however, poliovirus spreads from the intestines, through the blood, to the nervous system, where it can destroy nerve cells in the spinal cord and the base of the brain.

Polio infection in the nervous system leads to paralytic polio—the most feared type of the disease. The severity of paralytic polio depends on how many neurons are affected, but onset of paralysis can be very rapid. Commonly, a child might go to bed with minor symptoms and wake up being unable to walk.

There are three forms of paralytic polio. Spinal polio causes a flaccid (floppy) paralysis of one or more of the limbs, without any loss of feeling. Complete recovery is quite possible, however, and tends to happen within the first six months. Any weakness or paralysis remaining after a year is likely to be permanent and the patient is left with some degree of disability. Spinal polio accounted for 79% of all cases of paralytic polio during 1969 to 1979.

Another, less common, form of paralytic polio is so-called bulbar polio, where the poliovirus affects the cra-nial nerves in the upper spinal cord. This leads to paralysis of the pharynx (back of the throat), vocal cords, and respiratory (breathing) muscles. Bulbar polio is the most dangerous form of the disease, killing 75% of those affected. Pure bulbar polio accounted for only 2% of cases in the 1969–1979 period. The rest were bulbo-spinal polio, which is a combination of the two forms.

The complications of paralytic polio include urinary tract infection and pneumonia, which are common in any condition where a patient is immobilized. The overall death rate from paralytic polio is 2–5% for children and 15–25% for adults.

Most doctors will never see a case of polio. However, they may see a condition known as post-polio syndrome which affects 25–40% of those who had paralytic polio in childhood. The syndrome is characterized by fatigue, new muscle pain, and exacerbation of any existing weakness. It is more common with those left with residual disability by the original infection and among women. It is not clear what causes post-polio syndrome, but it may result from nerve damage occurring during the original recovery process. Post-polio syndrome has been shown not to be a re-activation of polio infection, and those affected are not infectious to others.

Poliovirus is transmitted by the fecal-oral route—that is, through consumption of contaminated food and water. It enters the body through the mouth and multi-plies in the throat and the gastrointestinal tract, the latter being confirmed through laboratory examination of the feces of people with polio. People with no symptoms, or

WORDS TO KNOW

ATTENUATED STRAIN: A bacterium or virus that has been weakened, often used as the basis of a vaccine against the specific disease caused by the bacterium or virus.

ENDEMIC: Present in a particular area or among a particular group of people.

ERADICATION: The process of destroying or eliminating a microorganism or disease.

INACTIVATED VACCINE: An inactivated vaccine is a vaccine that is made from disease causing microorganisms that have been killed or made incapable of causing the infection. The immune system can still respond to the presence of the microorganisms.

LIVE VACCINE: A live vaccine uses a virus or bacteria that has been weakened (attenuated) to cause an immune response in the body without causing disease. Live vaccines are preferred to killed vaccines, which use a dead virus or bacteria, because they cause a stronger and longer-lasting immune response.

WILD VIRUS: Wild - or wild-type - virus is a genetic description referring to the original form of a virus, first observed in nature. It may remain the most common form in existence but mutated forms develop over time and sometimes become the new wild type virus.

only mild symptoms, can still transmit the infection. They are most infections from 7–10 days before and the same period after the onset of symptoms (if these are present). The disease is highly infectious and, therefore, in communities where even one child remains unvaccinated, all are at risk of developing the disease.

Rarely, someone may contract polio—and pass it on to others—through vaccination. Vaccine-association paralytic polio (VAPP) occurs in around one person in two to three million following vaccination with the live vaccine.

■ Scope and Distribution

Children younger than five have always been most at risk of polio, although it can affect people of any age. For instance, American President Franklin D. Roosevelt con-

tracted the disease in 1921 at the age of 39. Polio was first described in England in 1789, and was only a sporadic disease during the eighteenth and nineteenth centuries.

However, from the turn of the nineteenth century polio became an epidemic disease around the world, although the first outbreak in the United States had occurred as early as 1843. It is not clear why the incidence of polio changed in this way. It is possible that improvements in standards of hygiene may have led to a loss of natural immunity against the disease, with children being less likely to be exposed to poliovirus in contaminated food or water. Such exposure may have led to mild or even asymptomatic infection that had no impact on health, but conferred a natural immunity against further attacks of polio.

In the early years of the twentieth century, Scandinavia, the United Kingdom, and North America were especially affected by polio. According to data released by the Health Section of the League of Nations (the forerunner of the United Nations), of 178,328 cases of polio occurring between 1919 and 1934, 54.3% were in the United States and Canada. However, the peak year for polio in the United States was 1952, with over 57,000 cases, including 21,000 paralytic cases.

In England, there were over 1,000 cases of polio in 1928 and in 1938, but between these years, the annual average was around 640. Polio became more of a problem in Britain after the World War II, with almost 8,000 cases being reported in 1947. There was also a very severe outbreak in 1952 that affected 238 per 100,000 of the population in Copenhagen, Denmark. The majority of these cases were bulbar polio, the most dangerous form of the disease.

The introduction of the polio vaccine in the 1950s began to bring the disease under control. However, in 1988, when the WHO declared a war on polio, the disease was still endemic in 125 countries around the world. Today polio is endemic only in four countries—Afghanistan, Pakistan, India, and Nigeria.

Polio has now been eradicated in the western world and in the western Pacific, including China. There have been occasional outbreaks, including one in the Netherlands in 1993, in areas where parents refused to have their children vaccinated. There are also very occasional cases linked with the vaccine itself.

■ Treatment and Prevention

There is no treatment for polio. During the 1930s and 1940s, it was common to immobilize the paralyzed limbs with splints to protect them. This was controversial, however, and some doctors recommended exercise instead, to build up the weakened limbs.

The need to support the breathing of those with paralytic polio led to the development of the Drinker

IN CONTEXT: SCIENTIFIC, POLITICAL, AND ETHICAL ISSUES

The eldest son of Orthodox Jewish-Polish immigrants, Jonas Salk (1914–1995) earned his medical degree in 1939. After his internship, and work on a flu vaccine, Salk devoted a considerable amount of his energies to writing scientific papers on a number of topics, including the polio virus. Some of these came to the attention of Daniel Basil O'Connor, the director of the National Foundation for Infantile Paralysis—an organization that had long been involved with the treatment and rehabilitation of polio victims. O'Connor eyed Salk as a possible recruit for the polio vaccine research his organization sponsored. When the two finally met, O'Connor was much taken by Salk—so much so, in fact, that he put almost all of the National Foundation's money behind Salk's vaccine research efforts.

Salk's first challenge was to obtain enough of the virus to be able to develop a vaccine in doses large enough to have an impact; this was particularly difficult since viruses, unlike culture-grown bacteria, need living cells to grow. The breakthrough came when the team of John F. Enders, Thomas Weller, and Frederick Robbins found that the polio virus could be grown in embryonic tissue—a discovery that earned them a Nobel Prize in 1954. Salk subsequently grew samples of all three varieties of polio virus in cultures of monkey kidney tissue, then killed the virus with formaldehyde. Salk argued that it was essential to use a killed polio virus (rather than a live virus) in the vaccine, as the live-virus vaccine would have a much higher chance of accidentally inducing polio in inoculated children. He therefore, exposed the viruses to formaldehyde for nearly 13 days. Though after only three days he could detect no virulence in the sample, Salk wanted to establish a wide safety margin; after an additional ten days of exposure to the formaldehyde, he reasoned that there was only a one-in-a-trillion chance of there being a live virus particle in a single dose of his vaccine. Salk tested it on monkeys with positive results before proceeding to human clinical trials.

Despite Salk's confidence, many of his colleagues were skeptical, believing that a killed-virus vaccine could not possibly be effective. His dubious standing was further compounded by the fact that he was relatively new to polio vaccine research; some of his chief competitors in the race to develop the vaccine—most notably Albert Sabin (1906–1993), the chief proponent for a live-virus vaccine—had been working for many years. As the field narrowed, the division between the killed-virus and the live-virus camps widened, and what had once been a polite difference of opinion became a serious ideological conflict. Salk and his chief backer, the National Foundation for Infantile Paralysis, were lonely in their corner. Salk failed to let his position in the scientific wilderness dissuade him and he continued, undeterred, with his research. To test his vaccine's

strength, in early 1952, Salk administered a type I vaccine to children who had already been infected with the polio virus. His results clearly indicated that the vaccine produced large amounts of antibodies. Buoyed by this success, the clinical trial was then extended to include children who had never had polio.

In May 1952, Salk initiated preparations for a massive field trial in which over 400,000 children would be vaccinated. The largest medical experiment that had ever been carried out in the United States, the test finally got underway in April 1954, sponsored by the National Foundation for Infantile Paralysis. More than one million children between the ages of six and nine took part in the trial, each receiving a button that proclaimed them a "Polio Pioneer." At the beginning of 1953, while the trial was still at an early stage, Salk's encouraging results were made public in the *Journal of the American Medical Association*. Predictably, media and public interest were intense. On April 12, 1955, the vaccine was officially pronounced effective, potent, and safe in almost 90% of cases. The meeting at which the announcement was made was attended by 500 of the world's top scientists and doctors, 150 journalists, and 16 television and movie crews.

Just two weeks after the announcement of the vaccine's discovery, however, eleven of the children who had received it developed polio; more cases soon followed. Altogether, about 200 children developed paralytic polio, eleven fatally. For a while, it appeared that the vaccination campaign would be railroaded. However, it was soon discovered that all of the rogue vaccines had originated from the same laboratory in California. Following a thorough investigation, it was found that the lab used faulty batches of virus culture, which were resistant to the formaldehyde. After furious debate and the adoption of standards that would prevent such a reccurrence, the inoculation resumed. By the end of 1955, seven million children had received their shots, and over the course of the next two years more than 200 million doses of Salk's polio vaccine were administered, without a single instance of vaccine-induced paralysis. By the summer of 1961, there had been a 96% reduction in the number of cases of polio in the United States, compared to the five-year period prior to the vaccination campaign.

After the initial inoculation period ended in 1958, Salk's killed-virus vaccine was replaced by a live-virus vaccine developed by Sabin; use of this new vaccine was advantageous because it could be administered orally rather than intravenously, and because it required fewer "booster" inoculations.

The battle between Sabin and Salk persisted well into the 1970s, with Salk writing an op-ed piece for the *New York Times* in 1973 denouncing Sabin's vaccine as unsafe and urging people to use his vaccine once more.

respirator or "iron lung" by physiologist Cecil Drinker (1887–1956) of the Harvard School of Public Health and his brother, chemical engineer Philip Drinker (1894–1972). Introduced in 1928, the iron lung was the forerunner of the modern intensive care unit, whose mission is to support the vital functions of dangerously

ill patients. Unfortunately, the existence of the iron lung forced doctors to have to make difficult decisions. Invariably, there would be more patients than iron lungs, and so they would have to decide which ones to treat.

Jonas Salk (1914–1995) introduced an inactivated polio vaccine (IPV) in 1955, following testing and trials.

This had to be given by injection. Then Albert Sabin (1906–1993) developed an attenuated (weakened) live vaccine (oral polio vaccine, OPV) that could be given by mouth, which was obviously much more convenient. Early experience with the Sabin vaccine was troubling, with some healthy volunteers developing paralytic polio (VAPP) after exposure. For instance, in 1962, there were 62 cases reported from non-epidemic areas of the United States, all occurring within 30 days of vaccination. It is unlikely that these cases arose from natural infection.

But Sabin persevered with his trials and the oral vaccine was introduced in the early 1960s and was used widely in the United States and in many developing countries. More advanced versions of OPV are now used where polio continues to be a threat. However, although OPV has been responsible for the elimination of wild poliovirus infection from the United States, the tiny risk of VAPP has meant that it has also been responsible for 95% of paralytic polio cases (the rest being imported cases).

For this reason, OPV has now been phased out and replaced by IPV, of which two versions are currently approved for use in the United States. A child should receive three doses of IPV within the first 18 months of life and a fourth dose at, or before, school entry. Travelers to the few remaining countries affected by polio, and certain laboratory workers, may need to have a booster dose of IPV vaccine to protect them. But a routine vaccination of adults is not necessary.

■ Impacts and Issues

Polio became a huge problem in North America. It affected children and cost them their lives or, if left disabled, could threaten their ability to lead a full and productive life. Therefore, the public exerted massive pressure on the government and scientists to find a solution in the form of a vaccine. In 1952, the number of cases of polio in the United States reached an unprecedented 57,268, and the debate over whether to release the vaccine that was being developed intensified. Organizations like the March of Dimes had raised substantial sums of money for research and called for trials of polio vaccine to begin without further delay, while researchers urged caution as they sought to perfect their lab experiments first. Testing of the Salk vaccine did, in fact, begin—albeit on a small scale—in 1952.

However, as with any vaccine, there were challenges to be met in terms of meeting demand and safety requirements, when it came to doing large scale vaccination against polio. There were problems in 1954, for example, when batches of vaccine were found to cause polio in experimental monkeys and were accordingly declared unfit for human use. Despite this, large scale testing of vaccine was finally able to begin in 1954. When successful

results from these trials were reported the following year, public excitement was such that church bells were set ringing in celebration in several towns.

The Salk vaccine reduced the rate of polio from 13.9 per 100,000 of the population in 1954 to 0.5 per 100,000 in 1961. However, some argued that the Sabin vaccine, which consisted of live, but attenuated, polio virus, might be even more effective. These arguments continued over the next few years. The two vaccines differ in that the former is made from killed poliovirus, while the latter is based on live virus. Put simply, a killed vaccine may be less effective, but may be safer. A live vaccine may, potentially, actually cause active disease if the virus it contains mutates into a form that could be infectious. However, a live vaccine may induce a more effective immune response and so confer better protection against the disease.

By 1985, the success of the polio vaccine gave the Pan American Health Organization the confidence to set the goal of eradicating polio from the Americas by 1990. Meanwhile, the WHO had declared the official eradication of smallpox in 1980 and decided to build on this success by launching the Global Polio Eradication Initiative in 1988. This was supported by Rotary International, the worldwide voluntary organization, the U.S. Centers for Disease Control and Prevention (CDC), and UNICEF, the United Nations Children's Fund.

The Initiative has had considerable success. Since 1988, the number of cases of polio worldwide has fallen by 99%. In 1994, the WHO Americas region, consisting of 36 countries, was declared polio-free, followed by the WHO Western Pacific region, consisting of 37 countries, in 2000, and the WHO European region (51 countries) in 2002.

This leaves four countries with endemic polio, down from 125 countries in 1988. Mass vaccination is the key to eradication of polio and, in 2005 alone, 400 million children received polio vaccine. Two billion children have been vaccinated since the campaign began, and it is estimated that five million have been saved from disabling paralysis.

However, the total eradication of polio remains a challenge. It can be difficult, even under normal conditions, to access children living in remote areas. Where war and poverty compromise or destroy a country's infrastructure, achieving vaccination goals is even more challenging. Currently, there are outbreaks in northern Nigeria, and a new outbreak in western Uttar Pradesh in India.

■ Primary Source Connection

The following report was issued by the World Health Organization (WHO) about a single-case outbreak of polio in China that occurred in October 1999. The government of China cooperated with the WHO and other international health agencies to contain the outbreak and determine whether the initial case was acquired from another world region where polio is endemic, or whether the virus was a "wild type" that emerged in the local area. Tracking the source of outbreaks is vital to eradication efforts.

Polio in China

18 JANUARY 2000

Disease Outbreak Reported

The following case report is from the WHO Polio Eradication Programme:

The case was first reported to the County EPS in Geizi Township, Xunhua County, Haidong Prefecture, Qinghai Province, on 13 October 1999, and reported to the Provincial EPS on the following day. The case was born on 13 June 1998, had onset of paralysis on 12 October, after a day of fever on 11 October. The parents took the boy to a local private clinic in a neighbouring township when a sudden onset of flaccid paralysis made him unable to stand or walk (both of which he had been capable of before). Two stool samples were taken, the first on 14 October and the second on 25 October. They were analyzed in the provincial laboratory. Both samples yielded poliovirus isolates, which were later typed and differentiated as P1 wild viruses at the national laboratory in Beijing. At the time that the second sample was taken five contacts were sampled, one of which, a four year old cousin of the infected child, was also positive for wild poliovirus. The case child was unregistered and had received zero doses of polio vaccine.

The case belongs to the Sala minority group, a Muslim group of Turkic speaking people whose ancestors migrated to Qinghai from the area of Turkmenistan about seven hundred years ago. There are around 80,000 Sala in China, 60,000 in Qinghai Province (nearly all of which live in Xunhua Sala Autonomous County) and nearly all of the remainder in neighbouring Gansu Province. Adult male Sala travel widely as traders and workers, within Qinghai province and outside to other provinces, including Gansu, Sichuan, Xinjiang, and particularly Tibet, even as far as the border area with Nepal.

Neither the case nor the direct family reported a history of travel outside the county in the two months prior to onset. No visit to the family by a traveler from outside the county was reported to occur during the same period. However, the family, including the case, attended a major festival of Sala people in the county capital during the period 25 to 28 September 1999. Up to 30,000 Sala are reported to have attended this gathering.

Despite intensive investigation in the area of the case, including searches of health facilities, no evidence of wide-scale circulation of wild poliovirus has yet been found. Surveillance quality including laboratory proficiency in Qinghai Province and in neighbouring provinces is in general good. Indications are therefore that the virus has been recently imported.

The Ministry of Health of China is actively collaborating with the global laboratory network including CDC Atlanta, NIID Tokyo and the national laboratories in India. Initial sequencing information on the wild poliovirus show a close similarity to viruses recently circulating in India. The virus is significantly different from those that have been circulating in China up to the last case in 1994. Further genomic sequencing work is proceeding.

A combined MOH/WHO/UNICEF/JICA mission visited Qinghai Province from 20–25 December 1999 to review the response to the case. Initial case response immunization has been carried out, achieving high coverage of the target group. Extensive additional activities are planned, including large scale immunization across several provinces, intensified surveillance, retrospective review of hospital records at all levels in several provinces, and active search for cases of acute flaccid paralysis.

World Health Organization.

"POLIO IN CHINA." *EPIDEMIC AND PANDEMIC ALERT AND RESPONSE (EPR), DISEASE OUTBREAK NEWS* (JANUARY 18, 2000).

SEE ALSO *Childhood Infectious Diseases, Immunization Impacts; Polio Eradication Campaign.*

BIBLIOGRAPHY

Books

Gould, Tony. *A Summer Plague: Polio and Its Survivors.* New Haven: Yale University Press, 1997.

Web Sites

Centers for Disease Control and Prevention (CDC). "Pink Book—Poliomyelitis." <http://www.cdc.gov/nip/publications/pink/polio.pdf> (accessed March 25, 2007).

World Health Organization. "Poliomyelitis." September 2006. <http://www.who.int/mediacentre/factsheets/fs114/en> (accessed March 25, 2007).

World Health Organization. Global Polio Eradication Initiative. "2005 Annual Report." May 2006. <http://www.polioeradication.org/content/publications/annualreport2005.asp> (accessed March 25, 2007).

Susan Aldridge

Polio Eradication Campaign

Introduction

Polio, short for poliomyelitis, is a viral disease, which primarily affects children under the age of five. It is highly infectious and can cause rapid paralysis of the limbs and the muscles used in breathing. In the twentieth century, polio began to reach epidemic proportions in the United States and elsewhere. The introduction of an effective vaccine in the 1950s finally began to reduce childhood deaths and disability from polio.

Inspired by the success of the polio vaccine, the World Health Organization (WHO) and its partners

launched the Global Polio Eradication Initiative in 1988. The campaign has led to a sharp drop in polio around the world—from around 350,000 cases in 1988 to fewer than 2,000 in the year 2005. Today polio is endemic in only four countries in the world, and the campaign is entering its final phases nearly everywhere. Eradication will prevent more than 10 million polio cases between today and the year 2040.

History and Scientific Foundations

In 1916, an epidemic of polio in the United States claimed around 6,000 lives and paralyzed 27,000 people. When vaccination began in the mid-1950s, there were around 20,000 cases per year. Five years later, the number had dropped to approximately 3,000. In 1979, there were only 10 cases of polio in the United States. Similarly dramatic reductions in polio cases were seen elsewhere.

The World Health Organization (WHO) declared the global eradication of smallpox in 1980. Given the success of the polio vaccine, the announcement of the Global Polio Eradication Initiative by the WHO in 1988 was a natural development. WHO was joined by Rotary International, a worldwide voluntary organization, the U.S. Centers for Disease Control and Prevention (CDC) and UNICEF, the United Nations Children's Fund. Rotary International had been involved in an earlier campaign to eliminate polio from the Americas and was committed to raising funds to protect all children from the disease.

The prime objective of the campaign is to interrupt the transmission of the wild poliovirus by mass vaccination and thereby achieve global eradication of the disease. In doing so, the WHO and its partners hope for the added and long-lasting benefit of strengthening health

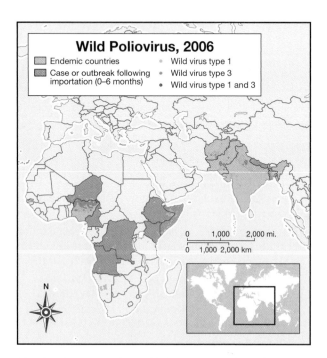

Map showing areas in the world that are impacted by wild poliovirus, January 16, 2006 to January 16, 2007. © Copyright World Health Organization (WHO). Reproduced by permission.

systems everywhere and promoting routine immunization against other infectious diseases.

The campaign relies upon vaccinating every child, however remote or poorly served by a country's health system. It has made significant progress. In the years since its launch, the number of polio cases has fallen by over 99%—from more than 350,000 in 1988 to 1,951 cases reported in 2005. Polio is now endemic in only four countries in the world—India, Pakistan, Afghanistan, and Nigeria. In 1988, the number of countries where polio was endemic totaled 125.

In 1994, the WHO region of the Americas, comprising 36 countries, was certified polio-free. Then, in 2000, the WHO Western Pacific Region, consisting of 37 countries and areas, including China, followed. In June 2002, the WHO European region, consisting of 51 countries, was finally also declared polio-free.

Two billion children around the world have been vaccinated against polio since the launch of the initiative, with 400 million vaccinations in 2005 alone. It appears that the campaign may now be entering its final phase, with Egypt and Niger having now achieved the goal of successfully interrupting polio transmission. Meanwhile, India and Pakistan are reporting their lowest ever number of cases. Type 3 polio can now be said to be on the verge of eradication in Asia.

However, the task that WHO and its partners set themselves is not yet complete. In parts of northern Nigeria, transmission of poliovirus is uncontrolled, with more than three times as many cases in that country in 2006 as in 2003. There have also been outbreaks in Uttar Pradesh, India, and in Somalia. Such pockets of transmission remain a threat to all. Polio is extremely infectious and it would take only one imported case to reintroduce the disease to a country which had worked to achieved polio-free status.

■ Applications and Research

The polio eradication strategy focuses primarily on high infant immunization coverage with four doses of oral polio vaccine (OPV) during the first year of life. Supplementary doses of OPV should also go to all children under five years in areas where they are especially at risk. Surveillance for the presence of polio infection is a vital part of the campaign. All cases of acute flaccid (floppy) paralysis, which might be polio, need to be reported and subjected to laboratory testing.

Once wild poliovirus transmission is limited to a specific area within a country, a targeted 'mop up' campaign is initiated. Ensuring every child is vaccinated can be very challenging. The involvement and commitment of the local community is essential. The main reason why there is still polio in Nigeria is that vaccination was suspended in 2003–2004 because of fears about the

---

WORDS TO KNOW

ENDEMIC: Present in a particular area or among a particular group of people.

ERADICATION: The process of destroying or eliminating a microorganism or disease.

MONOVALENT VACCINE: A monovalent vaccine is one that is active against just one strain of a virus, such as the one that is in common use against the poliovirus.

---

safety of the vaccine. Moreover, awareness of the benefits of vaccination may wane in communities where polio is in decline. Therefore, continual efforts to engage local people in the campaign are needed.

The Advisory Committee on Polio Eradication is an independent body that advises the campaign on science and policy. It has recommended the development of new and more effective vaccines to speed up the eradication effort. Therefore, monovalent OPVs are now being employed, and the use of this type of vaccine is set to increase in the coming years. A monovalent vaccine targets only one strain of the virus—polio has three (1, 2, and 3). Monovalent OPV1, against strain 1, was developed in a period of months and used for the first time in India and Egypt in April 2005 and May 2005, respectively.

Monovalent OPV1 was developed specifically for India and Egypt where dense populations and efficient virus transmission were presenting the greatest technical challenge to eradication. It has since been used to deal with outbreaks in Angola, Indonesia, and Yemen. This vaccine, along with its strain 3 equivalent, will likely become the main tool for polio eradication in the future.

■ Impacts and Issues

To be certified as polio-free, a region must have at least three years of zero polio cases due to wild poliovirus and show that it has a high standard of surveillance. It must also be able to show it can deal effectively with imported cases of polio. Many countries have achieved this status already, but in a few places, further work is still needed before the goal of polio eradication can be achieved.

At the start of 2006, five states in northern Nigeria accounted for over half of all polio cases worldwide. This is the only place in the world where polio incidence is continuing to rise, despite resumption in vaccination activity in 2004. Meanwhile, the Horn of Africa remains vulnerable, with an epidemic in Somalia having spread outwards from the capital, Mogadishu. It is hard to reach all children in this unstable area with its meager infrastructure, but vaccination is essential if the disease is not to spread to children in neighboring Ethiopia, Sudan, and Kenya.

The work of the Global Polio Eradication Initiative is ongoing and it needs substantial financial support. The money comes from a wide range of governments and organizations around the world. A funding "gap" of 85 million U.S. dollars was identified for 2006 and the shortfall for 2007–2008 is 400 million U.S. dollars, according to the WHO. Polio may seem remote in countries where it has been eradicated, but its continued existence in the world is a threat to all people because of the possibility of imported cases of this very infectious disease.

SEE ALSO *Polio (Poliomyelitis).*

BIBLIOGRAPHY

Web Sites

Centers for Disease Control and Prevention (CDC). "Pink Book—Poliomyelitis." <http://www.cdc.gov/nip/publications/pink/polio.pdf> (accessed March 25, 2007).

World Health Organization. "Poliomyelitis." September 2006. <http://www.who.int/mediacentre/factsheets/fs114/en> (accessed March 25, 2007).

World Health Organization. Global Polio Eradication Initiative. "2005 Annual Report." May 2006. <http://www.polioeradication.org/content/publications/annualreport2005.asp> (accessed March 25, 2007).

Susan Aldridge

Prion Disease

■ Introduction

The prion diseases are a group of rare and invariably fatal brain disorders that occur in both animals and humans. They are unusual in that the infective agent is neither a virus nor a bacterium, but an abnormal form of the prion protein (PrP) that is normally found in the brain. Prion disease leads to the development of tiny holes within brain tissue, giving it a characteristic "spongiform" appearance at post-mortem. Hence, prion diseases are also known as the transmissible spongiform encephalopathies (TSEs).

The best known of the human prion diseases is Creutzfeldt-Jakob disease (CJD), which affects about one person in one million. This rare disease came to public attention in 1996, with the announcement of a new form of CJD in the United Kingdom. Research has suggested that variant CJD is transmitted through exposure to beef contaminated by bovine spongiform encephalopathy (BSE), a prion disease of cattle.

■ Disease History, Characteristics, and Transmission

There are four forms of CJD, the major form of prion disease. Sporadic CJD accounts for around 85% of cases and familial CJD accounts for most of the rest. There have been about 200 cases of variant CJD around the world, and a few people have contracted so-called iatrogenic (caused by a treatment) CJD from prion contamination occurring through medical treatment. The other human prion diseases are Gerstmann-Straussler-Scheinker (GSS) syndrome and familial fatal insomnia (FFI), which resemble familial CJD, and kuru, an almost extinct disease confined to the Fore people of New Guinea.

Prion diseases are marked by progressive deterioration of brain function that is always fatal. Sporadic CJD affects mainly people over 50 years old and is marked by ataxia—a shakiness and unsteadiness caused by damage to the cerebellum at the base of the brain which controls

movement. Dementia (a deterioration of memory and other mental functions), swallowing difficulties, jerky movements, and blindness rapidly set in and the patient usually dies within six months.

In familial CJD, GGS, and FFI, the onset of the disease may be at a younger age and the disease's course measured in years rather than months. In FFI, as the name

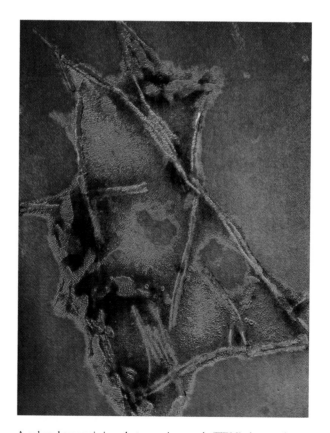

A colored transmission electron micrograph (TEM) shows prion fibrils in the brain of a cow infected with BSE (bovine spongiform encephalopathy) or "mad cow" disease. *Em Unit, VLA/Photo Researchers, Inc.*

WORDS TO KNOW

IATROGENIC: Any infection, injury, or other disease condition caused by medical treatment is iatrogenic (pronounced eye-at-roh-GEN-ik).

PRIONS: Any infection, injury, or disease condition caused by medical treatment is iatrogenic (pronounced eye-at-roh-GEN-ik).

SPONGIFORM: Spongiform is the clinical name for the appearance of brain tissue affected by prion diseases, such as Creutzfeld-Jakob disease or bovine spongiform encephalopathy. The disease process leads to the formation of tiny holes in brain tissue, giving it a spongy appearance.

PRION DISEASES

According to the National Center for Infectious Diseases at the Centers for Disease Control and Prevention (CDC), the following list represents prion-related diseases known as of May 2007.

Human Prion Diseases:

- Creutzfeldt-Jakob Disease (CJD)
- Variant Creutzfeldt-Jakob Disease (vCJD)
- Gerstmann-Straussler-Scheinker Syndrome
- Fatal Familial Insomnia
- Kuru

Animal Prion Diseases:

- Bovine Spongiform Encephalopathy (BSE)
- Chronic Wasting Disease (CWD)
- Scrapie
- Transmissible mink encephalopathy
- Feline spongiform encephalopathy

SOURCE: *Centers for Disease Control and Prevention, National Center for Infectious Diseases*

suggests, a major feature in a progressive and untreatable form of insomnia is caused by damage to the thalamus, the part of the brain regulating sleep-wake cycles.

Variant CJD has a younger age of onset than sporadic CJD and is marked by psychiatric problems and pain and odd sensations in the limbs. The time course of the disease is longer than in sporadic CJD with ataxia setting in at a later stage. In iatrogenic CJD and kuru, ataxia is the main feature and dementia is unusual.

All prion diseases are transmissible under laboratory conditions, yet only variant CJD, iatrogenic CJD, and kuru are infectious in the way this term is usually understood. The source of abnormal PrP in these disorders is either beef contaminated with BSE or exposure to brain tissue from someone with CJD.

In sporadic CJD and familial CJD, as well as in GGS and FFI, a spontaneous or inherited mutation in the PrP gene leads to the generation of abnormal PrP within the patient's brain—without any outside infection. This goes on to interact with normal PrP causing the characteristic spongiform damage within the brain.

■ Scope and Distribution

All prion diseases are very rare, occurring with a frequency of about one per one million of the population—or fewer—around the world. There have been about 200 cases of variant CJD in eleven countries, to date, most of which have occurred in the United Kingdom. Kuru has all but disappeared since the Fore people ceased the funeral practices that exposed them to the risk of the disease.

■ Treatment and Prevention

There are no proven cures for any of the prion diseases, although there are a number of drugs being developed for CJD. Drugs can be given to ease the symptoms, such as valproate or clonazepam for jerky movements.

■ Impacts and Issues

The American researcher Stanley Prusiner (1942–) was awarded the 1997 Nobel Prize for Medicine or Physiology for his work on prions. But there is still much more to be learned about how prions work. For instance, routes of transmission are not well understood. Prion diseases may be present without symptoms for many years, putting people at risk of infection. Therefore a better understanding of prions is an important challenge for neurology research.

The emergence of variant CJD in the 1980s in the United Kingdom among mostly young people sparked an epidemiological investigation that garnered worldwide attention. After the disease was linked with contaminated feed consumed by cattle in the U.K. that resulted in the cattle contracting bovine spongiform encephalopathy (BSE), the British beef industry suffered severe losses as over 150,000 cattle were slaughtered, many countries banned beef imports, and consumption of beef at home in the U.K. dropped dramatically. As other cases of variant CJD were linked to contaminated surgical instruments, stricter controls were put into place for decontamination and disposal of surgical instruments and tissues that could be infected with prions. In 2000, a British report titled "The BSE Inquiry" concluded that individual cattle were probably infected with BSE in the 1970s, that disease became epidemic as a consequence of an intensive farming practice (the recycling of animal protein, including prions, in ruminant feed), and that BSE had been transmitted to humans, enabling the new human prion disease (vCJD) to emerge.

SEE ALSO *Bovine Spongiform Encephalopathy ("Mad Cow" Disease); Creutzfeldt-Jakob Disease-nv; Kuru.*

BIBLIOGRAPHY

Books

Ridley, R.M., and H.F. Baker. *Fatal Protein: The Story of CJD, BSE and Other Prion Disease.* Oxford: Oxford University Press, 1998.

Web Sites

The BSE Inquiry Report. "Home Page." <http://www.bseinquiry.gov.uk/index.htm> (accessed May 15, 2007).

Centers for Disease Control and Prevention. "CJD (Creutzfeldt-Jakob Disease, Classic)." April 13, 2007 <http://www.cdc.gov/ncidod/dvrd/cjd/> (accessed February 21, 2007).

Centers for Disease Control and Prevention. "vCJD (Variant Creutzfeldt-Jakob Disease)." January 4, 2007 <http://www.cdc.gov/ncidod/dvrd/vcjd/index.htm> (accessed February 21, 2007).

U.K. Creutzfeldt-Jakob Disease Surveillance Unit. "National Creutzfeldt-Jakob Disease Surveillance Unit." February 5, 2007 <http://www.cjd.ed.ac.uk> (accessed February 21, 2007)

Susan Aldridge

ProMED

ProMED-mail, to give it its baptismal name, or ProMED, as everyone now calls it, was a happy accident. Barbara Hatch Rosenberg of the Federation of American Scientists organized a meeting in 1993 in Geneva, Switzerland, co-sponsored by the World Health Organization (WHO), to float the idea of a world-girdling chain of institutes capable of sending out teams to the site of any unusual disease outbreak in their neighborhood. The objective would be to determine whether it was of natural or unnatural origin. The conference itself was unusual in bringing together experts on not only human, but also animal and plant diseases, and on bioterrorism, which at the time was not high on anyone's priority list.

There were some 60 participants from 15 countries. The conclusion was that such a chain was highly desirable from the point of view of human health and food security. At a follow-up conference in the United States in 1994, further steps were outlined, and the late Dr. Robert Shope suggested the name ProMED, for Program for Monitoring Emerging Diseases. It was decided that an e-mail list be set up to enable discussion among the participating institutions. Charles Clemens of SatelLife offered to host the e-mail list, and I offered to run it, with the assistance of Stephen Morse, then of Rockefeller University. I was working for the New York State Health Department in Albany, New York, at the time, and was one of only a few of the conference participants who had access to e-mail then. Thus ProMED-mail, so called to distinguish it from its parent program, was launched in August 1994.

It turned out that absolutely no one in the program had anything to say to each other, so as we were supposed to be monitoring outbreaks, Steve and I started posting outbreak reports from the media. Then in May 1995, the Ebola epidemic in Kikwit, Zaire, hit the media, and people surfing the Web discovered that ProMED was posting information about it. I well remember the thrill when our mailing list, which had begun with 40 members in seven countries, hit 250. Later we were written up in the *Wall Street Journal* and our numbers went overnight to 500. Today, in mid-2007, we stand at over 40,000 in at least 180 countries, with many more accessing our Web site at <www.promedmail.org>. And, thanks to foundations and donations we still provide worldwide coverage, 7/365, without fee.

The uniqueness of ProMED is its stable of experts in the fields of clinical and veterinary medicine, microbiology, and plant pathology, all of whom serve on a part-time basis. It is the only free disease reporting system to cover human, livestock, wildlife, and food and feed crop diseases in one place, the latter because of the potential impact of animal and vegetable diseases on nutrition and therefore on human health. Since 2000, ProMED has been a program of the International Society of Infectious Diseases, which guarantees its freedom from political constraints that often cause delays in outbreak reporting. In fact, WHO has said that it uses ProMED reports to convince recalcitrant countries to report outbreaks officially, in view of the fact that a report has already appeared on ProMED.

During the anthrax-by-mail episode in the United States in 2001, the Science Advisor to the President told us that the White House's main sources of updates on the situation were CNN and ProMED. The Chief Veterinary Officers of Australia and New Zealand routinely copy livestock outbreak reports to ProMED at the same time as they send them to the World Animal Health Organization, and we get reports directly from hospitals and research institutes involved in outbreaks. We emphasize reports on outbreaks caused by select agents from the bioterrorism A list, such as anthrax and botulinum toxin, so that our readership understands that such natural outbreaks are not uncommon in some countries. We cover outbreaks due to biological toxins. Otherwise, we report on emerging diseases such as bird flu, using a rather broad definition of emerging that includes dengue but excludes most tuberculosis and HIV/AIDS reports.

ProMED has parallel lists in Spanish, Portuguese, and Russian, with a French version scheduled to launch shortly. These are not straight translations of the English reports, but are mainly reports of regional interest. Chinese and Japanese translations of many ProMED reports are found on the travel health Web sites of Hong Kong and Tokyo International Airport.

SEE ALSO *Emerging Infectious Diseases; GIDEON; Globalization and Infectious Disease; Re-emerging Infectious Diseases; SARS (Severe Acute Respiratory Syndrome); Virus Hunters.*

BIBLIOGRAPHY

Web Sites

International Society of Infectious Diseases. "ProMED." <http://www.promedmail.org> (accessed June 5, 2007).

World Health Organization. "Disease Outbreak News." <http://www.who.int/csr/don/en> (accessed June 8, 2007).

Jack Woodall

Psittacosis

■ Introduction

Psittacosis is a bacterial zoonotic (from animals) infection caused by the bacterium *Chlamydia psittaci*. This bacterium is present in birds and passed on to humans when they inhale airborne infectious particles such as feather dust, or bird secretions. Psittacosis causes acute symptoms of fever, headache, body aches, and a dry cough. Respiratory distress such as pneumonia may also arise. Psittacosis is not usually fatal, with approximately a 1% mortality (death) rate in the United States. Treatment using tetracycline antibiotics usually leads to a full recovery.

Psittacosis is a worldwide disease but outbreaks are rare. Importation of birds helps to spread the disease from one location to several. People in close contact with birds such as veterinarians, pet store owners, pet owners, and poultry producers are most at risk of contracting psittacosis. Psittacosis can be prevented through avoiding contact with infected birds or wearing protective gear such as gloves and masks when handling infected birds.

■ Disease History, Characteristics, and Transmission

Psittacosis was first identified in 1879 as a bacterial disease that infected birds and was later confirmed to also infect humans and other animals. During 1929 and 1930, a worldwide outbreak of psittacosis occurred when a shipment of infected parrots from Argentina spread the disease to numerous regions of the world. There were approximately 1,000 cases of which 200–300 were fatal. This resulted in a ban on importation in many major countries, including the United States, but this ban was lifted in 1973.

Psittacosis is a bacterial disease caused by the bacteria *Chlamydia psittaci* and is common in many bird species, both wild and tame. Humans become infected with *C. psittaci* if they inhale dried secretions from infected birds. This may include aerosolized (suspended in the air) feces, feather dust, and droplets from sneezing or coughing birds.

Psittacosis symptoms include fever, headache, body aches, and a dry cough. Pneumonia may also occur. Severe or untreated cases of psittacosis may develop complications such as a heart valve infection (endocarditis), liver inflammation (hepatitis), and neurologic complications. The mortality rate for psittacosis is approximately 1%.

■ Scope and Distribution

The organism that causes psittacosis occurs worldwide. Importation of birds exacerbates the chances of infection spreading from one region to another. Furthermore, the bird industry, including poultry farming and the pet trade, provide a route for the infection to spread.

In 2002, an outbreak in the Blue Mountains, Australia, involved 59 probable cases. The source of the infection was wild birds. The outbreak prompted the health department to raise public awareness about psittacosis. In Belgium in 1995, an outbreak occurred involving customs officers. The source of the infection was imported parakeets.

Most cases of psittacosis occur in people who have a close association with birds. This includes pet owners, pet store owners, bird fanciers, and poultry producers. In addition, young children, older adults, smokers, alcoholics, and immunocompromised people (people with a weakened immune system) tend to be more susceptible to infection.

■ Treatment and Prevention

Infection with *Chlamydia psittaci* is effectively treated using antibiotics. The most commonly prescribed antibiotics are tetracycline, doxycycline, and erythromycin. Treatment is normally administered for two weeks, after which a full recovery is expected.

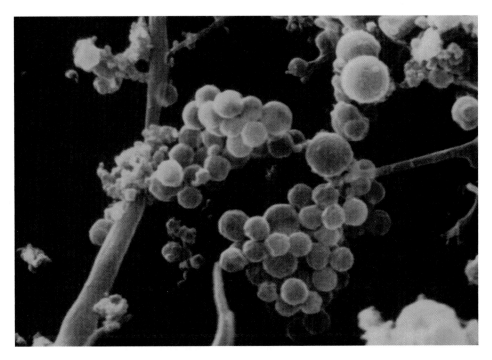

This false-color scanning electron micrograph (SEM) shows *Chlamydia psittaci*, a species of small, spherical bacteria causing lung disease (psittacosis) in humans. *Moredun Animal Health Ltd/Photo Researchers, Inc.*

The best prevention method against infection with *C. psittaci* is to avoid contact with infected birds, and to ensure birds are kept free from infection. Investigating the cause of sickness in ill birds will help determine whether *C. psittaci* is present. Once an infected bird is found, measures can be taken to prevent the disease spreading to other birds or to humans. Avoidance measures such as facemasks, gloves, and handwashing can help reduce the chance of inhaling or ingesting contaminated particles. No vaccine is available to prevent contraction of psittacosis.

■ Impacts and Issues

Some cases of psittacosis may go undiagnosed or be misdiagnosed as diagnosis can be difficult. The occurrence of pneumonia can mislead a practitioner to diagnose the illness as a case of pneumonia, rather than psittacosis. Therefore, the prevalence of psittacosis may currently be underestimated.

Another issue surrounding this disease is the difficulties associated with tracing the disease to its source. First, infected birds may be asymptomatic making it difficult to determine whether they are a source of infection. Secondly, the pet bird industry is not heavily regulated, making it difficult to track the exchange of birds. Therefore, tracing an infected bird back to its original origin may be impossible, making it difficult to prevent the spread of the disease. Wildlife trade, including exotic bird trade, also spreads the disease to new

areas. This makes it problematic to effectively control psittacosis and prevent outbreaks.

SEE ALSO *Animal Importation; Bacterial Disease; Pneumonia; Zoonoses.*

WORDS TO KNOW

AEROSOL: Particles of liquid or solid dispersed as a suspension in gas.

IMMUNOCOMPROMISED: A reduction of the ability of the immune system to recognize and respond to the presence of foreign material.

MORTALITY: Mortality is the condition of being susceptible to death. The term "mortality" comes from the Latin word *mors*, which means "death." Mortality can also refer to the rate of deaths caused by an illness or injury, i.e., "Rabies has a high mortality."

ZOONOSES: Zoonoses are diseases of microbiological origin that can be transmitted from animals to people. The causes of the diseases can be bacteria, viruses, parasites, and fungi.

BIBLIOGRAPHY

Periodicals

Karesh, W.B., R.A. Cook, E.L. Bennett, and J. Newcomb. "Wildlife Trade and Global Disease Emergence." *Emerging Infectious Diseases.* vol. 11, no. 7 (2005): 1000–1002.

Web Sites

American Museum of Natural History. "Some Facts about Psittacosis." 2003 <http://research.amnh.org/users/nyneve/psittacosis.html#hist> (accessed Mar. 7, 2007).

Centers for Disease Control (CDC). "Psittacosis." Oct. 13, 2005 <http://www.cdc.gov/ncidod/dbmd/diseaseinfo/psittacosis_t.htm> (accessed Mar. 7, 2007).

NSW Health Department. "Psittacosis: Questions and Answers." 2002 <http://www.health.nsw.gov.au/public-health/pdf/PsittacosisQA.pdf> (accessed Mar. 7, 2007).

Public Health and Infectious Disease

■ Introduction

An effective response to an infectious disease outbreak, epidemic, or pandemic requires a coordinated approach from all parts of the public health system. Public health units play an important role in disease control and response including planning for emergencies, surveillance, education, communication, case identification, case management, infection control, contact tracing, monitoring contacts in quarantine, border surveillance, epidemiological studies, and immunization.

The disease surveillance system must ensure that the first cases of the outbreak are quickly identified. Next, control strategies must be implemented to slow down the transmission of the pathogen while a vaccine or effective treatments are being developed. Surveillance would also detect the final case, indicating an end to the outbreak.

The Infectious Disease Surveillance System in the United States

Reporting of Communicable Diseases When a known "notifiable" disease or an unknown communicable disease is suspected to be a public health threat, clinicians should immediately notify the local health authority. Reporting requirements vary greatly from one region to another because of different conditions and different disease frequencies.

Communicable disease reporting is necessary to provide accurate and timely information for the initiation of investigation and control measures. It also encourages uniformity in morbidity and mortality reporting so that data among different health jurisdictions within a country and among nations will be consistent and comparable.

A reporting system functions at four levels:

- Collection of basic data on incidence, geographic dispersion, and patient outcomes in the local community where the disease occurs.
- Assembly of data at district, state, or provincial levels.
- Aggregation and analysis of the information at the national level.
- For certain designated diseases, the national public health agency reports data and analysis to the World Health Organization (WHO).

Reporting of Cases Each local health authority determines what diseases should be routinely reported. Physicians are required to report all notifiable illnesses that come to their attention. In addition, the statutes or regulations of many localities require reporting by hospital infectious disease officers, householders, or other persons having knowledge of a case of a reportable disease. These may be individual case reports or reports of groups of cases (collective reports).

Reporting of Epidemics For reporting purposes, diseases are usually classified into the following five classes, according to the advantages that can be derived from reporting. This classification provides a basis for inclusion in a local list of regularly reportable diseases. Case finding can be passive, i.e., the physician initiates the report as required, or active, when the public health officer regularly contacts clinicians, clinics, or hospitals to request the desired information.

Class 1: *Case Report Universally Required by International Health Regulations or as a Disease under Surveillance by the WHO.* This class can be divided into the following types:

- 1: Those diseases subject to the International Health Regulations (1969), 4th Annotated Edition 2005, WHO, Geneva: e.g., the internationally quarantinable diseases such as plague, cholera, and yellow fever.
- 1A: Diseases under Surveillance by WHO, established by the 22nd World Health Assembly: e.g., louse-borne typhus fever and relapsing fever, paralytic poliomyelitis, malaria, and influenza.

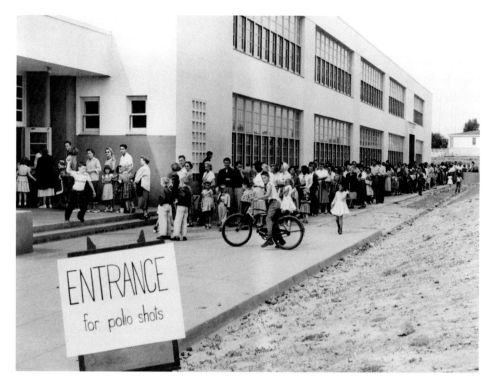

Students in San Diego, California, line up for a polio vaccination in 1955. In one of the most successful public health initiatives in U.S. history, mass inoculation campaigns largely wiped out polio in the nation. © *Bettmann/Corbis.*

The required case report is made to the health authorities by telephone, FAX, telegraph, or other rapid means; in an epidemic situation, collected reports of subsequent cases in a local area may be requested by the next superior jurisdiction on a daily or weekly basis. The local health authority forwards the initial report to the next superior jurisdiction by the most expeditious means.

Class 2: *Case report regularly required wherever the disease occurs.* Two subclasses are recognized, based on the relative urgency for investigation of contacts and source of infection, or for starting control measures. Examples include typhoid fever and diphtheria, brucellosis, and leprosy.

Class 3: *Selectively reportable in recognized endemic areas in many states and countries;* diseases of this class are not reportable. Reporting may be prescribed in particular regions, states, or countries if they recur with undue frequency or severity. Three subclasses are recognized, based on urgency of the investigation or control measures. Examples are scrub typhus, arenaviral hemorrhagic fever, bartonellosis, coccidioidomycosis, schistosomiasis, and fasciolopsiasis.

Class 4: *Obligatory report of epidemics—no case report required.* Pertinent data include number of cases, time frame, approximate population involved, and appa-

rent mode of transmission; e.g., staphylococcal foodborne intoxication, adenoviral keratoconjunctivitis, unidentified syndrome.

Class 5: *Official Report Not Ordinarily Justifiable.* Diseases of this class are of two general kinds: those typically sporadic and uncommon, often not directly transmissible from person to person (chromoblastomycosis), or those with an epidemiology that offers no special practical measures for control (common cold).

Diseases are often made reportable, but the information gathered is not put to practical use with no feedback to those who provided the data. This can lead to deterioration in the general level of reporting, even for diseases of critical importance. Better case reporting results when official reporting is restricted to those diseases for which control services are provided or potential control procedures are under evaluation, or epidemiologic information is needed for a definite purpose.

■ Impacts and Issues

Public Health Response to SARS

In 2003 the world experienced the sudden onset of an epidemic of the virulent disease severe acute respiratory syndrome or SARS. The response to this outbreak was the first opportunity for new global public health

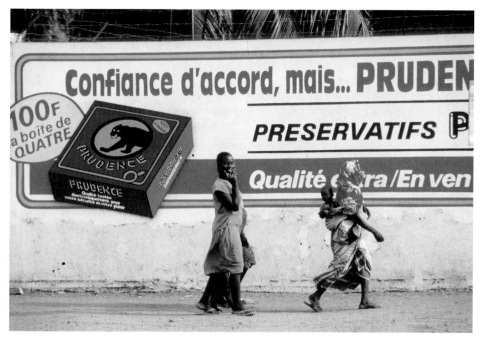

Women walk by a condom advertisement in Abidjan, Ivory Coast. Worldwide public health efforts to promote facts about the transmission of AIDS, to eliminate the social stigma associated with the disease, and to prevent the illness continue throughout the current AIDS pandemic. © *Karen Kasmauski/Corbis.*

surveillance and control agencies to act in anticipation of a potential avian influenza outbreak. The infectious agent was a highly pathogenic virus (in this case a coronavirus). Like the anticipated pattern for avian flu, the outbreaks spread from Asia to the rest of the world. Thus, the SARS epidemic was a trial run of emerging international public heath protocols to identify and respond to infectious disease threats.

The largest outbreak of SARS began in March 2003 in Beijing, China. This outbreak was resolved within six weeks of its peak in late April. Chinese public health agencies recorded case data from SARS cases observed in Beijing and their close contacts between March 5, 2003, and May 29, 2003 onto standardized surveillance forms, which were subsequently reviewed by epidemiologists. The epidemiological investigation focused on 1) the response of public health agencies to the SARS outbreak in terms of the timeline for implementing major control measures; 2) the number of reported cases and quarantined close contacts; 3) the calculated attack rates, with changes in infection control measures, management, and triage of suspected cases; and 4) the time lag between illness onset and hospitalization with information dissemination.

The investigation found that health care worker training in use of personal protective equipment and the isolation of patients with SARS, along with the establishment of fever clinics and designated hospital SARS wards, predated the steepest decline in cases. During the outbreak 30,178 exposed persons were quarantined in China. Attack rates among quarantined individuals were calculated by type of relationship to known victims and the age of the contact. Among 2,195 quarantined close contacts in five districts, the attack rate was 6.3%, with a range of 15% among spouses to less than 0.5% among work and school contacts. The attack rate among quarantined household members was found to increase with age from 5% in children younger than 10 years to 27% in adults aged 60 to 69 years.

Among nearly 14 million people screened for fever at airports, train stations, and roadside checkpoints, only 12 were found to have probable SARS. After initial reticence, the national and municipal governments adopted a policy of full disclosure, holding 13 press conferences about the SARS outbreak. Following the installation of strict screening and control procedures, the time interval between illness onset and hospitalization decreased from a median of five to six days on or before April 20, 2003, the day the outbreak was announced to the public, to two days after April 20. The rapid resolution of the SARS outbreak was due to multiple factors, including improvements in patient isolation and triage in both hospitals and communities of patients with suspected SARS and the propagation of information to health care workers and the public.

On the other side of the globe, the largest SARS outbreak in North America occurred in Toronto, Canada. Again, epidemiologists analyzed the patterns of transmission and the public health effects of control measures, and the findings and disease patterns closely

WORDS TO KNOW

INFECTION CONTROL: Infection control refers to policies and procedures used to minimize the risk of spreading infections, especially in hospitals and health care facilities.

MORBIDITY: The term "morbidity" comes from the Latin word "morbus," which means sick. In medicine it refers not just to the state of being ill, but also to the severity of the illness. A serious disease is said to have a high morbidity.

MORTALITY: Mortality is the condition of being susceptible to death. The term "mortality" comes from the Latin word *mors*, which means "death." Mortality can also refer to the rate of deaths caused by an illness or injury, i.e., "Rabies has a high mortality."

NOTIFIABLE DISEASE: A disease that the law requires must be reported to health officials when diagnosed; also called a reportable disease.

QUARANTINE: Quarantine is the practice of separating people who have been exposed to an infectious agent but have not yet developed symptoms from the general population. This can be done voluntarily or involuntarily by the authority of states and the federal Centers for Disease Control and Prevention.

PANDEMIC: Pandemic, which means all the people, describes an epidemic that occurs in more than one country or population simultaneously.

SURVEILLANCE: The systematic analysis, collection, evaluation, interpretation, and dissemination of data. In public health, it assists in the identification of health threats and the planning, implementation, and evaluation of responses to those threats.

paralleled those in China. Toronto Public Health examined 2,132 potential SARS cases, ascertained that 23,103 contacts of SARS patients required quarantine, and logged 316,615 calls on a hotline dedicated to SARS. According to the investigators, 225 Toronto residents met the case definition of SARS. Only three travel-related cases were not linked to the index patient, who came to Toronto from Hong Kong.

A resurgence of the outbreak occurred due to unrecognized SARS among hospitalized patients. This was eventually controlled using active surveillance of hospitalized patients. The control measures of Toronto Public Health brought about a reduction in the number of persons exposed to SARS in non-hospital and non-household settings from 20 before the control measures were implemented to zero after implementation. The number of patients exposed while in a hospital ward rose from 25 before the measures were taken to 68 afterwards, while the number exposed during a stay in the intensive care unit dropped from 13 to zero. The spread of the outbreak in the community (outside of hospital settings) was significantly reduced after instituting the control measures.

Toronto SARS transmission was mostly limited to hospitals and households where patients had contacts. Epidemiologists determined that for every case of SARS, public health authorities could expect to quarantine up to 100 patient contacts and investigate eight potential cases. Active in-hospital surveillance for SARS-like illnesses and heightened infection-control measures were essential in bringing the outbreak under control.

Although the public health response to SARS was successful within a short time-frame, it is far from clear that a similar response to an avian flu outbreak would be as successful, mainly because influenza mortality and infectivity could be much greater, while current treatments could be considerably less effective. For this reason, the production of an effective avian flu vaccine is seen as essential for controlling an avian flu outbreak.

Control of Infectious Disease Outbreaks

Once an outbreak of infectious disease has been detected, public health agencies must consider a range of disease control measures from the control of patient contacts and the immediate environment of the outbreak to mass vaccination programs or mass prophylaxis using anti-infective medication. Following are some examples of recent research and a discussion of the use of certain control measures in the context of public concern over the possibility of an avian flu pandemic.

Risks of Mass Vaccination and Prophylaxis as Disease Control Measures As public health experts consider the implications of serious infectious disease outbreaks, they must balance the potential benefits of control measures such as mass immunization. One consideration that leads to caution in implementing such measures is the occurrence of relatively rare but predictable adverse reactions or events due to vaccination or medication (medication-related adverse events or MRAEs). For example, it is generally considered unacceptable to incur predictable mortality by using vaccines that have a rate of adverse reactions, however low, unless there is an actual outbreak of a dangerous disease. Computer models for particular infectious diseases can calculate outbreak-specific predicted daily MRAE rates from model user inputs by applying a probability distribution to the reported timing of MRAEs. One such exercise modeled a hypothetical 2- to 10-day prophylaxis operation for one million people using recent data from both smallpox vaccination and anthrax antibiotic prophylaxis campaigns. It was found that the duration of a mass prophylaxis campaign is important in determining the ensuing amount of emergency services utilization due to actual or suspected adverse reactions. In a population of that size, a 2-day smallpox vaccination scenario would produce an estimated 32,000 medical encounters and 1,960 hospitalizations, peaking at 5,246 health care encounters six days after the start of the campaign. By contrast, a 10-day campaign would lead to a much lower peak surge, with a maximum of 3,106 encounters on the worst day, 10 days after campaign initiation.

Thus the duration of a mass prophylaxis campaign could have a significant impact on the timing and peak number of serious MRAEs, with very brief campaigns overwhelming existing emergency department (ED) capacity to treat real or suspected adverse reactions. Although these results could be refined by further study of adverse reaction rates, the results of modeling underline the necessity for coordinating public health and emergency medicine planning for infectious disease outbreaks in order to avoid preventable surges in ED use.

Travel Restrictions as a Disease Control Measure

Travel restrictions have often been suggested as an efficient way to reduce the spread of a communicable disease that threatens public health. Swedish researchers conducted a computer simulation of the effect of different levels of travel restrictions on the rapidity and geographical spread of an outbreak of a disease similar to SARS. They tested scenarios of travel restrictions in which travel over distances greater than 30 mi (50 km) and 12 mi (20 km) would be banned, taking into account different compliance levels. They found that a ban on journeys over 30 mi (50 km) would drastically reduce the speed and geographical spread of outbreaks, even when compliance is less than 100%. Their study supported the use of travel restrictions as an effective way to mitigate the effect of a future disease outbreak, at least when the infectivity of a disease is moderate as in the case of SARS. It is not known how effective they will be for airborne and animal borne infections with greater transmissibility such as a potential mutant H5N1 virus, discussed in more detail later.

Medication Stockpiles as a Potential Control Measure

As noted earlier, much of the discussion and research regarding infectious disease control measures has happened in the context of concern about a potential new worldwide influenza pandemic, such as happens about three times each century. The worst of these pandemics on record was the 1918 pandemic, which killed at least 20 million people. H5N1 flu has become endemic in Asian birds, and at least 74 human cases, including 49 deaths and probable human-to-human transmission, have occurred since the beginning of 2004. International health officials lack the resources to monitor avian flu in a population of hundreds of millions in the parts of Asia likely to become the epicenter of such a new pandemic, including some countries with rudimentary or no public health systems.

If such a pandemic reached the United States at the present time, it would be possible to manufacture only enough vaccine for perhaps a quarter of the population. The currently planned domestic stockpile of oseltamivir would leave over 99% of the country unprotected. In contrast, Great Britain's planned stockpile will be 25 times greater on a per-capita basis, and some authorities suggest that even that level is insufficient. To change the course of such a pandemic, vaccines and antiviral drugs will be needed in much greater quantities than current plans allow.

Most researchers agree that pandemic influenza will recur. The world's surveillance systems and countermeasures are likely inadequate, and current control measures may not significantly slow a pandemic once it has begun.

■ U.S. Case Example: Preparedness for Avian Flu in Massachusetts

In June 2006 in the Commonwealth of Massachusetts, a panel of national, state, and local experts met to assess the threat of an avian influenza pandemic. In particular, they discussed the readiness of state and local officials response to such a pandemic. The conference leaders suggested that political entities, the public health system, and the medical community need a "seamless network of protection" against this potentially lethal threat. Three major challenges to pandemic planning and preparedness were noted: 1) the scale of the challenge; 2) connectivity of communication; and 3) the danger of complacency.

The current threat posed by avian influenza was described at the conference as requiring monitoring for mutations in the virus and its ability to transmit efficiently among people, particularly since there is no immunity among human populations against H5N1. Also, the ease and frequency of international travel and transportation of goods means that an evolving threat anywhere in the world is a threat everywhere.

Attendees noted that the response to the SARS epidemic conveyed some valuable public health lessons. Among these was that travel advisories seemed to help to contain the SARS pandemic. Interventions such as social distancing (e.g., cancellation of large gatherings, quarantining persons infected with influenza, and the use of cough etiquette and masks) could be helpful in mitigating the effects of an influenza pandemic. Two scenarios of an avian flu epidemic in the United States were discussed. One was based upon the 1957–1958 (swine flu) pandemic, and one upon the more severe 1918 (Spanish flu) pandemic. Both scenarios assume that 30 percent of the current U.S. population will become ill; up to half of those who are ill will require outpatient medical care.

The major difference between the scenarios would be the severity of the illness. If the pandemic is moderately severe, as it was in 1957, then approximately 209,000 people in the United States could die. However, if the pandemic causes severe disease, estimates show that almost 10 million people would require hospitalization, with 1.5 million requiring ICU care. Data from the 1918 pandemic indicate that close to 2 million deaths could occur in the United States alone, and millions more worldwide.

The federal government has made it clear that, in the event of a pandemic, it will not be able to respond to every community. Rather, state and local jurisdictions must take responsibility for preparedness planning and response efforts. Basic public health tools, including good communication about risk, individual/family/community preparedness, identification and quarantine of confirmed cases, and social distancing could be most useful during the initial stages of a pandemic. Schools and businesses could choose to temporarily close and use technology to reduce direct contact between people.

Effective communication during a pandemic is essential. Since it is possible that the supply chain of services, goods, and food will be disrupted during a severe pandemic, it is recommended that individuals and families store at least a two-week supply of water and food, nonprescription drugs, and other health supplies including pain relievers, stomach remedies, cough and cold medicines, fluids with electrolytes, and vitamins. The CDC addresses these concerns and provides a number of preparedness checklists and other tools on their website, <www.pandemicflu.gov>.

In Massachusetts, the state's pandemic preparedness plan is "intended to ensure that essential services are maintained, there is minimal discomfort and loss of life, the most vulnerable are cared for and that individuals, families and first responders are protected." The plan addresses hospital and health care facility surge capacity and staffing issues, surveillance and identification of influenza, the health and safety of vulnerable populations, timely and effective communication, and continuity of government and essential services during a crisis.

Massachusetts executive branch agencies that oversee critical services have submitted mandatory "continuity of government" (COG) plans to ensure that critical operations will continue during a pandemic. Businesses, schools, colleges and universities, providers, and municipal governments should all be preparing "continuity of operations plans" (COOPs) in order to ensure contin-

gencies be made in the event of a pandemic. Educational outreach programs have begun and, to date, a number of impact estimates have been done in the state detailing the possible outcomes of an influenza pandemic. Legislation is pending that would indemnify emergency volunteer health workers and make them eligible for workers' compensation, which is important to recruiting needed staff. The administration will disseminate directives on how quarantine should be declared, what travel restrictions might result in the event of a pandemic, and where influenza specialty care clinics (ISCUs) are located. Simulation exercises have been conducted and public information campaigns have begun.

Five regional pandemic planning conferences have been held across Massachusetts that brought together representatives from public health and safety, business, healthcare, local government, primary and secondary schools, higher education, and the faith and human services communities. Among recommendations were improved hospital surge capacity, recruitment of volunteer healthcare staff, and increased state laboratory surveillance capabilities and stockpiles of antivirals.

Local Plans

Within Massachusetts there are a number of agencies and institutions that will be involved in the initial stages of a pandemic. Communities, businesses, schools, and individuals must be kept informed as a pandemic unfolds. A challenge at the local level is for public health officials to communicate effectively with other emergency responders that do not necessarily speak the same public health language.

Some critics assert that local public health officials are also being asked to conduct training, generate plans, and purchase supplies in preparation for a potential flu pandemic, but may lack the necessary resources and infrastructure to carry out their plans. Additionally, some community officials feel that they are not being included in federal and statewide planning.

To address these issues, the state has included each of the 351 local boards of health into one of 15 Emergency Preparedness Coalitions of contiguous municipalities in an effort to facilitate joint planning and resource distribution. The Coalition holds monthly planning meetings, allocates resources to local public health agencies, facilitates collaboration with area hospitals, evaluates training needs, and holds drills and regional flu clinics. These regional clinics were successful during the past influenza season and exemplified that collaboration within regions is possible.

Level of preparedness in Massachusetts

Many towns have created emergency plans, identified emergency dispensing sites, are running pandemic influenza drills, have a comprehensive response system in place, and are improving communication with other first responders. There is still insufficient long-term staffing, insufficient money to increase capacity, and the emergency personnel pool is inadequate. A clear definition of the role of local public health departments and joint planning strategies between towns are required, since there is tremendous variation across communities in terms of needs and resources.

■ Primary Source Connection

As increased migration and trade has heightened the threat of pandemic disease, cooperation among national governments and public health organizations worldwide has become essential. Since pandemic infectious diseases spread across national borders, disease prevention measures in one nation affect surrounding nations as well. The following article from the *New York Times* asserts that some pandemic influenza prevention measures disproportionately affect the poorest residents in regions where the disease is likely to emerge.

Ruth R. Faden is executive director and Patrick S. Duggan is research coordinator, both at the Berman Institute of Bioethics at Johns Hopkins. Ruth Karron is the director of the Center for Immunization Research at the Johns Hopkins Bloomberg School of Public Health.

Who Pays to Stop a Pandemic?

BIRD flu has not yet turned into a pandemic, but it is already killing the meager hopes of some of the world's poorest people for a marginally better life.

When poultry become infected with the deadly strain of avian influenza (H5N1), it is essential that all birds nearby be culled to prevent further spread. We all stand to benefit from this important pandemic prevention strategy, recommended by the World Health Organization and the United Nations Food and Agriculture Organization. Unfortunately, however, the world's poor are unfairly shouldering the burden of the intervention.

Last month officials in Jakarta, Indonesia, announced a ban on household farming of poultry there. The domestic bird population of Jakarta is estimated at 1.3 million. Thousands of families were given until Feb. 1 to consume, sell or kill their birds. Now inspectors are going door to door to destroy any remaining birds.

The Indonesian government pledged to pay about $1.50 for each bird infected with the H5N1 virus, a sum that may approximate the bird's fair market value. But most birds that have been killed under this policy are healthy, so their owners, most reports suggest, will receive nothing.

Moreover, it is not clear how Jakarta's poor will replace the income they once received from chickens and other birds. When officials impose widespread culling, industrial-scale poultry producers—like the company that owns the large British turkey farm where bird flu was found this month—usually have the resources to absorb the losses. But when the birds of small-scale poultry farmers are culled, entrepreneurs who were just beginning to move up the development ladder can be plunged right back into poverty. The most dependent and vulnerable members of the community become even more dependent and vulnerable. "Backyard birds" are the only source of income for many women and children.

Families whose birds are found to be infected with the virus may suffer even more. People in Cambodia, China and India whose poultry have been blamed for avian influenza outbreaks have often been subject to extreme stigma and isolation, and there have even been reports of suicides by desperate farmers.

It is inevitable that the world's poor will suffer most from a pandemic. A recent article in *The Lancet* predicted that if the next pandemic were to mimic the huge 1918 flu outbreak, 96 percent of an estimated 62 million deaths would occur in developing countries. But specific steps can and should be taken now to prevent or mitigate the injustices that are already occurring.

We are part of a group of 24 government officials, public health experts and scientists from 11 countries who recently met in Bellagio, Italy, with the support of the Rockefeller Foundation to call attention to how pandemic planning affects the world's disadvantaged. We created a checklist for avian influenza control that explicitly calls on the authorities to compensate people who suffer losses from bird-culling programs, regardless of whether the destroyed birds are infected with the avian influenza virus.

Such a program in Jakarta alone would be expensive. Just to compensate families for their culled birds would require nearly $2 million, not including the cost of administering the program. Indonesia's domestic bird population countrywide is estimated at 300 million, so if the culling program were to be expanded beyond Jakarta, the total compensation cost could run as high as $450 million.

Indonesia's avian influenza budget for the coming year is reported to be less than $50 million. Clearly, without donor assistance, the government cannot afford to compensate families and farmers fairly. So the burden of pandemic prevention must also fall on the world's wealthy nations.

Last year, the United States, the European Union and other nations pledged more than $2 billion to the global war chest for avian influenza response. Developing a program to compensate poor families in countries with limited resources is an enormous challenge. But it is time that the money pledged by the donor countries reach the people who are already the first victims of the next pandemic.

Ruth R. Faden, Patrick S. Duggan, and Ruth Karron

FADEN, RUTH R., PATRICK S. DUGGAN, AND RUTH KARRON. *NEW YORK TIMES ONLINE.* "WHO PAYS TO STOP A PANDEMIC?"

FEBRUARY 9, 2007. <HTTP://WWW.NYTIMES.COM/2007/02/09/
OPINION/09FADEN.HTML?_R=1&OREF=SLOGIN&
PAGEWANTED=PRINT> (ACCESSED JUNE 11, 2007).

SEE ALSO *Epidemiology; Food-borne Disease and Food Safety; Notifiable Diseases; Pandemic Preparedness.*

BIBLIOGRAPHY

Books

Heymann, David L. *Control of Communicable Diseases Manual*, 18 ed. Washington, D.C.: American Public Health Association, 2004, pp. 700.

World Health Organization. *International Health Regulations 2005*, 4th ed (annot.). New York: WHO, 2005.

Periodicals

Barry, John M. "The site of origin of the 1918 influenza pandemic and its public health implications." *Journal of Translational Medicine.* 2004.

Handel, A., I.M. Longini, Jr., and R. Antia. "What is the best control strategy for multiple infectious disease outbreaks?" *Proceedings of the Royal Society of London. Biological sciences.* 22; 274 (1611) March 2007: 833-7.

Lewis, Katharine Kranz. "The Pandemic Threat: Is Massachusetts Prepared? Findings from the Forum on Pandemic Flu, sponsored by the Massachusetts Health Policy Forum," June 2006. Policy Brief. The Massachusetts Policy Forum, August, 2006.

Web Sites

World Health Organization. "International Health Regulations." <http://www.who.int/csr/ihr/voluntarycompliancemay06EN%20.pdf> (accessed April 21, 2007).

Kenneth T. LaPensee

Puerperal Fever

Introduction

Puerperal (around the time if childbirth) fever is a highly infectious disease that resulted in significant maternal mortality (deaths) from the seventeenth to the nineteenth centuries, and still remains a potential threat in developing nations. It is caused most often by infection from Group A streptococcal bacteria during or immediately following childbirth and is transmissible between patients. During the historic epidemic periods, infection almost always proved fatal and mothers exhibited symptoms of fever, abdominal pain, and vaginal hemorrhage.

Puerperal fever was not prevalent in developed nations until the seventeenth century, when it became common for women to give birth and recover in hospitals. Hospital physicians were responsible for the examination and deliveries of many pregnant women each day. It was these routines that eventually indicated that doctors and nurses were responsible for transmitting the disease between patients. Physician and professor Oliver Wendell Holmes (1809–1894) and physician Ignaz Semmelweis (1818–1865) were each independently responsible for increasing awareness of this mode of transmission and implementing preventative measures against further spread of infection. In developed nations, puerperal fever poses little significant risk to expecting mothers.

Disease History, Characteristics, and Transmission

Puerperal fever, also referred to as childbed fever or puerperal sepsis, was a disease commonly affecting mothers during or shortly after childbirth up until the twentieth century. The first case of puerperal fever that was documented occurred in Paris in 1646, but it was not until 1879 that Louis Pasteur (1822–1895) identified the causative agent as bacteria belonging to the *Streptococcus* group.

Following childbirth, the placental attachment site in the uterus remains an open wound highly susceptible to infection from bacteria that occur normally on the skin, nose, throat, and vagina. Following infection by *Streptococcus* bacteria, the disease presents with rapid onset of fever, abdominal pain, abnormal vaginal discharge, and bleeding. Infection usually occurs within ten days of birth, and progresses to septicemia (bacterial infection in the blood) or peritonitis (generalized infection of the lining of the abdomen). During periods of epidemics, puerperal fever carried a fatality rate of up to 100 percent.

The significant prevalence of puerperal fever began only after the establishment of lying in hospitals, where physicians were completing many deliveries each day and treating many

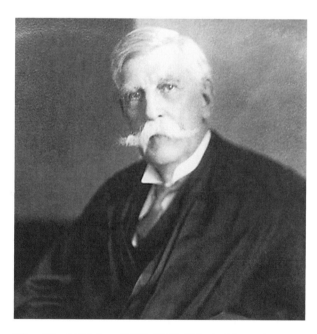

Oliver Wendell Holmes (1809–1894), U.S. physician and poet, prepared an 1843 paper on puerperal fever, a post-natal infection of the womb. *Rutgers University Library.*

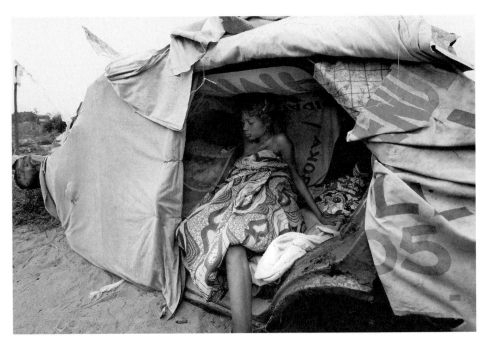

One of many street people in the Democratic Republic of Congo, this young woman gave birth in the rusting wreckage of a car in an old cemetery-turned-garbage dump. She was later taken to a clinic to treat major infections following the birth of her child. Lack of a skilled attendant during childbirth is a major risk factor for maternal mortality, often arising from infection. *AP Images.*

WORDS TO KNOW

MORTALITY: Mortality is the condition of being susceptible to death. The term "mortality" comes from the Latin word *mors*, which means "death." Mortality can also refer to the rate of deaths caused by an illness or injury, i.e., "Rabies has a high mortality."

PUERPERAL: An interval of time around childbirth, from the onset of labor through the immediate recovery period after delivery.

SEPTICEMIA: Prolonged fever, chills, anorexia, and anemia in conjunction with tissue lesions.

women who had given birth each day. Practitioners at that time were attending a number of patients each day without using sterilization procedures between patients. In 1843, Oliver Wendell Holmes concluded that physicians and nurses were responsible for transmitting the infection through their hands and clothing.

Unaware of this prior conclusion, physician Ignaz Semmelweis of Hungary noticed that one ward of physicians in his hospital had a 16 percent fatality rate compared with the midwife wards, which had a 2 percent fatality rate. Semmelweis recognized that the physicians had been performing autopsies on puerperal fever patients prior to deliveries, and concluded that the physicians were spreading the infection from patient to patient. Semmelweis then introduced mandatory washing with chlorinated lime at the beginning of shifts and prior to vaginal examination. Mortality was subsequently reduced to less than 3 percent.

■ Scope and Distribution

Although puerperal fever had a relatively recent period of significant endemicity during the eighteenth and nineteenth centuries, it has been recognized for thousands of years that delivering women may be at risk of a fever that could be fatal. However, the mortality rates of puerperal fever in ancient and medieval times were lower, as women generally gave birth at home and were therefore not at risk of exposure to infection carried by attending medical staff.

Today, in developed countries, deaths from puerperal fever are rare and the mortality rate is about 0.1 per 10,000 births. This significant reduction in fatalities is largely attributed to improvements in sanitation and hygiene during birth, as well as the use of antibiotics to treat bacterial infections. Those at increased risk of developing puerperal fever are women with compromised immunity, women who are anemic, and women who endure a long labor.

In developing nations, childbirth-related fatalities remain a considerable threat to women, with 95 percent of maternal deaths occurring in Africa and Asia. In developing countries, around 1 in 16 births are fatal compared to 1 in 2,800 among developed countries. The exact causes of these deaths are often not determined, but puerperal fever is often a significant contributing factor. This substantial risk is due to a lack of healthcare training and facilities, which increases the risk of patients developing puerperal fever. Poor health care facilities also reduce the chances that the infection will be effectively treated.

■ Treatment and Prevention

During periods when puerperal fever was epidemic, the rapid onset of infection, the ease of transmission between patients, and the lack of knowledge regarding causation made both treatment and prevention impossible. Until the causative agent and mode of transmission could be understood, puerperal fever remained an almost certain threat among maternity wards.

The discovery by Oliver Wendell Holmes and Ignaz Semmelweis that medical birthing attendants were responsible for transmitting infection between patients was revolutionary in the fight against puerperal fever. Due to these realizations, practices were established to ensure physicians did not spread the infection. These practices included changing clothing between births, washing of hands with chlorinated solutions before and after attending to patients, and sterilizing implements used during childbirth. These practices are still followed as a defense against childbirth infections.

Once it was established that puerperal fever was a result of infection by *Streptococcus* bacteria, treatment of infection also became possible. The use of intravenous antibiotic regimes from the onset of labor through to delivery, especially in prolonged and complicated labors, can effectively treat mothers at risk for puerperal fever.

■ Impacts and Issues

Although the impacts of puerperal fever have been diminished in the developed world since physicians gained an appreciation of the nature of the disease, it remains a significant threat to expecting mothers in developing nations.

One of the main issues of this disease is that the *Streptococcus* bacteria responsible for causing infection are part of the normal flora of the skin, nose, throat, and vagina. This means that potentially every woman is at risk of developing infection during or following childbirth even in the absence of an outside reservoir of the contagion. In developed countries, problematic births are often predicted prior to the event and physicians can take a suitable course of action to prevent

IN CONTEXT: BIRTHS ATTENDED BY SKILLED HEALTH PERSONNEL

The list below reflects data from countries reporting that less than half (50%) of all births are attended by skilled health personnel as reported by the World Health Organization in February 2007. Data was not available or published for all countries, including Sudan and Congo.

- Ethiopia: 5.6 % (2000)
- Nepal: 10.9 % (2001)
- Bangladesh: 13.4 % (2004)
- Afghanistan: 14 % (2003)
- Chad: 14.4 % (2004)
- Niger: 15.7 % (2000)
- Lao People's Democratic Republic: 19.4 % (2001)
- Yemen: 21.6 % (1997)
- Pakistan: 23 % (2001-02)
- Timor-Leste: 23.6 % (2002)
- Bhutan: 23.7 % (2000)
- Haiti: 23.8 % (2000)
- Burundi: 25.2 % (2000)
- Eritrea: 28.3 % (2002)
- Rwanda: 31.3 % (2000)
- Cambodia: 31.8 % (2000)
- Somalia: 34.2 % (1999)
- Guinea-Bissau: 34.7 % (2000)
- Guinea: 34.8 % (1999)
- Nigeria: 35.2 % (2003)
- Uganda: 39 % (2000)
- Mali: 40.6 % (2001)
- Guatemala: 41.4 % (2002)
- Kenya: 41.6 % (2003)
- Sierra Leone: 41.7 % (2000)
- India: 42.5 % (2000)
- Zambia: 43.4 % (2001-02)
- Central African Republic: 44 % (2000)
- United Republic of Tanzania: 46.3 % (2004-05)
- Angola: 47.1 % (2000)
- Ghana: 47.1 % (2003)
- Mozambique: 47.7 % (2003)
- Togo: 48.6 % (2000)

SOURCE: *World Health Organization, WHO Database on Skilled Attendant at Delivery. World Health Organization (http://www.who.int/reproductive-health/global_monitoring/data.html).*

further complications associated with such infections. Such measures are not available to the majority of women in developing nations.

There is also a lack of healthcare training among developing countries, including medical personnel who do not entirely understand the mechanisms of disease. This can lead to medical personnel passing the infection from patient to patient. This makes it more likely for women in developing nations to develop puerperal fever, while reduced health care resources also makes it more likely that the infection will be fatal.

Further issues exist for the children born from maternally fatal deliveries as they are often instantly subject to disadvantage. Until they reach a certain age, they are unable to contribute to labor and productivity but remain a strain on essential resources such as food and water. The society may view them as a liability rather than a member of the community, which results in significant social impact.

At the United Nations Millennium Summit in 2000, world leaders established a set of goals to combat certain sources of poverty, illness, illiteracy, hunger, and environmental problems. These goals are commonly referred to as the U.N. Millennium Goals. One of the primary development and health goals is to reduce the maternal mortality ratio by 75 percent by 2015. Worldwide, maternal mortality is highest among poor and rural women in developing nations.

While noticeable improvements in the maternal mortality ratio have occurred since the inception of the Millennium Development Goals in 2000, maternal mortality remains high in the regions where women are most likely to die from childbearing, especially sub-Saharan Africa and Southern Asia. Puerperal sepsis continues to be a significant problem. Researchers and health care providers found that women who had a skilled attendant during childbirth—along with access to emergency care if needed—were less likely to die or suffer debilitating complications. Overall, only 56% of women in developing regions have a skilled health care attendant during childbirth. In sub-Saharan Africa, only 36% of women have a skilled attendant assist their birth, compared to 88 percent of women in Latin America.

SEE ALSO *Bacterial Disease; Contact Precautions; Disinfection; Handwashing; Sterilization.*

BIBLIOGRAPHY

Books

Mandell, G. L., J. E. Bennett, and R. Dolin. *Principles and Practice of Infectious Diseases, Volume 2.* Philadelphia, PA: Elsevier, 2005.

Mims, C., H. Dockrell, R. Goering, I. Roitt, D. Wakelin, and M. Zuckerman. *Medical Microbiology.* St. Louis, MO: Mosby, 2004.

Nuland, S. B. *The Doctors' Plague: Germs, Childbed Fever, and the Strange Story of Ignc Semmelweis.* New York: W. W. Norton & Company, 2004.

Web Sites

Internet Modern History Sourcebook. "Oliver Wendell Holmes: Contagiousness of Puerperal Fever, 1843." August, 1998 <http://www.fordham.edu/halsall/mod/1843holmes-fever.html> (accessed March 8, 2007).

World Health Organization (WHO). "Maternal Deaths Disproportionately High in Developing Countries." October 20, 2003 <http://www.who.int/mediacentre/news/releases/2003/pr77/en/index.html> (accessed March 8, 2007).

Q Fever

Introduction

Q fever is a disease of humans and some animals that is caused by a bacterium called *Coxiella burnetii*. The infection is a zoonosis—it is passed to humans by contact with infected animals that are not usually harmed by the organism. The animals typically affected are sheep, cattle, and goats. Q fever can occur and clear quickly (this type is called an acute infection), or can persist for a much longer time (this is called a chronic infection).

Disease History, Characteristics, and Transmission

Q fever was first described in Australia in 1935 by the physician Edward H. Derrick (1898–1976) in people working in an Australian slaughterhouse. At the time, the cause for the illnesses was unknown; hence the term Q, which was short for Query. In 1937, *C. burnetii* was isolated and identified. The following year, the same organism was isolated from ticks in Montana, leading researchers to suspect a tick-mediated animal-human connection. The U.S. researchers also showed that the microbe was a type of bacterium called a rickettsia. Rickettsia are important from the standpoint of infectious diseases. As an example, other rickettsia are responsible for the potentially serious diseases called Rocky Mountain spotted fever and trench fever.

C. burnetti is a gram-negative organism, meaning it has two membranes surrounding the inner contents of the cell. In addition, the bacterium requires a host cell in order to grow and divide. This is similar to viruses. However, unlike viruses, which are not considered to be alive, *C. burnetii* is living and can survive, but cannot grow and divide, when not in a host cell.

The bacteria can survive for a long time in the natural environment, as they are not easily killed by heat, dryness, and even chemical compounds that readily kill other bacteria. This makes it more likely that the bacteria will be spread to those who come into contact with them.

Q fever results from inhalation of the bacteria. Infections have been traced to the inhalation of bacteria dislodged into the air from dry hay or a dusty barnyard. Only a few living organisms need be inhaled to establish an infection. This route of infection is different from other rickettsial diseases, where the bacteria are transferred from animal to human by tick bites. People who are most at risk of acquiring Q fever are those who are around animals like goats, sheep, and cattle, since these animals can naturally harbor the bacterium. The bacteria can be present in the milk, urine, amniotic fluid, and feces of the animals. Also, bacteria can be present in amniotic fluid and the placenta, and so can be spread to people who help in the birth of animals. Veterinarians, processing plant workers, and livestock farmers are more susceptible to Q fever than the general population.

For reasons that are not clear, only about 50% of those people who inhale the bacteria display symptoms. The symptoms include a sudden and high fever, a flulike sickness, severe headache, nausea with vomiting, abdominal

---

WORDS TO KNOW

ACUTE: An acute infection is one of rapid onset and of short duration, which either resolves or becomes chronic.

GRAM-NEGATIVE BACTERIA: All types of bacteria identified and classified as a group that does not retain crystal-violet dye during Gram's method of staining.

ZOONOSES: Zoonoses are diseases of microbiological origin that can be transmitted from animals to people. The causes of the diseases can be bacteria, viruses, parasites, and fungi.

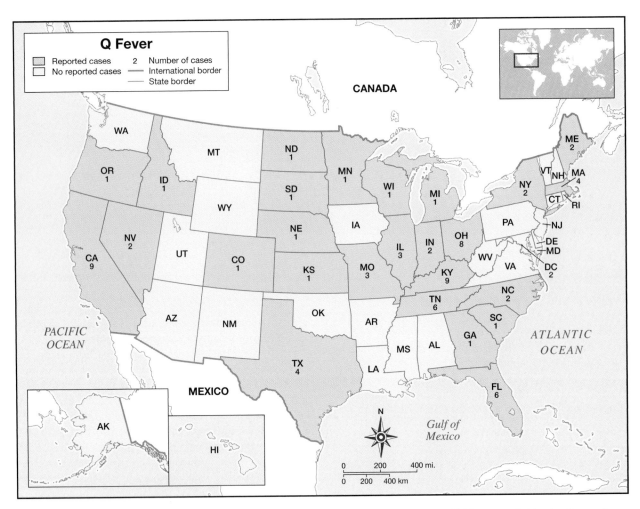

Map showing the number of reported cases of Q fever in the United States and U.S. territories in 2003, as recorded by the Centers for Disease Control and Prevention (CDC). *Data courtesy of Centers for Disease Control.*

pain, and a general feeling of being unwell. People can lose weight during their illness, which can take some time to regain following their recovery. Only 1–2% of those with the milder form of Q fever die of the illness.

A serious lung infection (pneumonia) can develop in 30–50% of people with Q fever. Liver damage including hepatitis can also occur. These symptoms usually ease in several months. However, a more persistent form of Q fever can develop, resulting in debilitating damage to heart valves due to the longer-lasting infection that kills up to 60% of those who acquire the chronic infection.

There are two different forms of *C. burnetii* that differ in the types of molecules present on the outer surfaces of their cells. The two forms have been designated phase I and phase II. The phase I form is associated with the chronic form of Q fever.

The short-term form of Q fever does not always immediately lead to the longer form; indeed, the chronic form of Q fever can develop in the absence of the milder form of the

disease. The time lag between the short-term and chronic forms of Q fever can be as long as several decades.

■ Scope and Distribution

The bacterium responsible for Q fever occurs worldwide. Countries such as Australia and the United States with a heavier emphasis on livestock agriculture, or which have a greater prevalence of animals that naturally harbor the bacterium, have a higher occurrence of the disease.

■ Treatment and Prevention

Diagnosis of Q fever most typically involves the detection of antibodies to *C. burnetii* or genetic material from the bacterium. Growing the organism is difficult, so detection of the bacterium itself is not typically accomplished. Following diagnosis, treatment consists of antibiotic therapy.

Typically, this is effective, although the therapy will be necessary for years when the infection is chronic. Heart valve damage can require replacement of the defective tissue.

A vaccine for Q fever exists. As of 2007, it is available in Australia and parts of Europe, but is not yet widely available in North America. Beginning in 2001, people at risk in Australia could be vaccinated. North Americans identified at higher risk of Q fever can also now be vaccinated. Similarly, a vaccine for animals exists, but is not yet in widespread use in North America.

Prevention of the transmission of the bacterium to humans involves wearing masks when around domestic livestock and the prompt disposal of the placenta and other tissues resulting from the birth process.

■ Impacts and Issues

Q fever can be a potentially serious disease because it can be spread from animals to people. In the United States, cases of the illness have been required to be reported to the Centers for Disease Control and Prevention since 1999. Imported livestock are also monitored for the presence of the bacterium, since transfer to other domestic animals could occur unknowingly in the absence of development of any symptoms in these hosts.

Why only about 50% of infected people display symptoms of infection is still unclear, but is important to learn if vaccines are to be fully protective. Research is underway to try and distinguish factors associated with people, the bacterium, or both that help some people ward off the consequences of infection. Additionally, it is not clear why Q fever does not persist for a long time in some people, but becomes a chronic, destructive, and potentially life-threatening condition in others.

SEE ALSO *Animal Importation; Bioterrorism; Opportunistic Infection; Zoonoses.*

BIBLIOGRAPHY

Books

Tierno, Philip M. *The Secret Life of Germs: What They Are, Why We Need Them, and How We Can Protect Ourselves Against Them.* New York: Atria, 2004.

Periodicals

Anderson, Alicia D. "Q Fever and the U.S. Military." *Emerging Infectious Diseases.* 11:1320–1323 (2005).

Web Sites

Centers for Disease Control and Prevention. "Q Fever." <http://www.cdc.gov/ncidod/dvrd/qfever/index.htm> (accessed May 1, 2007).

Brian Hoyle

IN CONTEXT: SOCIAL AND PERSONAL RESPONSIBILITY

The Division of Viral and Rickettsial Diseases at the Centers for Disease Control and Prevention (CDC) states that the following measures should be used in the prevention and control of Q fever:

- Educate the public on sources of infection.
- Appropriately dispose of placenta, birth products, fetal membranes, and aborted fetuses at facilities housing sheep and goats.
- Restrict access to barns and laboratories used in housing potentially infected animals.
- Use only pasteurized milk and milk products.
- Use appropriate procedures for bagging, autoclaving, and washing of laboratory clothing.
- Vaccinate (where possible) individuals engaged in research with pregnant sheep or live *C. burnetii*.
- Quarantine imported animals.
- Ensure that holding facilities for sheep should be located away from populated areas. Animals should be routinely tested for antibodies to *C. burnetii*, and measures should be implemented to prevent airflow to other occupied areas.
- Counsel persons at highest risk for developing chronic Q fever, especially persons with pre-existing cardiac valvular disease or individuals with vascular grafts.

SOURCE: *Centers for Disease Control and Prevention, National Center for Infectious Diseases, Division of Viral and Rickettsial Diseases*

Rabies

■ Introduction

Rabies, from the Latin word *rabies* for mad, has long been one of the most-feared of diseases. It was described by the Greek philosopher Aristotle (384–322 BC) who realized that humans could contract rabies through being bitten by infected dogs, which is still the most common way the disease is transmitted. Rabies claims the lives of around 55,000 people around the world each year, mainly in rural parts of Africa and Asia.

Rabies is an acute viral illness which affects the brain and nervous system. Left untreated, it is invariably fatal. The symptoms are dramatic, including seizures, hallucinations, foaming at the mouth, and violent throat spasms. Rabies is a zoonosis—a disease of animals which can affect humans. Wild mammals are the reservoir of the rabies virus and they can, in turn, affect domestic animals like cats and dogs. Humans usually become infected through a bite from a wild or domestic animal with rabies. Fortunately, an effective vaccine against rabies is available and this can be used either before or after exposure to the virus.

■ Disease History, Characteristics, and Transmission

The rabies virus belongs to the rhabdovirus group and is a bullet-shaped enveloped RNA virus (that is, its genetic material is RNA, rather than DNA). The incubation period of the virus is between ten days and as long as one year. Early symptoms are vague and may resemble flu—and include fatigue, headache and nausea.

Once the rabies virus reaches the brain and nervous system, dramatic neurological symptoms set in. These include hallucinations, agitation, muscle spasm, paralysis, and seizures. Foaming at the mouth is a classic symptom of rabies and is a combination of increased salivation and difficulty in swallowing. The latter produces another classic symptom—hydrophobia, or fear of water, where extreme throat spasms may be induced by even the sight of water. Sometimes rabies dominated by agitation is known as furious rabies, while that dominated by paralysis is called dumb rabies.

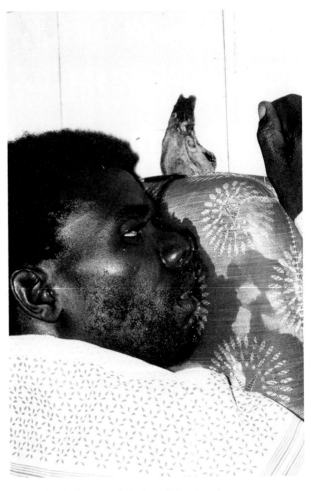

A man drools due to an infection of the virus that causes rabies. *Dr. M.A. Ansary/Photo Researchers, Inc.*

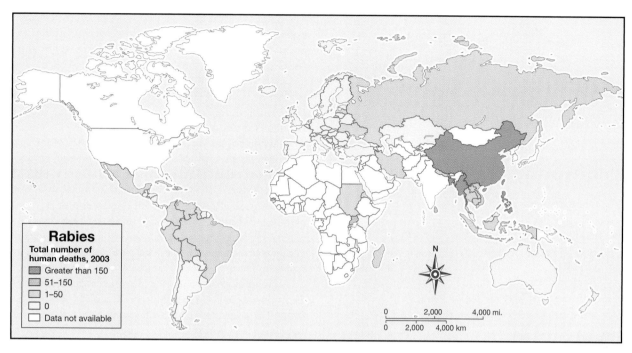

World map showing where human deaths due to rabies were reported, 2003. © *Copyright World Health Organization (WHO). Reproduced by permission.*

Within days of the onset of symptoms, a person with rabies will enter a coma and death is usually by paralysis of the respiratory muscles. Survival is extremely rare—there have been only six documented cases and all of these individuals had been protected to some extent by vaccination before or after exposure to the rabies virus.

The rabies virus eventually passes through the nervous system to the salivary glands and it is the saliva of an infected animal which transmits the disease to other animals and to humans. Exposure to the rabies virus usually occurs from a bite by an infected animal, although the virus might also sometimes be transmitted through a scratch or lick from the animal. Infections have also occurred through inhaling aerosols from the droppings of infected bats.

Wild carnivorous mammals, including skunks, foxes, wolves, jackals, raccoons and coyotes, act as a reservoir for rabies virus. The infection may be passed to domestic animals—that is, dogs and cats. Humans can be infected by direct contact with either wild or domestic mammals. The former is sometimes known as sylvatic rabies, the latter as urban rabies. An animal with rabies virus will not be infectious all the time—only when the virus is in their saliva which can happen late on in the incubation period, because it has to pass from the muscle, where infection occurs, through the nervous system to the salivary glands.

Insectivorous and vampire bats can also transmit rabies. Rodents, such as rats, mice, and hamsters, and lagomorphs, such as rabbits and hares, hardly ever get infected with rabies and have never been shown to transmit it to humans. However, woodchucks and groundhogs were responsible for 86 per cent of 368 cases of rabies among rodents reported to the Centers for Disease Control and Prevention (CDC) between 1985 and 1994. Other herbivorous mammals including cattle, horses, and deer can become infected with rabies but very rarely infect humans.

Human to human transmission of rabies is rare, but not unknown. There have been eight cases recorded among recipients of transplanted corneas and three in recipients of solid transplanted organs. In theory, bites could also transmit rabies from one person to another, although no such cases are known. Casual contact, such as touching or contact with non-infectious fluids, does not carry a risk of infection with rabies virus.

■ Scope and Distribution

Rabies is a global problem which has been recognized for at least 3,000 years. At the turn of the twentieth century, there were over one hundred cases of rabies in the United States each year. Now that number is fewer than five. The disease is notifiable to the CDC and states also collect data on cases. According to a survey carried out by the World Health Organization (WHO) in 2004, there are around 55,000 deaths from rabies each year worldwide, most of them in rural Africa and Asia. Around half of all

WORDS TO KNOW

INCUBATION PERIOD: Incubation period refers to the time between exposure to disease causing virus or bacteria and the appearance of symptoms of the infection. Depending on the microorganism, the incubation time can range from a few hours (an example is food poisoning due to *Salmonella*) to a decade or more (an example is acquired immunodeficiency syndrome, or AIDS).

NOTIFIABLE: By law, occurrences of some diseases must be reported to government authorities when observed by health-care professionals. Such diseases are called notifiable diseases or reportable diseases. Cholera and yellow fever are examples of notifiable diseases.

RESERVOIR: The animal or organism in which the virus or parasite normally resides.

SYLVATIC: Sylvatic means pertaining to the woods and refers to diseases such as plague that are spread by animals such as ground squirrels and other wild rodents.

ZOONOSES: Zoonoses are diseases of microbiological origin that can be transmitted from animals to people. The causes of the diseases can be bacteria, viruses, parasites, and fungi.

cases of rabies from dog bites occur among children under the age of 15.

There is marked geographical variation in the mammal species that pose a threat of rabies. In the United States, sylvatic rabies accounts for most cases and urban rabies is rare; the reverse is true in developing countries. Bats are the most common reservoirs of the disease in Latin America and the wolf in Eastern Europe.

■ Treatment and Prevention

There is no specific treatment for rabies once the symptoms have begun. A rabies vaccine was first developed by Louis Pasteur in the late 1880s. This was a crude preparation made from the dried spinal cord of infected rabbit. Similar vaccines are still in use in some countries, although WHO does not recommend them. Rabies vaccines made in cell culture are preferred for safety reasons.

Rabies vaccine can be given either before or after exposure to the virus. Pre-exposure vaccine should be given where a person's occupation brings them into contact with wild animals or with the virus itself—for instance, veterinarians, animal handlers, and certain laboratory workers. Travelers to regions where rabies is common and children living in these countries should also be vaccinated.

Post-exposure vaccination is needed if someone has been potentially exposed to rabies virus through an animal bite or other contact. Each year, over one million Americans receive an animal bite and these must always be taken seriously. But only a few of these will pose any risk of rabies infection, so each case must be carefully evaluated. An important part of this is having an expert examine the animal involved for symptoms and signs of rabies.

Vaccination of domestic animals against rabies plays an important role in keeping the disease at bay. Some European countries, such as France, Switzerland, and Belgium, have eliminated rabies in their wildlife through vaccination campaigns, and this is being tried in places where the disease is more common such as India and South Africa.

■ Impacts and Issues

In 2004, WHO was informed of a case of rabies in a dog owned by a resident of the city of Bordeaux, in France. Many people had handled this dog over a five-week period when the animal was potentially infectious. WHO had to put out a call for these individual to come forward for assessment and possible post-exposure vaccination. The dog had been imported illegally from Morocco and had not been vaccinated against rabies.

This incident shows the importance of taking animal import and quarantine regulations seriously. By flouting these on entry to France, the dog's owner put many people's lives at risk. Responsible owners get their pets vaccinated against rabies. And, when it comes to wildlife, it is best to admire from afar and never to handle or touch an animal that you do not know.

Wisconsin teenager Jeanna Giese became the first person known to have survived symptomatic rabies without vaccination. In September 2004, Giese contracted rabies after being bitten on the finger by a bat. One month after the bite, she was admitted to the hospital. Rabies was considered always fatal in unvaccinated patients, but physicians and Giese's family chose an experimental treatment. Physicians put Giese into a drug-induced coma for a week, at the same time giving her several strong antiviral drugs (amantadine and ribavirin). Giese's immune system fought the infection. She returned to school the following academic year after several months of recovery and intense physical therapy. Physicians and medical researchers continue to debate whether Giese survived because of the experimental treatment, or whether other factors, such as a stronger-than-average immune system or a weaker-than-average strain of rabies, played a larger role.

Following the Giese case, there was an increased focus on bats as potentials vectors of disease. Though bats are beneficial in controlling mosquito and insect populations, researchers estimate that 1% of bats in the United States carry rabies. Bats rarely bite humans and cause only minor injury at the location of the bite. It is possible for bites on sleeping victims to go undetected. In August 2006, over 1,000 young girls were advised to obtain rabies vaccinations after attending a Girl Scout camp where bats were present in sleeping quarters. Not all of families opted for vaccination, but none of the girls have developed rabies.

Cases of rabies are increasing, even in developed urban environment. In 2006, the Chinese government passed a law that forbid dogs in many in public places and limited dog ownership to one animal per household. Rabies is endemic in China, and is one of the nation's leading causes of death from infectious disease. However, officials cited the popularization of pet ownership and the failure of many pet owners to vaccinate dogs as primary causes for the resurgence of rabies, especially in the nation's cities.

SEE ALSO *Animal Importation; Zoonoses.*

BIBLIOGRAPHY

Books

Wilson, Walter R. and Merle A. Sande. *Current Diagnosis & Treatment in Infectious Diseases.* New York: McGraw Hill, 2001.

Web Sites

Center for Diseases Control and Prevention (CDC) National Center for Infectious Diseases. "Rabies." January 7, 2005 <http://www.cdc.gov/ncidod/dvrd/rabies> (accessed Apr 19, 2007).

World Health Organization. "Rabies." <http://www.who.int/mediacentre/factsheets/fs099/en> (accessed April 19, 2007).

Susan Aldridge

LOUIS PASTEUR AND THE RABIES VACCINE

By 1880 French scientist Louis Pasteur (1822–1895) had shown that vaccination against anthrax worked in animals. He used a weakened, or attenuated, form of a culture of the anthrax bacterium as the vaccine and found it protected animals against the disease, compared to control animals that had not been vaccinated. In 1880, he decided to turn his attention to rabies a feared disease with a high mortality rate. Pasteur showed that a vaccine made from an attenuated form of the rabies virus could protect dogs that had been bitten by rabid animals. He hesitated, however, before trying his vaccine on humans.

Pasteur's first human patient was a young boy called Joseph Meister who was brought to him from Alsace on July 6, 1885. Joseph had been bitten fourteen times by a rabid dog on his hands, legs, and thighs. Clearly, his life was in danger and Pasteur administered the first dose of vaccine the next day. He used the dried-out spinal cord from a rabid rabbit as the source of vaccine. The drying process allowed the virus to lose much of its virulent character and helped allay safety fears. The boy was given increasingly strong doses of vaccine over the next twelve days and was soon able to return to Alsace in good health, having developed no symptoms of rabies, nor any ill effects from the vaccination.

The development of an effective rabies vaccine was the final, and most dramatic, success of Pasteur's long and distinguished career in medicine, chemistry, and microbiology. Pasteur's work on rabies led to the establishment of the now world-famous Pasteur Institute in Paris. The Institute was funded through public contributions and was initially devoted to rabies vaccination. Since its launch in 1888, the Institute has been home to many distinguished scientists, including several Nobel Prize winners.

Rapid Diagnostic Tests for Infectious Diseases

■ Introduction

Before the era of molecular biology, determination of the identity of the cause of an infectious disease—the process of diagnosis—involved the observation of the symptoms of the disease, the culturing (growing and identifying) of the responsible bacteria, virus, or protozoa (which still is not always possible or may require a long time), and the results of a variety of biochemical tests. Diagnosis typically took days or weeks.

Beginning in the 1970s, the ability to detect target regions of bacterial and viral deoxyribonucleic acid (DNA) or ribonucleic acid (RNA) has made it possible to both demonstrate the presence of microorganisms in blood, urine, and tissue samples from an infected person, and now to identify the microorganism even to the species level. Some of these molecular-based tests can be done in minutes.

Other rapid diagnostic tests are based on the presence of an antibody that is produced by the human immune system in response to the presence of a certain bacterial or viral component, usually a protein, that is generically termed an antigen. These immunotests are based on the detection of the binding of the sample antigen to the antibody.

■ History and Scientific Foundations

Rapid molecular tests rely on the detection of target regions of the microbial genetic material. Once the genetic sequence—the arrangement of the building blocks (nucleotides) of the DNA or RNA—of a variety of important microbial pathogens has been determined, target regions that are unique to a given organism or a gene that codes for the presence of an important disease-causing contributor such as a toxin can be identified. The detection of these target regions can be proof of the presence of the microbe even in the absence of the actual isolation of the organism. Furthermore, compar-ison of the genetic sequence with sequences that have been saved in databases can identify the genus and some-times even the species of the infecting microorganism.

The target genetic region may only be present in low quantities. A technique called polymerase chain reaction (PCR)—which was developed in the 1980s and which earned its discoverer, Kary Mullis, the 1993 Nobel Prize in Chemistry—enables the amplification of bits of DNA. Because each PCR cycle doubles the amount of the genetic material and because cycles can be done quickly (sometimes in minutes), literally billions of copies of the target DNA can be made in a few hours.

Immuno-based tests rely on the binding of a particular sample antigen to its corresponding antibody that is bound to a support such as a paper strip. Antigen-antibody bind-ing is a specific reaction. Other antigens in a sample will not bind to the bound antibody unless they are almost identical both in the arrangement of amino acids that makes up the protein but in the three-dimensional shape adopted by the protein molecules in solution. As well, commercially available immunostrips contain controls that verify that the observed antigen-antibody binding, which is detected by the development of a color, is not a mistake.

■ Applications and Research

Rapid diagnostic tests have become popular in the diag-nosis of infectious diseases. Since the 1980s, various antigen-antibody binding tests have been available for the examination of fluid specimens that include whole blood, the serum, and plasma components of blood, saliva, urine, and even fluid recovered from tissues.

The various tests, which can be capable of detecting as little as one nanogram of an antigen in the sample, include hepatitis B, human immunodeficiency virus (HIV), malaria (based on detection of an antigen of the malaria-causing microbe, *Plasmodium falciparum*), syphilis (based on detection of a *Treponema pallidum* antigen), *Streptococcus* (a common cause of a throat

WORDS TO KNOW

ANTIBODY: Antibodies, or Y-shaped immunoglobulins, are proteins found in the blood that help to fight against foreign substances called antigens. Antigens, which are usually proteins or polysaccharides, stimulate the immune system to produce antibodies. The antibodies inactivate the antigen and help to remove it from the body. While antigens can be the source of infections from pathogenic bacteria and viruses, organic molecules detrimental to the body from internal or environmental sources also act as antigens. Genetic engineering and the use of various mutational mechanisms allow the construction of a vast array of antibodies (each with a unique genetic sequence).

ANTIBODY-ANTIGEN BINDING: Antibodies are produced by the immune system in response to antigens (material perceived as foreign). The antibody response to a particular antigen is highly specific and often involves a physical association between the two molecules. Biochemical and molecular forces govern this association.

ANTIGEN: Antigens, which are usually proteins or polysaccharides, stimulate the immune system to produce antibodies. The antibodies inactivate the antigen and help to remove it from the body. While antigens can be the source of infections from pathogenic bacteria and viruses, organic molecules detrimental to the body from internal or environmental sources also act as antigens. Genetic engineering and the use of various mutational mechanisms allow the construction of a vast array of antibodies (each with a unique genetic sequence).

CULTURE: A culture is a single species of microorganism that is isolated and grown under controlled conditions. The German bacteriologist Robert Koch first developed culturing techniques in the late 1870s. Following Koch's initial discovery, medical scientists quickly sought to identify other pathogens. Today bacteria cultures are used as basic tools in microbiology and medicine.

IMMUNO-BASED TEST: An immuno-based test is a medical technology that tests for the presence of a disease by looking for reaction between disease organisms that may be present in a tissue or fluid sample and antibodies contained in the test kit.

PCR (POLYMERASE CHAIN REACTION): The Polymerase Chain Reaction, or PCR, refers to a widely used technique in molecular biology involving the amplification of specific sequences of genomic DNA.

infection known as "strep throat"), urinary tract infections (based on the enhanced production of several enzymes during an infection), and influenza.

The rapid detection of influenza is noteworthy since influenza viruses are characterized by their changing outer surface, and so their antigenic composition, from year to year. The rapid test targets a viral component that has proven to be more stable over time.

Research continues to refine the molecular and immuno-based rapid diagnostic tests, both in terms of their accuracy and the spectrum of microbial diseases that can be detected. For example, research published in 2006 reported on a PCR-based system that allows different types of hemorrhagic fevers to be distinguished. Since speed is vital is the treatment of people suffering from hemorrhagic diseases such as Ebola, this advance will help increase the survival rate of this traditionally lethal suite of diseases.

■ Impacts and Issues

Being able to rapidly diagnose infectious diseases can help initiate treatment faster, which can be key in com-

bating a swiftly spreading infection. Furthermore, for diseases such as influenza that are caused by a virus, a rapid diagnosis curtails the misuse of antibiotics, which are useless against viral infections but which can stimulate the development of antibiotic resistance in resident bacteria. Such antibiotic misuse has been a key factor in the development of bacterial antibiotic resistance, which is increasingly making diseases such as tuberculosis more difficult and expensive to treat.

Molecular techniques require specialized (and expensive) equipment and trained personnel. This can be a limitation for smaller clinics in developed countries and can be completely impractical for rural clinics in developing and underdeveloped countries. Immuno-based tests are less expensive, the test strips are easier to transport and store as refrigeration is usually not required, and the results are clear and do not require interpretation.

The use of immuno-based strip tests has brought rapid diagnostic testing to rural clinics in underdeveloped and developed regions. Staff at these clinics can be easily trained to carry out and interpret the test results. The tests are also useful to field staff of agencies

IN CONTEXT: TERRORISM AND BIOLOGICAL WARFARE

The Advanced Diagnostics Program is funded by the Defense Advanced Research Projects Agency of the United States government (DARPA). Its objective is to develop tools and medicines to detect and treat biological and chemical weapons in the field at concentrations low enough to prevent illness. Challenges to this task include minimizing the labor, equipment, and time for identifying biological agents. One area of interest includes development of field tools that can identify many different agents. To accomplish this goal, several groups funded under the advanced diagnostics program have developed field-based biosensors that can detect a variety of analytes including fragments of DNA, various hormones and proteins, bacteria, salts, and antibodies. These biosensors are portable, run on external power sources, and require very little time to complete analyses.

A second focus of the advanced diagnostics project is the identification of known and unknown or bioengineered pathogens and development of early responses to infections. A final goal is to develop the ability to continuously monitor the body for evidence of infection. Researchers are addressing this goal in two ways. The first involves engineering monitoring mechanisms that are internal to the body. In particular, groups funded under the initiative are developing bioengineered white blood cells to detect infection from within the body. Often genetic responses to infection occur within minutes of infection so analysis of blood cells provides a very quick indication of the presence of a biological threat. The second method involves the development of a wearable, non-invasive diagnostic device that detects a broad-spectrum of biological and chemical agents.

including the World Health Organization and the United States Centers for Disease Control and Prevention, which respond to illness outbreaks. The rapid detection of a disease and its geographical scope can be vital in combating an outbreak.

Rapid diagnostic tests are also being increasingly used to detect microbial contamination of food and water, especially since the deliberate release of anthrax-laden letters in the autumn of 2001 in the United States. The realization that the nation's food and drinking water supplies are vulnerable to malicious contamination has spurred efforts to establish safeguards.

SEE ALSO *Food-borne Disease and Food Safety.*

BIBLIOGRAPHY

Books

Brunelle, Lynn, and Barbara Ravage. *Bacteria.* Milwaukee, WI: Gareth Stevens Publishing, 2003.

DeGregori, Thomas R. *Bountiful Harvest: Technology, Food Safety, and the Environment.* Washington, DC: Cato Institute, 2002.

Periodicals

Greenwald, Jeffrey L., Gale R. Burstein, Jonathan Pincus, and Richard Branson. "A Rapid Review of Rapid HIV Antibody Tests." *Current Infectious Disease Reports* 8 (2006): 125–131.

Palacios, Gustavo, et al. "Masstag Polymerase Chain Reaction for Differential Diagnosis of Viral Hemorrhagic Fevers." *Emerging Infectious Diseases* 12 (2006): 692–695.

Brian Hoyle

Rat-bite Fever

Introduction

Rat-bite fever (RBF) is an acute infectious disease in humans caused by the scratch or bite of rodents, mostly rats, infected with one of two bacteria, *Streptobacillus moniliformis* or *Spirillum minus*. It is not transmitted from person to person. Scratches and bites are not necessarily the only way to contract the infection. Both bacteria are also able to be passed from rodents to humans through urine or mucous secretions from the eyes or nose of infected rats.

Rat-bite fever occurs most often among biomedical laboratory technicians, pet store employees who handle rodents, and people who have rodents as pets. It also occurs among people who live in rat-infested conditions. Children are more likely to be infected, both from their time spent inside and outdoors. Other animals that can carry the infectious bacteria are cats, dogs, gerbils, mice, squirrels, and weasels. The disease is also known as Haverhill fever and epidemic arthritic erythema (redness).

Disease History, Characteristics, and Transmission

Symptoms from the bacteria *Streptobacillus moniliformis* begin two to 22 days (usually within 10 days) after an initial bite or scratch. The infection can also be acquired by drinking contaminated milk or water (this form of the disease is sometimes referred to as Haverhill fever).

Symptoms are similar to severe influenza (flu), with a moderate fever (101–104°F [38.3–40.0°C]), chills, nausea, vomiting, headache, joint and back pain, gastrointestinal problems, and a reddish-pink rash (usually erupting about three days after initial contact with the bacteria) made of tiny bumps located generally on the palms of the hands and the soles of the feet.

Infections from the bacterium *Spirillum minus* are more common than infections with the other bacterium that causes rat-bite fever. With this bacterium, the infection is called spirillary rat-bite fever, or is sometimes known as sodoku. Symptoms do not begin until four to 28 days (usually less than 10 days) after exposure, and after the wound made by the bite or scratch has already healed. After the wound appears to initially heal, it suddenly becomes swollen and chronically inflamed.

Symptoms include fever, chills, and headache. The fever lasts longer than with *Streptobacillus moniliformis*, and may also reoccur over a period of months. Gastrointestinal symptoms are less severe than with the Haverhill-type fever. The rash is a light rosy color, causes itching, and covers most or all of the body. Joint and muscle pain does not usually occur or, if it does, it is much less severe than with the Haverhill-type fever.

WORDS TO KNOW

ABSCESS: An abscess is a pus-filled sore, usually caused by a bacterial infection. It results from the body's defensive reaction to foreign material. Abscesses are often found in the soft tissue under the skin, such as the armpit or the groin. However, they may develop in any organ, and they are commonly found in the breast and gums. Abscesses are far more serious and call for more specific treatment if they are located in deep organs such as the lung, liver, or brain.

ERYTHEMA: Erythema is skin redness due to excess blood in capillaries (small blood vessels) in the skin.

SEPTIC: The term "septic" refers to the state of being infected with bacteria, particularly in the bloodstream

■ Scope and Distribution

The infection caused by the bacterium *Streptobacillus moniliformis* has been found in the past to occur in the United States. With this bacterium, the infection is commonly called streptobacillary rat-bite fever. According to the Division of Bacterial and Mycotic Diseases, of the U.S. Centers for Disease Control and Prevention (CDC), it is rarely reported in the United States today and, consequently, accurate statistics on the incidence of the disease are not known.

The infection caused by the bacterium *Spirillum minus* is usually found in Asia and Africa, and its prevalence is much more common.

■ Treatment and Prevention

The bacterium *Streptobacillus moniliformis* is identified by a culture of blood or fluid that is taken from one of the affected joints of the infected human. The culture is then analyzed in a laboratory.

Antibiotics including procaine penicillin G or penicillin V by mouth (orally) are the most common treatments for streptobacillary rat-bite fever. If the patient is allergic to penicillin, erythromycin can be provided orally. Treatment is usually successful, although the infection can be sometimes eliminated by the human body itself, given sufficient time. However, if left untreated and when the body is unable to eliminate the disease, it can develop into serious complications such as septic (infectious) arthritis, abscesses (infections) to any tissue or organ of the body, endocarditis (inflammation of the heart's lining); meningitis (inflammation of the lining surrounding the brain and spine); and pneumonia (inflammation of the lungs). Without treatment, death can result from complications about 13% of the time.

The disease caused by the bacterium *Spirillum minus* is identified by examining blood or tissue removed from the wound of the infected human. Spirillary rat-bite fever is usually treated with procaine penicillin G or penicillin V by mouth. If the patient is allergic to penicillin, tetracycline can be given orally. If it is not treated, the fever usually subsides, but returns again in cycles of two to four days, which can continue for up for one year. In most circumstances, the illness, even without treatment, will resolve itself within four to eight weeks.

With both forms of rat-bite fever, the CDC Division of Bacterial and Mycotic Diseases recommends that humans avoid contact with animals capable of passing on the bacterial organisms. If contact cannot be avoided with rodents, recommendations include wearing gloves, regularly washing hands, and avoiding hand-to-mouth contact while handling rodents and cleaning their cages. With streptobacillary rat-bite fever, drinking only pasteurized milk and water from safe sources can help prevent the disease.

■ Impacts and Issues

Rat-bite fever and other types of rodent infestations contribute greatly to the decline of already poor communities. Rodents cause extensive losses of food and destruction of property when they are present in large numbers. They can cause damage and loss of revenue to grocery stores, warehouses, cargo carriers, and homes. Rodents can also cause loss of property due to fires from the gnawing of electrical wiring.

Sometimes rodents are controlled improperly with poisons, which exaggerates the problems already present. Health and safety problems can occur, especially among children, domesticated animals and pets, and the environment with improper poison use.

Along with rat-bite fever, large populations of rats within communities can increase the chance of contracting diseases such as hantavirus, leptospirosis (also called Weil's disease, canicola fever, and 7-day fever), plague, salmonella, and typhoid. These diseases can be potentially deadly, especially among the young and elderly.

SEE ALSO *Bacterial Disease; Vector-borne Disease; Zoonoses.*

BIBLIOGRAPHY

Books

Committee on Infectious Diseases of Mice and Rats, Institute of Laboratory Animal Resources, Commission on Life Sciences, National Research Council. *Infectious Diseases of Mice and Rats.* Washington, DC: National Academy of Sciences, 1991.

Richardson, V.C.G. *Diseases of Small Domestic Rodents.* Oxford, UK, and Malden, MA: Blackwell Publishing, 2003.

Periodicals

Elliott, S.P. "Rat Bite Fever and *Streptobacillus moniliformis.*" *Clinical Microbiology Reviews.* January 1, 2007: 20 (1): 13–22.

Web Sites

Centers for Disease Control and Prevention. "Rat-bite Fever." October 26, 2006 <http://www.cdc.gov/ncidod/dbmd/diseaseinfo/ratbitefever_g.htm#whatisrbf> (accessed March 18, 2007).

Re-emerging Infectious Diseases

■ Introduction

In the mid-twentieth century, the development of highly effective antibiotics and implementation of successful disease prevention and global vaccination programs led to the control or eradication of serious diseases such as polio and smallpox. At the time, it was widely assumed that infectious disease would ultimately become a minor problem. However, both newly emergent and re-emergent infectious diseases now present a growing public health threat worldwide.

According to the World Health Organization (WHO), infectious and parasitic diseases constitute the second most lethal cause of mortality (death) globally after cardiovascular diseases, implicated in 26% of deaths in 2002. Re-emergent infections have gained renewed virulence (the degree to which an organism can cause disease) due to other emerging or chronic diseases that impair the immune system (e.g., HIV/AIDS, diabetes, cancer) or the spread of antibiotic, antiviral, and anti-fungal medication resistance. In addition, there is the threat of re-emergent infectious disease that is intentionally spread in connection with bioterrorism, as occurred in the United States in the anthrax attacks of 2001. Although the numbers of people infected and killed were small in these attacks, the potential for widespread

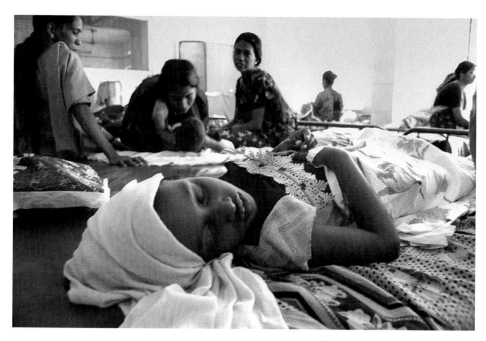

A child with chikungunya symptoms sleeps at a government medical center in southern India in October 2006. During an outbreak, Indian Health Minister Ambumani Ramadoss maintained that there had been no deaths due to the viral infection in the country. However, the Kerala government claimed 86 people had died due to the infections, according to a news agency. *AP Images.*

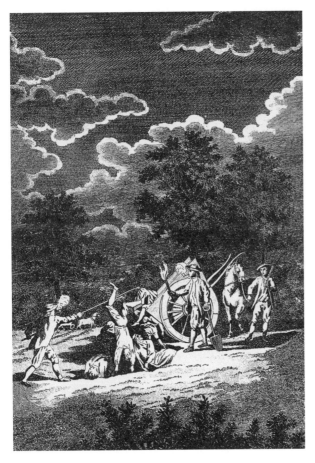

In London, workers bury the victims of the plague at night in mass graves in 1665. Two of the workers are smoking pipes, partly to combat the stench of the corpses, and partly in the hope that tobacco smoke will prevent them from becoming infected. *HIP/Art Resource, NY.*

targeted assaults make the use of bioterrorism agents especially disturbing to consider.

■ History and Scientific Foundations

In the United States, the National Institute of Allergy and Infectious Diseases (NIAID) and the Centers for Disease Control and Prevention (CDC) have expanded research funding, information sharing, and clinical support to fight emerging and re-emerging infectious disease. Focusing on re-emerging diseases, the CDC journals *Emerging Infectious Disease* and the *Morbidity and Mortality Weekly Report (MMWR)* now feature frequent reports of re-emergent infections such as coccidioidomycosis, the incidence of which began to dramatically increase as a consequence of the HIV/AIDS pandemic.

In the past decade, epidemiologists have confronted the re-emergence of West Nile fever, human monkey-

pox, dengue, tuberculosis, and malaria, at times in populations for which these diseases had not previously been a problem. Furthermore, certain infections such as *Staphylococcus aureus* and *Mycobacterium tuberculosis* have developed increasing resistance to drug agents that were previously effective treatments.

Malaria

The resurgence of the ancient plague of malaria, due to rising rates of resistance to chloroquine and other drugs, currently affects more than 300 million people and results in the deaths of more than one million victims worldwide each year, the majority occurring among children in sub-Saharan Africa. Recently, epidemiologists have discovered a connection between resurgent malaria and the HIV/AIDS epidemic.

According to a study sponsored by the Millennium Fund, HIV has major effects on the incidence of malaria. HIV-induced immunodeficiency may decrease the immune response against malarial infection and the risk of parasitemia, and illness with malaria has been inversely correlated to CD4 cell counts, which are adversely affected by AIDS.

HIV infection in regions where malaria transmission is endemic (naturally occurring) mainly increases the risk of clinical malaria in adults and malarial fever in children. In regions in which malaria transmission is not yet endemic, high HIV prevalence results in considerably higher than expected malaria morbidity and mortality. Infection with HIV also affects the treatment and prophylaxis of malaria. Antimalarial therapy is most effective in individuals with some previous immunity to malaria, so immunosuppression due to HIV infection can decrease antimalarial treatment response.

The failure so far to develop an effective vaccine for malaria has sometimes been ascribed to the low prevalence of the disease among industrialized nations. However, the disease poses formidable scientific and technical hurdles to vaccine development, including issues regarding the appropriateness and accessibility of animal models. Other difficulties are due to the need to develop assays (analyses) for ongoing validation of candidate antigens through process development and scale-up production, as well as assays predictive of protection for assessment of immunogenicity (ability to provoke an immune response) and efficacy in clinical trials. Furthermore, the clinical trials themselves are difficult to design because the ultimate measure of efficacy is the interruption of malaria transmission. In spite of these challenges, pharmaceutical companies are currently beginning clinical development of a variety of vaccine candidates that show promise.

Tuberculosis

Another resurgent disease with connections to the HIV/AIDS epidemic is tuberculosis (TB), which according to the WHO is endemic to regions inhabited by one third of the world's population and results in some eight million new cases and two million deaths annually. Tuberculosis rates are extremely high among the HIV-infected population. The one currently available vaccine for tuberculosis offers some protection, but its effectiveness diminishes over time. Effective pharmaceutical treatment exists, but the treatment regimen is lengthy and it is difficult for patients to maintain adherence, which gives rise to multidrug-resistant TB strains. This in turn has added impetus to programs to develop novel vaccines, some of which are now in the pre-clinical investigation stage.

Although more than a billion people have dormant tuberculosis infections, the disease becomes symptomatic when immune systems are weakened by HIV. TB risk doubles shortly after infection with HIV, and increases further over time. A recent study estimates that 9% of the 8.3 million new adult TB cases worldwide in 2000 were directly attributable to HIV. Furthermore, HIV infection makes treating active TB much more difficult, leading to an increase in TB rates in high-HIV-prevalence areas, particularly sub-Saharan Africa. The spread of HIV in sub-Saharan Africa is primarily responsible for driving the number of active TB cases upward by 6% each year.

In 2005, a virulent strain of tuberculosis killed all but one of 53 infected patients at the Church of Scotland Hospital in South Africa's rural KwaZulu-Natal Province. The strain of TB, named XDR for "extensively drug-resistant," cannot be treated effectively with most tuberculosis drugs, and may be incurable.

Since the detection of XDR, more cases have been found at other South African hospitals. Some epidemiologists and TB experts argue that XDR TB has probably moved beyond the borders of South Africa into Lesotho, Swaziland, Mozambique, and perhaps to Zimbabwe. At least two in three South African TB sufferers are HIV-positive. If XDR TB becomes established in the HIV-positive population, it could devastate tens of millions of HIV-infected people throughout sub-Saharan Africa.

HIV-negative people have a low probability of contracting tuberculosis, even if they are already infected with the TB bacillus. However, since tuberculosis is spread through the air, people in close contact with an active TB victim have some risk of contracting the disease.

It seems likely that all of the 52 people who died in the initial outbreak of XDR-TB in the South African hamlet of Tugela Ferry in 2005 and early 2006 had AIDS. Most of the patients died within a few weeks of infection with drug-resistant tuberculosis, an unprecedented TB mortality rate according to epidemiologists.

WORDS TO KNOW

ADAPTIVE IMMUNITY: Adaptive immunity is another term for acquired immunity, referring to the resistance to infection that develops through life and is targeted to a specific pathogen. There are two types of adaptive immunity, known as active and passive. Active immunity is either humoral, involving production of antibody molecules against a bacterium or virus, or cell-mediated, where T-cells are mobilized against infected cells. Infection and immunization can both induce acquired immunity. Passive immunity is induced by injection of the serum of a person who is already immune to a particular infection.

EMERGING INFECTIOUS DISEASE: New infectious diseases such as SARS and West Nile virus, as well as previously known diseases such as malaria, tuberculosis, and bacterial pneumonias that are appearing in forms that are resistant to drug treatments, are termed emerging infectious diseases.

ENDEMIC: Present in a particular area or among a particular group of people.

ERADICATION: The process of destroying or eliminating a microorganism or disease.

IMMUNOGENICITY: Immunogenicity is the capacity of a host to produce an immune response to protect itself against infectious disease.

INNATE IMMUNITY: Innate immunity is the resistance against disease that an individual is born with, as distinct from acquired immunity that develops with exposure to infectious agents.

PATHOGEN: A disease causing agent, such as a bacteria, virus, fungus, etc.

VIRULENCE: Virulence is the ability of a disease organism to cause disease: a more virulent organism is more infective and liable to produce more serious disease.

The WHO has requested to establish a program in South Africa to deal with the outbreak, but South African officials insist that they have the capabilities to handle the issue and should maintain control of any such program.

West Nile Virus

West Nile Virus (WNV) has been endemic in Africa, West Asia, Europe, and the Middle East for centuries, but has only re-emerged in the United States since 1999. The first WNV infections occurred in the New York metropolitan area and have continued to spread throughout the United States during the summer season, infecting increasingly larger populations. The inexorable spread of the virus has prompted vaccine and drug therapy development, with some candidates currently showing some prevention or treatment effectiveness in animals. Currently the most immediately promising approach to slowing the spread of WNV is the control of insect vectors. New methods of controlling mosquitoes and countering mosquito resistance to insecticides are under development for use in areas where WNV threatens to become endemic.

Potential bioterrorism agents

The use of anthrax in terroristic attacks can be seen as a deliberate effort to promote the re-emergence of infectious agents that have otherwise been either eradicated, as in the case of smallpox, or largely controlled, as in the case of anthrax itself. Bioterrorism could also promote the emergence of a pathogen such as the Ebola virus in a setting such as the urban United States that is radically different and distant from the rural African regions in which such infections have occurred to-date. Since a wide variety of dangerous and virulent pathogens could potentially be used as bioweapons, defensive strategies must rely on research at a very broad and basic level in terms of understanding how human immune systems react to them and how infections can be detected, prevented, and treated.

■ Applications and research

Currently, a wide variety of scientific and industrial biodefense research infrastructure projects are underway in the United States, including the development of Regional Centers of Excellence for Biodefense and Emerging Infectious Disease Research, in addition to the building of secure facilities, including two National Biocontainment Laboratories and nine Regional Biocontainment Laboratories.

Research projects recently completed or underway include the gene sequencing of pathogens considered to be the most potent threats, the screening of chemical compounds that could provide potential treatments, and development of animals to test promising drugs. Immunologists are also investigating ways to boost human innate immunity.

Innate immunity is the immune system's first line of defense and is represented by monocytes and neutrophils (white blood cells), which react to any and all foreign substances and organisms in the body. This innate immune system is distinct from adaptive immunity, the second line of defense represented by T cells and B cells (lymphocytes), which are influenced by the innate immune system to recognize specific pathogens and foreign organisms and destroy them in a focused attack. Finally, as with the other types of re-emergent infections, vaccine development is being fostered under the nation's biodefense program.

■ Impacts and Issues

Clearly, vaccine development is central to the control of re-emerging infections, particularly development of an effective vaccine for HIV, which is key to preventing the spread of tuberculosis and a number of other infections that otherwise would not have been able to regain virulence after decades of effective treatment and prevention. The HIV epidemic, the rapid growth of international travel and commerce, and the danger of deliberate spread of pathogens into vulnerable new populations will continue to foster or threaten the re-emergence of dangerous pathogens. This threat will pose an ongoing and permanent challenge to public health agencies that must be dealt with by intensified basic biological and clinical research.

The best strategy for dealing with the threat of emerging and re-emerging infections alike is the funding, implementation, and staffing of an excellent global public health infrastructure, which will require international cooperation on an unprecedented scale.

SEE ALSO *Emerging Infectious Diseases; Lyme Disease; Malaria; Pandemic Preparedness; Tuberculosis; War and Infectious Disease; West Nile.*

BIBLIOGRAPHY

Books

Brower, Jennifer, and Peter Chalk. *The Global Threat of New and Reemerging Infectious Diseases: Reconciling U.S. National Security and Public Health Policy.* Santa Monica, CA: Rand, 2003.

Periodicals

Corbett, E., et al. "The Growing Burden of Tuberculosis: Global Trends and Interactions with the HIV Epidemic." *Archives of Internal Medicine* 163, 9 (May 12, 2003): 1009–1021.

Hecht, R., et al. "Putting It Together: AIDS and the Millennium Development Goals." *PLoS Medicine* 3, 11 (2006).

Kirkland, T.N., and J. Fierer. "Coccidioidomycosis: A Reemerging Infectious Disease." *Emerging Infectious Diseases* 2, 3 (July-September 1996).

Web Sites

Fauci, Anthony S. *Millbank Memorial Fund.* "Emerging and Re-emerging Infectious Diseases: The Perpetual Challenge." January 2006. <http://www.milbank.org/reports/0601fauci/0601fauci.html> (accessed June 4, 2007).

World Health Organization. "The World Health Report 2004—Changing History." <http://www.who.int/whr/2004/en/> (accessed June 4, 2007).

Kenneth LaPensee

Relapsing Fever

Introduction

Relapsing fever is an acute infectious disease caused by various bacteria within the genus *Borrelia*. The disease is commonly recognized by repetitious bouts of fever. Relapsing fever is a zoonotic (acquired from animals) disease that is transmitted to humans primarily from parasitic insects called body lice (louse-borne relapsing fever), which enter the inside of the body, and by the bites of soft-bodied ticks (tick-borne relapsing fever), which occur on the outside of the body.

The louse-borne relapsing fever (LBRF) is transmitted to humans from lice (specifically, *Pediculus humanus*) that are infected with the bacterium *Borrelia recurrentis*. The lice enter the human body through mucous membranes and then invade the bloodstream. They eventually multiply inside the abdomen of the host.

The tick-borne relapsing fever (TBRF) is transmitted to humans from bites of ticks infected with *Borrelia* bacteria species such as *Borrelia hermsii* and *Borrelia Parkeri*. The ticks spread from hosts such as rodents and other animals. *B. hermsii* and *B. recurrentis* cause similar symptoms, but *B. hermsii* causes more relapses and is responsible for more deaths. *B. recurrentis* infection, on the other hand, results in longer periods with fever and without fever, and with more extended incubation periods.

Disease History, Characteristics, and Transmission

For both forms of the disease, the first symptoms occur five to 15 days after the bite of an infected vector (an organism such as the tick or louse that transmits a disease-causing organism). Symptoms include, initially, a high and sudden fever, followed by chills, shakes, neck stiffness, sweating, low body temperature, low blood pressure, nausea, vomiting, rash, headache, and muscle and/or joint pains.

When these symptoms become serious, many patients develop central nervous system (CNS) problems such as stupor, seizure, facial droop, weakness, and coma. Heart and liver tissues that are invaded by the bacteria often result in hepatitis (inflammation of the liver), meningitis (inflammation of the meninges), or myocarditis (inflammation of the heart muscle). Bleeding and pneumonia are other problems associated with the disease. Death

WORDS TO KNOW

INCUBATION PERIOD: Incubation period refers to the time between exposure to disease causing virus or bacteria and the appearance of symptoms of the infection. Depending on the microorganism, the incubation time can range from a few hours (an example is food poisoning due to *Salmonella*) to a decade or more (an example is acquired immunodeficiency syndrome, or AIDS).

HOST: Organism that serves as the habitat for a parasite, or possibly for a symbiont. A host may provide nutrition to the parasite or symbiont, or simply a place in which to live.

VECTOR: Any agent, living or otherwise, that carries and transmits parasites and diseases. Also, an organism or chemical used to transport a gene into a new host cell.

ZOONOSES: Zoonoses are diseases of microbiological origin that can be transmitted from animals to people. The causes of the diseases can be bacteria, viruses, parasites, and fungi.

occurs in up to 10% of untreated persons with these serious symptoms of relapsing fever.

In LBRF, the first round of symptoms lasts from three to six days and is followed by other milder rounds of symptoms, with each episode lasting up to three days. Fever may be absent for up to two weeks before another round occurs. Generally, the patient has symptoms when the organism is within the host's blood and, then, the symptoms disappear when the organism leaves the blood.

The effects of LBRF become critical to the patient when severe jaundice (yellowing of the skin and mucous membranes due to impaired liver function), changes in mental status, bleeding, and prolonged QT interval on an ECG (the measure on an electrocardiogram between the beginning of the Q wave and the end of the T wave within the heart's electrical cycle). According to the Centers for Disease Control and Prevention (CDC), LBRF has a mortality rate of 1% with treatment and between 30–70% without treatment.

■ Scope and Distribution

LBRF occurs primarily in Ethiopia and Sudan in northern Africa. It is also found in Europe and India. The disease is often the cause of epidemics within areas of poor living conditions and regions where famine and war are prevalent. During World War I (1914–1918) and World War II (1939–1945), millions of people died from LBRF.

TBRF is found in Africa, Asia, Saudi Arabia, South America, Spain, and certain areas in the western section of the United States and Canada. In the United States, it usually occurs west of the Mississippi River, predominately in the mountains of the West and the high-elevation deserts and plains of the Southwest. There are now signs of TBRF infecting people in the southeastern parts of the United States. According to the CDC, there are about 25 cases in the U.S. annually.

■ Treatment and Prevention

According to the CDC, treatment of TBRF usually involves a one-week course of antibiotics. When treated properly, most people recover and death only rarely occurs. Tetracycline is often used as the antibiotic of choice; however, up to one-half of all persons with relapsing fever have negative reactions to tetracycline, including anxiety, fever, sweating, rapid heart rate, and low blood pressure. Chloramphenicol, doxycycline, erythromycin, and penicillin are also used to treat the disease.

The duration for antibiotic treatment of LBRF, according to the CDC's Division of Vector-Borne Infectious Diseases (DVBID), is one single dose of antibiotics. The death rate for untreated LBRF ranges from 10 to 70% and for TRBF the death rate is between 4 and 10%. With early treatment, death rates are reduced to between 2 to 5%. However, people with liver dysfunc-

tion, myocarditis, and pneumonia have a higher risk of death than others.

Both forms of relapsing fever can be prevented by wearing protective clothing and using insect repellent. Comprehensive lice and tick control should be used in areas hardest hit with the infections.

■ Impacts and Issues

Relapsing fever was once a global concern. However, with antibiotic treatment, it is now restricted mostly to areas of the developing world. Circumstances such as increased worldwide travel by humans and wide movements by animals, however, and even the trend toward washing clothes in cold and warm water rather than hot water, are causing a re-emergence of relapsing fever.

In addition, according to the CDC, since the 1980s, increased numbers of *Borrelia* species have been discovered to be associated with relapsing fever.

The most recent cases of tick-borne relapsing fever have occurred in mountainous areas of the western United States, primarily among vacationers to forests or cabins in higher-elevations (above 8,000 feet, or 2,438 meters). Campers and other persons rarely realize that they are bitten by the soft ticks that carry TBRF, as the ticks feed for a few minutes, then fall off. When experiencing a fever after vacationing in the mountains, therefore, it is advisable to seek medical treatment. TBRF remains on the list of modifiable diseases for health officials in many western states, in order to track the prevalence of the disease and the ticks that cause it.

All of these situations demonstrate that the potential for relapsing fever, as it is with other re-emerging infectious diseases, is unpredictable. The potential for it to emerge in areas where not recognized earlier is great. People who are very young, old, pregnant, or have weakened physical conditions have increased risk of the affects and complications of relapsing fever.

SEE ALSO *African Sleeping Sickness (Trypanosomiasis); Bacterial Disease; Emerging Infectious Diseases; Travel and Infectious Disease.*

BIBLIOGRAPHY

Books

Edlow, Jonathan A., ed. *Tick-borne Diseases.* Philadelphia, PA: W.B. Saunders Company, 2002.

Goodman, Jesse L., David T. Dennis, and Daniel E. Sonenshine. *Tick-borne Diseases of Humans.* Washington, DC: ASM Press, 2005.

Web Sites

Cutler, Sally J., Veterinary Laboratories Agency (Surrey, United Kingdom), U.S. Centers for Disease Control and Prevention. "Possibilities for Relapsing Fever Reemergence." March 2006 <http://www.cdc.gov/ncidod/eid/vol12no03/05-0899.htm> (accessed April 27, 2007).

Centers for Disease Control and Prevention. "Relapsing Fever: Introduction." November 10, 2004 <http://www.cdc.gov/ncidod/dvbid/RelapsingFever/index.htm> (accessed April 27, 2007).

Centers for Disease Control and Prevention. "Treatment of Tick-Borne Relapsing Fever." November 10, 2004 <http://www.cdc.gov/ncidod/dvbid/RelapsingFever/RF_Treatment.htm> (accessed April 27, 2007).

Resistant Organisms

◼ Introduction

Resistant organisms are microbes—bacteria, fungi, viruses, or parasites—that have evolved immunity to one or more of the drugs used to kill them. Drugs that kill microbes are called antimicrobials. Resistance threatens human health because it reduces or eliminates the efficacy of drugs used to treat infections. If organisms evolve resistance to drugs faster than new drugs can be discovered, doctors' choices for treating infections by those organisms dwindle. This has happened for many real-world bacteria, viruses, fungi, and parasites. Resistance to a drug is more likely to evolve when the drug is widely used. Antibiotic resistance, in particular, has arisen in part because of chronic overuse of antibiotics in medical and agricultural settings. Antibiotics are often prescribed for viral, not bacterial, infections (antibiotics have no effect on viruses), and millions of pounds of antibiotics are given to livestock each year. Most experts agree that in the early twenty-first century, antimicrobial resistance has reached a crisis stage.

◼ Disease History, Characteristics, and Transmission

History

Resistant organisms did not arise before the mid-twentieth century because antimicrobials potent enough to force the evolution of resistance were not known. Penicillin, for example, was discovered in 1928 and was first widely used during World War II (1939–45). Penicillin-resistant *Escherichia coli* bacteria were first observed in 1940. Penicillin-resistant staphylococcus bacteria were reported in 1944, and, by the 1950s, a penicillin-resistant strain of *Staphylococcus aureus* became a worldwide problem in hospitals. By the 1960s, most staphylococci were resistant to penicillin.

Another example of resistance development is the malaria parasite and the antimalarial drug chloroquine.

Chloroquine was introduced in the 1940s. Ten years later, resistance to chloroquine evolved independently in Asia and South America but remained rare. After another twenty years, resistance appeared in East Africa and spread rapidly thereafter. Today, chloroquine-resistant malaria is found in several regions across the globe. Malaria infects 300 to 500 million people yearly, killing about 1 million, almost all in developing nations.

Since the late 1980s, pathogens resistant to more than one drug—which are even more difficult to treat than organisms with single-drug resistance—have emerged at an accelerating pace. However, development of new antimicrobials has slowed.

Characteristics

In any wild population of microorganisms, whether bacteria or viruses, there will be small, random, heritable differences—genetic differences—between individuals. The protein recipe for a microorganism is not rigid and exact; its many proteins can take on slightly different forms without compromising its ability to survive. When a population of microorganisms is exposed to a drug designed to destroy it, the genetic differences between individuals sometimes allow microorganisms to survive. Thus, the entire next generation of microorganisms will tend to be more resistant to that drug. If this evolutionary process of variation and selection is repeated, resistance can evolve.

In general, the more often a drug is used, the more quickly resistance may evolve. However, resistance can also evolve when insufficient quantities of a drug are used and some microorganisms survive. The fewer survivors there are, the more resistant they may be. Thus dosing to the threshold of elimination can be worse than drastically underdosing (which does not select so strongly for resistance).

Resistance may still evolve even if drugs are dosed appropriately. This has been the case with antivirals, antifungals, and antiparasitics. However, needless or

WORDS TO KNOW

ANTIBACTERIAL: A substance that reduces or kill germs (bacteria and other microorganisms but not including viruses). Also often a term used to describe a drug used to treat bacterial infections.

ANTIBIOTIC: A drug, such as penicillin, used to fight infections caused by bacteria. Antibiotics act only on bacteria and are not effective against viruses.

ANTIFUNGAL: Antifungals (also called antifungal drugs) are medicines used to fight fungal infections. They are of two kinds, systemic and topical. Systemic antifungal drugs are medicines taken by mouth or by injection to treat infections caused by a fungus. Topical antifungal drugs are medicines applied to the skin to treat skin infections caused by a fungus.

ANTIMICROBIAL: A material that slows the growth of bacteria or that is able to kill bacteria. Includes antibiotics (which can be used inside the body) and disinfectants (which can only be used outside the body).

BACTERIA: Single-celled microorganisms that live in soil, water, plants, and animals that play a key role in the decay of organic matter and the cycling of nutrients. Some bacteria are agents of disease. Microscopic organisms whose activities range from the development of disease to fermentation. Bacteria range in shape from spherical to rod-shaped to spiral. Different types of bacteria cause many sexually transmitted diseases, including syphilis, gonorrhea, and chlamydia. Bacteria also cause diseases ranging from typhoid to dysentery to tetanus. Bacterium is the singular form of bacteria.

COHORT: A cohort is a group of people (or any species) sharing a common characteristic. Cohorts are identified and grouped in cohort studies to determine the frequency of diseases or the kinds of disease outcomes over time.

DRUG RESISTANCE: Drug resistance develops when an infective agent such as a bacterium, fungus or virus, develops a lack of sensitivity to a drug that would normally be able to control or even kill them. This tends to occur with over-use of anti-infectives, which selects out populations of microbes most able to resist them, while killing off those organisms that are most sensitive. The next time the anti-infective agent is used, it will be less effective, leading to the eventual development of resistance.

MICROORGANISM: Microorganisms are minute organisms. With the single yet-known exception of a bacterium that is large enough to be seen unaided, individual microorganisms are microscopic in size. To be seen, they must be magnified by an optical or electron microscope. The most common types of microorganisms are viruses, bacteria, blue-green bacteria, some algae, some fungi, yeasts, and protozoans.

PATHOGEN: A disease causing agent, such as a bacteria, virus, fungus, etc.

VIRUS: Viruses are essentially nonliving repositories of nucleic acid that require the presence of a living prokaryotic or eukaryotic cell for the replication of the nucleic acid. There are a number of different viruses that challenge the human immune system and that may produce disease in humans. In common, a virus is a small, infectious agent that consists of a core of genetic material (either deoxyribonucleic acid (DNA) or ribonucleic acid (RNA) surrounded by a shell of protein. Very simple microorganisms, viruses are much smaller than bacteria that enter and multiples within cells. Viruses often exchange or transfer their genetic material (DNA or RNA) to cells and can cause diseases such as chickenpox, hepatitis, measles, and mumps.

---

inadequate use of antimicrobials encourages more rapid evolution of resistance.

The features that make an organism resistant to a drug vary widely because the precise ways in which antimicrobials attack organisms vary widely. Any mutation that interferes with the harmful action of the drug on the organism will confer resistance. For example, some bacteria have become resistant to the antibiotic penicillin by evolving the ability to produce beta-lactamases, which are enzymes (a type of protein) that deactivate the antibiotic. In other cases, microorganisms utilize several methods of antibiotic resistance: learning how to keep drugs from passing into the cell or accumulating there; altering surface molecules that antimicrobial drugs bind to; or evolving alternatives to series of chemical reactions in the cell (metabolic pathways) that are blocked by antimicrobials.

Transmission

Transmission of resistant organisms occurs by the same mechanisms as for their non-resistant relatives, but is more likely to occur in certain settings. For example, infection by methicillin-resistant *Staphylococcus aureus* happens more commonly in hospital intensive-care units and long-term care facilities. Methicillin-resistant *S. aureus* has also been detected on pets, having probably been transmitted to them by humans, and may be transmitted back to humans from these animals. It has not been detected in food animals.

■ Scope and Distribution

Resistant organisms are most common in settings where antimicrobial drugs are most widely used. They are therefore most often encountered in industrialized countries. In the United States, for example, about a third of all *Staphylococcus aureus* infections are now methicillin-resistant. Certain organisms that are found and treated almost exclusively in developing countries, such as the malaria parasite, have evolved resistant varieties in those regions.

■ Treatment and Prevention

When doctors find that they are trying to treat an infection by a resistant organism, they use trial and error to find a drug to which the organism is not resistant. This process usually involves trying one drug after another, starting with those that are least toxic for the patient and most specific for the target organism, and working towards drugs that are less desirable or potentially produce greater side effects. Even when a drug that works is found—and some organisms are now resistant to all the agents used against them—the delay involved in this process is dangerous to the patient.

The U.S. Centers for Disease Control (CDC) has stated that antibiotic resistance is a key microbial threat to health in the United States. The CDC launched a National Campaign for Appropriate Antibiotic Use in the Community in 1995, which was renamed in 2003 as Get Smart: Know When Antibiotics Work. This campaign seeks to slow the evolution of antibiotic resistance primarily by discouraging the unnecessary use of antibiotics for upper respiratory infections. Seventy-five percent of antibiotics prescribed by office-based physicians are for upper respiratory infections, most of which are viral and therefore unaffected by antibiotics.

IN CONTEXT: REAL-WORLD RISKS

Acquired adaptation of bacteria to many antibiotics has become a problem since the early 1990s. For example, many hospitals now must cope with the presence of methicillin-resistant *Staphylococcus aureus* (MRSA), which displays resistance to almost all currently used antibiotics. Dealing with infections caused by MRSA and other resistant organisms requires increased hospital staff hours, increased supplies, and can restrict the availability of hospital beds when cohorting (grouping together patients with the same disease) or isolation is necessary.

The few antibiotics to which antibiotic-resistant bacteria do respond tend to be expensive, with few options for delivery. For example, the drug meropenum is sometimes prescribed for persons with pneumonia, meningitis, or serious skin infections that are caused by organisms that are resistant to common antibiotics. Meropenum can be delivered by intravenous injection or infusion only, and is two to three times more expensive than the commonly prescribed antibiotics for these conditions.

Additionally, disease-causing organisms can sometimes adapt so that they are able grow and multiply on solid surfaces. This mode of growth is called a biofilm. A biofilm environment induces many changes in growing bacteria, some of which involve the expression of previously unexpressed genes and deactivation of actively expressing genes. The structure of the biofilm and these genetic changes often make the bacteria extraordinarily resistant to many antibiotics. Biofilms sometimes occur on some hospital surfaces and in implanted devices such as artificial joints and long-term intravenous access catheters.

■ Impacts and Issues

Antimicrobial resistance has become a major public health concern in recent years. According to the U.S. National Institute of Allergies and Infectious Diseases, tuberculosis, gonorrhea, malaria, and childhood ear infections are all more difficult to treat today, because of antimicrobial resistance, than they were a few decades ago. Chloroquine resistance evolved by the malaria parasite threatens millions of lives: since 1978, chloroquine resistance has been reported in all tropical African countries, becoming more common in recent decades. The impact on public health has been major, with malaria deaths doubling or tripling in some African countries. In Senegal, child deaths from malaria have increased by up to a factor of 6 with the growth of chloroquine resistance. All alternatives to chloroquine are more expensive and have comparatively severe side effects.

One of the most contentious aspects of antimicrobial resistance today is the use of antibiotics in agriculture. Millions of pounds of antibiotics are fed to livestock annually in the United States and elsewhere, mostly as growth promoters. Studies over the last several decades have shown that this promotes the evolution of resistant organisms. In 2005, the U.S. Food and Drug Administration banned the use enrofloxacin (an antibacterial) in poultry. The European Union has banned the use of a range of almost all growth-promoting hormones and antimicrobials in agriculture.

Some experts also warn that the nearly universal use of antimicrobial household soaps may contribute to the evolution of resistant organisms. Ordinary soap and water wash bacteria away rather than killing them directly and so do not provide selective pressure for evolution of resistance. Moreover, studies in India have found that antimicrobial soaps do not improve health any more than old-fashioned soaps.

Phage therapy—the use of certain viruses to infect and kill bacteria—shows some promise as an alternative strategy for treating infections by multiply resistant organisms, and research continues in this area.

SEE ALSO *Antibiotic Resistance; Antimicrobial Soaps; Antiviral Drugs; Nosocomial (Healthcare-Associated) Infections; Vancomycin-resistant Enterococci.*

BIBLIOGRAPHY

Books

Salyers, Abigail A. and Dixie D. Whitt. *Revenge Of The Microbes: How Bacterial Resistance Is Undermining The Antibiotic Miracle*. Washington, DC: ASM Press, 2005.

Periodicals

Cunha, Burke A. "Effective Antibiotic-Resistance Control Strategies." *The Lancet* 357 (2001): 1307.

Lipsitch, Marc, and Matthew H. Samore. "Antimicrobial Use and Antimicrobial Resistance: A Population Perspective." *Emerging Infectious Diseases* 8 (2002): 347-354.

Shea, Katherine M. "Antibiotic Resistance: What is the Impact of Agricultural Uses of Antibiotics on Children's Health?" *Pediatrics* 112 (2003): 253-258.

Smith, David L., et al. "Agricultural Antibiotics and Human Health" *PloS Medicine* 2 (2005): 731-735.

Web Sites

Centers for Disease Control (U.S. Government). "A Public Health Action Plan to Combat Antibiotic Resistance." February 9, 2005. <http://www.cdc.gov/drugresistance/actionplan/aractionplan.pdf> (accessed February 26, 2007).

Centers for Disease Control (U.S. Government). "About Antibiotic Resistance." April 21, 2006. <http://www.cdc.gov/drugresistance/community/anitbiotic-resistance.htm> (accessed February 26, 2007).

RSV (Respiratory Syncytial Virus) Infection

■ Introduction

Respiratory Syncytial virus (RSV) is a ribonucleic acid (RNA)-containing virus that causes a lung infection (pneumonia) that affects the oxygen- and carbon dioxide-carrying tubes called the bronchioles. These tubes are very tiny and are located deep within the lungs. Because of this, the infection, which is also known as bronchiolitis, can hamper the function of the lungs.

RSV infections can be spread easily from person-to-person and can occur repeatedly in infants. Indeed, RSV infections are the most common cause of bronchiolitis and pneumonia in newborns and infants under one year of age.

■ Disease History, Characteristics, and Transmission

The first symptoms of an RSV lung infection are often mistaken for a cold. A child can have a fever and a runny nose. The involvement of the lungs can be evident as a cough and sometimes a wheezing type of breathing.

A lung infection that involves the bronchioles may not occur the first time someone is infected by RSV. However, up to 40% of infants do experience the more severe lung infection; this can require hospitalization, especially in infants under six months of age.

Most children recover from the infection within a few weeks. However, repeated cold-like infections can then occur throughout life. In addition, the lung infection can be more serious, especially in elderly people or those whose immune systems are less capable of fighting off infections.

The virus is spread in the tiny drops of mucus and other fluids that are expelled from the nose during a sneeze and from the lungs when someone coughs. If another person is close by, these drops can be inhaled and the virus may then be able to establish an infection

in the new host. Alternatively, the virus-laden droplets can land on inanimate objects such as a doorknob or can be transferred to a hand when the nose is wiped. Touching an object before the hands are washed can also transfer the virus. If the contaminated object is touched within a few hours, the virus can picked up on the hands and transfer to the new host can occur.

This route of transmission makes RSV infection especially prevalent in more northern climates during colder months when people are indoors more often and the chances of person-to-person spread is greater. This sort of a pattern is known as a community outbreak. Illness in warmer climates shows less of a seasonal pattern.

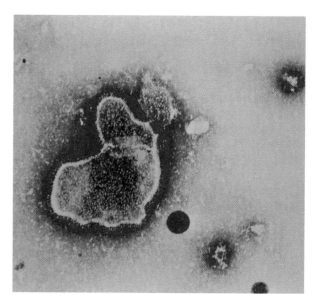

This colored transmission electron micrograph (TEM) shows a Respiratory Syncytial virus (RSV). This pneumovirus, a type of paramyxovirus, is a major cause of human respiratory tract infections in temperate climates, especially in winter. *CDC/Photo Researchers, Inc.*

WORDS TO KNOW

ATTENUATED STRAIN: A bacterium or virus that has been weakened, often used as the basis of a vaccine against the specific disease caused by the bacterium or virus.

BRONCHIOLITIS: Inflammation (-itis) of the bronchioles, the small air passages in the lungs that enter the alveoli (air sacs), is bronchiolitis.

■ Scope and Distribution

RSV infection tends to be more prevalent in climates that have colder seasons, since people are in closer indoor contact for part of the year. However, the infection can occur virtually anywhere. Because infants and the elderly are the most susceptible, RSV infection is associated with hospitals, daycare centers, and retirement or elder-care settings.

■ Treatment and Prevention

Spread of RSV can be minimized or even prevented by common-sense hygiene. Covering the nose and mouth with a tissue when sneezing or coughing can prevent the spread of virus-laden droplets in the air. Washing the hands with regular hand soap will inactivate any RSV on the skin.

The presence of the virus can be detected by isolation of the virus. In addition, molecular techniques can be used to detect protein components of the virus by the presence of antibodies to these proteins (antibodies are proteins produced by the immune system in response to the presence of a component that is foreign to the host) and by the presence of viral genetic material. These tests are fairly specialized and require trained staff and a laboratory with the necessary equipment. Tests to monitor the antibody levels are the more common molecular approach.

Diagnosis is usually confirmed only for severe illnesses in hospitalized patients. For most people who have RSV infection, no specific treatment is administered, since the illness is limited. In infants and children, treatment typically is aimed at reducing the discomfort due to fever, and acetaminophen is most commonly used for this purpose.

More severe disease can require the use of supplemental oxygen or even mechanical ventilation (when a tube is inserted down the patient's trachea to deliver oxygen directly to the lungs), since the lungs may not be functioning efficiently. Antiviral drugs such as ribavirin are also administered. The drug is structurally similar to the viral RNA and so can interfere with the process used by the virus to make new copies of itself.

Another treatment option for more severe RSV infection is the use of immune globulin, a compound produced by the immune system. This strategy is especially useful for people whose own immune systems are malfunctioning and so not as capable of producing the compound. Immune globulin is usually given intravenously.

■ Impacts and Issues

The fact that RSV infections predominantly affect the very young and the elderly makes it a concern for these age groups. In some cases, lung function can be affected by RSV infection to the point that hospitalization and mechanical breathing assistance is necessary. In the United States, about 80,000 children are hospitalized with RSV infections every year.

Almost half of otherwise healthy babies who are hospitalized with RSV develop asthma later in childhood. Asthma is the number one reason for school absences in children due to a chronic illness, resulting in about 14 million lost school days per year in the United States. In several studies, researchers are tracking healthy newborns who develop RSV as they grow to determine genetic and environmental factors that may link RSV with asthma.

RSV infections also highlight the potential for an infectious disease to spread more easily in a crowded indoor environment and the importance of common-sense hygiene. Such hygienic measures as cleaning toys and equipment in daycare centers and frequent handwashing can help to significantly minimize the risk of infection.

Efforts are ongoing to develop a vaccine against RSV. Researchers at Vanderbilt University are pursuing one approach that involves using genetic technologies to manipulate genes in the RSV virus. By causing small mutations or deletions in the genes of the virus, an improved attenuated (weakened) form of the RSV virus is produced that could lead to the development of a safe, efficient vaccine. As of 2007, a vaccine for RSV is not yet available.

SEE ALSO *Public Health and Infectious Disease.*

BIBLIOGRAPHY

Books

Cane, Patricia, ed. *Respiratory Syncytial Virus.* Vol. 14 of *Perspectives in Medical Virology.* New York: Elsevier Science, 2006.

Hart, Tony. *Microterrors: The Complete Guide to Bacterial, Viral and Fungal Infections That Threaten Our Health.* Tonawanda, NY: Firefly Books, 2004.

Sears, William, and Martha Sears. *The Baby Book: Everything You Need to Know About Your Baby from Birth to Age Two.* New York: Little, Brown, 2003.

Web Sites

Centers for Disease Control and Prevention. "Respiratory Syncytial Virus." January 1, 2005. <http://www.cdc.gov/ncidod/dvrd/revb/respiratory/rsvfeat.htm> (accessed March 1, 2007).

Brian Hoyle

Retroviruses

■ Introduction

Retroviruses are viruses that contain ribonucleic acid (RNA) as their genetic material. This contrasts with the majority of other microorganisms that instead contain deoxyribonucleic acid (DNA). Like other viruses, retroviruses create new copies of themselves by infecting a host cell and using the hosts' genetic replication machinery. To accomplish this, early in the infection process of retroviruses an enzyme called reverse transcriptase is produced. The enzyme can transform the viral RNA into DNA, which is then inserted into the host DNA. The inserted viral DNA can be replicated along with the host DNA during growth and division of the host cell, and the manufactured viral components assemble to form new copies of the virus.

Retroviruses cause a number of serious infections in humans and other creatures. The most infamous is acquired immunodeficiency syndrome (AIDS, also cited as acquired immune deficiency syndrome), which is considered by most scientists to be caused by several versions of a retrovirus called the human immunodeficiency virus (HIV). Other retroviruses can stimulate abnormal cell growth; these retroviruses can also be termed oncogenic viruses.

■ History and Scientific Foundations

The first known retrovirus, the Rous sarcoma virus, was discovered in 1911. It was subsequently shown that the virus was a cause of cancer in some species of chickens. The demonstration of the ability of retroviruses to cause human diseases did not come until almost 70 years later.

In 1980, researchers at the National Cancer Institute discovered the first human retrovirus. They found the virus within leukemic T cells of patients with an aggressive form of T cell cancer. These patients were from the southern United States, Japan, and the Caribbean. Almost all patients with this form of cancer were found to have antibodies (immune system proteins made in response to an infection) to HTLV.

HTLV and HIV infect and replicate inside of T cells, which are vital to the human immune response. As more T cells are disabled, the immune system becomes progressively less efficient and microorganisms not normally capable of causing disease are able to do so. These infections are called opportunistic infections. HTLV also causes a lethal cancer called adult T cell leukemia.

Retroviruses are spherical. An outer structure called a capsule surrounds either one or two strands of RNA. The capsule also contains proteins that can recognize target protein sites on the host cell. The association of the viral and host proteins enables the virus to attach to the host cell, which is necessary before the virus can enter the host. For example, in the case of the HIV retrovirus, the viral proteins bind to T cell proteins called CD4 receptors.

Once inside the host cell, the retrovirus begins to make more copies. Retroviruses are an exception to the general order of replication, which involves the use of DNA as a template to make a type of RNA called messenger RNA, which in turn provides the information to make proteins. Instead, retroviruses have a preliminary step in which the viral RNA is used to manufacture DNA. From then on, the replication process occurs as in other cells.

Retroviruses contain an enzyme called reverse transcriptase that produces DNA from the viral RNA. The viral-derived DNA can then be integrated into the host's DNA. When the host cell replicates, the viral DNA is read along with the host DNA. The manufactured viral components are then assembled to produce new virus particles. Reverse transcriptase is unique to retroviruses. This is their Achilles' heel. Drugs that impair this enzyme can interrupt the production of new retrovirus. As a result, therapies to treat HIV infections usually include a reverse transcriptase inhibitor.

WORDS TO KNOW

DEOXYRIBONUCLEIC ACID (DNA): Deoxyribonucleic acid (DNA) is a double-stranded, helical molecule that forms the molecular basis for heredity in most organisms.

GENE THERAPY: Gene therapy is the name applied to the treatment of inherited diseases by corrective genetic engineering of the dysfunctional genes. It is part of a broader field called genetic medicine, which involves the screening, diagnosis, prevention, and treatment of hereditary conditions in humans. The results of genetic screening can pinpoint a potential problem to which gene therapy can sometimes offer a solution. Genetic defects are significant in the total field of medicine, with up to 15 out of every 100 newborn infants having a hereditary disorder of greater or lesser severity. More than 2000 genetically distinct inherited defects have been classified so far, including diabetes, cystic fibrosis, hemophilia, sickle-call anemia, phenylketonuria, Down syndrome and cancer.

HUMAN IMMUNODEFICIENCY VIRUS (HIV): The human immunodeficiency virus (HIV) belongs to a class of viruses known as the retroviruses. These viruses are known as RNA viruses because they have RNA (ribonucleic acid) as their basic genetic material instead of DNA (deoxyribonucleic acid).

HUMAN T-CELL LEUKEMIA VIRUS: Two types of human T-cell leukemia virus (HTLV) are known. They are also known as human T-cell lymphotrophic viruses. HTLV-1 often is carried by a person with no obvious symptoms. However, HTLV-I is capable of causing a number of maladies. These include abnormalities of the T cells and B cells, a chronic infection of the myelin covering of nerves that causes a degeneration of the nervous system, sores on the skin, and an inflammation of the inside of the eye. HTLV-II infection usually does not produce any symptoms. However, in some people a cancer of the blood known as hairy cell leukemia can develop.

ONCOGENIC VIRUS: An oncogenic virus is a virus that is capable of changing the cells it infects so that the cells begin to grow and divide uncontrollably.

OPPORTUNISTIC INFECTION: An opportunistic infection is so named because it occurs in people whose immune systems are diminished or are not functioning normally; such infections are opportunistic insofar as the infectious agents take advantage of their hosts' compromised immune systems and invade to cause disease.

REVERSE TRANSCRIPTASE: An enzyme that makes it possible for a retrovirus to produce DNA (deoxyribonucleic acid) from RNA (ribonucleic acid).

RIBONUCLEIC ACID (RNA): Any of a group of nucleic acids that carry out several important tasks in the synthesis of proteins. Unlike DNA (deoxyribonucleic acid), it has only a single strand. Nucleic acids are complex molecules that contain a cell's genetic information and the instructions for carrying out cellular processes. In eukaryotic cells, the two nucleic acids, ribonucleic acid (RNA) and deoxyribonucleic acid (DNA), work together to direct protein synthesis. Although it is DNA (deoxyribonucleic acid) that contains the instructions for directing the synthesis of specific structural and enzymatic proteins, several types of RNA actually carry out the processes required to produce these proteins. These include messenger RNA (mRNA), ribosomal RNA (rRNA), and transfer RNA (tRNA). Further processing of the various RNAs is carried out by another type of RNA called small nuclear RNA (snRNA). The structure of RNA is very similar to that of DNA, however, instead of the base thymine, RNA co

ROUS SARCOMA VIRUS: Rous sarcoma virus, named after American doctor Francis Peyton Rous (1879–1970), is a virus that can cause cancer in some birds, including chickens. It was the first virus known go to be able to cause cancer.

T CELL: Immune-system white blood cells that enable antibody production, suppress antibody production, or kill other cells. When a vertebrate encounters substances that are capable of causing it harm, a protective system known as the immune system comes into play. This system is a network of many different organs that work together to recognize foreign substances and destroy them. The immune system can respond to the presence of a disease-causing agent (pathogen) in two ways. Immune cells called the B cells can produce soluble proteins (antibodies) that can accurately target and kill the pathogen. This branch of immunity is called humoral immunity. In cell-mediated immunity, immune cells known as the T cells produce special chemicals that can specifically isolate the pathogen and destroy it.

Retroviruses that cause cancer do so when the reverse transcribed-viral DNA is integrated into the DNA of the host. In some cases, the viral DNA can insert itself within a gene. This will alter the sequence of the gene, which can, in turn, alter or completely destroy the genetic information. This sort of disruption may occur in a gene that codes for a molecule that helps regulate cell division. When this happens, the result can be the uncontrolled cell growth and division that is the hallmark of cancer.

■ Applications and Research

Retroviral research has focused on understanding how the viruses infect cells, with the aim of blocking or even preventing the infection. Blocking the attachment of the virus to the host cell by binding an added molecule either to the viral protein involved in binding or to the target site on the host surface can prevent infection. Within the human body, this sequence is not as straightforward as it is in the laboratory, but progress is being made.

A powerful potential application of retroviruses involves their use as vehicles to get genes inside of other cells. This technique has been explored in gene therapy, where host genes can be disrupted or their activity increased, depending on the aim of the therapy. When the retroviral genetic material enters the host cell and, in turn, enters the host DNA, the target gene is also inserted. This can allow the target gene to be expressed. In another approach, the insertion of the retrovirus can disrupt a host gene. For example, insertion of the viral genetic material can disable a bacterial gene that codes for the manufacture of a destructive toxin. However, as discussed below, the trials of retroviral gene therapy in humans have been plagued with problems.

■ Impacts and Issues

Retroviruses that cause human diseases sickened and killed millions of people in the twentieth century alone. While the best known of these diseases is AIDS, other retroviruses cause paralysis, physical and mental deterioration, at least one type of muscular dystrophy, multiple sclerosis, and arthritis.

Multiple sclerosis and arthritis are examples of autoimmune diseases, in which the body's immune system malfunctions and reacts against it own tissues. There is evidence that such autoimmune diseases may be caused by inserted retroviral genetic material. The original insertion, which produced the genetic changes that underlie the immune difficulties, may have occurred thousands of years ago, with the inserted DNA being passed from generation to generation ever since. Studies have shown that this ancient retroviral genetic material makes up almost 10 percent of the human genome.

Retroviral diseases are global and affect people in wealthy and poorer nations. The consequences are particularly severe in developing countries, since these diseases can disrupt family life (since care for the afflicted person is necessary), and cause absences from school and the workplace that impair the national economies.

Retroviruses that are used in gene therapy are altered to cripple their ability to establish an infection in host cells. These disabled retroviruses are able to incorporate their genetic material into the host cell genome, but are not able to produce new viruses. These retroviruses have been used in disease therapy in animals. But retroviral gene therapy in humans is still experimental.

In 1999, 18-year-old Jesse Gelsinger died of multiple organ failure days after beginning retroviral gene therapy. A severe immune reaction to the retrovirus used is argued to have been responsible for his death. In 2003, the U.S. Food and Drug Administration banned gene therapy trials using retroviruses in a type of cells called blood stem cells. The ban continues as of 2007.

SEE ALSO *HIV; Pneumocystis carinii Pneumonia; Viral Disease.*

BIBLIOGRAPHY

Books

Lyon, Maureen, and Lawrence J. D'Angelo. *Teenagers, HIV, and AIDS: Insights from Youths Living with the Virus.* Washington, DC: Praeger Publishers, 2006.

Mader, Sylvia. *Biology.* 8th ed. New York: McGraw-Hill, 2003.

Whiteside, Alan. *HIV/AIDS: A Very Short Introduction.* Oxford: Oxford University Press, 2007.

Brian Hoyle

Rickettsial Disease

Introduction

Bacteria from the genus *Rickettsia* give rise to rickettsial diseases. These bacteria are transmitted from infected mammals to humans via arthropod vectors. Once the bacteria are in the body, they infect the cells lining blood vessels and cause cell death. This results in complications relating to the blood. There are numerous types of rickettsial diseases caused by different species of these bacteria. Common symptoms of rickettsial diseases include fever, headache, depression, and fatigue. In some cases, a rash forms on the body, either around the site of infection, or on random areas.

Rickettsial diseases occur worldwide. Some diseases remain limited to certain geographic regions, while others are present on almost all continents. The distribution of the arthropod that carries the infectious bacteria determines the distribution of the disease. Rickettsial diseases are generally treated with a course of antibiotics. However, delayed administration of treatment can lead to more serious illness, and even death. While no vaccine is available to prevent contracting rickettsial diseases, prevention is achieved by avoiding contact with arthropods. This involves using repellents or wearing protective clothing.

Disease History, Characteristics, and Transmission

Rickettsial diseases are caused by bacteria from the genus *Rickettsia*. These bacteria are named after Howard Taylor Ricketts (1871–1910) who died from typhus, one type of rickettsial disease. Rickettsial disease should not to be confused with another disease called rickets, which is caused by a deficiency of vitamin D.

Rickettsial bacteria cause illness in hosts by infecting the cells and causing cell destruction or death. They tend to infect vascular cells, that is, cells lining the blood vessels, and thus cell death leads to increased permeability of these vessels. This causes changes in blood volume, concentration, and pressure, which is debilitating for the host.

Rickettsial bacteria are present in arthropods and mammals. Transmission usually occurs when an arthropod feeds on an infected mammal, sometimes becoming the intermediate host, and then feeds on a human. Humans may also become infected if they come in direct contact with the blood or feces of an infected arthropod. One rickettsial disease, Q fever, is transmitted not by arthropods, but by airborne droplets containing the bacteria.

There are many different types of rickettsial diseases. The main types are grouped into the spotted fever group, the typhus group, or with scrub typhus. Most of the diseases share similar symptoms. In general, acute symptoms of fever, headache, depression, and fatigue occur within two weeks of exposure to a bacterium. A rash also often appears a few days after the onset of fever. This rash can appear on various regions of the body, as in Rocky Mountain spotted fever, or may occur specifically as skin lesions that develop at the site of the arthropod bite. Other complications of infection include blood vessel damage and organ damage, but these symptoms depend on the severity and type of infection.

Scope and Distribution

Rickettsial diseases occur worldwide. However, not all rickettsial diseases are present in all countries. Endemic (naturally occurring at a steady rate) and epidemic typhus occur worldwide, whereas North Asian tick typhus, Queensland tick typhus, and scrub typhus have particular distributions that limit them to certain locations. The distribution of rickettsial diseases is determined by the distribution of their arthropod vectors.

However, cases of specific rickettsial diseases sometimes occur in areas not known to harbor the bacterium. This is a consequence of travel. Travelers infected in one

WORDS TO KNOW

ARTHROPOD: A member of the largest single animal phylum, consisting of organisms with segmented bodies, jointed legs or wings, and exoskeletons.

INTERMEDIATE HOST: An organism infected by a parasite while the parasite is in a developmental form, not sexually mature.

VECTOR: Any agent, living or otherwise, that carries and transmits parasites and diseases. Also, an organism or chemical used to transport a gene into a new host cell.

country may not exhibit symptoms until they are in another country due to the long incubation period for these bacteria.

In the United States, endemic rickettsial diseases include Rocky Mountain spotted fever, rickettsial pox, and cat-flea transmitted infection. Rickettsial diseases tend to be less prevalent during modern times than when they were first discovered. This is most likely a result of both improved prevention methods and the introduction of effective treatments. However, despite effective treatments, some rickettsial diseases can still be fatal, including Rocky Mountain spotted fever, which has an approximate mortality rate of 4%, or epidemic typhus, which has a mortality rate of approximately 10% in young adults and 60–70% in older patients. In Rocky Mountain spotted fever a late diagnosis can lead to more serious complications, which contributes to higher mortality rates. In the case of epidemic typhus, increased age can decrease a patient's chance of survival.

■ Treatment and Prevention

Effective treatment of rickettsial disease is usually involves a course of antibiotics. The best results are achieved when treatment is administered within the first week of illness. The longer the illness goes without treatment, the less chance there is of a good recovery. Tetracycline antibiotics effectively destroy rickettsial bacteria and thus derivatives from this group are most often used for treatment. The preferred tetracycline is doxycycline, since it has few negative side effects when used for short periods in low doses. Another form of tetracycline used is chloramphenicol. For patients older than 18 years of age, fluoroquinolones may be used, and have been shown to be effective against some forms of rickettsial bacteria.

Antibiotic treatment usually takes less than a week. Fever generally disappears 1–3 days after treatment begins. If the fever does not begin to subside, misdiagnosis is likely. Once a patient no longer has a fever, treatment is stopped. Other treatment, based on treating the complications caused by the bacteria, such as hypotension, coagulation, and fluid leakage, is usually given with the antibiotics. This treatment usually lasts about two weeks.

Rickettsial diseases cannot yet be prevented by vaccination. Research is underway to determine a possible vaccination for certain infections. Currently, the best prevention method is avoidance or elimination of arthropod vectors in order to decrease the chance of being bitten. Avoidance measures include using repellents when outdoors, avoiding long grass or woodlands, wearing clothing that completely covers the arms and legs, wearing boots, and thoroughly checking the body after walking through arthropod-inhabited areas. Often, quick removal of ticks that have become attached to the body can prevent infection. Elimination of arthropod vectors involves using pesticides in arthropod-inhabited areas.

■ Impacts and Issues

One of the greatest issues surrounding rickettsial diseases is the impact that late diagnosis has on recovery. The treatments currently used for cases of rickettsial disease usually result in a successful recovery. However, the later treatment is given, the less chance there is of a good recovery. Late diagnosis may occur when patients do not visit their doctor, or when medical personnel misdiagnose the disease. Some types of rickettsial disease, such as Rocky Mountain spotted fever, sometimes feature a characteristic red rash. In the absence of this rash, the symptoms of this infection are similar to a multitude of other infections. Therefore, Rocky Mountain spotted fever may be misdiagnosed and the wrong treatment administered. Despite effective treatment for this disease, the mortality rate still stands at almost 4%, and this mortality rate is largely due to misdiagnosis and, thus, delayed administration of proper treatment.

SEE ALSO *Arthropod-borne Disease; Bacterial Disease; Host and Vector; Q Fever; Rocky Mountain Spotted Fever; Typhus; Zoonoses.*

BIBLIOGRAPHY

Books

Arguin, P.M., P.E. Kozarsky, and A.W. Navin. *Health Information for International Travel 2005–2006.*

Washington, DC: U.S. Department of Health and Human Services, 2005.

Beers, M.H. *The Merck Manual of Diagnosis and Therapy.* 18th ed. Whitehouse Station, NJ: Merck, 2006.

Mandell, G.L., J.E. Bennett, and R. Dolin. *Principles and Practice of Infectious Diseases.* 6th ed. Philadelphia: Elsevier, 2004.

Web Sites

Centers for Disease Control and Prevention. "Rocky Mountain Spotted Fever." May 20, 2005. <http://www.cdc.gov/ncidod/dvrd/rmsf/index.htm> (accessed March 7, 2007).

WebMD. "Rickettsial Infection." March 27, 2006. <http://www.emedicine.com/ped/topic2015.htm> (accessed March 7, 2007).

Rift Valley Fever

■ Introduction

Rift Valley fever (RVF) is a viral disease usually associated with outbreaks among livestock animals, but also affects humans. It is caused by a virus from the family *Bunyaviridae* and is endemic in areas of Africa, but can spread to surrounding regions.

The virus is passed to animals and humans via mosquitoes. The virus is naturally occurring in some mosquitoes and the highest incidence of infection is associated with periods of heavy rain and flooding when mosquito populations are at peak numbers. Mortality rates among animals are high, but typically only 1% of human cases prove fatal. Symptoms generally resolve within a week of illness onset and include fever, headache, and weakness. In some cases, complications occur including inflammation of the eyes, meningoencephalitis, and hemorrhagic fever.

There are currently no preventative treatments available. However, researchers are developing vaccines and treatments for the disease among humans and animals. Increasing evidence of human fatalities has led to Rift Valley

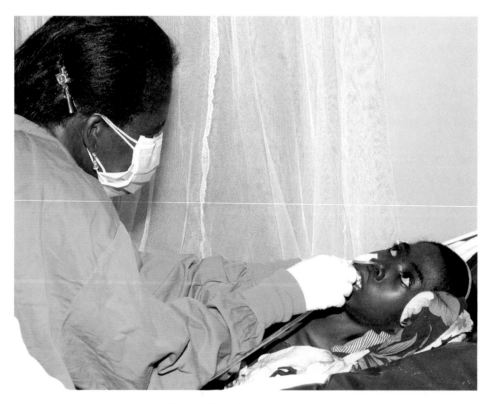

A nurse attends to a person with Rift Valley fever during an outbreak of the disease in Kenya in January 2007. *AP Images.*

710

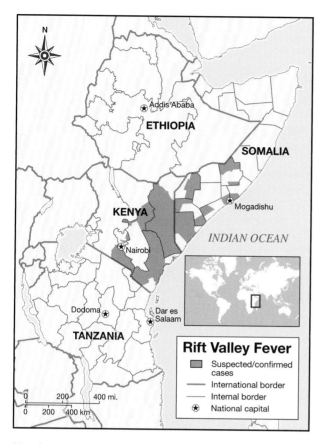

Map showing Rift Valley Fever outbreak in Kenya and Somalia, January 2007.   © *Copyright World Health Organization (WHO). Reproduced by permission.*

fever being termed an emerging virus and one that is considered to pose significant potential threat to communities.

Disease History, Characteristics, and Transmission

Rift Valley fever (RVF) is a viral disease primarily affecting domestic livestock (such as cattle, sheep, buffalo, goats, and camels), but one that can also be passed on to humans. The disease is caused by the RVF virus, which is a member of the genus *Phlebovirus* in the family Bunyaviridae. RVF was first reported among livestock in Kenya around 1915. The Rift Valley virus was first isolated in Kenya in 1931.

The Rift Valley fever virus is naturally occurring in some species of mosquitoes such as the *Aedes*. The virus may lay dormant in the eggs, which are capable of surviving for several years in dry conditions. During periods of heavy rain and flooding, these eggs will hatch and cause a significant increase in the mosquito population. The mosquitoes transfer the virus to the animals on which they feed. The disease can be transmitted to

humans via mosquitoes, or by exposure to the blood or organs of infected animals.

In humans, the virus is symptomatic in 90% of those infected. Incubation of the infection is usually 2 to 6 days, after which symptoms commonly present as a flulike illness including fever, headache, muscle pain, generalized weakness, dizziness, and weight loss. In less than 2% of cases, the illness progresses and develops into a severe form. In less than 2% of cases, eye disease occurs and involves ocular swelling and retinal inflammation. This can lead to permanent vision loss, including blindness. In less than 1% of cases, RVF leads to meningoencephalitis. The most severe complication is hemorrhagic fever, and this occurs in less than 1% of cases. The hemorrhagic fever complication is responsible for most RVF deaths, with around 50% of cases of hemorrhagic fever proving fatal.

Scope and Distribution

Rift Valley fever was initially limited to the regions of eastern and southern Africa where sheep and cattle are raised. Prior to 2000, RVF was limited to Africa. In late 2000, cases of Rift Valley occurred in Saudi Arabia and Yemen. This spread of the virus indicates a potential threat of the virus spreading further into Europe or Asia.

People at risk of contracting the disease include people in contact with animals such as animal herdsman, veterinarians, and abattoir (slaughterhouse) workers. Frequent exposure to mosquito bites in areas where outbreaks occur will also increase risk of contracting the virus. Travelers to areas where the Rift Valley fever virus is endemic are also under threat of infection, particularly during times of viral outbreak.

Epidemics are almost always associated with heavy rainfall periods and localized flooding, which creates breeding grounds for the mosquitoes. The first RVF outbreak was reported in Egypt in 1977–1978 where human infection rates in some parts were as high as 35% and 598 deaths resulted from hemorrhagic fever. An epidemic occurred in 1987 in West Africa due to flooding caused from construction of the Senegal River Project. In 1997, Kenya and Somalia suffered an epidemic that resulted in 300 human fatalities with much higher rates for livestock. In 2006, an epidemic occurred in Kenya following flooding.

Treatment and Prevention

Diagnosis of Rift Valley fever in humans is performed through laboratory blood analysis identifying antibodies to the virus. In the majority of cases, the causative agent is obvious due to the epidemic nature of outbreak. There is no treatment available for the infection except for supportive therapy for the symptoms. Researchers are investigating the potential for the use of an antiviral drug in humans. However, as of 2006, it is still in developmental stages.

WORDS TO KNOW

ENDEMIC: Present in a particular area or among a particular group of people.

EPIDEMIC: From the Greek *epidemic*, meaning "prevalent among the people," is most commonly used to describe an outbreak of an illness or disease in which the number of individual cases significantly exceeds the usual or expected number of cases in any given population.

EPIZOOTIC: The abnormally high occurrence of a specific disease in animals in a particular area, similar to a human epidemic.

Many animal vaccines have been developed to protect against RVF infection, but are often subject to limitation. One such vaccine was found to deliver immunity to mice for up to three years, but led to spontaneous abortion when administered to pregnant ewes. It was found that multiple doses of vaccines may be required to provide immunity. This would prove problematic in areas of endemicity where successful immunity would be subject to resource availability. Human vaccines are also under trial, but as of 2006, are in the early phases and require significant testing.

Preventative measures may be taken by people to avoid contracting the disease. These include reducing possible contact with mosquitoes. This may be achieved by wearing protective clothing such as long pants and long sleeved shirts in addition to the use of insect repellents and bed nets while sleeping. People in contact with animal blood or tissue can avoid infection by wearing gloves and other protective equipment.

■ Impacts and Issues

Rift Valley fever poses significant economical impacts on communities due to the fatality rates among livestock and the permanent threat of epidemics in certain areas. In an outbreak of RVF in Kenya in the 1950s, over 100,000 sheep were killed. This devastated the community and it took several years to recover. In pregnant livestock, infection by this virus results in abortion of almost all fetuses. This raises the issues of herd sustainability and growth. The mode of transmission of the Rift Valley fever virus makes it virtually impossible for farmers to protect their herds or themselves. With the natural occurrence of the virus in some mosquitoes, a rainy season or flood will almost certainly leave some communities devastated.

The complications associated with infection from RVF among humans can be quite severe and as such, this disease can also be considered a high risk. Spreading of the disease from Africa to Yemen and Saudi Arabia has raised concern that the disease could spread to new areas. It is considered that stock, mosquitoes, and travelers could all potentially act as carriers of the virus and introduce it into new regions. Various species of mosquitoes act as vectors for the RVF virus, suggesting that the virus could be maintained once in a new region. This may potentially cause animal and human epidemics.

In addition to being spread by mosquitoes, the virus can also be spread by aerosols. This suggests that the virus could be introduced to a new area and spread rapidly within the area. These concerns have led the United States to list Rift Valley fever as a significant biological warfare threat.

Rift Valley fever remains a health threat, especially in Africa's developing nations and at-risk areas following natural disasters. From December 2006 through February 2007, an epidemic of Rift Valley in Kenya fever killed 155 people. There were nearly 700 suspected cases associated with the outbreak. The epidemic hit most acutely in several regions already strained by severe flooding and food shortages. Health officials instituted a quarantine of animals and humans in disease-affected areas, but the disease spread across national borders, infecting 90 and killing 19 in neighboring Tanzania.

SEE ALSO *Airborne Precautions; Antiviral Drugs; Bioterrorism; Emerging Infectious Diseases; Viral Disease.*

BIBLIOGRAPHY

Books

Fong, I.W., and K. Alibek. *Bioterrorism and Infectious Agents: A New Dilemma for the 21st Century.* New York: Springer Science, 2005.

Mandell, G.L., J.E. Bennett, and R. Dolin. *Principles and Practice of Infectious Diseases.* Vol. 2. Philadelphia, PA: Elsevier, 2005.

Web Sites

Centers for Disease Control and Prevention (CDC). "Rift Valley Fever Fact Sheet." <http://www.cdc.gov/ncidod/dvrd/spb/mnpages/dispages/Fact_Sheets/Rift_Valley_Fever_Fact_Sheet.pdf> (accessed March 9, 2007).

Directors of Health Promotion and Education. "Rift Valley Fever." 2005 <http://www.dhpe.org/infect/rift.html> (accessed Mar. 9, 2007).

World Health Organization (WHO). "Rift Valley Fever." September, 2000 <http://www.who.int/mediacentre/factsheets/fs207/en/> (accessed March 9, 2007).

Ringworm

Introduction

Ringworm, also known medically as *Tinea* and dermatophytosis, is a group of contagious, very common cutaneous (skin) infections, which can also involve the scalp, hair, or nails. It is caused by various moldlike fungi called dermatophytes, which live on dead tissues of the body. Because many different fungi species cause ringworm, an infection with one species will not make a person immune to infection from other species.

Moist areas of the body such as the groin, between the toes, and in the armpits are generally infected the most frequently. The infected area often looks inflamed and feels itchy. These symptoms are caused by sensitivity to the fungus or by a secondary bacterial infection. Ringworm, in its most serious forms, causes an acute infection with blisters on the feet or lesions on the scalp.

Disease History, Characteristics, and Transmission

The most common symptom of ringworm is flat, nearly round lesions. They may be dry and scaly, or moist and crusty. Eventually, they turn red and become extended, itchy bumps with edges that blister and secrete fluid. As the infection continues, the color sometimes becomes nearly clear in the center and redder on the outside. This pattern causes the patch to look ringlike in appearance, which gives ringworm its common name.

The incubation period is generally not known. However, ringworm of the scalp (*tinea capitis*) usually appears 10–14 days after contact and ringworm of the body (*tinea corporis*) usually appears in 4–10 days.

Ringworm infection is most often spread during human-skin-to-human-skin contact. It becomes contagious to another person even before the infection is evident on the first person. Ringworm is sometimes spread when humans touch infected cats and dogs; when humans care for other domestic animals such as cows and pigs; and when humans touch contaminated clothes, towels, hairbrushes, combs, headgear (such as hats), or other infected objects.

The most contagious form—ringworm of the scalp—is seen primarily in children. Symptoms include growing pimples, itching of scalp, and breaking off of hair. The scalp may temporarily become bald in patches.

Ringworm can also occur on the arms, legs, and trunk. It causes raised, round patches on the skin. The inner parts heal first, while the outer parts further spread the infection. When ringworm infection reaches other areas of the body, such as the armpit and groin, the shape

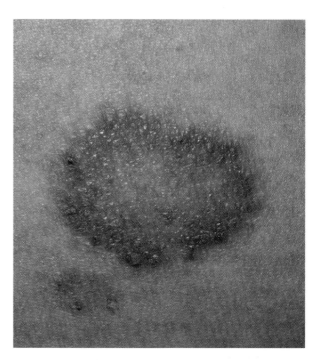

A characteristic ringworm rash, caused by a fungal infection of the skin, is shown on a woman's abdomen. *Dr P. Marazzi/Photo Researchers, Inc.*

IN CONTEXT: CULTURAL CONNECTIONS

Ringworm-causing fungi affect various parts of the body and give rise to alternative names and conditions. In the scalp ring worm is known as *tinea capitis*, on the body, ringworm is known as *tinea corporis*). In the groin region ringworm is known as *tinea cruris*, more commonly called "jock itch," and on the feet ringworm is known as *tinea pedis*, more commonly known as athlete's foot.

Over one million children (about 0.3% of the 2006 population) are infected with scalp ringworm annually in the United States. It is a highly contagious, and the number of children infected each year is increasing. Ringworm of the scalp represents over 90% of all skin fungal infections in U.S. children aged ten years or younger. About 7% of the U.S. population suffers from ringworm of the scalp. It is most frequently caught in overcrowded conditions such as medical facilities, nursing homes, and educational institutions. Elderly people and people with weak immune systems are at increased risk for acquiring ringworm because of their susceptibility to infections.

Jock itch and athlete's foot are important economically because they are targets of several commercial products and generate millions of dollars in advertising revenues spent to market the over-the-counter products designed to fight the fungal infections.

often changes to resemble butterfly wings or it may be completely irregular in shape. The condition is called *tinea cruris*, or jock itch, when it affects the groin area.

The fingernails and toenails may also be infected. This condition is called *tinea unguium*. When this happens, the nails become yellowish, thickened, and deformed. They may crumble and fall off. When the infection spreads to the feet, ringworm is often called athlete's foot (*tinea pedis*). When ringworm affects facial hair it is called *tinea*

barbae; when it affects the face, *tinea faciei*; and when it affects hands and palms, *tinea manuum*.

■ Scope and Distribution

Ringworm can occur almost anywhere in the world. Because the fungi that cause *tinea cruris* and *tinea pedis* thrive in moist and humid areas, they occur most frequently in the tropical and subtropical areas of the world.

■ Treatment and Prevention

Doctors often identify ringworm visually. If not recognizable, it is often diagnosed by scraping off or plucking some material from the infected area. The sample is examined under a microscope to confirm the presence of fungal growth. Ringworm of the scalp is diagnosed with an ultraviolet light under which the fungus appears to be a bright, yellowish green color.

Ringworm treatment includes topical antifungal medications. Common antifungal creams, lotions, or powders that contain miconazole, econazole, or clotrimazole are often used either by prescription or over-the-counter.

Infected children are sometimes isolated from others, especially other children, to prevent further spreading of the infection. Griseofulvin is commonly used to treat animals and humans. It usually eliminates the infection, but side effects can be pronounced. Undecylenic acid is sometimes used as a fungicide. Antibiotics may be necessary to cure bacterial infections.

According to the Mayo Clinic, although ringworm is unpleasant, it is not serious except for people with weak immune systems. Ringworm usually resolves itself without a visit to the doctor within four weeks. Bed linens and pajamas should be washed daily. A person should seek medical treatment if the infection becomes severe or persistent. Antifungal drugs, including fluconazole, itraconazole, ketoconazole, and terbinafine, are sometimes taken by mouth for persistent infections.

The National Institutes of Health recommends a variety of measures to prevent ringworm including:

- Shampoo hair regularly, especially after it is cut.
- Wear shoes in shower stalls, gym locker rooms, pools, and other moist areas.
- Keep skin and feet clean and dry.
- Do not share personal care items or items of apparel, such as towels, hairbrushes, shoes, or hats.
- Avoid touching pets or other domestic animals that have bald spots.

■ Impacts and Issues

Anyone can get ringworm. Children are more susceptible to certain types of ringworm fungi, while other types occur equally in all age groups. Children become more susceptible to ringworm when they are malnourished, live in a warm climate, practice poor hygiene, come into contact other children or pets with ringworm, or have weak immune systems due to medicines or disease. Complications of ringworm include spreading the infection to other areas than the initial site; bacterial skin infections; skin irritations, such as contact dermatitis; and side effects from drugs used for treatment.

SEE ALSO *Mycotic Disease.*

BIBLIOGRAPHY

Books

Brock, David. *Infectious Fungi.* Philadelphia: Chelsea House Publishers, 2006.

Yosipovitch, Gil, et al., eds. *Itch: Basic Mechanisms and Therapy.* Oxford: Taylor & Francis, 2004.

Periodicals

Weinstein, A. "Topical Treatment of Common Superficial Tinea Infections." *American Family Physician.* 65 (May 15, 2002): 2095–2102.

Web Sites

Mayo Clinic. "Ringworm of the Body." October 4, 2006. <http://www.mayoclinic.com/health/ringworm/DS00489/DSECTION=1> (accessed March 22, 2007).

MedlinePlus. "Ringworm." June 16, 2005. <http://www.nlm.nih.gov/medlineplus/ency/article/001439.htm> (accessed March 28, 2007).

River Blindness (Onchocerciasis)

Introduction

Onchocerciasis (on-kough-sir-KY-A-sis) is caused by a type of parasitic worm called a helminth and occurs mainly in Africa. The worms are spread by the bite of infected black flies, which live mainly near fast-running rivers and streams. Hence, the alternative name—river blindness—for the condition.

Once they have invaded the body, the worms reproduce and millions of microscopic offspring migrate to the eye. When they die, the toxic effects cause severe and chronic inflammation of the cornea and related areas of the eye that lead to loss of vision. The threat of river blindness led to mass migration of people in West Africa away from areas infested with the black fly. This had severe economic consequences, since they settled in less productive upland areas. Fortunately, the anti-parasitic drug ivermectin can be used to treat river blindness. Mass treatment programs have decreased the burden of river blindness in recent years.

Disease History, Characteristics, and Transmission

River blindness, known clinically as oncocerciasis, is caused by a tiny parasitic worm called *Onchocerca volvulus*. The vector of the disease is a black fly belonging to the *Simulium* genus. These flies breed near fast moving rivers and streams in the savannas and rainforests in several African countries. Therefore, people living in such areas are prone to infection. The incubation time of the parasite varies between nine and 24 months.

River blindness does not always cause any symptoms. But the parasitic worms, known as microfiliae, may accumulate in characteristic nodules under the skin. Dermatitis, with severe itching, is common and the skin may become wrinkled and thickened. The resulting disfigurement is sometimes called "leopard" or "lizard" skin. More seriously, the parasites may migrate to the eyes. The microfiliae have been found in all parts of the eye except the lens and, when they die, they cause toxic effects, such as inflammation and bleeding, which can ultimately lead to blindness.

Transmission of river blindness occurs when someone is bitten by an infected black fly. This introduces the parasitic worms in a larval form under the skin where they mature. Then the mature female worm releases millions of microfiliae, which migrate towards the eyes. The microfiliae may also move to the surface of the skin, where they may be ingested by other black flies, which may go on and bite someone else, thereby spreading the infection.

Unlike malaria, which can be transmitted by just a single mosquito bite, it usually takes several black fly bites to transmit river blindness. The intensity of infection in an individual depends upon the number of microfiliae they are carrying, which, in turn, depends upon how many bites they have sustained. Blindness usually occurs in people with intense infection.

Scope and Distribution

River blindness is the second leading cause of preventable blindness worldwide. (Trachoma is the leading cause of blindness.) According to the World Health Organization (WHO), around 120 million people worldwide are at risk of river blindness. There are nearly 18 million actual cases of the disease, with about 270,000 cases of blindness and 6.5 million cases of severe itching and dermatitis resulting. The vast majority of these cases occur in Africa, with the remainder occurring in Yemen and in Central and South America.

In Africa, 30 countries in equatorial West, Central, and East Africa are affected by river blindness—areas where there are the fast-running rivers and streams frequented by *Simulium* black flies. In Central and South America, the affected countries are Mexico, Guatemala, Ecuador, Colombia, and Venezuela. Because infection

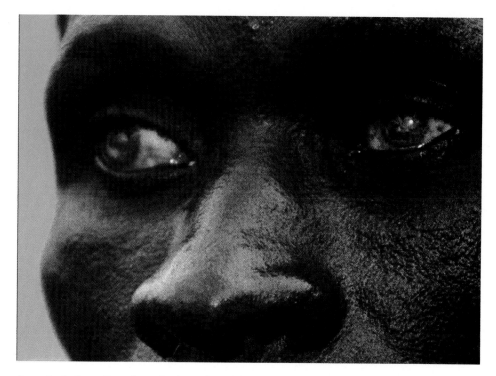

A man in the Ivory Coast shows the signs of river blindness. The disease causes an expressionless stare of the eyes, which is referred to as "dead eyes" or *Mara* ("the look of the lion") in the Malinke dialect.   *AP Images.*

with river blindness normally requires several bites, it is the populations of these countries, rather than visitors, who are most affected. However, there have been cases among adventure travelers, missionaries, and Peace Corps volunteers.

■ Treatment and Prevention

The oral anti-parasitic drug ivermectin is effective against the microfilariae, but is less effective against the adult worms. An annual dose, for two years, should clear the infection and relieve dermatitis as well as prevent blindness. Previously, the drug diethylcarbamazine was used, but this drug has severe side effects and the WHO no longer recommends it.

There are no vaccines against river blindness. Insecticides can help control black flies in areas where river blindness is a problem. The flies bite during the day and those at risk should wear long sleeved shirts and pants to avoid being bitten.

■ Impacts and Issues

Blindness has a profound impact on someone's earning capacity and quality of life. River blindness has therefore proved a severe obstacle to socioeconomic development in many African countries. According to the WHO, in the 1970s, around 50% of all men under the age of 40 in

some West African communities had been blinded by onchocerciasis. This caused migration away from fertile river valleys infested by black fly to less productive upland country. The resulting economic losses were around $30 million.

Clearly the world had to take action to halt the economic and social toll of river blindness in the world's poorest countries. Over the last 30 years, there have been various coordinated efforts to control the disease. In 1974, the Oncocerciasis Control Program (OCP) began in West Africa. This program was based on vector control—treating the breeding sites of the black fly with larvicides, that is, insecticides that kill fly larvae. The OCP expanded over the next several years to cover many river systems in seven countries, and it eventually doubled in size to cover 11 countries. The program ended in 2002, by which time river blindness had been virtually eliminated as a public health problem in 11 West African countries.

In 1989, a second strategy was added, involving the distribution of drugs to treat river blindness. Then, in the mid-1990s, the African Program for Oncocerciasis (APOC) began, with the aim of covering a further 19 countries, which comprised the rest of Africa affected by river blindness. In these countries, vector spraying was not a viable option because of environmental conditions. Therefore APOC is based upon the distribution of ivermectin, donated by Merck & Co, the company that discovered the drug. To date, the APOC has protected

WORDS TO KNOW

HELMINTH: A representative of various phyla of worm-like animals.

MICROFILIAE: Live offspring produced by adult nematodes within the host's body.

VECTOR: Any agent, living or otherwise, that carries and transmits parasites and diseases. Also, an organism or chemical used to transport a gene into a new host cell.

more than 600,000 people from blindness and reclaimed more than 61 million acres (25 million hectares) of previously infested land for resettlement and agricultural cultivation.

APOC is based in Burkina Faso, in West Africa, and aims to eliminate oncocheriasis throughout the African continent. It works by placing communities themselves at the heart of ivermectin distribution, supported by a number of partners, such as international agencies and national governments. It is financed by voluntary contributions via The World Bank and run by the WHO. APOC aims to prevent one million cases of blindness each year and hopes to achieve its goals by the year 2010. The program may also be a model for other health care interventions in developing countries.

Meanwhile, oncocheriasis is also covered by the WHO initiative, VISION 2020: The Right to Sight, which aims to eliminate preventable blindness worldwide by the year 2020. It is a partnership between the WHO and the International Agency for the Prevention of Blindness (IAPB), a coalition of eye-care professional groups and nongovernmental organizations involved in eye care. The initiative grew from the positive experience of APOC, recognizing that river blindness is just one of five preventable conditions causing 75% of cases of blindness. The other four are cataracts, refractive errors and low vision, trachoma, and a group of conditions that cause childhood blindness. Poor communities are disproportionately affected by these conditions, and there is a cost-effective solution for each of them. The strategy of VISION 2020 is to bring these solutions to as many people as possible.

SEE ALSO *Developing Nations and Drug Delivery; Economic Development and Infectious Disease; Parasitic Diseases; Trachoma.*

BIBLIOGRAPHY

Books

Wilson, Walter R., and Merle A. Sande. *Current Diagnosis & Treatment in Infectious Diseases.* New York: McGraw Hill, 2001.

Web Sites

Centers for Disease Control and Prevention. "Oncocerciasis (River Blindness)." September 27, 2004. <http://www.cdc.gov/ncidod/dpd/parasites/onchocerciasis/factsht_onchocerciasis.htm> (accessed April 20, 2007).

The World Bank. "Defeating Onchocerciasis (Riverblindness) in Africa." <http://www.worldbank.org/afr/gper/defeating.htm> (accessed April 22, 2007).

World Health Organization. "Magnitude and Causes of Visual Impairment." November 2004. <http://www.who.int/mediacentre/factsheets/fs282/en/> (accessed April 22, 2007).

Susan Aldridge

Rocky Mountain Spotted Fever

■ Introduction

Rocky Mountain spotted fever is a bacterial disease caused by *Rickettsia rickettsii*. This bacterium causes holes in blood vessels, which allows to blood leak into tissues and organs, causing damage to these areas. Humans become infected with Rocky Mountain spotted fever following a bite from an infected tick. Infection can also occur following contact with the blood or feces of infected ticks. Rocky Mountain spotted fever is present in most of the United States and has a yearly infection rate of about 800 cases. It is also found in some regions in South America. Similar strains of *Rickettsia* bacteria cause spotted fevers worldwide.

This disease usually results in fever, nausea, vomiting, headache, muscle aches, lack of appetite, diarrhea, abdominal pains, and, in some cases, a characteristic red rash. While recovery is likely for patients who receive early treatment, delayed treatment can result in complications, including death. Treatment involves a course of antibiotics for the duration of the fever. Since there is no vaccine available, the best prevention method is avoidance of ticks. This reduces the chance that a tick bite will lead to transmission of *R. rickettsii*.

■ Disease History, Characteristics, and Transmission

Rocky Mountain spotted fever was first identified as a tick-borne bacterial disease by Howard T. Ricketts

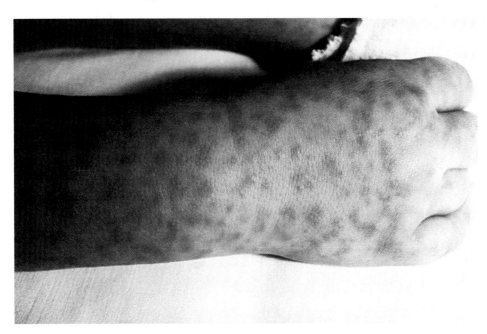

A child's right hand and wrist display the characteristic rash of Rocky Mountain spotted fever. The most severe and frequently reported rickettsial illness in the United States, the disease is caused by *Rickettsia rickettsii*, a species of bacteria that is spread to humans by ticks. *Science Source.*

WORDS TO KNOW

ACARACIDES: A chemical that kills mites and ticks is an acaracide.

TICK: A tick is any blood-sucking parasitic insect of suborder *Ixodides*, superfamily *Ixodoidea*. Ticks can transmit a number of diseases, including Lyme disease and Rocky Mountain spotted fever.

VECTOR: Any agent, living or otherwise, that carries and transmits parasites and diseases. Also, an organism or chemical used to transport a gene into a new host cell.

(1871–1910) shortly before his death. Prior to its identification, this disease was first recognized in 1896 in the Snake River Valley of Idaho where it affected hundreds of people and was often fatal. Although it was first found in the Rocky Mountains, this disease occurs all over the United States, except for Hawaii, Vermont, Maine, and Alaska. Rocky Mountain spotted fever is a potentially fatal disease, and prior to 1940, had a mortality rate of 30%. This rate decreased to 3–5% following introduction of an effective antibiotic treatment.

Rocky Mountain spotted fever is caused by the bacterium *Rickettsia rickettsii*. Infection occurs when a tick vector bites an infected animal and then bites a human. Infection can also occur if human skin is contaminated with tick blood or feces. The most common ticks to spread this infection to humans are the American dog tick (*Dermacentor variabilis*) and the Rocky Mountain wood tick (*Dermacentor andersoni*). *R. rickettsii* lives and reproduces within cells lining blood vessels. The bacteria cause cell death, which leads to gaps forming in the surface of the blood vessel. Blood leaks through these gaps into surrounding tissue and causes tissue and organ damage. Blood leakage also causes a red rash that is present in some cases.

Various symptoms may arise over the course of a week. Initial symptoms include fever, nausea, vomiting, headache, muscle aches, and lack of appetite. A faint rash may also appear within 2–5 days after fever. Later symptoms include abdominal pain, joint pain, and diarrhea. In addition, usually around six days after the onset of fever, a red, spotted rash occurs in 35–60% of patients. Complications can arise in patients suffering severe cases when the respiratory, central nervous, gastrointestinal, and renal systems are affected. Long-term effects of Rocky Mountain spotted fever can include paralysis, amputation of limbs due to gangrene, loss of hearing

and bowel or bladder control, and development of movement disorders.

Scope and Distribution

Rocky Mountain spotted fever occurs in almost all regions of the United States. It is dominant in the south-Atlantic regions, particularly in North Carolina. This fever also occurs in South America, particularly in Argentina, Brazil, Colombia, Costa Rica, Panama and, also, in Mexico. Bacterial strains (types) closely related to *Rickettsia rickettsii* also cause spotted fevers worldwide. The type of *Rickettsia* bacterium present in a region determines which type of spotted fever occurs in the area.

In the United States, the Centers for Disease Control and Prevention (CDC) recorded 250–1,200 cases of Rocky Mountain spotted fever annually from 1955 to 2005. This fever predominantly occurs during warm weather when ticks are more active. The summer months in the United States, from April through to September, mark the highest levels of infection throughout the year.

All people can potentially contract Rocky Mountain spotted fever. However, males, Caucasians, and children are infected most often. Increased exposure to ticks increases the likelihood of infection. Therefore, people who live with dogs or people who reside near tick-inhabited areas, such as woodlands, are at risk of infection.

Treatment and Prevention

A course of antibiotics is used to treat Rocky Mountain spotted fever. Doxycycline is recommended by the CDC as an effective drug to eradicate this infection. However, for pregnant women, chloramphenicol should be used as an alternative to doxycycline, since doxycycline is associated with the risk for malformations of the teeth and bones in unborn children. Treatment administered immediately provides the best results. Fever usually subsides within 1–3 days following antibiotic treatment given within 4–5 days after the onset of the disease. However, recovery from fever will take longer in patients who receive treatment later, or who are suffering a severe illness.

There is no vaccine available for Rocky Mountain spotted fever. Therefore, the best prevention method is to avoid contact with ticks. This can be achieved in several ways. Areas inhabited by ticks, such as long grasslands and woodlands, may be avoided. If these areas can't be avoided, repellents on clothing or skin can help repel ticks and prevent them from biting. In addition, protective clothing, such as long-sleeved shirts, boots, and hats, can be worn to prevent ticks coming in contact with the skin. It is also important to thoroughly check the body for ticks following any activity in tick habitats. This may prevent ticks from biting, or, in the cases when ticks have already attached to the skin, will ensure early removal and reduce the chances of infection.

Large-scale prevention methods include the use of acaricides (insecticides that kill ticks) in tick-infested areas in order to reduce the number of ticks. If there are fewer ticks in an area, it is less likely that humans will be bitten.

■ Impacts and Issues

Rocky Mountain spotted fever is a potentially life-threatening disease. Late diagnosis and delayed treatment increase the chances of complications, such as kidney failure and even death. As this disease infects approximately 800 people a year in the United States and is potentially fatal, increased awareness and reminders about prevention are recommended by the Directors of Health Promotion and Education.

This disease can be difficult to diagnose during the initial stages due to its wide range of symptoms and the fact that not all cases exhibit the characteristic red rash. This is a problem, since late diagnosis increases the chances of severe complications and possible fatalities. To address this problem, treatment is usually given before conclusive evidence confirms the disease. This approach ensures that patients with the disease receive treatment as soon as possible.

Despite prevention methods, such as the use of aracicides, the wearing of protective clothing, and the use of repellents, ticks can still come in contact with humans. When people find ticks on their bodies, removal is vital, and the earlier it is done, the less chance there is of infection. However, incorrect removal of ticks can cause complications. If the mouthparts of the tick remain in the body, infection can still occur. Furthermore, handling ticks with bare hands also increases the risk of exposure as infection can occur when blood or feces come in contact with open skin. The best technique for removing a tick involves grabbing the tick with tweezers as close to the skin as possible and pulling it away from the skin. Coating ticks with petroleum jelly or burning them with a match are not effective techniques for tick removal, despite the popularity of these methods with the general public.

SEE ALSO *Bacterial Disease; Rickettsial Disease; Zoonoses.*

BIBLIOGRAPHY

Books

Mandell, G. L., J. E. Bennett, and R. Dolin. *Principles and Practice of Infectious Diseases.* 6th ed. Philadelphia: Elsevier, 2004.

Periodicals

Parola, P., C. D. Paddock, and D. Raoult. "Tick-Borne Rickettsioses Around the World: Emerging Diseases Challenging Old Concepts." *Clinical Microbiology Reviews* 18 (October 2005): 719–756. Also available online at <http://cmr.asm.org/cgi/content/full/18/4/719>.

Web Sites

Centers for Disease Control and Prevention. "Rocky Mountain Spotted Fever." May 20, 2005. <http://www.cdc.gov/ncidod/dvrd/rmsf/index.htm> (accessed March 6, 2007).

Directors of Health Promotion and Education. "Rocky Mountain Spotted Fever." <http://www.astdhpphe.org/infect/rms.html> (accessed March 6, 2007).

Illinois Department of Public Health. "Rocky Mountain Spotted Fever." <http://www.idph.state.il.us/public/hb/hbrmsf.htm> (accessed March 6, 2007).

Rotavirus Infection

■ Introduction

Rotavirus is one of the primary causes of gastroenteritis among children around the world and the most common cause of severe diarrhea. There are approximately 130 million cases worldwide annually and over 500,000 deaths. In the United States, about 55,000 children are hospitalized each year due to gastroenteritis caused by rotavirus.

There are eleven different strains of rotavirus, of which four are known to cause diarrhea in humans. The disease has an incubation period of up to two days, after which symptoms such as fever, stomach ache, vomiting, and diarrhea appear. The disease is usually self-limiting within eight days. However, dehydration is a severe complication and may prove fatal if untreated.

Rotavirus is very stable in the environment and while transmission usually occurs through ingestion of fecally contaminated food or water, people may also become infected following contact with contaminated surfaces, such as toys and benches. Prior infection by rotavirus may reduce the severity of subsequent infections and, due to this fact, trials of a vaccine are being conducted. It is thought that this vaccine could lessen the impact of infection among children and significantly reduce mortality rates around the world.

■ Disease History, Characteristics, and Transmission

Rotavirus is the causative agent for most cases of gastroenteritis among children globally. It was first shown to cause diarrhea in 1972 and was named the following year based on the wheel-like appearance of the virus. Of the several strains identified, Group A is associated with childhood gastroenteritis, while Groups B and C most often occur in adults. The disease is also called infantile diarrhea and winter diarrhea because outbreaks most commonly occur in infants and during the cooler months of winter.

Symptoms usually appear within 48 hours of infection and include fever, abdominal cramping, vomiting, and watery diarrhea, lasting up to eight days. Chronic conditions may result in severe fluid loss leading to dehydration, which is a common complication associated with gastroenteritis. Signs of dehydration include dry lips, a dry tongue, dry skin, and sunken eyes. While dehydration is readily treatable, it is responsible for the fatalities associated with infections of this kind.

Rotavirus infections are highly contagious and are transmitted via the fecal-oral route. The highest incidence is among infants and children, where good hygiene is difficult to maintain. Following ingestion, the viral particles imbed in the mucosal layers of the small intestine and may be passed in excretions. The virus is very stable in the environment and infection may result from ingestion of contaminated food and water or from contact with contaminated surfaces, such toys or tables. Prior infection does not produce complete immunity, but subsequent infections are usually less severe than the primary infection.

■ Scope and Distribution

Rotavirus is responsible for an estimated 130 million cases of diarrhea worldwide annually and over 500,000 deaths. In the United States, over 3 million cases occur annually and over 55,000 children are hospitalized as a result. The availability of health care makes fatal cases of rotavirus rare in the United States.

The ability of the virus to persist in the environment enhances the threat of infection among all societies. In the United States, the disease is usually seen in the winter with annual epidemics most often occurring between the months of November and April. In developing nations, the virus circulates all year as a result of poorer access to clean water and health care. Outbreaks

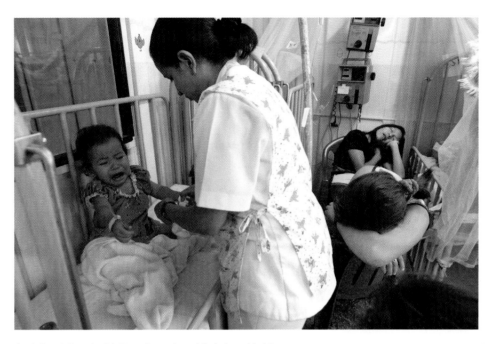

An infant infected with Rotavirus cries while being aided by a nurse.   *AP Images.*

are common due to the way in which the virus is transmitted and to the fact that contamination of a major water source often results in infection for everyone using that supply.

The highest rates of infection occur among infants and children. In developed nations, rotavirus is most likely to occur before a child's second birthday. Children between the ages of 6 and 24 months who attend day care are at higher risk for rotavirus infection. This is due to the fact that these locations commonly harbor diseases transmitted by the fecal-oral route, and the fact that it is difficult to ensure the maintenance of good hygiene practices, such as handwashing, at this young age.

Adults tend not to develop the disease and adults in contact with the virus typically only develop a mild infection. Most instances of adult infection occur in elderly people and those with compromised immunity, such as transplant patients, chemotherapy patients, and people with human immunodeficiency virus (HIV).

■ Treatment and Prevention

In persons with intact immunity, the infection is self-limiting and symptoms will resolve within a few days of onset. While there is no specific treatment for the infection itself, oral rehydration therapy is essential and acts to restore the fluid lost as a result of severe dehydration. In developed countries, electrolyte and fluid replacement solutions are readily available over-the-counter, although serious cases of dehydration may require hospitalization for intravenous treatment. Substantial rehydration options are much more limited in developing nations and, in cases

of contaminated water supply, drinking the contaminated water further contributes to the infection rather than helping to treat the symptoms of the infection.

The environmental stability of rotavirus means that basic hygiene is often not enough to prevent infection. Improvements in food, water, and sanitation do not often reduce disease incidence, although they may be employed to limit the spread of the infection. In day care settings, monitoring children to ensure that they are correctly washing hands after toilet use and during food preparation can reduce the spread of the disease.

A combined vaccine of all four strains of rotavirus known to cause severe gastroenteritis was approved for use in 1998. However, the vaccine was later withdrawn due to potentially fatal side effects involving blocking or twisting of the intestine. In 2006, the U.S. Food and Drug Administration approved a vaccine for use in the United States. A second vaccine was approved for use in Europe in 2006. The Rotavirus Vaccine Program (RVP) was established in 2003 by PATH with the support of the World Health Organization and the Centers for Disease Control and Prevention. The goal of RVP is to make the vaccines available in developing countries.

■ Impacts and Issues

Rotavirus is responsible for 20–70% of hospitalizations and up to 800,000 of the 3 million deaths per year from diarrhea in developing nations. Within these communities of limited resources, these infections almost always result in severe symptoms and carry a significant mortality rate.

WORDS TO KNOW

DEHYDRATION: Dehydration is the loss of water and salts essential for normal body function. It occurs when the body loses more fluid than it takes in. Water is very important to the human body because it makes up about 70% of the muscles, around 75% of the brain, and approximately 92% of the blood. A person who weights about 150 pounds (68 kilograms) will contain about 80 quarts (just over 75 liters) of water. About two cups of water are lost each day just from regular breathing. If the body sweats more and breathes heavier than normal, the human body loses even more water. Dehydration occurs when that lost water is not replenished.

FECAL-ORAL ROUTE: The transmission of minute particles of fecal material from one organism (human or animal) to the mouth of another organism.

REHYDRATION: Dehydration is excessive loss of water from the body; rehydration is the restoration of water after dehydration.

STRAIN: A subclass or a specific genetic variation of an organism.

In developed countries, the fatalities associated with rotavirus infection are significantly lower, with only around 100 of the 3 million cases resulting in death. However, in these areas, the rate of infection is still quite high and therefore poses other issues for communities. The economic impact of the disease is significant, since infected children account for over 500,000 physician visits, over 50,000 hospitalizations, and an estimated $300 million in medical costs each year.

Recognition of the impacts associated with diarrhea caused by rotavirus led to extensive research to develop vaccines against this disease. The development of the vaccine against rotavirus is expected to reduce the incidence and severity of rotavirus infections in developed countries. However, the successful development of a vaccine brings with it numerous issues regarding not only affordability, but also availability to communities in developing countries. Immunization at a cost of $10–20 per dose may be cost effective in industrialized countries, but is generally impractical in developing nations where per capita health care expenditure is less. This suggests that the global defense against rotavirus infection will require the cooperation of national governments and international agencies.

SEE ALSO *Childhood Infectious Diseases, Immunization Impacts; Handwashing; Vaccines and Vaccine Development; Viral Disease; Water-borne Disease.*

BIBLIOGRAPHY

Books

Mandell, G.L., J.E. Bennett, and R. Dolin. *Principles and Practice of Infectious Diseases.* 6th ed. Philadelphia: Elsevier, 2004.

Periodicals

World Health Organization. "Rotavirus Vaccines." *Weekly Epidemiological Record* 81 (January 6, 2006): 8 Also available online at: <http://www.who.int/wer/2006/wer8101.pdf> (accessed May 10, 2007).

Web Sites

Centers for Disease Control and Prevention. "Rotavirus Home Page." March 26, 2007. <http://www.cdc.gov/rotavirus/> (accessed May 10, 2007).

National Institute of Allergy and Infectious Disease (NIAID). "Rotavirus Vaccine: Preventing Severe Diarrheal Disease in Infants." May 25, 1999 <http://www.niaid.nih.gov/Publications/discovery/rotav.htm> (accessed March 12, 2007).

Rotavirus Vaccine Program (RVP). "About RVP." 2007. <http://www.rotavirusvaccine.org/about.htm> (accessed March 12, 2007).

Roundworm (Ascariasis) Infection

Introduction

Ascariasis (as-kuh-RYE-uh-sis), or roundworm infection, is an infection caused by the parasitic helminth, or roundworm *Ascaris lumbricoides*. It is considered to be the largest roundworm that infects the intestines of humans. *A. lumbricoides* infects humans and other mammals when embryonated eggs are ingested with contaminated food or water.

The parasite, which is commonly called the giant intestinal roundworm, can grow up to a length of 6–12 in (15–30 cm) by a diameter of 0.12–0.32 in (0.3–0.8 cm) in males and 8–14 in (20–35 cm) by 0.2 in (0.5 cm) in females. The embryonated eggs are the infectious part of the disease.

It is estimated that up to one-fourth of the world's population is infected with the roundworm *A. lumbricoides*. The National Institutes of Health (NIH) estimates that, generally, over one billion people are infected worldwide, with children being affected more seriously and more frequently than adults.

Disease History, Characteristics, and Transmission

Infection occurs via the fecal-oral route, most often when contaminated food is eaten that contains fertilized eggs within fecal material. The larvae hatch and burrow into the moist lining (mucosa) of the intestines. They then travel to the lungs where they further mature—usually for 10 to 14 days. They eventually travel through the respiratory tract and up into the throat where they are swallowed and sent to the small intestines. They mature as worms while attached to the walls of the small intestines.

A mature female can produce about 200,000 eggs per day. Roundworms live approximately one to two years. The time from egg ingestion to egg egression with feces is between two and three months. Upon egress from a host, the eggs become infectious within 18 days

to several weeks—with the range dependent on soil conditions such as temperature.

Symptoms are usually few, and sometimes not even evident, especially when the worms are immature and small. Noticeable symptoms usually occur between four and 16 days of ingestion. Common symptoms include diarrhea, fever, inflammation, wheezing, and nonproductive cough. Other serious problems develop whenever the worms live within the lungs (pulmonary symptoms) or throughout the body (neurological disorders). The final symptoms are gastrointestinal distress, nausea, vomiting, fever, nutritional insufficiencies, peritonitis (inflammation of abdominal wall), enlargement of the liver or spleen, and observation of live worms in stools. In rare cases, worms may obstruct the intestines, cause pneumonitis (inflammation of the lungs), or cause eosinophilia (increase in white blood cells).

Humans become infected by direct contact of the worms to skin and through the ingestion of soil and vegetation that contain fecal matter contaminated with eggs. Transmission can also occur when wastewater is recycled onto crop fields as fertilizer—a practice that is common in developing countries.

Scope and Distribution

Roundworm infection is found throughout the world, but especially in tropical regions and among the poorest areas with the worst of hygiene conditions. It is pronounced along the rural areas of the Gulf Coast within the United States; in Africa, especially Nigeria; and in Southeast Asia, especially Indonesia. About 2 percent of people in the United States are estimated to be infected with roundworms. High-risk groups include visitors and travelers to third-world countries.

Treatment and Prevention

The diagnosis is easily made when the infected person actually observes worms in his/her stool or vomit. If that does not happen, stool samples can be taken to medically

WORDS TO KNOW

EMBRYONATED: When an embryo has been implanted in a female animal, that animal is said to be embryonated.

HELMINTH: A representative of various phyla of worm-like animals.

FECAL-ORAL-ROUTE: The spread of disease through the transmission of minute particles of fecal material from one organism to the mouth of another organisms. This can occur by drinking contaminated water, eating food that was exposed to animal or human feces (perhaps by watering plants with unclean water), or by the poor hygiene practices of those preparing food.

PARASITE: An organism that lives in or on a host organism and that gets its nourishment from that host. The parasite usually gains all the benefits of this relationship, while the host may suffer from various diseases and discomforts, or show no signs of the infection. The life cycle of a typical parasite usually includes several developmental stages and morphological changes as the parasite lives and moves through the environment and one or more hosts. Parasites that remain on a host's body surface to feed are called ectoparasites, while those that live inside a host's body are called endoparasites. Parasitism is a highly successful biological adaptation. There are more known parasitic species than nonparasitic ones, and parasites affect just about every form of life, including most all animals, plants, and even bacteria.

■ Impacts and Issues

Ascariasis dominates in areas with poor sanitation. According to the Office of Laboratory Security at the Public Health Agency of Canada, roundworm infection is concentrated in moist tropical areas of the world. Within these regions, its incidence can be over 50 percent. The highest group infected in these areas is children aged three to eight years. It adds to iron-deficiency anemia, malnutrition, and impairment of growth and intelligence among the people it affects.

Complications that occur as a direct result of roundworm infection occur in many cases. The most common complication is intestinal tract obstruction. Although complications are only fatal in a small number of cases, according to the NIH, an estimated 8,000 to 10,000 deaths occur annually in the world, primarily in children. Male children are thought to more likely get the disease because of amount of time that they play in dirt.

The disease has generally been neglected in the past because it occurs primarily in poor, rural areas of the world. The affliction has been around for thousands of years. However, aggressive treatment has been recently attempted in some regions.

According to a 2005 paper published in the journal *PLoS Medicine*, ascariasis is considered one of thirteen neglected tropical diseases in Africa. The authors contend that even though HIV (human immunodeficiency virus), TB (tuberculosis), and malaria are the most serious of the tropical diseases, others such as ascariasis are also major medical problems in need of attention throughout the world. Even though neglected in the past, recent attempts to remedy the affects of ascariasis have been successful though affordable and effective means.

SEE ALSO *Food-borne Disease and Food Safety; Globalization and Infectious Disease; Handwashing; Helminth Disease; Travel and Infectious Disease.*

BIBLIOGRAPHY

Books

Handbook of Diseases. Philadelphia, Penn.: Lippincott Williams & Wilkins, 2004.

Holland, Celia V., and Malcolm W. Kennedy. *The Geohelminths: Ascaris, Trichuris, and Hookworm.* Boston, Mass.: Kluwer Academic Publishers, 2002.

Infectious Diseases Sourcebook, edited by Karen Bellenir. Detroit, Mich.: Omnigraphics, 2004.

Tamparo, Carol D. *Diseases of the Human Body.* Philadelphia, Penn.: F.A. Davis Co., 2005.

Web Sites

MedlinePlus, National Institutes of Health. "Ascariasis." October 9, 2006. <http://www.nlm.nih.gov/medlineplus/ency/article/000628.htm> (accessed May 21, 2007).

Office of Laboratory Security, Public Health Agency of Canada. "Ascaris lumbricoides." January 23, 2001.

show the presence of eggs. Blood counts can also diagnosis eosinophilia; and respiratory samples can find pneumonitis and other pulmonary diseases.

Treatment involves medicines that commonly combat parasitic worms such as albendazole (Albenza®), mebendazole (Ovex®, Vermox®), piperazine (Entacyl®), pyrantel pamoate (Antiminth®, Pin-Rid®, Pin-X®), and thiabendazole (Mintezol®). Corticosteroid medicine is sometimes given to counter inflammation.

Roundworm infection is prevented by using careful and comprehensive hygiene techniques such as protecting food from soil and dirt, thoroughly washing vegetables and fruits, washing hands especially after using the toilet, and other similar sanitary measures.

<http://www.phac-aspc.gc.ca/msds-ftss/
msds9e.html> (accessed May 21, 2007).

PLoS Medicine, Public Library of Science. "Rapid-Impact
Interventions: How a Policy of Integrated Control
for Africa's Neglected Tropical Diseases Could
Benefit the Poor." October 11, 2005. <http://
medicine.plosjournals.org/perlserv/?request=get
-document&doi=10.1371/journal.pmed.
0020336#JOURNAL-PMED-0020336-T001>
(accessed May 21, 2007).

Rubella

Introduction

The word rubella comes from the Latin word for "little red" and refers to the characteristic rash that accompanies the disease. It was first described in the early nineteenth century, when it was thought to be a type of either scarlet fever or measles. German doctors then decided that rubella was a disease in its own right—which is why it is sometimes called German measles.

People of any age can contract rubella, and there were many epidemics in the first half of the twentieth century. Rubella only poses a real risk to the developing fetus. Infection during the first three months of pregnancy can cause the child to be born with congenital rubella syndrome, which may be accompanied by deafness, mental retardation, and blindness. Vaccination has greatly reduced the rate of rubella in the United States, and it is especially important that women of child-bearing age are protected from the disease.

Disease History, Characteristics, and Transmission

The rubella virus belongs to the togavirus family and is a single-stranded RNA virus—that is, its genetic material is RNA, not DNA. It only naturally infects humans although other animals can be infected in experimental conditions. The incubation period of rubella virus is around 14 days, and infections are most common in late winter and early spring.

Most people with rubella infection have no, or only mild, symptoms. A rash, which is sometimes the only symptom, appears around 14–17 days after exposure to the virus. This rash is fainter than a measles rash and consists of tiny red spots. The rubella rash typically begins on the face and then spreads down the trunk to the rest of the body. Sometimes the rash is preceded by fever and swollen glands, while tiny red spots may appear on the soft palate. Generally the rash clears up in 3–4 days.

Adults are more prone to complications and more severe symptoms of rubella than children. Arthritis in the fingers, wrists, and knees affects 70% of adult females with rubella. Encephalitis (inflammation of the brain) is

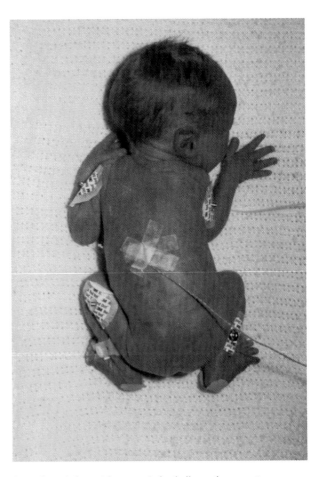

A newborn infant with congenital rubella syndrome. *James Stevenson/Photo Researchers, Inc.*

a rare complication, affecting one in 6,000 rubella cases, and clinical studies have suggested a mortality rate varying between zero and 50%.

Congenital rubella syndrome (CRS) occurs among babies born to a mother who was infected with the virus during early pregnancy. Rubella can affect all the organs of a developing fetus. Deafness is the most common symptom, but cataract and other visual defects, and neurological abnormalities may also occur. The problems may not appear until the child is two to four years old. Other complications arising from CRS include diabetes and autism. Maternal infections occurring after 20 weeks of pregnancy are far less likely to lead to CRS.

Rubella is transmitted by the respiratory route—through coughs and sneezes. It is only moderately contagious. People without symptoms may still be infectious. Those with symptoms are at their most infectious when the rash appears.

■ Scope and Distribution

Rubella has been known since the nineteenth century and was long thought to be a trivial disease. Then, in 1941, the Australian ophthalmologist Norman Gregg reported a worrying trend—78 cases of severe cataracts among newborns, all of which could be traced back to rubella infection among the mothers in early pregnancy. Later, other problems such as heart defects, deafness, and mental retardation were noted in such babies. CRS is now diagnosed in around 85% of babies who have been exposed to rubella in the womb.

Epidemics of rubella were the norm every 7–10 years throughout the first half of the twentieth century and were always followed by an increase in the number of cases of CRS. The last major epidemic in the United States was in 1964 when there were 20,000 resulting cases of CRS and many deaths of babies in the womb.

Rubella and CRS became notifiable diseases in the United States in 1966 and a peak of 57,686 cases was noted in 1969, the year in which a vaccine was first introduced. Since then, cases have fallen to around 0.5 per 100,000 of the population, although there have been outbreaks in California, in 1990, and among the Amish people of Pennsylvania, in 1991. Following these outbreaks, California reported 25 new cases of CRS, Pennsylvania reported 33. The National Congenital Rubella Registry, which is managed by the National Immunization Program, carries out the national surveillance of CRS.

In 2004, the Centers for Disease Control and Prevention declared that rubella was no longer endemic in the United States. Cases that do occur tend to be among Hispanic people who have been born in the Caribbean or in Latin America.

Rubella occurs around the world and it can affect people of any age. However, only around 10% of cases

WORDS TO KNOW

MEASLES: Measles is an infectious disease caused by a virus of the paramyxovirus group. It infects only man and the infection results in life-long immunity to the disease. It is one of several exanthematous (rash-producing) diseases of childhood, the others being rubella (German measles), chickenpox, and the now rare scarlet fever. The disease is particularly common in both pre-school and young school children.

MMR VACCINE: MMR (measles, mumps, rubella) vaccine is a vaccine that is given to protect someone from measles, mumps, and rubella. The vaccine is made up of viruses that cause the three diseases. The viruses are incapable of causing the diseases but can still stimulate the immune system.

NOTIFIABLE DISEASE: A disease that the law requires must be reported to health officials when diagnosed; also called a reportable disease.

RIBONUCLEIC ACID (RNA): Any of a group of nucleic acids that carry out several important tasks in the synthesis of proteins. Unlike DNA (deoxyribonucleic acid), it has only a single strand. Nucleic acids are complex molecules that contain a cell's genetic information and the instructions for carrying out cellular processes. In eukaryotic cells, the two nucleic acids, ribonucleic acid (RNA) and deoxyribonucleic acid (DNA), work together to direct protein synthesis. Although it is DNA (deoxyribonucleic acid) that contains the instructions for directing the synthesis of specific structural and enzymatic proteins, several types of RNA actually carry out the processes required to produce these proteins. These include messenger RNA (mRNA), ribosomal RNA (rRNA), and transfer RNA (tRNA). Further processing of the various RNAs is carried out by another type of RNA called small nuclear RNA (snRNA). The structure of RNA is very similar to that of DNA, however, instead of the base thymine, RNA co

TOGAVIRUS: Togavirus are a type of virus. Rubella is caused by a type of togavirus.

IN CONTEXT: SCIENTIFIC, POLITICAL, AND ETHICAL ISSUES

With regard to a potential connection between the measles, mumps, and rubella Vaccine (MMR Vaccine) and autism, scientists at the National Immunization Program (NIP) at Centers for Disease Control and Prevention (CDC) state that "the weight of currently available scientific evidence does not support the hypothesis that MMR vaccine causes autism. CDC recognizes there is considerable public interest in this issue, and therefore supports additional research regarding this hypothesis. CDC is committed to maintaining the safest, most effective vaccine supply in history."

As of May 2007 the CDC further states that, "there is no convincing evidence that vaccines such as MMR cause long term health effects. On the other hand, we do know that people will become ill and some will die from the diseases this vaccine prevents. Measles outbreaks have recently occurred in the UK and Germany following an increase in the number of parents who chose not to have their children vaccinated with the MMR vaccine. Discontinuing a vaccine program based on unproven theories would not be in anyone's best interest. Isolated reports about these vaccines causing longterm health problems may sound alarming at first. However, careful review of the science reveals that these reports are isolated and not confirmed by scientifically sound research. Detailed medical reviews of health effects reported after receipt of vaccines have often proven to be unrelated to vaccines, but rather have been related to other health factors. Because these vaccines are recommended widely to protect the health of the public, research on any serious hypotheses about their safety are important to pursue. Several studies are underway to investigate still unproven theories about vaccinations and severe side effects."

SOURCE: *Centers for Disease Control and Prevention, National Immunization Program*

given in combination with mumps and measles as the MMR vaccine. It is recommended that a child be vaccinated with MMR between the age of 12 and 15 months, and he or she should receive another dose before school entry. Women of childbearing age should be checked for their immunity to rubella, or offered vaccination, if they do not already have evidence of having received the vaccine earlier. This can be done as part of regular gynecologic care, that is, at the family planning clinic, at a sexual health clinic, or in the doctor's office.

The rubella vaccine is very safe and confers lifelong immunity. Any adverse effects from MMR are likely due to the measles component, not the rubella component. However, there is a small theoretical risk that an unborn child could be affected by rubella vaccine, so it is not recommended for pregnant women, or for women who might become pregnant within four weeks of receiving the vaccine.

■ Impacts and Issues

Despite mass vaccination efforts, there are still an average of five to six cases of CRS per year in the United States. The numbers are tiny, in comparison to the size of the population. Yet each case represents a family tragedy and is costly in terms of health care for the child involved. In the United States, it is estimated that the lifetime health care costs for a person with CRS are more than $200,000. The mothers of most of the babies born with CRS in the United States were themselves born in countries where rubella vaccine was not readily available. Therefore, such vulnerable women should be targeted for rubella vaccination before they become pregnant. In addition, vaccination with MMR ought to be made universally available to reduce the burden of CRS worldwide.

SEE ALSO *Measles (Rubeola); Mumps; Scarlet Fever.*

BIBLIOGRAPHY

Books

Wilson, Walter R., and Merle A. Sande. *Current Diagnosis & Treatment in Infectious Diseases.* New York: McGraw Hill, 2001.

Web Sites

Centers for Disease Control and Prevention Pink Book. "Rubella." <http://www.cdc.gov/nip/publications/pink/rubella.pdf> (accessed April 23, 2007).

Susan Aldridge

occur in people over 40 years old. In recent years, adults between 15 and 39 have accounted for about half of all cases, so rubella is no longer considered to be a childhood disease.

■ Treatment and Prevention

There is no treatment for rubella infection. The first live vaccines were introduced in 1969 and were replaced by an improved version in 1979. Rubella vaccine is now

St. Louis Encephalitis

Introduction

St. Louis encephalitis is a serious viral disease, affecting the brain and nervous system. It is the most common human disease spread by mosquitoes in the United States. The virus that causes the disease was discovered during an outbreak in St. Louis, Missouri, in 1933, giving the disease its common name. Encephalitis is an inflammation of the brain that can lead to serious symptoms and complications, such as convulsions and paralysis. The mortality rate from the disease can be as high as 30%.

The virus that causes St. Louis encephalitis is an arbovirus—short for arthropod-borne virus. Arboviruses are spread by invertebrates, of which the most important are blood-sucking insects, such as mosquitoes. There is no treatment or vaccine for St. Louis encephalitis and prevention depends upon controlling mosquitoes or avoiding their bites. Creating new habitats for mosquitoes, through deteriorating urban conditions, encourages the spread of the disease, as does global warming.

Disease History, Characteristics, and Transmission

The St. Louis encephalitis virus is a flavivirus, related to the Japanese encephalitis virus. It is spread by mosquitoes of the *Culex* genus. In temperate areas of the United States, cases tend to occur during late summer and early fall. In the southern states, the infection may occur throughout the year.

Mild cases of St. Louis encephalitis virus infection have no symptoms other than fever and headache. More serious infections are accompanied by a severe headache, high fever, neck stiffness, stupor, disorientation, tremor, convulsions, and paralysis. The patient may enter a coma and the mortality rate is 3–30 percent.

St. Louis encephalitis is transmitted through the bite of the infected *Culex* mosquito, which acquires the virus by feeding on birds such as finches, sparrows, blue jays, doves, and robins. There is no person-to-person transmission and neither birds nor mosquitoes become ill by being infected with the virus.

Scope and Distribution

St. Louis encephalitis occurs in North, Central, and South America and in the Caribbean. It is mainly a public health problem in the United States, with 4,478 cases being reported since 1964—an average of 128 cases each year. Outbreaks have occurred in Mississippi, the western states, and Florida. The last major outbreak was in the Midwest in 1974–1977, when there were 2,500 cases in 35 states. Outbreaks have been smaller since then, with the last one being in New Orleans, Louisiana, in 1999 where 20 cases were reported.

The elderly, and those living in low-income and crowded conditions, are especially at risk of St. Louis encephalitis. Those working outdoors in certain areas, where they may come into contact with infectious mosquitoes, are also at risk.

Treatment and Prevention

There is no treatment for St. Louis encephalitis and no vaccine. Prevention relies upon public health measures to control mosquitoes. People in areas where there have been cases should avoid going out during dusk and dark, when the mosquitoes are most active. It is important to cover up with long pants and long-sleeved tops to avoid bites, and to use mosquito repellent.

Impacts and Issues

There is potential for further epidemics of St. Louis encephalitis in the United States, because mosquitoes will always create new habitats given the right conditions. In urban areas, conditions, such as poor waste

WORDS TO KNOW

ARTHROPOD-BORNE VIRUS: A virus carried caused by one of a phylum of organisms characterized by exoskeletons and segmented bodies.

ENCEPHALITIS: A type of acute brain inflammation, most often due to infection by a virus.

VECTOR: Any agent, living or otherwise, that carries and transmits parasites and diseases. Also, an organism or chemical used to transport a gene into a new host cell.

disposal, may allow new breeding sites for mosquitoes to develop. A major concern is whether global warming will create new favorable habitats for the *Culex* mosquitoes that are the vector for the transmission of St. Louis encephalitis.

Since there is no effective treatment or vaccine for St. Louis encephalitis, and the disease could increase in the coming years, more research is needed. There is potential for a better understanding of the mosquito life cycle, especially with respect to its overwintering, and for better control of this vector. Research leading to development of a vaccine and an antiviral treatment for the disease is also desirable. On a global level, St. Louis encephalitis is currently rare, but it is a disease that could increase in importance, if global warming expands the range of its vector.

SEE ALSO *Eastern Equine Encephalitis; Encephalitis; Japanese encephalitis; Mosquito-borne Diseases.*

BIBLIOGRAPHY

Web Sites

Centers for Disease Control and Prevention. "Arborial Encephalitides." November 7, 2005. <http://www.cdc.gov/ncidod/dvbid/arbor/index.htm> (accessed April 28, 2007).

Directors of Health Promotion and Education. "St. Louis Encephalitis." <http://www.dhpe.org/infect/sle.html> (accessed April 28, 2007).

Salmonella Infection (Salmonellosis)

■ Introduction

Salmonellosis refers to a human infection that is caused by bacteria in a genus called *Salmonella*. Contamination of food by the bacteria is a common cause of salmonellosis.

Salmonellosis due to the contamination of food can be a food infection or a food intoxication, depending on the antigenic type (serotype) of *Salmonella* involved. A food infection relies on the growth of the bacteria to levels capable of causing symptoms. Growth of the contaminating strain is not necessary for a food intoxication since it is a toxin that has already been produced by the contaminating bacteria that cause the illness. Salmonellosis is most often a food infection, but if enough toxin-loaded bacteria are ingested, salmonellosis can be an intoxication.

Salmonellosis is common and widespread. Of particular concern, *Salmonella* have emerged that are resistant to many commonly used antibiotics.

■ Disease History, Characteristics, and Transmission

Salmonella is a Gram-negative, rod-shaped bacterium. It is named after Daniel Salmon (1850–1914), who, with Theobald Smith (1859–1934), isolated the bacterium from pigs in 1885. Since then, over 2,500 different serotypes of the bacterium have been found; the term serotype indicates the protein composition of the bacterial surface, which produces a distinct immune response by the host. The many different serotype indicates that the surface of *Salmonella* is highly variable.

The bacterium is commonly found in the gastrointestinal tract of humans and other animals. In this environment it is of no concern. However, if food or water contaminated with *Salmonella*-containing feces are ingested, illness can result. Like other fecal bacteria, food contamination most often occurs when the food is handled by someone who has not properly washed their hands after having a bowel movement. Good hygiene is important in minimizing the risk of salmonellosis.

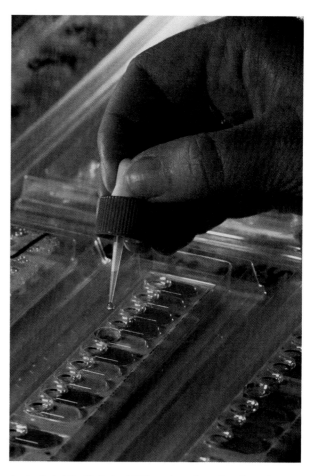

An Analytical Profile Index (API) test is performed to detect bacteria responsible for disorders related to *Salmonella* infections and other food poisoning. This method is used to identify bacteria based on biochemical reactions between the bacteria and various chemicals placed in the API wells. *G.Tompkinson/Photo Researchers, Inc.*

WORDS TO KNOW

CONTAMINATED: The unwanted presence of a microorganism or compound in a particular environment. That environment can be in the laboratory setting, for example, in a medium being used for the growth of a species of bacteria during an experiment. Another environment can be the human body, where contamination by bacteria can produce an infection. Contamination by bacteria and viruses can occur on several levels and their presence can adversely influence the results of the experiments. Outside the laboratory, bacteria and viruses can contaminate drinking water supplies, foodstuffs, and products, causing illness.

ENTEROTOXIN: Enterotoxin and exotoxin are two classes of toxin that are produced by bacteria.

LIPOPOLYSACCHARIDE (LPS): Lipopolysaccharide (LPS) is a molecule that is a constituent of the outer membrane of Gram-negative bacteria. The molecule can also be referred to as endotoxin. LPS can help protect the bacterium from host defenses and can contribute to illness in the host.

SEROTYPES: Serotypes or serovars are classes of microorganisms based on the types of molecules (antigens) that they present on their surfaces. Even a single species may have thousands of serotypes, which may have medically quite distinct behaviors.

TOXIN: A poison that is produced by a living organism.

Salmonellosis is caused most often by two strains: *S. typimurium* and *S. enteritidis.* Other serotypes of the bacterium usually cause disease in animals such as cattle and pigs. If these serotypes infect humans, the infection can be severe and even life-threatening.

Poultry carcasses can be contaminated with intestinal contents during slaughter of the bird. The bacteria can remain alive long enough for the carcass to be shipped to a grocery store and sold. The bacteria are readily killed by heat. But, if cooking is inadequate, the surviving organisms are capable of causing illness. Eggs can also be contaminated if the shell has a crack or break, which allows the bacteria to enter the inside of the egg. Other foods that are often involved in salmonellosis are raw meat (if it is undercooked), processed meat, dairy

products, custards and cream-based desserts, and sandwich filling such as tuna salad or chicken salad.

Symptoms of salmonellosis develop within a few hours of eating contaminated food. The symptoms include abdominal cramping, nausea with vomiting, fever, headache, chills and sweating, a feeling of weakness, and loss of appetite. Some people also develop watery diarrhea or—if cells lining the intestine are damaged—bloody diarrhea. The rapid loss of fluids due to diarrhea can be dangerous to infants and the elderly. As well, less commonly the infection spreads to the bloodstream. Some people can develop a painful condition called Reiter's syndrome, which can persist for years and which can lead to arthritis.

For most people, the infection lasts 4–7 days, and most people recover without needing medical attention. However, severe diarrhea usually results in hospitalization.

Outbreaks of salmonellosis can occur, due to the consumption of contaminated food in a restaurant or at a social gathering. In recent example, an outbreak due to *S. typhimurium* that occurred in 21 of the United States in September, 2006 was traced to the consumption of contaminated tomatoes at restaurants. However, a number of studies have indicated that more than 80% of cases occur individually. This is unfortunate, according to the World Health Organization (WHO), as it diverts media attention from a serious global problem, especially in developing and underdeveloped countries.

The *Salmonella* that cause salmonellosis possess what are termed virulence factors; molecules that enable the bacteria to establish an infection. One important virulence factor is called adhesin. This is a molecule that can recognize a target site on the host cell and help the bacterium adhere to the host cell target. An example of a *Salmonella* adhesin are tubes called fimbriae that stick out from the bacterial surface. The end of each fimbriae contains a protein that can bind with a specific host cell surface protein.

Another virulence factor is called lipopolysaccharide (LPS). There are many different structures of LPS. Those that are longer can help shield the bacterial surface from host compounds that can damage or kill the bacteria. Furthermore, a part of LPS called lipid A is a toxin.

Some strains of *Salmonella* also produce a toxin called enterotoxin. This toxin is located inside the bacteria, so as the numbers of *Salmonella* increase, the concentration of the enterotoxin in the food increases. Ingesting the food releases the enterotoxin in the intestine, where it ruptures the intestinal cells by forming a hole in their cell membrane.

■ Scope and Distribution

Salmonellosis is global in occurrence and common. According to data from the United States Centers for Disease Control and Prevention (CDC), more than 40,000 cases of salmonellosis are reported each year in the United States.

Since many more cases are never reported, the actual total is much higher—1.4 million cases, according to CDC. Approximately 1,000 people in the United States die of salmonellosis-related complications every year.

■ Treatment and Prevention

Diagnosis of salmonellosis relies on recognition of its symptoms and the identification of *Salmonella* from a stool (fecal) sample. Current tests that detect certain *Salmonella* proteins do not require growth of the bacteria, and thus can be completed within hours.

Identification of the type of *Salmonella* involved usually helps in determining which antibiotics to use. Salmonellosis usually responds well to antibiotics, however, serotypes of *Salmonella* that are resistant to a variety of antibiotics exist and are becoming more common.

Prevention involves good hygiene including handwashing and the cleaning of cooking utensils and equipment that have been used with foods such as poultry and ground meat before their re-use. Foods containing raw eggs should not be eaten; even if the eggs appeared intact, cracks that are not visible to the eye are large enough to allow bacteria to contaminate the egg.

Researchers are exploring the production of a vaccine against salmonellosis. The most promising strategy is to block the adhesion of the bacteria to the intestinal cells. This strategy has proven successful in developing a vaccine that appeared on the market in 2006 for another intestinal bacterium called *Escherichia coli* O157:H7 (*E. coli* O157:H7).

■ Impacts and Issues

Salmonellosis has major economic impacts. Millions of people each year miss work and school because of the illness. Health care dollars are spent looking after those who become hospitalized. Exact figures are difficult to obtain, especially from developing countries, as they do not report on salmonellosis. But, in the United States, the estimated 1.4 million annual number of cases of salmonellosis results in the hospitalization of 15,000 people. The annual total medical cost of dealing with salmonellosis in the U.S. is estimated to be $1 billion. Other costs due to lost productivity and lost wages push the total cost to an estimated $3 billion. In Denmark, food-related salmonellosis cost the economy $14 million in lost wages and health care costs in 2001.

In February 2007, *Salmonella*-contaminated peanut butter was responsible for a nationwide salmonellosis outbreak in the United States. The FDA warned consumers not to purchase or eat certain brands of peanut butter manufactured at a facility in Georgia. Companies with brands associated with the salmonellosis outbreak recalled all potentially contaminated products, including peanut butter for home use and commercial peanut

> ## *IN CONTEXT*: EFFECTIVE RULES AND REGULATIONS
>
> According to the Division of Bacterial and Mycotic Diseases at Centers for Disease Control and Prevention (CDC), the CDC "monitors the frequency of *Salmonella* infections in the country and assists the local and State Health Departments to investigate outbreaks and devise control measures. CDC also conducts research to better identify specific types of Salmonella. The Food and Drug Administration inspects imported foods, milk pasteurization plants, promotes better food preparation techniques in restaurants and food processing plants, and regulates the sale of turtles. The FDA also regulates the use of specific antibiotics as growth promotants in food animals. The US Department of Agriculture monitors the health of food animals, inspects egg pasteurization plants, and is responsible for the quality of slaughtered and processed meat. The US Environmental Protection Agency regulates and monitors the safety of drinking water supplies."
>
> SOURCE: *Centers for Disease Control and Prevention (CDC), Coordinating Center for Infectious Diseases, Division of Bacterial and Mycotic Diseases.*

butter products used by some fast-food chains. The *Salmonella*-contaminated foods associated with outbreak affected approximately 370 people in over 40 states. While salmonellosis is typically associated with poultry products, the 2007 outbreak was not the first associated with peanut butter. A similar salmonellosis event that occurred in Australia in the mid–1990s was traced to contaminated peanut butter.

The human suffering and economic consequences of salmonellosis is likely to increase with the continuing spread of *Salmonella* serotypes that are resistant to a variety of commonly used antibiotics. The WHO is trying to determine the global prevalence and antibiotic resistance patterns of the multi-drug resistant *Salmonella* through its Global Salm-Surv program.

SEE ALSO *Food-borne Disease and Food Safety.*

BIBLIOGRAPHY

Books

Prescott, Lansing M., John P. Harley, and Donald A. Klein. *Microbiology.* New York: McGraw-Hill, 2004.

Tortora, Gerard J., Berell R. Funke, and Christine L. Case. *Microbiology: An Introduction.* New York: Benjamin Cummings, 2006.

United States Food & Drug Administration. *Bad Bug Book: Foodborne Pathogenic Microorganisms and Natural Toxins Handbook.* McLean: International Medical Publishing, 2004.

Brian Hoyle

Sanitation

Introduction

Poor sanitation permits infectious diseases to spread as fecal matter contaminates drinking water. In the developed world, water treatment has practically eliminated cholera, typhoid, and dysentery. In the third world, however, the absence of safe drinking water and latrines is associated with high rates of diarrheal illness. Unimproved sanitation includes public or shared latrines, pit latrines without slabs or open pits, hanging toilets or hanging latrines, bucket latrines, and an absence of facilities that forces people to use any area for defecation.

At the start of the twenty-first century, there were about 2.6 billion people in the world without adequate sanitation facilities. A lack of proper sanitation killed about 4,500 children per day while sentencing their neighbors to sickness and squalor. The elderly are more susceptible and more likely to die from diseases related to sanitation than other adults.

History and Scientific Foundations

Before the development of microbiology, the specific causes of diseases were unknown. Diseases such as cholera, typhoid, and dysentery were common in the United States, Europe, and other parts of the world. In 1854, during an Asiatic cholera epidemic in London, physician John Snow linked a contaminated well to deaths. A house privy emptying into a cesspool overflowed to a drain passing close to the well. Feces infected with the bacterium *Vibrio cholerae* contaminated the water and produced a toxin that caused diarrhea, vomiting, and severe fluid and electrolyte loss. Snow's discovery tied poor sanitation directly to disease and death.

In subsequent years, links between sanitation and typhoid, typhus, and dysentery were established. Dehydration is the outstanding characteristic of these diseases and the main cause of death. Typhoid is caused by a

bacterium called *Salmonella typhi*. A different pathogen (disease-causing organism), *Salmonella paratyphi*, causes

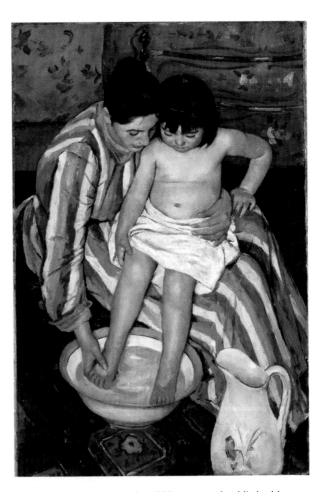

Cholera epidemics during the 1880s prompted public health officials to promote personal hygiene, including regular bathing, as a way to prevent the spread of cholera. *Mary Cassatt, American, (1844-1926), The Child's Bath, 1893, Oil on canvas, 39 1/2 x 26 in., Robert A. Waller Fund, 1910.2 Reproduction, The Art Institute of Chicago.*

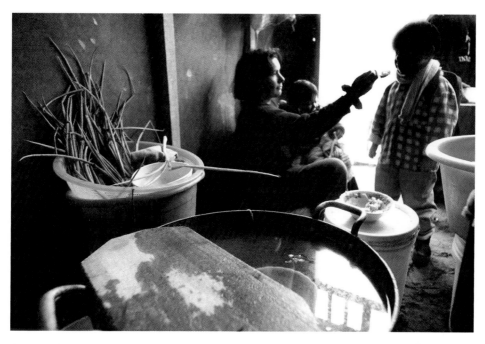

A woman feeds her son next to a pot of dirty water in a community soup kitchen in Lima, Peru, in August 2002. Many community kitchens like this one lack potable water, leading them to recycle the same water for washing dishes and preparing food. As a result, hygiene is poor, and disease afflicts many residents. *AP Images.*

paratyphoid fever. *S. typhi* and *S. paratyphi* are passed in the feces and, occasionally, in the urine of infected people. Most cases of typhoid result from contaminated drinking water and poor sanitation. Typhoid causes fever, rash, delirium, and diarrhea.

Dysentery is also known as traveler's diarrhea. The two most common causes of dysentery are *Shigella* bacteria or amebic infection by the *Entamoeba histolytica*. Both forms of dysentery are spread by fecal contamination of food and water. Amebic dysentery is prevalent in regions where human excrement or "night soil" is used as fertilizer. Cysts (inactive amebas) are excreted in the feces of an infected person. When cysts are ingested with contaminated water, they become active amebas in the intestine and dysentery results. Dysentery was once known as "the bloody flux" because in produced blood in the feces.

Poor sanitation and hygiene are also prime contributors to the spread of schistosomiasis and soil-transmitted helminthiasis (worms). Children are particularly prone to infections because their high level of activity brings them into regular contact with contaminated water and soil.

■ Impacts and Issues

Diarrhea resulting from inadequate sanitation and a lack of clean drinking water affected the daily life of 42% of the world's population in 2000 according to the World Health Organization (WHO). In sub-Saharan Africa, about 769,000 children under five years of age died annually from diarrheal diseases between 2000 and 2003. Of the 57 million children under five years old in the developed nations, about 700 died annually from diarrheal diseases in the same period. A baby in sub-Saharan Africa has almost a 520 times greater chance of dying from diarrhea than an American or European child.

With so few families in the developing nations having access to a latrine or to water for hygiene, many people live in a environment that permits disease to spread rapidly. Chronic poor health robs children of the cognitive development necessary for schooling and takes earning power away from adults.

Oral rehydration therapy (ORT) is an inexpensive and effective way of saving lives. The widespread availability of oral hydration salts has contributed to significant reductions in infant deaths from diarrhea in the third world. However, ORT does not address the root causes of diarrhea.

Improved sanitation reduces deaths from diarrhea by an average of 32%. Accordingly, the WHO advises the construction of flush/pour-flush facilities to piped sewer systems, septic tanks, or pit latrines; pit latrines with slabs; and composting toilets. Communal facilities for groups of homes are not, as a rule, maintained in a clean and sanitary condition. They are not recommended. WHO further advises that the political environment in

WORDS TO KNOW

FECAL-ORAL ROUTE: The transmission of minute particles of fecal material from one organism (human or animal) to the mouth of another organism.

PATHOGEN: A disease causing agent, such as a bacteria, virus, fungus, etc.

SENTINEL: Sentinel surveillance is a method in epidemiology where a subset of the population is surveyed for the presence of communicable diseases. Also, a sentinel is an animal used to indicate the presence of disease within an area.

TOXIN: A poison that is produced by a living organism.

IN CONTEXT: DISEASE IN DEVELOPING NATIONS

According to the World Health Organization (WHO):

- "In 2002, 2.6 billion people lacked access to improved sanitation, which represented 42% of the world's population.
- Over half of those without improved sanitation—nearly 1.5 billion people—live in China and India.
- In sub-Saharan Africa sanitation coverage is a mere 36%.
- Only 31% of the rural inhabitants in developing countries have access to improved sanitation, as opposed 73% of urban dwellers.
- In order to meet the sanitation Millennium Development Goals target, an additional 370 000 people per day up to 2015 should gain access to improved sanitation."

tionally, accidentally swallowing small amounts of fecally contaminated water can cause illness. Pools that contain chlorinated water are considered safe places to swim if the disinfectant levels and pH are properly maintained. All travelers who have diarrhea are advised to refrain from swimming to avoid contaminating recreational water. Travelers with open cuts or abrasions that might serve as entry points for pathogens are warned to avoid swimming and wading in areas with poor sanitation.

Improvements in sanitation bring immediate and enduring benefits in health and dignity. However, these improvements can be beyond the financial means of some governments, particularly those in third world nations. In the 1980s, Brazil developed a condominial sewer system. Condominial systems provide less expensive, localized hookups for poor neighborhoods by connecting groups of houses, rather than individual houses, to the larger grid and by using cheaper materials. However, they have not been adapted in other developing countries as quickly as is needed. Bolivia built condominial systems only after it received assistance from the Swedish International Development Cooperation Agency and the World Bank's Water and Sanitation Program. These support agencies provided technical skills as well as funds. Other developing nations require the same sort of help.

China has used tightly sealed excreta vats for years to store human excrement for use as fertilizer. The vats produce ammonia and albuminoid nitrogen under anaerobic (without oxygen) conditions, which is reported to kill parasite eggs and reduce transmission of parasitic and infectious diseases. Chinese scientists have developed a biogas tank that is likely the future means of dealing with excrement. The tanks are tightly sealed to permit the fermentation and settling of excreta, livestock manure, crop stalks, weeds, and tree leaves. The tight seal prevents contamination of nearby water sources. About 60% of the gas produced in the tanks is methane. The methane from a family unit is used for cooking. This solution is both locally and globally environmentally friendly.

In 2004, Lee Jong-wook, then Director-General of the WHO, declared that sanitation is still a major sentinel (marker) for public health worldwide. Lee prefaced the 2004 "Water, Sanitation, and Hygiene Links to Health: Facts and Figures," with "I often refer to it as 'Health 101,' which means that once we can secure access to clean water and to adequate sanitation facilities for all people, irrespective of the difference in their living conditions, a huge battle against all kinds of diseases will be won." Included in the United Nations Millennium Goals is a specific target aiming to halve the number of people without access to safe drinking water and basic sanitation by the year 2015.

developing nations needs to be changed to support improved sanitation. WHO seeks legislation and regulations in support of sanitation; an increase in national capacity in the form of sanitation engineers and stronger institutions; governmental allocation of financial resources; educational programs that link sanitation, hygiene, health, and economic development; and improved information flow from producers to users.

The Centers for Disease Control recommends that travelers avoid raw food in areas where sanitation is inadequate. The only foods safe to consume in these regions are either cooked or fruit that has been washed in clean water and then peeled by the traveler personally. Addi-

BIBLIOGRAPHY

Salvato, Joseph A., Nelson L. Nemerow, and Franklin J. Agardy. *Environmental Engineering.* Hoboken, NJ: John Wiley, 2003.

World Health Organization/UNICEF Joint Monitoring Program for Water Supply and Sanitation. *Water for Life: Making it Happen.* Geneva: WHO, 2005.

Web Sites

Centers for Disease Control. "Travelers's Health." April 25, 2007 <http://www.cdc.gov/travel/index.htm> (accessed April 26, 2007).

World Health Organization. "Water, Sanitation, and Health." <http://www.who.int/water_sanitation_health/en/> (accessed May 5, 2007).

Caryn E. Neumann

SARS (Severe Acute Respiratory Syndrome)

■ Introduction

Severe acute respiratory syndrome (SARS) is the first emergent and highly transmissible viral disease to appear among humans during the twenty-first century. Patients with SARS develop flulike fever, headache, malaise, dry cough, and other breathing difficulties. Many patients develop pneumonia, and in 5–10% of cases, the pneumonia and other complications are severe enough to cause death. SARS is caused by a virus that is transmitted usually from person to person—predominantly by the aerosolized droplets of virus infected material.

■ Disease History, Characteristics, and Transmission

Many flu causing viruses have previously originated from Guangdong province in China because of cultural and exotic cuisine practices that bring animals, animal parts, and humans into close proximity. In such an environment, pathogens can more easily genetically mutate and make the leap from animal hosts to humans. The first cases of SARS showed high rates among Guangdong food handlers and chefs.

Chinese health officials initially remained silent about the SARS outbreak, and no special precautions were taken to limit travel or prevent the spread of the disease. The world health community, therefore, had no chance to institute testing, isolation, and quarantine measures that might have prevented the subsequent global spread of the disease.

Although not discovered until epidemiologists began to probe the subsequent 2003 outbreak, epidemiologists traced the first known case of what was eventually known as SARS to a November 2002 case in Guangdong province. By mid-February 2003, Chinese health officials tracked more than 300 cases, including five deaths in Guangdong province from what was at the time described as an acute respiratory syndrome.

On February 21, 2003, Liu Jianlun, a 64-year-old Chinese physician from Zhongshan hospital (later determined to have been a "super-spreader," a person capable of infecting unusually high numbers of contacts) traveled to Hong Kong to attend a family wedding despite

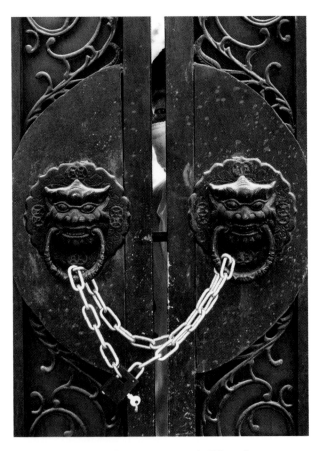

A Chinese worker, under quarantine at a building where investigators suspect other employees caught and spread SARS, peers through a gap in a gate in Beijing in April 2004. © China Photos/Reuters/Corbis.

740

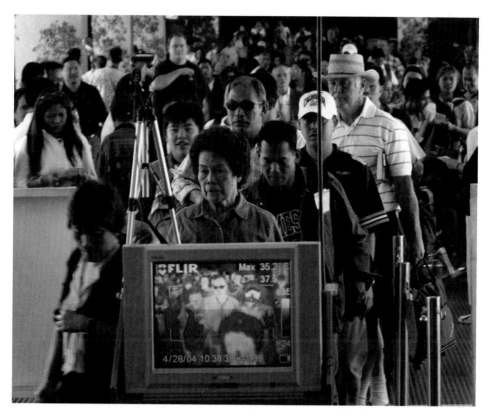

Tourists walk past a thermal scanner used to detect passengers with fevers at Manila International airport. The Philippines has tightened its watch on arriving passengers at all international airports after China reported suspected cases of the potentially deadly severe acute respiratory syndrome (SARS) in Beijing. *© Romeo Ranoco/Reuters/Corbis.*

the fact that he had a fever. Epidemiologists subsequently determined that Jianlun passed on the SARS virus to other guests at the Metropole Hotel where he stayed—including American businessman Johnny Chen, who was en route to Hanoi, three women from Singapore, two Canadians, and a Hong Kong resident. Jianlun's travel to Hong Kong and the subsequent travel of those he infected allowed SARS to spread from China to the infected travelers' destinations.

Chen, the American businessman, grew ill in Hanoi, Viet Nam, and was admitted to a local hospital. Chen infected 20 health care workers at the hospital including noted Italian epidemiologist Carlo Urbani who worked at the Hanoi World Health Organization (WHO) office. Urbani provided medical care for Chen and first formally identified SARS as a unique disease on February 28, 2003. By early March, 22 hospital workers in Hanoi were ill with SARS.

Unaware of the problems in China, Urbani's report drew increased attention among epidemiologists when coupled with news reports in mid-March 2003 that Hong Kong health officials had also discovered an outbreak of an acute respiratory syndrome among health care workers. Unsuspecting hospital workers admitted

the Hong Kong man infected by Jianlun to a general ward at the Prince of Wales Hospital because it was assumed he had a typical severe pneumonia—a fairly routine admission.

The first notice that clinicians were dealing with an usual illness came—not from health notices from China of increasing illnesses and deaths due to SARS—but from the observation that hospital staff, along with those subsequently determined to have been in close proximity to the infected persons, began to show signs of illness. Eventually, 138 people, including 34 nurses, 20 doctors, 16 medical students, and 15 other health-care workers, contracted pneumonia.

One of the most intriguing aspects of the early Hong Kong cases was a cluster of more than 250 SARS cases that occurred in a cluster of high-rise apartment buildings—many housing health care workers—that provided evidence of a high rate of secondary transmission. Epidemiologists conducted extensive investigations to rule out the hypothesis that the illnesses were related to some form of local contamination (e.g., sewage, bacteria on the ventilation system, etc.). Rumors began that the illness was due to cockroaches or rodents, but no scientific evidence supported the hypothesis that the disease pathogen was carried by insects or animals.

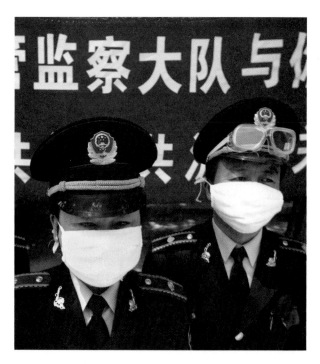

Chinese security guards wear masks to ward off SARS as they monitor the quarantined dormitory buildings of Beijing's Northern Jiaotong University in April 2003. About 400 students and workers were isolated or quarantined after SARS cases were found there. © *Reuters/Corbis.*

Hong Kong authorities then decided that those suffering the flulike symptoms would be given the option of self-isolation, with family members allowed to remain confined at home or in special camps. Compliance checks were conducted by police.

One of the Canadians infected in Hong Kong, Kwan Sui-Chu, return to Toronto, Ontario, and died in a Toronto hospital on March 5, 2003. As in Hong Kong, because there were no alerts from China about the SARS outbreak, Canadian officials did not initially suspect that Sui-Chu had been infected with a highly contagious virus, until Sui-Chu's son and five health care workers showed similar symptoms. By mid-April 2003 Canada reported more than 130 SARS cases and 15 fatalities.

Increasingly faced with reports that provided evidence of global dissemination, on March 15, 2003, the World Health Organization took the unusual step of issuing a travel warning that described SARS as a "worldwide health threat." WHO officials announced that SARS cases, and potential cases, had been tracked from China to Singapore, Thailand, Vietnam, Indonesia, Philippines, and Canada. Although the exact cause of the "acute respiratory syndrome" had not, at that time, been determined, WHO officials issuance of the precautionary warning to travelers bound for South East Asia about the potential SARS risk served notice to public health officials about the potential dangers of SARS.

Within days of the first WHO warning, SARS cases were reported in United Kingdom, Spain, Slovenia, Germany, and in the United States.

WHO officials were initially encouraged that isolation procedures and alerts were working to stem the spread of SARS, as some countries reporting small numbers of cases experienced no further dissemination to hospital staff or others in contact with SARS victims. However, in some countries, including Canada, where SARS cases occurred before WHO alerts, SARS continued to spread beyond the bounds of isolated patients.

WHO officials responded by recommending increased screening and quarantine measures that included mandatory screening of persons returning from visits to the most severely affected areas in China, Southeast Asia, and Hong Kong.

On March 29, 2003, Dr. Urbani, the scientist who initially reported a SARS case, died of complications related to SARS contracted while investigating the outbreak.

Mounting reports of SARS showed an increasing global dissemination of the virus. By April 9, 2003, the first confirmed reports of SARS cases in Africa reached WHO headquarters, and, eight days later, a confirmed case was discovered in India.

WHO took the controversial additional step of recommending against non-essential travel to Hong Kong and the Guangdong province of China. The recommendation, sought by infectious disease specialists, was not controversial within the medical community, but caused immediate concern regarding the potentially widespread economic impacts.

In China, fear of a widespread outbreak in Beijing caused a late, but intensive, effort to isolate SARS victims and halt the spread of the disease. By the end of April 2003, schools in Beijing were closed as were many public areas. Despite these measures, SARS cases and deaths continued to mount. According to the World Health Organization, by the end of the outbreak in July 2003, 8098 people worldwide had contracted SARS, and 774 had died from complications of the disease. In the United States eight people had laboratory evidence of SARS infection and all of the patients had recently traveled out of the country to places with SARS outbreaks.

The 2003 SARS outbreak then subsided almost as quickly as it arose.

In 2004, Chinese officials reported new cases of possible SARS in Beijing and in Anhui Province with at least one confirmed death. Almost 100 contacts were placed under medical observation. Chinese authorities reported outbreaks of SARS affecting laboratory workers who were exposed to the virus. In late 2004, four more unlinked, community-acquired cases of SARS were found in Guangdong province, and, although the source of this outbreak was unconfirmed, it is suspected to have

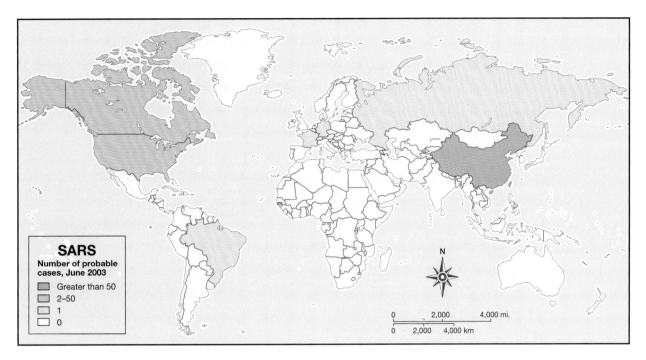

Map showing the number of probable cases of SARS as of June 26, 2003. *© Copyright World Health Organization (WHO). Reproduced by permission.*

originated in wild animals, most likely those found in food markets.

Scope and Distribution

At the end of April 2003, SARS public health officials expressed concern that SARS had the potential to become a global pandemic. Scientists, public health authorities, and clinicians around the world struggled to both treat and investigate the disease.

Global efforts at isolation, quarantine, and observation proved effective and a pandemic did not occur, however, and the last SARS infection in humans was reported in China in 2004.

As of May 2007, the Centers for Disease Control and Prevention (CDC) and World Health Organization reported no current cases of SARS anywhere in the world.

Treatment and Prevention

Scientists scrambled to isolate, identify, and sequence the pathogen responsible for SARS. Modes of transmission characteristic of viral transmission allowed scientists to place early attention on a group of viruses termed coronaviruses—some of which are associated the common cold. There was a global two-pronged attack on the SARS pathogen, with some efforts directed toward a positive identification and isolation of the virus and other efforts directed toward discovering the genetic molecular structure and sequence of genes contained in

the virus. The development of a genomic map of the precise nucleotide sequence of the virus would be key in any subsequent development of a definitive diagnostic test, the identification of effective anti-viral agents, and perhaps a vaccine.

The development of a reliable and definitive diagnostic test was considered of paramount importance in keeping SARS from becoming a global pandemic. A definitive diagnostic test would not only allow physicians earlier treatment options, but would also allow the earlier identification and isolation of potential carriers of the virus.

Without advanced testing, physicians were initially forced to rely upon less sensitive tests that were unable to identify SARS prior to 21 days of infection, in most cases too late to effectively isolate the patient.

In mid-April 2003, Canadian scientists at the British Columbia Cancer Agency in Vancouver announced that they had sequenced the genome of the coronavirus most likely to be the cause of SARS. Within days, scientists at the Centers for Disease Control (CDC) in Atlanta, Georgia, offered a genomic map that confirmed more than 99% of the Canadian findings. Both genetic maps were generated from studies of viruses isolated from SARS cases. The particular coronavirus mapped had a genomic sequence of 29,727 nucleotides—average for the family of coronavirus that typically contain between 29,000 and 31,000 nucleotides.

Proof that the coronavirus mapped was the specific virus responsible for SARS would eventually come from

Published Date 10-FEB-2003

    Subject PRO/EDR> Pneumonia - China (Guangdong): RFI

PNEUMONIA - CHINA (GUANGDONG): RFI
****
A ProMED-mail post
<http://www.promedmail.org>
ProMED-mail is a program of the
International Society for Infectious Diseases
<http://www.isid.org>

[1]
Date: 10 Feb 2003
From: Stephen O. Cunnion, MD, PhD, MPH

This morning I received this e-mail and then searched your archives
and found nothing that pertained to it. Does anyone know anything
about this problem?

"Have you heard of an epidemic in Guangzhou? An acquaintance of mine
from a teacher's chat room lives there and reports that the
hospitals there have been closed and people are dying."

--
Stephen O. Cunnion, MD, PhD, MPH
International Consultants in Health, Inc
Member ASTM&H, ISTM

******
[2]
Date: 10 Feb 2003
From: Jack Soo
Source: Hong Kong's Information Services Department [edited]
<http://www.news.gov.hk/en/category/healthandcommunity/030210/html/030210en05017.htm>

Take precautions when traveling abroad

The public should take precautions when traveling abroad and tell
doctors if there are signs of fever or infections that do not abate
and are unusual, says Secretary for Health, Welfare & Food Dr Yeoh
Eng-kiong.

Commenting on the problem of pneumonia on the Mainland, Dr Yeoh said
the Department of Health has already touched base with the Guangdong
authorities to learn more about the type of infection prevalent
there. The department will also determine whether there is any
particular risk of that infection coming to Hong Kong.

He assured the public that the Government is always on the alert, as
the Department of Health has a very good communicable disease
surveillance system.

Coupled with the network of reporting sources both from the public
and private sectors, as well as communication channels with
authorities on the Mainland and Macau, the Government is informed of
any infections that may spread to Hong Kong.

He called on the public not to be unduly concerned.

"We'll certainly be doing our part as the health authorities, but
individuals should always take precautions when they travel aboard,"
he added.

--
Jack Soo

[ProMED-mail appreciates the preliminary information above from Jack
Soo and would be grateful for any additional information. The
etiology and extent of this apparent outbreak of pneumonia are
unclear, as is whether the outbreak is secondary to influenza. -
Mod.LM]

This e-mail is a request for information about the disease that was later identified as SARS. Stephen O. Cunnion, a retired U.S. Navy epidemiologist, posted the e-mail to ProMED, an Internet site for infectious disease reporting, after he had heard from a friend that fear was gripping the city of Guangzou in China, where people were dying of an unidentified disease. *Courtesy, Dr. Stephen O. Cunnion and Dr. Jack Soo.*

animal testing. Rhesus monkeys were exposed to the virus via injection and inhalation and then monitored to determine whether SARS-like symptoms developed, and then if sick animals exhibited a histological pathology (i.e., an examination of the tissue and cellular level pathology) similar to findings in human patients. Other tests, including polymerase chain reaction (PCR) testing, helped positively match the specific coronavirus present in the lung tissue, blood, and feces of infected animals to the exposure virus.

Identification of a specific pathogen can be a complex process, and positive identification requires thousands of tests. All testing is conducted with regard to testing Koch's postulates—the four conditions that must be met for an organism to be determined to the cause of a disease. First, the organism must be present in every case of the disease. Second, the organism must be able to be isolated from the host and grown in laboratory conditions. Third, the disease must be reproduced when the isolated organism is introduced into another, healthy host. The fourth postulate stipulates that the same organism must be able to be recovered and purified from the host that was experimentally infected.

SARS has an incubation period range of 2–7 days, with an average incubation of about four days. In some cases incubation has taken 10 days, and, in a very rare number of cases, as long as 14 days. Much of the inoculation period allows the virus to be both transported and spread by an asymptomatic carrier. With air travel, asymptomatic carriers can travel to anywhere in the world. The initial symptoms are non-specific and common to the flu. Infected cases then typically spike a high fever 100.4°F (38°C) as they develop a cough, shortness of breath, and difficulty breathing. SARS often fulminates (reaches it maximum progression) in a severe pneumonia that can cause respiratory failure and results in death in about 10% of its victims.

No definitive therapy has been demonstrated to have clinical effectiveness against the virus that causes SARS. Antibiotics, antiviral medications, corticosteroids, and supportive therapies such as fluids and ventilation are the mainstays of treatment for SARS.

Isolation and quarantine remain potent tools in the modern public health arsenal. Both procedures seek to control exposure to infected individuals or materials. Isolation procedures are used with patients with a confirmed illness. Quarantine rules and procedures apply to individuals who are not currently ill, but are known to have been exposed to the illness (e.g., been in the company of a infected person or come in contact with infected materials).

Isolation and quarantine both act to restrict movement and to slow or stop the spread of disease within a community. Depending on the illness, patients placed in isolation may be cared for in hospitals, specialized health care facilities, or, in less severe cases, at home. Isolation

is a standard procedure for TB patients. In most cases, isolation is voluntary; however, isolation can be compelled by federal, state, and some local law.

■ Impacts and Issues

Before the advent of vaccines and effective diagnostic tools, isolation and quarantine were the principal tools to control the spread of infectious disease. The term "quarantine" derives from the Italian *quarantine* and *quaranta giorni* and dates to the plague in Europe. As a precautionary measure, the government of Venice restricted entry into the port city and mandated that ships coming from areas of plague—or otherwise suspected of carrying plague—had to wait 40 days before being allowed to discharge their cargos. The legal basis of quarantine in the United States was established in 1878 with the passage of Federal Quarantine Legislation in response to continued outbreaks of yellow fever, typhus, and cholera.

During the later years of the nineteenth century and throughout the twentieth century, the law bent toward protecting the greater needs of society. Quarantine was often used for political, as well as medical, reasons; it was implemented to contain and discourage immigration. In other cases, such as with tuberculosis (TB), quarantine, proved effective and courts wielded wide authority to isolate, hospitalize, and to force patients to take medications.

The public discussion of SARS-related quarantine in the United States and Europe renewed tensions between the needs for public heath precautions that safeguard society at large and the liberties of the individual.

States governments within the United States have a general authority to set and enforce quarantine

IN CONTEXT: REAL-WORLD RISKS

With regard to severe acute respiratory syndrome (SARS) the Centers for Disease Control and Prevention (CDC) states that "available information suggests that persons with SARS are most likely to be contagious only when they have symptoms, such as fever or cough. Patients are most contagious during the second week of illness. However, as a precaution against spreading the disease, CDC recommends that persons with SARS limit their interactions outside the home (for example, by not going to work or to school) until 10 days after their fever has gone away and their respiratory (breathing) symptoms have gotten better."

"To date, no cases of SARS have been reported among persons who were exposed to a SARS patient before the onset of the patient's symptoms. If transmission of SARS recurs, there are some common-sense precautions that you can take that apply to many infectious diseases. The most important is frequent handwashing with soap and water or use of an alcohol-based hand rub. You should also avoid touching your eyes, nose, and mouth with unclean hands and encourage people around you to cover their nose and mouth with a tissue when coughing or sneezing."

SOURCE: *Centers for Disease Control and Prevention*

conditions. At the federal level, the CDC's Division of Global Migration and Quarantine is empowered to detain, examine, or conditionally release (release with restrictions on movement or with a required treatment protocol) individuals suspected of carrying certain listed communicable diseases.

In 2003 the CDC recommended SARS patients be voluntarily isolated, but did not recommend enforced isolation or quarantine. Regardless, CDC and other public health officials, including the Surgeon General, sought and secured increased powers to deal with SARS. On April 4, 2003, U.S. President George W. Bush signed Presidential Executive Order 13295 that added SARS to a list of quarantinable communicable diseases. The order provided health officials with the broader powers to seek "... apprehension, detention, or conditional release of individuals to prevent the introduction, transmission, or spread of suspected communicable diseases ..."

Other diseases on the U.S. communicable disease list, specified pursuant to section 361(b) of the Public Health Service Act, include "Cholera; Diphtheria; infectious Tuberculosis; Plague; Smallpox; Yellow Fever; and Viral Hemorrhagic Fevers."

Canada, hit early and much harder by SARS than the United States, responded by closing schools and some hospitals in impacted areas. Canadian health offi-

cials advised seemingly healthy travelers from areas with known SARS cases to enter into a 10-day voluntary quarantine. Once in isolation, individuals were asked to frequently take their temperature and remain separated from other family members. Within a month, almost 10,000 people were in some form of quarantine. Canadian government officials, including then Prime Minister Jean Chrétien, publicly complained when, on April 23, the WHO recommended a three-week postponement of non-essential travel to Toronto. After criticism and intense lobbying of WHO by Chrétien's government and Canadian public health officials, WHO discontinued the recommendation on April 30, 2003. When Canada's cases of SARS spiked, Toronto was returned to the WHO list and was not removed until July 2, 2003. WHO officials kept in place similar warnings about travel to Beijing and Hong Kong.

Faced with a more immediate danger and larger numbers of initial cases, an authoritarian government in Singapore was less hesitant in ordering quarantine of victims and those potentially exposed to the virus. One of the three Singapore women initially infected in Hong Kong was later identified as a super-spreader who infected more than 90 people. She recovered, but both her mother and father died of SARS.

During the 2003 outbreak, passengers arriving in Singapore coming from other countries with SARS were required to undergo questioning by nurses in isolation garb and then required to walk through a thermal scanner calibrated to detect an elevated body temperature. Soldiers immediately escorted those with elevated temperatures into quarantine facilities. Those subsequently allowed to remain in their homes were monitored by video cameras and electronic wristbands.

Health authorities assert that the emergent virus responsible for SARS will remain endemic (part of the natural array of viruses) in many regions of China, and that outbreaks could continue on a seasonal basis.

In the aftermath of the 2003 SARS outbreak, a Chinese official publicly apologized for a slow and inefficient response to the 2003 SARS outbreak. Allegations that officials covered up the true extent of the spread of the disease caused the dismissal of several local administrators including China's public health minister and the mayor of Beijing. This admission was politically significant for the new leadership in China, and encouraging to many in the public health services. Reporting procedures and compliance to international health regulations still, however, show wide differences and sensitivities to political issues not only for China but many other nations and or local regions.

The 2003 SARS outbreak provided a test of recent reforms in International Health Regulations designed to increase surveillance and reporting of infectious diseases—and to enhance cooperation in preventing the international spread of disease. Although not an act of bioterrorism, because the same epidemiologic principles and isolation protocols might be used to both initially determine and initially respond to an act of bioterrorism, intelligence and public heath officials closely monitored the political, scientific, and medical responses to the SARS outbreak. In many regards, the SARS outbreak provided a real and deadly test of public health responses, readiness, and resources.

■ Primary Source Connection

Dr. Carlo Urbani, an Italian physician and specialist in infectious diseases, was among the first to recognize SARS as a new infectious disease threat. Along with other virus hunters, Dr. Urbani's skill, bravery and dedication helped save lives, but cost him his own. The following is an report of his death as published in the *New England Journal of Medicine.*

SARS and Carlo Urbani

On February 28, the Vietnam French Hospital of Hanoi, a private hospital of about 60 beds, contacted the Hanoi office of the World Health Organization (WHO). A patient had presented with an unusual influenza-like virus. Hospital officials suspected an avian influenza virus and asked whether someone from the WHO could take a look. Dr. Carlo Urbani, a specialist in infectious diseases, answered that call. In a matter of weeks, he and five other health care professionals would be dead from a previously unknown pathogen.

We now know that Hanoi was experiencing an outbreak of severe acute respiratory syndrome (SARS). Dr. Urbani swiftly determined that the small private hospital was facing something unusual. For the next several days, he chose to work at the hospital, documenting findings, arranging for samples to be sent for testing, and reinforcing infection control. The hospital established an isolation ward that was kept under guard. Dr. Urbani worked directly with the medical staff of the hospital to strengthen morale and to keep fear in check as SARS revealed itself to be highly contagious and virulent. Of the first 60 patients with SARS, more than half were health care workers. At a certain moment, many of the staff members made the difficult decision to quarantine themselves. To protect their families and community, some health care workers put themselves at great personal risk, deciding to sleep in the hospital and effectively sealing themselves off from the outside world.

In some ways, the SARS outbreak in Hanoi is a story of what can go right, of public health's coming before politics. First-line health care providers quickly alerted the WHO of an atypical pneumonia. Dr. Urbani recognized the severity of the public health threat. Immediately, the WHO requested an emergency meeting on Sunday,

---

IN CONTEXT: EFFECTIVE RULES AND REGULATIONS

The 2003 severe acute respiratory syndrome (SARS) outbreak did not spread within the United States. In response to the 2003 SARS outbreak, the Centers for Disease Control and Prevention (CDC) states that its responses to the outbreak were as follows: That the "CDC:

- Worked closely with WHO and other partners in a global effort to address the SARS outbreak of 2003.
- Activated its Emergency Operations Center to provide round-the-clock coordination and response.
- Committed more than 800 medical experts and support staff to work on the SARS response.
- Deployed medical officers, epidemiologists, and other specialists to assist with on-site investigations around the world.
- Provided assistance to state and local health departments in investigating possible cases of SARS in the United States.
- Conducted extensive laboratory testing of clinical specimens from SARS patients to identify the cause of the disease.
- Initiated a system for distributing health alert notices to travelers who may have been exposed to cases of SARS."

SOURCE: *Centers for Disease Control and Prevention*

March 9, with the Vice Minister of Health of Vietnam. Dr. Urbani's temperament and intuition and the strong trust he had built with Vietnamese authorities were critical at this juncture. The four-hour discussion led the government to take the extraordinary steps of quarantining the Vietnam French Hospital, introducing new infection-control procedures in other hospitals, and issuing an international appeal for expert assistance. Additional specialists from the WHO and the Centers for Disease Control and Prevention (CDC) arrived on the scene, and Médecins sans Frontiéres (MSF, or Doctors without Borders) responded with staff members as well as infection-control suits and kits that were previously stocked for outbreaks of Ebola virus. The Vietnam French Hospital has been closed temporarily, and patients with SARS are cared for in two wards of the public Bach Mai Hospital, with the assistance of a team from MSF. No new cases in health care workers have been reported, and the outbreak in Vietnam appears to be contained. By dealing with the outbreak openly and decisively, Vietnam risked damage to its image and economy. If it had decided to take refuge in secrecy, however, the results might have been catastrophic.

Dr. Urbani would not survive to see the successes resulting from his early detection of SARS. On March 11, he began to have symptoms during a flight to Bangkok. On his arrival, he told a colleague from the CDC who greeted him at the airport not to approach him. They sat down at a distance from each other, in silence, waiting for an ambulance to assemble protective gear. He fought SARS for the next 18 days in a makeshift isolation room in a Bangkok hospital. Dr. Carlo Urbani died on March 29, 2003.

SARS is a pandemic of our global age. In just a few weeks, SARS had spread through air travel to at least three continents. Conversely, in the same amount of time, researchers working in no fewer than 10 countries have collaborated to identify the virus, sequence its genome, and take steps toward rapid diagnosis. It is now hoped that the large strides taken in basic research will quickly lead to therapeutic advances or a vaccine.

Health care workers continue to be on the front line. Apart from the index patient, all the patients in the Vietnamese outbreak who died were doctors and nurses. In Hong Kong, approximately 25 percent of patients with SARS have been health care professionals, including the chief executive of the hospital authority. The intensive care wards are full—a situation that is exacerbated by the staffing difficulties presented by the hundreds of SARS cases affecting medical personnel. It is becoming difficult to import additional infection-control equipment, since countries where the suits are manufactured are holding onto their stocks as they brace themselves for outbreaks of SARS within their own borders. Once effective drug therapy has been found, similar problems may arise with availability and distribution, especially if the effective treatment turns out to involve a relatively rare and expensive drug, such as ribavirin.

It remains to be seen whether the number of new SARS outbreaks will ebb or whether what we have seen to date is indeed the leading edge of a much larger pandemic. Currently, the attack rate in Hong Kong is approximately 2 cases per 10,000 population over the course of two months. This rate compares favorably with the seasonal attack rates of influenza-like illness, which reached 50 cases per 10,000 population in one week this winter in Europe.

In 1999, Dr. Urbani was president of MSF-Italy and a member of the delegation in Oslo, Norway, that accepted the Nobel Peace Prize. Although he would be gratified that so much has been accomplished with respect to SARS in such a short time, he would certainly point out that the other diseases he worked with—such as the human immunodeficiency virus and AIDS, tuber-culosis, and malaria, which kill millions of people each year—deserve to be treated with similar urgency. Whatever the future direction of SARS, it is clear that Dr. Urbani's decisive and determined intervention has bought precious time and saved lives. We remember Dr. Urbani with a mixture of pride in his selfless devotion to medicine and unspeakable grief about the void his departure has left in the hearts of his colleagues around the world.

Source Information: From Médecins sans Frontiéres (Doctors without Borders) U.S.A. (B.R.), Belgium (M.V.H.), Vietnam (D.S.), and Italy (N.D.)

Brigg Reilley, M.P.H., Michel Van Herp, M.D., M.P.H., Dan Sermand, Ph.D., and Nicoletta Dentico, M.P.H.

"SARS AND CARLO URBANI." *NEW ENGLAND JOURNAL OF MEDICINE.* MAY 15, 2003. <HTTP://CONTENT.NEJM.ORG/CGI/ CONTENT/FULL/348/20/1951> (ACCESSED JUNE 11, 2007).

SEE ALSO *Contact precautions; Developing Nations and Drug Delivery; Emerging Infectious Diseases; Influenza; Influenza Pandemic of 1918; Influenza, Tracking Seasonal Influences and Virus Mutation; Isolation and Quarantine; Notifiable Diseases; Pandemic Preparedness; Personal Protective Equipment; Standard Precautions; Vaccines and Vaccine Development.*

BIBLIOGRAPHY

Periodicals

Ksiazek T.G., et al. "A Novel Coronavirus Associated with Severe Acute Respiratory Syndrome." *New England Journal of Medicine.* 10.1056. April 10, 2003.

Rosenthal, E. "From China's Provinces, a Crafty Germ Spreads." *New York Times.* April 27, 2003.

Web Sites

Centers for Disease Control and Prevention (CDC). "Severe Acute Respiratory Syndrome (SARS)." <http://www.cdc.gov/ncidod/sars/index.htm> (accessed May 30, 2007).

World Health Organization. "Investigation into China's Recent SARS Outbreak Yields Important Lessons for Global Public Health." <http:// www.wpro.who.int/sars/docs/update/update_ 07022004.asp> (accessed May 30, 2007).

Brenda Wilmoth Lerner

Scabies

Introduction

Scabies is an infestation of the skin by the human itch mite, which is known as *Sarcoptes scabiei*. It occurs all around the world and is one of the most common skin problems reported to dermatologists. The word scabies comes from the Latin *scabere*, which means to scratch. There is a variant known as Norwegian scabies, which is very infectious and can lead to epidemics in places such as nursing homes, homeless shelters, and prisons. Scabies is caused by close human contact, including sexual contact, and leads to intense itching because of an immune response to the infestation.

Most healthy people can ward off an attack of scabies. But in those whose immunity is compromised because of HIV/AIDS or other factors, such as old age, the mites can take hold. Poor hygiene, malnutrition, and overcrowding are strong risk factors for an outbreak of scabies. Treatment is usually by a skin cream or tablets containing a drug that kills the mites.

Disease History, Characteristics, and Transmission

Mites are tiny organisms, barely visible to the human eye at around 0.4 millimeters in length. *S. scabiei* mate on human skin, after which the male dies. The fertilized female burrows through the epidermis—the outer layer of skin—and lays eggs in her "burrow." Typically, around 10–15 organisms are found in an infestation giving rise to symptoms, although there can be many more in immunocompromised hosts, such as people with HIV/AIDS. Scabies arises from human contact, including sexual intercourse.

The symptoms of scabies come from the human immune response to the feces of the female mite in her burrow. There is severe itching—known clinically as pruritis—which is especially intense at night or after a hot shower or bath. This can occur in any part of the body, but is most common between the fingers, in the genitalia, and around the waist or other areas constricted by clothing. Among adults, scabies tends not to cause symptoms on the face, arm, neck, or soles of the feet, but these areas may be affected in children. Pustules—pimples filled with pus, a yellow fluid made up of dead white blood cells, bacteria, and bits of dead tissue—and blisters might occur in areas affected by scabies.

The so-called Norwegian variant of scabies, sometimes also called crusted scabies, often affects the face, scalp, palms of the hands, and soles of the feet. It may be mistaken for eczema or psoriasis, two other

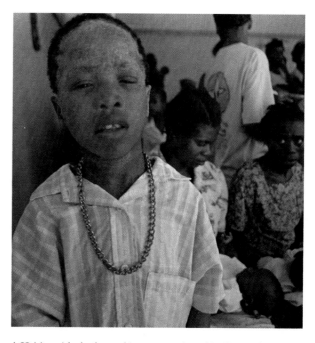

A Haitian girl who has scabies, a contagious skin disease that causes intense itching, waits for the U.S. Support Group medical team at the Brothers of Charities in a slum in Port-au-Prince, Haiti. *AP Images.*

WORDS TO KNOW

ATOPY: Atopy is an inherited tendency towards hypersensitivity towards immunoglobulin E, a key component of the immune system, which plays an important role in asthma, eczema and hay fever.

MITE: A mite is a tiny arthropod (insect-like creature) of the order *Acarina*. Mites may inhabit the surface of the body without causing harm, or may cause various skin ailments by burrowing under the skin. The droppings of mites living in house-dust are a common source of allergic reactions.

PRURITIS: Pruritis is the medical term for itchiness.

PUSTULES: A pustule is a reservoir of pus visible just beneath the skin. It is usually sore to the touch and surrounded by inflamed tissue.

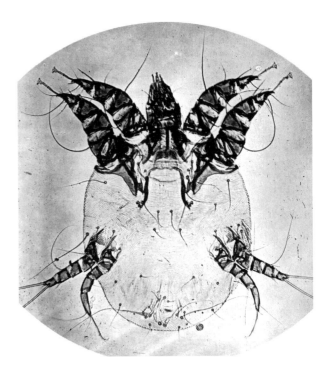

This photo of the microscopic mite *Sarcoptes scabei* that causes the skin condition scabies was taken in France around 1930. Long persistent in the developing world, scabies mites are also showing a modern-day resurgence in the developed world, especially in areas where people reside in close quarters, such as nursing homes and cruise ships. *Boyer/Roger Viollet/Getty Images.*

inflammatory skin conditions. Norwegian scabies is very contagious.

Scope and Distribution

Scabies is a worldwide problem, affecting 300–500 million people each year. It is more likely to occur where conditions of crowding, poor hygiene, and malnutrition are found. Accordingly, scabies is often seen in hospitals, nursing homes, prisons, and mental institutions.

Those with reduced immunity, such as patients with HIV/AIDS, are more prone to scabies and thousands to millions of *S. scabiei* eggs may be found under the skin of these individuals. Those with known atopy—that is, with hereditary, allergy-related symptoms such as asthma or eczema—may be more vulnerable to scabies, because of their sensitivity to the house dust mite, which is related to *S. sabiei*.

Treatment and Prevention

Scabies is treated by a 5% cream of permethrin, which is applied from the neck down to cover the whole body. Among young children, treatment of the face might also be needed. The treatment is left for several hours to kill the mites and is then washed away. This cures 90% of those infested. Oral ivermectin may also be useful, especially if the all-body topical treatment is hard to administer, as in nursing home residents. Meanwhile, clothing,

bedding, and other items that might have been in touch with the mites should be washed.

Treatment of close contacts is also a good idea, to prevent reinfestation. Those treated may find their symptoms persist afterwards for four weeks or so because of the time needed to clear the body of the mite feces that cause the inflammatory response. The itching can be treated in all those affected by an antihistamine drug.

Impacts and Issues

Scabies is an uncomfortable disease that is largely a product of poor hygiene or crowded living conditions. It also targets those with compromised immunity, such as people with AIDS or the elderly. Therefore, those at risk need to be aware of the problem of scabies and take action to avoid close and prolonged contact with those who could already be infested.

SEE ALSO *Lice Infestation (Pediculosis).*

BIBLIOGRAPHY

Books

Gates, Robert H. *Infectious Disease Secrets.* 2nd ed. Philadelphia: Hanley and Beltus, 2003.

Wilson, Walter R., and Merle A. Sande. *Current Diagnosis & Treatment in Infectious Diseases.* New York: McGraw Hill, 2001.

IN CONTEXT: SOCIAL AND PERSONAL RESPONSIBILITY

The Division of Parasitic Diseases at Centers for Disease Control and Prevention (CDC) states the scabies is contracted by "direct, prolonged, skin-to-skin contact with a person already infested with scabies. Contact must be prolonged (a quick handshake or hug will usually not spread infestation). Infestation is easily spread to sexual partners and household members. Infestation may also occur by sharing clothing, towels, and bedding."

The CDC further states that "anyone who is diagnosed with scabies, as well as his or her sexual partners and persons who have close, prolonged contact to the infested person should also be treated. If your health care provider has instructed family members to be treated, everyone should receive treatment at the same time to prevent reinfestation."

SOURCE: *Centers for Disease Control and Prevention, National Center for Infectious Diseases, Division of Parasitic Diseases*

Scarlet Fever

■ Introduction

In the nineteenth century, scarlet fever was one of the most feared of all childhood diseases, with a mortality of up to 35%. The causative agent is the bacterium *Streptococcus pyogenes*. Today scarlet fever still exists, but tends to be a very mild disease in developed countries, although serious complications are still common in developing nations.

The modern, milder, form of scarlet fever is sometimes called pharyngitis (throat infection) with rash, or scarlatina. It is not clear why this disease has lost its virulence. Unlike other childhood diseases, vaccination has not played a role in reducing its toll. The microbe itself may have mutated into a milder pathogen, or improvements in hygiene may have contributed. The advent of antibiotics and drugs to treat seizures and fever has certainly helped deal with the cause and symptoms of scarlet fever.

■ Disease History, Characteristics, and Transmission

The *S. pyogenes* bacteria causing scarlet fever is known as Group A streptoccoccus (GAS); the "A" refers to a characteristic antigen protein that exists on the surface of the microbe. GAS also causes strep throat (sometimes called bacterial sore throat) and impetigo. It is also responsible for necrotizing fasciitis, which involves the soft tissue under the skin, and toxic shock syndrome, both of which are potentially fatal. Around 40% of the population are asymptomatic carriers of GAS and the bacterium does not have an animal reservoir (an organism that maintains the infective agent). The main symptoms of scarlet fever are a very sore, red throat, possibly with visible white or yellow patches, and the bright red rash that gives the disease its name.

The rash is caused by production of a toxin by the bacteria that spreads into the bloodstream via infected tissue in the throat. It begins as small spots on the neck and upper chest, it then spreads to the rest of the body. When the skin is pressed, it goes pale and the rash feels like sandpaper. The cheeks are flushed while the mouth remains pale, as if the patient had a white moustache. The tongue is often coated with a white fur, with tiny

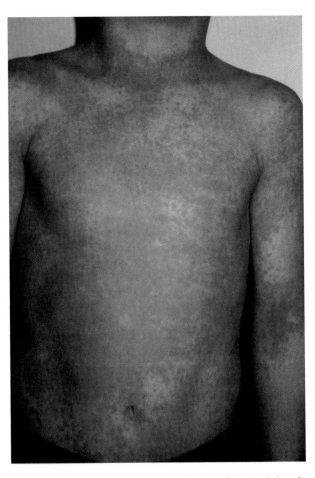

Scarlet fever, a contagious disease, produces a rash in its victims. It is transmitted mainly in childhood through coughing or drinking contaminated milk. *Biophoto Associates/Photo Researchers, Inc.*

projections called papillae poking through. Doctors sometimes call this a "strawberry" tongue, from its appearance. After a few days, it turns into a "raspberry" tongue, becoming red with prominent papillae.

Other symptoms of scarlet fever include headache, vomiting, swollen glands, and poor appetite. As the rash fades, within three to four days of onset, the skin of the face, palms, and tips of the fingers and toes may begin to peel. More serious cases of scarlet fever—rare in the West, more common in the developing world—are divided into two types, known as toxic and septic. In the toxic form, fever can be extreme, accompanied by delirium, convulsions, and rapid pulse, leading to death within 24 hours. In the septic form, the course of the disease is more prolonged, causing death in two to three weeks.

The complications of scarlet fever include upper airway obstruction, meningitis, pneumonia, mastoiditis, and otitis media (a severe ear infection). Later complications, such as kidney disease and rheumatic fever—which weakens the heart in the long term—may also occur.

Scarlet fever is transmitted by coughs and sneezes, as the saliva and nasal fluids are infectious. Coming into contact with items contaminated with these fluids therefore carries a risk of infection. Sharing cups and utensils can transmit infection.

■ Scope and Distribution

Scarlet fever used to cause pandemics with high mortality in the nineteenth century in the United States, Western Europe, and in Scandinavia. Often, because of a lack of understanding of how the disease was transmitted, all the patient's belongings would be burned for fear of contamination. Long periods of convalescence were common, perhaps because of complications due to rheumatic fever.

Because scarlet fever is now a mild disease in the West, it is no longer notifiable (tracked through mandaory reporting) in many countries. The United Kingdom (UK), however, still collects data on scarlet fever cases and noted 2,200 cases occurring in England and Wales in 2004. Ten years previously, the number of cases was around 6,000, which suggests the disease is on the decline.

Ninety percent of cases of scarlet fever occur among children between the ages of two years and eight years. In temperate regions, the number of cases peaks in the winter months. Complications, such as rheumatic fever, ear infections, and pneumonia, are relatively common in developing countries.

■ Treatment and Prevention

Scarlet fever is treated with antibiotics, with penicillin being the most common drug used. For those allergic to penicillin, erthryomycin or clindamycin are often pre-

WORDS TO KNOW

GROUP A STREPTOCOCCUS (GAS): A type (specifically a serotype) of the streptococcus bacteria, based on the antigen contained in the cell wall.

NOTIFIABLE DISEASE: A disease that the law requires must be reported to health officials when diagnosed; also called a reportable disease.

RASH: A rash is a change in appearance or texture of the skin. A rash is the popular term for a group of spots or red, inflamed skin that is usually a symptom of an underlying condition or disorder. Often temporary, a rash is only rarely a sign of a serious problem.

RESERVOIR: The animal or organism in which the virus or parasite normally resides.

TOXIN: A poison that is produced by a living organism.

scribed instead. Completing the course of treatment is essential to prevent the onset of rheumatic fever or other complications. The majority of patients make an uneventful recovery after treatment.

Paracetamol or ibuprofen are useful for treating the symptoms of scarlet fever. Cold liquids, like milkshakes and popsicles, and warm soup are useful for soothing throat pain, while a humidifier placed in the room will help ease dryness of the throat. In general, the patient should be kept very well hydrated, and get plenty of rest.

Good hygiene, including thorough handwashing, is very important in preventing the transmission of scarlet fever. Therefore, children with the illness, even if the case is mild, should be kept away from school or child care centers. Utensils belonging to a child who is sick at home should always be kept separate from those used by the rest of the family.

■ Impacts and Issues

When an infectious disease is notifiable, it allows public health authorities to mount an investigation and stop an outbreak from spreading. In 2006, the UK Health Protection Agency dealt with an outbreak of scarlet fever in the southern county of Wiltshire, where 50 cases were reported during January and February.

There were clusters of cases in two child care centers—16 in one, four in the other. Six of the 50 cases were in adults aged 18 years or more, while the rest occurred in children aged between eight months and ten years. Eleven cases had been reported during the same period of 2004 and only four in the same period of 2005. Therefore, this outbreak was unusual. In the first center, all children with symptoms received penicillin and were excluded for five days after beginning their treatment. The center closed down for several days. The second outbreak was reported on January 26, but no new cases were reported after January 31 in this child care center.

The local health protection team sent letters to all doctors in the area, informing them of the outbreaks. All suspected cases were to have throat swabs taken to test for the presence of GAS. This resulted in reports of 30 other cases of scarlet fever. The team also sent letters to the parents of all the children at the center to ask them to be on the alert for symptoms. However, they decided not to screen the children for GAS unless more serious scarlet fever cases were reported. Although they wanted to break the chain of transmission through asymptomatic carriers, they did not want to expose young children to antibiotics unnecessarily.

Samples from the throat swabs that had been taken were sent to the Health Protection Agency Centre for Infections for detailed analysis. These actions were taken because previous experience showed that outbreaks of scarlet fever can have serious consequences for the young patients if the infection is not treated promptly and adequately.

SEE ALSO *Impetigo; Necrotizing Fasciitis; Strep Throat; Toxic Shock.*

BIBLIOGRAPHY

Books

Wilson, Walter R., and Merle A. Sande. *Current Diagnosis & Treatment in Infectious Diseases.* New York: McGraw Hill, 2001.

Periodicals

Health Protection Agency. "Scarlet Fever Outbreak in Two Nurseries in South West England." *CDR Weekly* 16 (March 2, 2006): 1–2.

Marshall, S. "Scarlet Fever: the Disease in the UK." *The Pharmaceutical Journal* 277 (July 22, 2006): 115–116.

Web Sites

Centers for Disease Control and Prevention. "Scarlet Fever." October 13, 2005. <http://www.cdc.gov/ncidod/dbmd/diseaseinfo/scarletfever_g.htm> (accessed April 28, 2007).

Scrofula: The King's Evil

■ Introduction

Scrofula is a form of extrapulmonary (outside the lungs) tuberculosis, a bacterial infection of *Mycobacterium tuberculosis*.

■ Disease History, Characteristics, and Transmission

The disease has a long and interesting history, first mentioned by Herodotus in 400 BC who recommended that sufferers be quarantined. Scrofula has also had a long association with royalty. It became known as the King's Evil as early as 491 A.D, and was thought to be cured by the "king's touch." French monarchs claimed the ability to heal the disease from the time of Clovis in 481 AD through Louis XVI, who was beheaded in 1793, as did English kings beginning with Edward the Confessor (1042-66), ending with the Hanoverian dynasty in the eighteenth century.

Since antiquity, monarchs claimed a quasi-divine status, often asserting that the royal family had a divine right to rule. Various ceremonies of royal courts may have lead to the association of royalty with magical powers of healing. Perhaps because the lesions appeared and reappeared, people who were "touched" may have experienced an illusion of cure.

Politics also played a role in kings claiming they could heal scrofula. When the legitimacy of royal power was threatened, for instance among early Norman kings who ruled England by conquest, "healing ceremonies" became predominant. Usually in these rituals, the physician would hold the head of the patient as the king would pronounce, "The king touches you, and God cures you," making the sign of the cross touching forehead to chin and cheek to cheek. After the ceremony, French kings would distribute alms, and in England, the king would cross the sore of the sick person with a stamp of gold called an angel, worth ten shillings. The angel had a hole bored through it for a ribbon to be drawn, so the sufferer could wear it around his neck.

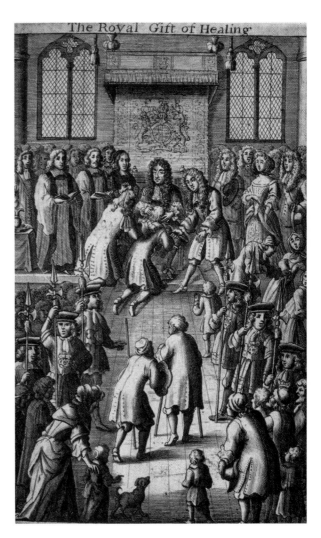

"The Royal Gift of Healing," an engraving, shows King Charles II (1630–1685) of England healing the sick. It was believed that the royal touch could cure diseases such as epilepsy and scrofula (also known as the king's evil). *HIP/Art Resource, NY.*

WORDS TO KNOW

ANTIBIOTIC RESISTANCE: The ability of bacteria to resist the actions of antibiotic drugs.

BROAD-SPECTRUM ANTIBIOTICS: Broad-spectrum antibiotics are drugs that kill a wide range of bacteria rather than just those from a specific family. For, example, Amoxicillin is a broad-spectrum antibiotic that is used against many common illnesses such as ear infections.

ENDEMIC: Present in a particular area or among a particular group of people.

LESIONS: The tissue disruption or the loss of function caused by a particular disease process.

QUARANTINE: Quarantine is the practice of separating people who have been exposed to an infectious agent but have not yet developed symptoms from the general population. This can be done voluntarily or involuntarily by the authority of states and the federal Centers for Disease Control and Prevention.

IN CONTEXT: PRE-SCIENTIFIC PRACTICE AND BELIEF

Samuel Johnson, an eighteenth-century author who wrote the first comprehensive English dictionary, suffered from scrofula as a child, and proudly wore his angel around his neck his entire life.

The true reason why scrofula was contracted was not known until the late nineteenth century. Because scrofula seemed to affect whole families, it was assumed that it was a hereditary, rather than an infectious disease. One of the common ways it spreads is though infected milk—either from an infected mother's or wet nurse's breast milk, or through contaminated cow's milk fed to infants or children. Before Koch's postulates of disease or pasteurization of milk in the 1880s, there was little understanding of the connection between bacteria and illness. During the mid-to-late nineteenth century in the United States, clean and inexpensive milk was also difficult to get; milk was often watered down, chalk or dye could be added to whiten dirty milk, and "swill milk," produced by cows fed distillery waste was common. These cows often carried bovine tuberculosis, and milk bottles were not sterilized.

It was also not until regulations about food safety were standardized, milk was regularly pasteurized, and dairy cleanliness maintained that scrofula ceased to be a health threat in industrialized nations.

■ Disease History, Characteristics, and Transmission

The term "scrofula" comes from the Latin "scrofulae" or a breeding sow, as pigs were thought to be susceptible to the disease, and the glandular swellings on the neck were compared to little pigs.

Scrofula results in an inflammation of the lymph glands and an enlargement of the lymph nodes in the neck. The nodes often ulcerate causing draining sores, and the sufferer also has fevers, chills, sweats, and sometimes weight loss. Lesions often subside, and then reappear as the disease takes its course and spreads through the skin, mucous membranes, bones and joints.

The disease can be contracted either through person-to-person contact, or via contaminated milk, or even via household objects that come into contact with the mouth.

■ Scope and Distribution

Though in developed countries, scrofula is now quite rare, lowered immune function resulting from HIV infection increases the risk of contracting the disease. As antibiotic resistance to tuberculosis has increased, scrofula has been making its reappearance, particularly in underdeveloped countries.

■ Treatment and Prevention

Though the king's touch is no longer considered effective, new challenges have arisen in the treatment of scrofula.

Treatment is largely through broad-spectrum antibiotics in a nine-to-twelve month course, and recovery is usually complete though there can be scarring around the lymph nodes.

Other treatments include short-course chemotherapy for tuberculosis patients, and increased detection protocols. In severe cases, surgery is done to remove the infected lymph nodes, but surgery alone tends to have disappointing results as it does not remove the underlying infection and it can cause scarring.

■ Impacts and Issues

Since 1985, scrofula has made a comeback in the United States largely due to immigration from endemic countries, rising rates of HIV infection, antibiotic resistance, and the abandonment of aggressive tuberculosis screening and control programs.

In sub-Saharan Africa, and increasingly in Asia and South American, scrofula is also posing a threat, particularly as a form of HIV-related tuberculosis. In its TB/IV Clinical Manual, the World Health Organization reports that growing rates of HIV-infections increase demands on programs to control tuberculosis, and there is more tuberculosis recurrence in AIDS patients.

SEE ALSO *Tuberculosis.*

BIBLIOGRAPHY

Books

Bloch, Marc *The Royal Touch. Sacred Monarchy and Scrofula in England and France.* London: Routledge and Kegan Paul; Monteal: McGill-Queen's University Press, 1973.

Periodicals

Barlow, Frank. "The King's Evil," *The English Historical Review*, 95, 374 (January 1980), pp. 3-27.

Harries, Anthony and Dermot Maher. "Introduction," *TB/HIV: A Clinical Manual* World Health Organization, 1996.

Lomax, Elisabeth. "Hereditary of Acquired Disease? Early Nineteenth Century Debates on the Cause of Infantile Scrofula and Tuberculosis," *Journal of the History of Medicine and Allied Sciences* October 1977, pp. 356-374.

Wheeler, Susan. "Henry IV of France Touching for Scrofula by Pierre Firens." *Journal of the History of Medicine and Allied Sciences* 58 (2003), pp. 79-81.

Jacqueline Wolf, *Don't Kill Your Baby: Public Health and the Decline of Breastfeeding in the 19th and 20th Centuries* Columbus: Ohio University Press, 2001.

Web sites

McClay, John E. "Scrofula," E-medicine from WebMD <http://www.emedicine.com/Ent/topic524.htm> (accessed March 2, 2006.

SCROFULA: THE KING'S EVIL

'tis call'd the Evil:
A most miraculous work in this good King;
Which often, since my here-remain in England,
I have seen him do. How he solicits heaven,
Himself best knows: but strangely-visited people,
All swoln and ulcerous, pitiful to the eye,
The mere despair of surgery he cures
Shakespeare, *Macbeth*, Act IV, scene 3

Anna Marie Roos

Sexually Transmitted Diseases

■ Introduction

Sexually transmitted diseases (STDs), also called sexually transmitted infections (STI), are passed on through intimate sexual contact. The most important STDs are HIV/AIDS, *Chlamydia*, syphilis, and gonorrhea. These are very different diseases in their infective causes, symptoms and health consequences. What they have in common is that people often do not realize that they are infected and may pass their disease onto others through sexual contact. Moreover, having one STD can put people at greater risk of contracting another—for instance, people with syphilis are more likely to become infected with HIV.

People at risk of STDs need to come forward for testing and treatment. The stigma attached to attending a sexual health clinic is less than it used to be, but there is still a need for greater awareness. Prevention of STDs is challenging, for it involves people's sexual behavior—whether they choose to use condoms, be selective about their sexual partners, or even abstain from sex.

■ Disease History, Characteristics, and Transmission

STDs are a diverse group of conditions, ranging from HIV/AIDS and syphilis, to scabies and thrush. In the past, they were known as venereal diseases (VD), the term venereal deriving from Venus, the goddess of love. AIDS and syphilis can be life threatening, *Chlamydia* infection can lead to infertility, and human papilloma virus (HPV) can lead to cervical cancer. Some STDs, like thrush and non-specific urethritis (infection of the urethra), are not usually medically serious, but can cause a great deal of discomfort. The symptoms of STDs vary, but often include itching, swelling, or redness around the vagina or penis, and unusual discharge or pains in the lower abdomen.

Perhaps the most feared of the STDs is HIV/AIDS. HIV is the human immunodeficiency virus, which as the name suggests, attacks the immune system, rendering the infected person powerless against opportunistic infections, such as *Pneumocystis carinii* pneumonia,

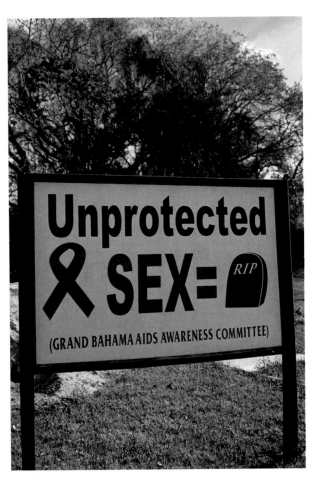

An AIDS awareness sign in the Bahamas warns of the dangers of unprotected sex. © *Nik Wheeler/Corbis.*

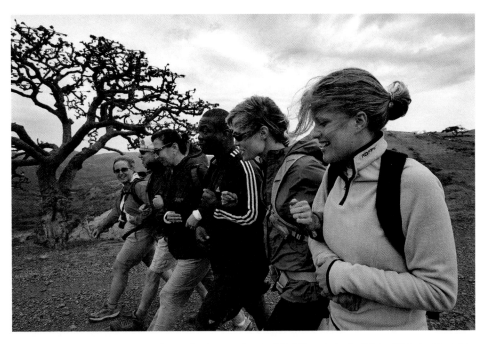

Walkers raise money during the Elizabeth Glaser Pediatric AIDS Foundation's "Africa Walk for Hope" in South Africa, 2004. The walk is intended to raise money to prevent mother-to-child transmission of HIV and extend care and treatment to people already infected. © *Jon Hrusa/epa/Corbis.*

Candida, and cytomegalovirus—all caused by microbes that are harmless in a healthy person. A rare skin cancer called Kaposi's sarcoma may also occur during the later stages of HIV/AIDS.

It can take ten years or more between first being infected with HIV, usually during sexual contact, before AIDS develops. At first, the immune system fights back against the infection and the person seems well. However, they can still infect others during this time. Eventually, the immune system breaks down, and opportunistic infections and other complications set in.

The first stage of HIV/AIDS lasts from first exposure to the appearance of antibodies in the person's blood, which may take up to three months. Antibodies are proteins made by the immune system as part of its response to infection. Some people display symptoms resembling a feverish illness, sore throat, or headache soon after they have been infected with HIV. This is a sign of the immune system fighting the infection. Sometimes the dentist is the first person to discover symptoms of HIV infection because mouth problems are quite common.

After this first stage, HIV infection enters a second, silent phase with few, if any, symptoms, which can last for as long as 15 years. The immune system is keeping the infection in check, but the person is still infectious to others through sexual contact or by other contact with infected blood. In the third stage, the immune system finally begins to show the signs of damage done by HIV. A common symptom at this time is swollen lymph glands, or lymphadenopathy.

In the final stage, classified as AIDS, the virus becomes more active than before and there are many symptoms such as malaise (a general feeling of being unwell), night sweats, weight loss, diarrhea. This is when opportunistic infections set in and Kaposi's sarcoma take hold. AIDS, in its final stages, may also affect the brain causing a gradual deterioration in mental faculties called dementia.

Chlamydia trachomatis infection is probably the most common of the sexually transmitted diseases that are caused by bacteria. When *C. trachomatis* infects the genital tract it often produces no symptoms, although women may report a burning sensation on urination and a vaginal discharge. Men may experience a discharge from the penis, as well as itching and a burning sensation.

Chlamydia infection must be taken seriously because, if left untreated, can cause serious damage to the female reproductive system, leading to pelvic inflammatory disease and infertility. A major complication is ectopic pregnancy, a potentially fatal condition where a fertilized egg starts to develop within one of the Fallopian tubes instead of in the womb. Women with *Chlamydia* are also up to five times more likely to become infected with HIV if exposed to it.

Gonorrhea is another important bacterial STD and is caused by infection with *Neisseria gonorrhoeae*. It causes urethritis (inflammation of the lining of the urethra) among men and cervicitis (inflammation of the cervix) in women. In men, the first symptom of

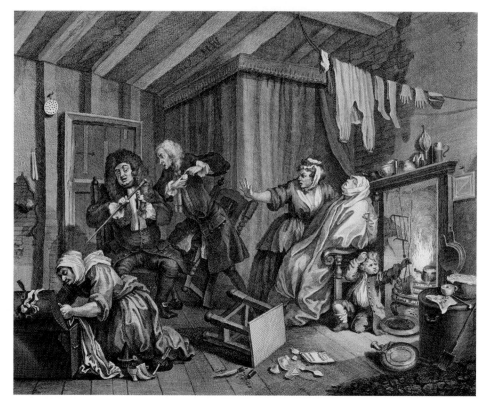

In this 1732 engraving by William Hogarth (1697–1764), a prostitute is shown dying from venereal disease in the sick room of a prison. *HIP/Art Resource, NY.*

gonorrhea is usually painful urination, followed by a thick prurulent (pus-containing) discharge from the urethra. However, many men have no symptoms. In women, painful urination is also the first symptom of gonorrhea. This is followed by a vaginal discharge and, sometimes, bleeding. Occasionally, the symptoms in women are so vague that they are mistaken for a vaginal or urinary infection. Most women with gonorrhea have no symptoms at all.

Gonorrhea may lead to various complications. In men, the epididymis (the coiled tube leading sperm from the testicles) may become inflamed, which can lead to infertility. Gonorrhea in women can lead to salpingitis, which is inflammation of the Fallopian tubes and it is also a leading cause of pelvic inflammatory disease (PID), a chronic condition that is often accompanied by severe abdominal pain and fever, long-lasting pelvic pain, and infertility.

Syphilis is caused by the bacterium *Treponema pallidum* and progresses through an infectious and a non-infectious stage over many years. The infectious stage lasts for a few months during which time symptoms may cause little or no illness. The non-infectious stage, which follows if syphilis is not treated early on, may also be without symptoms, or it may be accompanied by major heart or neurological damage.

Infectious syphilis starts with the appearance of a single sore, known as a chancre, either on or inside the genitals or elsewhere on the body, such as on the eyelid or lip. Those affected may be completely unaware of the presence of the chancre, which lasts for three to six weeks and heals without treatment, but is infectious to sexual contacts.

A skin rash and mucous membrane lesions are the prime symptoms of the secondary stage of syphilis. Sometimes the rash from secondary syphilis is so faint as to be unnoticeable. There may be other symptoms such as fever, swollen glands, weight loss, headaches, loss of appetite, and fatigue. However, this stage also resolves within a few weeks without any treatment.

Latent or tertiary syphilis is untreated disease past the primary and secondary stage. It has no obvious symptoms and may or may not be infectious. Complications, which may occur many years after the original infection, can affect the brain and the heart. A pregnant woman with syphilis might pass the disease onto her unborn child. Congenital syphilis can lead to stillbirth, death shortly after birth, physical deformity, or neurological problems.

Genital herpes, often known solely as herpes, is caused by the Herpes Simplex virus (HSV) and may cause no symptoms, remaining undiagnosed for a long time. Possible symptoms of HSV infection include itchiness, burning, and pain in the genital area, pain when passing urine, and the presence of small fluid-filled blisters developing into sores. People with herpes have an increased risk of becoming infected with HIV, and pregnant women may pass the infection onto their babies during childbirth. Neonatal (the newborn period) herpes can have a mortality rate as high as 60%.

The human papillomavirus (HPV) causes both genital warts and cervical cancer. While HPV infection often causes no symptoms, it sometimes triggers benign tumors known as papillomas, or warts on the hands and feet or in the genital area. Most HPV infections clear up on their own, but they are also capable of causing cancers in the cervix and, more rarely, in the vagina, vulva, penis, and anus.

Other STDs include non-specific urethritis, which affects men and causes discomfort in the urethra, the tube leading from the bladder to the tip of the penis. A discharge from the urethra is also common. Trichomoniasis is caused by the bacterium *Trichomonas vaginalis* and may have no symptoms or may produce a yellow or green discharge from the vagina and be accompanied by soreness. Men usually act as carriers of trichomoniasis and often do not show symptoms themselves. Thrush is a yeast infection of the vagina or penis, which can result in intense itching and a thick white discharge. Finally, both pubic lice and scabies are passed on by close contact, including sexual contact, and may cause intense itching.

STDs are generally transmitted through intimate sexual contact with another person. This can occur through unprotected vaginal, oral, or anal sex, or having genital contact with an infected partner. The relative risks of various kinds of sexual activity tend to vary with the disease. For instance, the risk of contracting gonorrhea and syphilis through oral sex appears to be greater than that of contracting HIV.

The risk of becoming infected with HIV is elevated between two and five times by having another STD, maybe because these can involve breaks in the skin in the genital area, making it easier for the virus to enter the body. Non-ulcerative STDs like trichomoniasis may increase HIV risk through increasing the number of white blood cells that can be infected by the virus.

■ Scope and Distribution

Most major public health organizations, such as the Center for Disease Control and Prevention (CDC), the World Health Organization (WHO) and the United Kingdom's Health Protection Agency (HPA), collect data on STDs in order to plan policy and educate and inform the population of the risks.

WORDS TO KNOW

ANTIBODIES: Antibodies, or Y-shaped immunoglobulins, are proteins found in the blood that help to fight against foreign substances called antigens. Antigens, which are usually proteins or polysaccharides, stimulate the immune system to produce antibodies. The antibodies inactivate the antigen and help to remove it from the body. While antigens can be the source of infections from pathogenic bacteria and viruses, organic molecules detrimental to the body from internal or environmental sources also act as antigens. Genetic engineering and the use of various mutational mechanisms allow the construction of a vast array of antibodies (each with a unique genetic sequence).

CHANCRE: A sore that occurs in the first stage of syphilis at the place where the infection entered the body.

HARM-REDUCTION STRATEGY: In public health, a harm-reduction strategy is a public-policy scheme for reducing the amount of harm caused by a substance such as alcohol or tobacco. The phrase may refer to any medical strategy directed at reducing the harm caused by a disease, substance, or toxic medication.

LYMPHADENOPATHY: Any disease of the lymph nodes (gland like bodies that filter the clear intercellular fluid called lymph to remove impurities) is lymphadenopathy.

NOTIFIABLE DISEASE: A disease that the law requires must be reported to health officials when diagnosed; also called a reportable disease.

OPPORTUNISTIC INFECTION: An opportunistic infection is so named because it occurs in people whose immune systems are diminished or are not functioning normally; such infections are opportunistic insofar as the infectious agents take advantage of their hosts' compromised immune systems and invade to cause disease.

PRURULENT: Containing, discharging, or producing pus.

According to the WHO, there are 340 million new cases of curable STDs around the world each year, along with five million cases of new HIV infections. The CDC's National Surveillance Data for *Chlamydia*, gonorrhea, and syphilis for 2005 suggests that there are

19 million new infections each year in the United States, of which almost half occur among young people aged 15 to 24. Many notifiable (state health departments mandate reporting of certain diseases) STDs go unreported, and HPV and genital herpes, which are probably extremely common, are not reported at all.

The HPA reports a continual rise in STDs in the United Kingdom since the 1990s. Between 2004 and 2005, there was a three percent increase to a total of 790,387 confirmed cases. The largest increase was in cases of syphilis, up by 23 percent to a total of 2,807 cases. There were also rises in *Chlamydia*, genital warts and herpes, which are reported to the HPA. As in the United States, the biggest increases have been noted in the 16 to 24 year age group.

Treatment and Prevention

Most STDs are treatable by either a single dose or course of antibiotics, when the cause is bacterial. Antiviral drugs are used to treat genital herpes, although they cannot actually cure the infection. Genital warts do eventually disappear without treatment, although some people may chose to have them removed by liquid nitrogen or treatment with caustic agents. HIV/AIDS is treatable with antiretroviral drugs, which stop the virus from reproducing. The treatment regimes are complex, but enable the patient to live with HIV rather than dying from AIDS.

Informing current and past sexual partners of a positive diagnosis of an STD, so they can also be diagnosed and treated, is key to reducing the risk of spreading and re-infection. A sexual health clinic will normally help the patient do this.

Among those who are sexually active, practicing safer sex is the most effective way of preventing STDs. This involves using a male condom for each occasion of penetrative sex and considering the choice of sexual partner carefully. That is, there is no guarantee that any prospective partner does not already have an STD—and therefore, the more sexual partners a person has, the higher their chance of exposure to infection, even with the use of condoms, as they do not provide 100% effective protection. Abstinence from sex or monogamous sex with a healthy partner are behavioral choices that may afford the highest level of protection from STDs. Healthcare workers advising in this area attempt to exercise sensitivity and take care not to make judgments on their patient's behaviors, while providing them with the information they need to reduce their risk of contracting an STD.

Impacts and Issues

The increase in STDs in the United States and elsewhere can partly be attributed to an increase in awareness of the issue, better diagnostic techniques, and an increase in the number of sexual health clinics carrying out tests. Other reasons include earlier age of first sexual activity, people having more partners, and increased mobility of groups such as tourists, immigrants, and armed forces who may be more likely to have partners outside of a primary relationship.

Anyone who is sexually active—whatever their age or sexual orientation—is at risk of contracting an STD and should be aware of the attendant risks and symptoms. Not only do STDs cause direct health problems, such as infertility or cervical cancer, they also have the indirect consequence of increasing the risk of HIV infection. Moreover, people tend to have more than one STD at a time. Often, the symptoms are not apparent, which means the person remains infectious and passes the disease onto others without modifying their sexual behavior.

STDs are lifestyle diseases, where the risk of transmission is related directly to the number of sexual partners a person has. Conversely, celibacy is the best way not to become infected. However, the situation is usually more complex than this—merely counseling people not to have sexual contact with others is one approach to prevention, but is not generally effective if it is the only approach taken. Instead, a "harm reduction" strategy can also be applied, where persons are advised about safer sex, using condoms, and these are made readily available. One of the largest worldwide public health efforts in history began after the advent of AIDS in the 1980s, and used a harm-reduction strategy to teach how HIV is transmitted and prevented, distribute condoms, deliver care for those infected, and change cultural attitudes necessary for bringing the discussion of AIDS prevention to the forefront.

In 2006, a vaccine was approved in the United States to guard against four types of HPV infection, the cause of genital warts and ultimately, most cases of cervical cancer. The vaccine is recommended for girls and young women from age nine to 26. Research has shown that it affords the highest level of protection against genital warts and cervical cancer among those who have not been exposed to HPV infection already—that is, those who have not become sexually active. Girls and women who have been exposed to HPV may gain some protection with the vaccine, but it cannot cure any existing HPV infection. In Texas, Governor Rock Perry mandated that all schoolgirls entering sixth grade receive the vaccine beginning in 2008. Citing the high cost (around $300 for the series of injections) and some parental objections, the state legislature overruled the mandate, at least until the year 2011. Eventually, the HPV vaccine could prevent not only the common STD caused by the human papilloma virus, but most cases of cervical cancer, the second leading cause of cancer death among women worldwide.

SEE ALSO *AIDS (Acquired Immunodeficiency Syndrome); Chlamydia Infection; Gonorrhea; Herpes Simplex 1 Virus; HIV; HPV (Human Papillomavirus) Infection; Syphilis.*

BIBLIOGRAPHY

Books

Adler, Michael, et al. *ABC of Sexually Transmitted Diseases.* London: BMJ, 2004.

Wilks, D., M. Farrington, and D. Rubenstein. *The Infectious Disease Manual,* 2nd. ed. Malden: Blackwell, 2003.

Periodicals

Weinstock H., et al. "Sexually transmitted diseases among American youth: incidence and prevalence estimates, 2000." *Perspectives on Sexual and Reproductive Health* 2004; 36(1):6–10.

Web Sites

Centers for Disease Control and Prevention (CDC). "Trends in Reportable Sexually Transmitted Diseases in the United States, 2005." December 2006 <http://www.cdc.gov/std/stats> (accessed May 16, 2007).

NHS Direct. "Sexually Transmitted Infections." <http://www.nhsdirect.nhs.uk/articles/> (accessed May 16, 2007).

World Health Organization. "Sexually Transmitted Infections." <http://www.who.int/reproductive-health/stis/index.htm> (accessed May 16, 2007).

Susan Aldridge

Shigellosis

■ Introduction

Shigellosis is an infection of the gastrointestinal tract that arises when a person is infected with bacteria in the genus *Shigella*. These bacteria are transmitted among a human population when people ingest food or drink contaminated with fecal matter from an infected person. Following a 24-hour incubation period, most patients experience nausea, diarrhea, fever, and stomach cramps. While most people recover from shigellosis within a week without treatment, severe cases require antibiotics in order to recover.

Shigellosis occurs worldwide. It is most prevalent in developing nations in which epidemics often occur. Anyone can get shigellosis, but it is more common among people with poor hygiene, such as young children, as well as people living or traveling through areas with dense living conditions and poor sanitation. Since there is no vaccine against shigellosis, prevention is achieved through improving sanitation and hygiene, washing hands prior to handling food, washing food prior to eating, and boiling drinking water. Shigellosis can become a major issue during emergency situations, such as mass evacuations when many people temporarily live together in poor conditions. There is also potential for *Shigella* bacteria to be used for biological warfare.

■ Disease History, Characteristics, and Transmission

Shigellosis is a gastrointestinal infection caused by bacteria from the genus *Shigella*. There are four species of

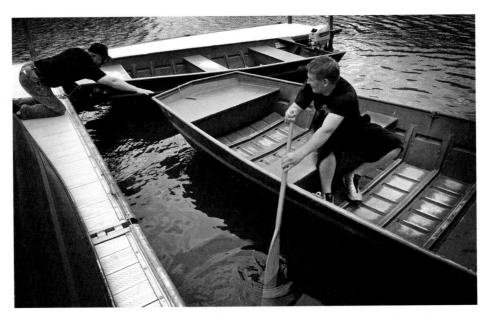

Park officials closed this lake for swimming after some visitors tested positive for shigellosis, which could have been spread through contact with lake water containing shigella bacteria. *AP Images.*

Shigella, S. dysenteriae, S. flexneri, S. boydii, and *S. sonnei. Shigella* infect humans and other primates. Bacteria from this genus were first identified by the Japanese scientist Kiyoshi Shiga (1871–1957) in 1897 after he isolated *S. dysenteriae,* which was causing dysentery, a gastrointestinal disease, in infected people.

Shigellosis is usually transmitted via the fecal-oral route, that is, people become infected after ingesting food or water contaminated with infected feces. Inadequate handwashing after using the toilet, or changing a baby diaper, followed by food or water handling leads to contamination of food and drink. This is a very common method for person-to-person transmission of the *Shigella* bacteria. Flies are also a source of transmission as they travel between infected fecal matter and food or drink. Food and water may also become contaminated when vegetables are grown in soil containing sewage, or when people defecate in bodies of water.

Shigellosis leads to the development of gastrointestinal symptoms, such as dysentery. Symptoms include diarrhea, fever, stomach cramps, and nausea. Symptoms generally begin a day or two after the bacteria is contracted, although it may take up to a week for a person to fall ill. Although recovery is usual in most cases, infection with *S. flexneri* may result in long-term problems such as arthritis, eye irritation, and painful urination. This is known as Reiter's syndrome and may continue for months to years.

■ Scope and Distribution

Shigellosis occurs worldwide. It is particularly common in developing countries in which the bacteria are present in almost all communities most of the time. Furthermore, *S. dysenteriae* type 1, although rare in the United States, is a major health concern for many developing countries. In the United States, the most common forms of *Shigella* are *S. sonnei,* which causes over two-thirds of shigellosis infections, and *S. flexneri,* which causes most of the remaining cases. The annual number of cases of shigellosis in the United States ranges from as few as 1,000 to as many as 18,000, although this number is likely to be underestimated, since many mild cases go undiagnosed.

Although anyone is capable of contracting shigellosis, some people are more susceptible. This includes toddlers who usually aren't fully toilet trained. In addition, childcare facilities provide a setting in which the bacteria can spread through a number of children in a short period of time. Foreign travelers are also more susceptible to infection, if they travel through regions in which the disease is prevalent and sanitation methods are poor. Persons living together in crowded conditions or institutions, such as prisons, are also more susceptible to developing the disease, most likely as a result of poor hygiene.

The transmission of shigellosis is enhanced in conditions of poor sanitation and close human contact. These conditions are common in developing countries where funding for sanitation may be lacking and residents may not be educated about the need for hygiene. In addition, these conditions are also common in emergency situations, for example, after a hurricane or earthquake, when many people are often housed together temporarily.

■ Treatment and Prevention

Shigellosis is a bacterial disease and is treated with antibiotics. However, mild cases of shigellosis do not require antibiotics, since a full recovery usually occurs within a week. However, people suffering from severe infections, or those who have a compromised immune system that prevents them fighting the infection themselves, usually require a course of antibiotics. The most common antibiotics used are ampicillin, trimethoprim/sulfamethoxazole, nalidixic acid, or ciprofloxacin. However, *Shigella* bacteria are beginning to develop resistance to antibiotics, which reduces the effectiveness of treatment. In order to combat this problem, health officials are trying to reduce the reliance on antibiotics by limiting their use.

Other treatments are aimed at the symptoms of the infection. These may include administering fluids to prevent or reverse dehydration and medicines to reduce temperature and prevent convulsions. Antidiarrheal agents are not recommended by the Centers for Disease Control and Prevention (CDC), since they are likely to make the illness worse.

While research on the development of a vaccine against shigellosis has been underway since 1940, no vaccine is currently available. As a result, preventative measures center around avoiding ingestion of *Shigella* bacteria. In developed countries, in which sanitation is usually good and water is clean, prevention is best achieved through handwashing and improving personal hygiene. However, in developing countries, in which sanitation is often poor and clean water is not readily available, improvements in sanitation methods and increased availability of clean water are necessary to prevent community-wide spread of the bacteria. In addition, people with shigellosis can best prevent spreading the disease to others by washing their hands after going to the toilet, avoiding preparing food for others, and avoiding public swimming areas.

■ Impacts and Issues

Shigellosis is common in developing countries due to poor sanitation and, in some cases, overcrowding. However, situations such as this can arise in developed nations when natural disasters, such as hurricanes, tornadoes, and floods, cause mass evacuation of people. Often mass evacuations result in a large number of people having to live in close quarters. Since these living quarters are often temporary and are usually not made to house large numbers of people, sanitation standards tend to be lower than normal. The combination of high density living with poor sanitation increases the risk of shigellosis within the population.

Another potential issue concerning *Shigella* bacteria is its use as a biological weapon. *Shigella* has been considered a potential agent of biological warfare since at least 1932 when the Japanese investigated its potential. Biological warfare involves using pathogens or toxins to cause mass death and disease among humans, animals, or plants during war. Biological terrorism is similar, except the pathogens and toxins are used for terrorist purposes. In addition to *Shigella*, other bacterial agents, such as *Salmonella* and *Escherichia coli*, are considered potential biological threats. *Shigella* can potentially be spread via a community's water supply, which could cause many cases of shigellosis. In 1996, one case of *S. dysenteriae* caused an outbreak of shigellosis. A worker from Dallas contaminated muffins and doughnuts with *Shigella* prior to feeding coworkers. This resulted in a number of the workers developing shigellosis, and the perpetrator was jailed.

SEE ALSO *Antibiotic Resistance; Bacterial Disease; Bioterrorism; Childhood Infectious Diseases, Immunization Impacts; Cohorted Communities and Infectious Disease; Dysentery;* Salmonella *Infection (Salmonellosis).*

BIBLIOGRAPHY

Books

Fong, I. W., and K. Alibek. *Bioterrorism and Infectious Agents: A New Dilemma for the 21st Century.* New York: Springer Science, 2005.

Mandell, G. L., J. E. Bennett, and R. Dolin. *Principles and Practice of Infectious Diseases.* 6th ed. Philadelphia: Elsevier, 2004.

Web Sites

Baylor College of Medicine. "Potential Bioterrorism Agents." July 5, 2006. <http://www.bcm.edu/molvir/eidbt/eidbt-mvm-pbt.htm> (accessed March 12, 2007).

Centers for Disease Control and Prevention. "Hurricane Recovery Information." September 16, 2005. <http://www.bt.cdc.gov/disasters/hurricanes/katrina/shigella.asp> (accessed March 12, 2007).

Centers for Disease Control and Prevention. "Shigellosis." October 13, 2005. <http://www.cdc.gov/ncidod/dbmd/diseaseinfo/shigellosis_g.htm> (accessed March 12, 2007).

New York State, Department of Health. "Shigellosis." June 2004. <http://www.health.state.ny.us/diseases/communicable/shigellosis/fact_sheet.htm> (accessed March 12, 2007).

Shingles (Herpes Zoster) Infection

■ Introduction

Shingles is a disease that arises when the varicella-zoster virus (VZV), which causes chickenpox when it initially infects a human, reactivates after lying dormant in nerve cells. Shingles develops first as localized pain after which a rash, composed of fluid-filled blisters, forms. Fever, headache, chills, and a general feeling of sickness often accompany the pain. The rash develops within a few days and it may take several weeks for the blisters to break open and crust over. A person is infectious until the rash crusts over. Some cases of shingles result in serious complications, the most common being post-herpetic neuralgia, a type of nerve pain.

Treatment for shingles involves oral administration of an antiviral treatment. In addition, the symptoms and any complications also are treated. Treatment for post-herpetic neuralgia is aimed primarily at controlling the pain.

Shingles is a worldwide disease, but is most common in older adults, usually those aged 50 year old or older. Immunocompromised people are also at a greater risk of developing shingles. Prevention is achieved by preventing exposure of non-immune individuals to the fluid from rash blisters. In addition, a vaccine has been developed that is aimed at preventing shingles in patients 60 years old and older.

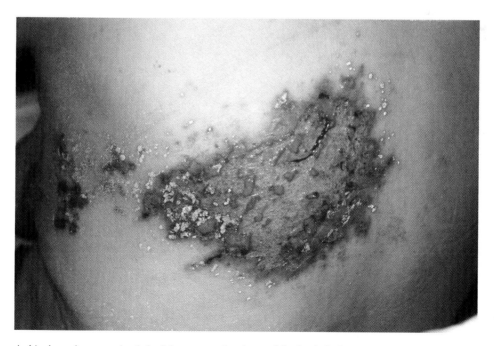

A shingles rash on a patient's back has ruptured and caused further infection.   *DR M.A. Ansary/Photo Researchers, Inc.*

WORDS TO KNOW

CHICKENPOX: Chickenpox (also called varicella disease and sometimes spelled chicken pox) is a common and extremely infectious childhood disease that can also affect adults. It produces an itchy, blistery rash that typically lasts about a week and is sometimes accompanied by a fever.

IMMUNOCOMPROMISED: A reduction of the ability of the immune system to recognize and respond to the presence of foreign material.

POSTHERPETIC NEURALGIA: Neuralgia is pain arising in a nerve that is not the result of any injury. Postherpetic neuralgia is neuralgia experienced after infection with a herpesvirus, namely *Herpes simplex* or *Herpes zoster*.

VARICELLA-ZOSTER VIRUS (VZV): Varicella zoster virus is a member of the alpha herpes virus group and is the cause of both chickenpox (also known as varicella) and shingles (herpes zoster).

■ Disease History, Characteristics, and Transmission

Shingles, which is also known as herpes zoster, is caused by a virus known as varicella-zoster virus (VZV). This virus also causes chickenpox. Shingles arises in people who have already had chickenpox, since the virus remains in the body.

Usually, VZV remains dormant in the body. It settles in nerve roots, and when activated, causes the development of shingles. Shingles is characterized by the development of pain, itching, or tingling in a region on the body where a rash will develop a few days later. This pain is often accompanied by fever, headache, chills, or an upset stomach, making patients feel unwell. The rash develops blisters filled with fluid. These blisters break open and crust over. Infection normally lasts for four to five weeks, and, in most individuals, the skin heals and recovery is complete.

Some cases of shingles develop serious complications. Skin may be damaged due to scratching of the rash, and some cases of skin damage result in scarring. Deafness and blindness also can occur when the virus spreads to nerves within the ear or eye regions. This may be temporary, but in some cases is permanent. Brain inflammation (encephalitis) and death may also occur in rare cases. More commonly, pain may occur following recovery from the rash.

Approximately 20% of people with shingles develop this pain, known as post-herpetic neuralgia. The pain is often severe and most likely is caused by nerve damage.

The varicella-zoster virus is transmitted when humans come in contact with airborne respiratory droplets or with fluid from rash blisters. When a person is first infected with this virus, they develop chickenpox. Once a person has contracted this virus, they retain it, and shingles develops when the virus reactivates. Exposure to fluid from shingles blisters does not cause people to become infected with shingles, but it can cause a person with no prior infection to contract chickenpox.

■ Scope and Distribution

Varicella-zoster virus occurs worldwide and causes the development of both chickenpox and shingles. Within the United States, the Centers for Disease Control and Prevention (CDC) reports an estimated one million cases of shingles annually. Anyone who has had chickenpox, and thus retains VZV, can potentially develop shingles. However, the majority of shingles cases occur in people older than 50 years of age. While children and adults under 50 do develop shingles, the risk of developing shingles increases with age.

Shingles is also more likely to develop in people who are immunocompromised. People with medical conditions, such as cancer or HIV, or those who have received organ transplants, have a compromised immune system that is less able to fight off infections. Therefore, these individuals are more likely to develop shingles.

While shingles cannot be spread from one person to another, people who have not previously been infected by VZV can contract the virus if they come in contact with infectious fluid from shingles blisters. However, this will result in chickenpox, not shingles.

While the majority of shingles patients recover fully after an infection, the CDC reports a fifth of U.S. patients suffer from post-herpetic neuralgia. This amounts to 200,000 people who develop this condition annually.

■ Treatment and Prevention

Treatment is available for shingles and recovery is more likely the sooner treatment is administered. Shingles is treated using antiviral medications that are administered orally. These include acyclovir, famciclovir, and valacyclovir. Treatment does not cure the viral disease. Instead, it acts to hinder the progression of the disease throughout the nerves.

To treat the symptoms of shingles, in particular, the pain from the rash, pain-relieving medications, such as ibuprofen, naproxen, indomethacin, and nonsteroidal anti-flammatory drugs, are administered. For more intense pain, stronger analgesics, such as codeine or oxycodone, may be prescribed.

Treatment for post-herpetic neuralgia varies. The treatments tend to focus on treating the pain. Some treatments include: patches that release the pain-relieving medication lidocaine directly into the affected area; analgesics, which have sedating properties; opioids, which control pain; and antidepressants, which help patients tolerate severe pain. Some patients also receive electrical nerve stimulation or have the affected nerve cells blocked. However, the pain experienced often differs from patient to patient, and treatments that work for one patient do not necessarily work for another.

The spread of VZV from shingles patients to previously non-infected people can be prevented by covering the rash, avoiding touching the rash, and washing hands often to prevent contaminating items with fluid from the rash. Once the rash crusts over, the virus is no longer contagious.

A vaccine has been developed that causes people to develop immunity to VZV. This has been found to decrease the number of people developing chickenpox, and is thought to lessen the risk of the virus remaining dormant and possibly reactivating as shingles. A new vaccine, Zostavax, was developed in 2006. This vaccine prevents shingles and, in 2006, the vaccine was approved for use in patients 60 years old and over.

■ Impacts and Issues

Shingles usually affects older people and, in 20% of cases, the patient develops post-herpetic neuralgia. Post-herpetic neuralgia is nerve pain that lasts for three months or more. The pain can vary from mild to severe, and patients may experience burning, stabbing, or gnawing sensations. This side effect of the varicella-zoster virus is a serious issue for a number of reasons. The pain experienced by persons with shingles can often be persistent and debilitating. Furthermore, the treatments used for nerve pain tend to work for some people, while having no effect for other people, making pain management difficult. The number of people in the United States suffering from post-herpetic neuralgia is significant and while some may be relieved of the pain in a few months, many suffer severe pain for years following recovery from shingles.

Shingles can also be a dangerous disease when it infects immunocompromised persons. People with medical conditions, such as cancer or HIV, or those who have received organ transplants, have weakened immune systems and they are less capable of fighting off the disease. Therefore, more serious complications such as post-herpetic neuralgia, meningitis, and even death, are more likely in these persons if they contract shingles. Furthermore, vaccination is not a viable option, since even small doses of the virus may cause complications for these people. Therefore, avoidance of the virus, or rapid treatment, is vital for patients who are immunocompromised in order to prevent serious complications.

SEE ALSO *AIDS (Acquired Immunodeficiency Syndrome); Cancer and Infectious Disease; Chickenpox (Vari-*

IN CONTEXT: PERSONAL AND SOCIAL RESPONSIBILITY

The National Immunization Program (NIP) at Centers for Disease Control and Prevention (CDC) states that "Shingles cannot be passed from one person to another. However, the virus that causes shingles, VZV, can be spread from a person with active shingles to a person who has never had chickenpox through direct contact with the rash. The person exposed would develop chickenpox, not shingles. The virus is not spread through sneezing, coughing or casual contact. A person with shingles can spread the disease when the rash is in the blister-phase. Once the rash has developed crusts, the person is no longer contagious. A person is not infectious before blisters appear or with post-herpetic neuralgia (pain after the rash is gone)."

With regard to what can be done to prevent the spread of shingles, the CDC states that "the risk of spreading shingles is low if the rash is covered. People with shingles should keep the rash covered, not touch or scratch the rash, and wash their hands often to prevent the spread of VZV. Once the rash has developed crusts, the person is no longer contagious."

SOURCE: *Centers for Disease Control and Prevention, National Immunization Program (NIP)*

---

cella); HIV; Vaccines and vaccine development; Viral Disease.

BIBLIOGRAPHY

Periodicals

Kimberlin, D.W., and R.J. Whitley. "Varicella-Zoster Vaccine for the Prevention of Herpes Zoster." *New England Journal of Medicine* 356 (March 29, 2007): 1338–1343.

Web Sites

Centers for Disease Control and Prevention. "Shingles (Herpes Zoster)." October 19, 2006. <http://www.cdc.gov/nip/diseases/shingles/faqs-disease-shingles.htm> (accessed March 7, 2007).

Centers for Disease Control and Prevention (CDC). "Varicella Disease (Chickenpox)." May 26, 2005. <http://www.cdc.gov/nip/diseases/varicella/> (accessed Mar. 7, 2007).

U.S. Department of Health and Human Services. "Shingles: An Unwelcome Encore." June 2005. <http://www.fda.gov/FDAC/features/2001/301_pox.html> (accessed March 7, 2007).

World Health Organization. "Varicella Vaccine." May 2003. <http://www.who.int/vaccines/en/varicella.shtml> (accessed March 7, 2007).

Smallpox

■ Introduction

Smallpox is a infectious disease caused by a virus. It was eradicated by 1980 thanks to a global vaccination program, but stocks of variola virus are still held by at least two governments, those of the United States and the Russian Federation. The smallpox virus, also called the variola virus or simply variola, is most often spread by ingestion of virus particles in saliva, either by direct contact or through inhaling droplets dispersed in the air by coughing. When ingested, the smallpox virus first infects the tissues of the throat and nasal cavities, followed by the blood and lymph nodes. About 12 days after infection, a variety of flulike symptoms appear, including fever. Pustules (pus-filled lumps) develop on the skin and are painful at first, then itchy. The more deadly of variola's two varieties, *Variola major*, kills about 30% of the people that it infects. Sixty-five percent to 80% of those that do survive the disease are disfigured by pitted scars (pockmarks). Some survivors are also blinded by scarring of the retina. Before a vaccine was developed, smallpox was one of the most common causes of blindness worldwide.

■ Disease History, Characteristics, and Transmission

History

The evolutionary origin of the variola (smallpox) virus, a member of the genus *Orthopoxvirus*, family Poxviridae, is still obscure. It probably began as a virus in rodents and first infected humans in Africa about 12,000 years ago. The oldest historical reference is in a Chinese document dating to the fourth century. The name "variola," from the Latin for "spotted," dates to the sixth century. The term "smallpox" dates to the 1400s, when it was used to distinguish smallpox from syphilis (the "great pox").

North and South America were free of smallpox until European explorers arrived in the late 1400s. The disease soon spread to the Native American population, which had a much higher mortality rate than the Old World

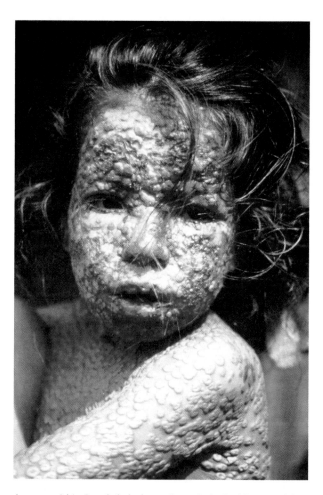

A young girl in Bangladesh shows the typical raised bumps of the smallpox infection, which she contracted in 1973. In 1977, the World Health Organization announced that smallpox, a potentially fatal disease, had been eradicated from the country. By 1980, it was eliminated in the rest of the world. © *CDC/PHIL/Corbis.*

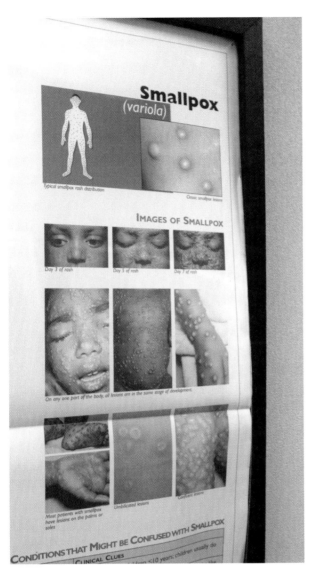

Information on smallpox is shown at the U.S. Public Health Service Quarantine Station in Atlanta's Hartsfield Jackson International Airport in 2005. Built before the 1996 Olympics, it is one of 18 such facilities located in major airports. Ten of the 18 quarantine stations have become operational since 2003 in response to threats of disease importation and bioterrorism. *Barry Williams/Getty Images.*

population, probably because there had been no history of natural selection for resistance to the disease. Some historians estimate that 90% of the population of the New World was killed by smallpox. For example, the Aztec population in South America fell from 25 million in 1519 to only 3 million in 1569. Smallpox was not originally spread deliberately by the Europeans, although in the French and Indian wars of the mid-1700s British military forces gave smallpox-infected blankets to Indians who were cooperating with the French—one of the earliest recorded efforts at biological warfare.

In 1796, English physician Edward Jenner (1749–1823) showed that inoculating a person with pus from a cowpox lesion could prevent smallpox. Inoculation had been discovered before—the earliest known use of smallpox inoculation dates to about 1000 BC, in India—but the idea of inoculation with the harmless cowpox virus had not yet been put forward in Europe by somebody with the professional and class standing to establish it as a known medical fact.

At the time of Jenner's work, smallpox was killing about 400,000 people a year in Europe and millions worldwide. The practice of variolation had already been used to fight smallpox for some decades in Europe and for centuries in Asia. Variolation (named after the disease, variola—the existence of viruses was not yet understood) involved infecting a healthy person with smallpox from a mild case of the disease, either by inserting smallpox-scab material into the nostrils or by rubbing it onto a scratch on the skin. People inoculated in this way were far less likely to die from the more severe form of smallpox than were un-inoculated people. However, there was still a significant death rate from smallpox contracted through variolation (1–2%). Jenner's method of inoculation with cowpox virus was much safer. Although his views were not accepted for a few years, they did catch on. Over 100,000 inhabitants of Britain had been vaccinated with cowpox by 1800 and the British Parliament passed the Vaccination Act in 1840 to make vaccination of infants mandatory and to outlaw variolation. Mandatory smallpox vaccination of children soon became the standard in industrialized countries.

So successful was vaccination that the disease was eradicated from prosperous countries. The last case of smallpox in the United States occurred in 1949. At that time, smallpox was still infecting about 50 million people every year worldwide, about 30% of whom died. Thanks to vaccination, the number of infections dropped to about 15 million per year by 1967. In that year, the World Health Organization (WHO) of the United Nations started a program—the WHO Intensified Smallpox Eradication Program—to eliminate smallpox completely. In 1972, the United States began phasing out mandatory vaccination of schoolchildren. In 1977, the last natural case of smallpox on Earth was seen in Somalia, and in 1980, WHO declared that the eradication campaign had been a success. Smallpox had become the first (and, as of 2007, still the only) major infectious disease to be completely eradicated by human effort.

Characteristics

Smallpox occurs in two forms, variola major and variola minor. Both forms cause similar symptoms, but variola minor is fatal only about 1–2% of the time, compared to 30% or higher for variola major. These two varieties of variola have been recognized for centuries, even before the viral nature of the disease was understood. The two varieties of virus are similar enough that immunity to one confers immunity to the other. Variolation with scabs or pus from mild smallpox cases—an ancient method of immunizing people against smallpox—usually involved infected people with variola minor, granting them immunity from variola major with a fairly low risk of death from the treatment.

The variola virus is most often caught by inhalation of saliva droplets coughed out by a person who already has the disease. Virus particles lodge in the nasal cavities or throat and infect those tissues first, then grow in the lymph nodes nearest the site of infection. (Lymph nodes are small, bean-shaped organs that filter lymph, a clear fluid that is drained from tissues through the system of lymphatic vessels and then returned to the blood.) The patient has no symptoms during this phase of the disease. After three or four days, virus particles spread through the bloodstream to the bone marrow, spleen, and other parts of the lymphatic system, where they multiply. The smallpox virus, like all viruses, multiplies by tricking body cells into manufacturing more virus particles, using genetic material supplied by the virus itself. More smallpox virus particles appear in the blood 8–10 days after infection. During these initial phases—termed the incubation period—the patient feels healthy and cannot infect other persons. About 12–14 days after infection (with a range of 7–17 days), the incubation period ends and the next phase of the illness—termed the prodrome, prodromal stage, or preeruptive stage—begins suddenly. In this stage, symptoms appear, but do not yet include the skin eruptions or lesions that make the patient capable of spreading the infection. Prodromal symptoms may include fever and last 2–4 days. After the prodromal stage, the disease can next show four distinct courses or clinical presentations. These are termed ordinary smallpox, modified smallpox, flat smallpox, and hemorrhagic smallpox.

Ordinary Smallpox

Ordinary smallpox accounts for about 90% of cases. After the prodromal stage, the fever may drop and the patient feels less sick. The smallpox rash then appears as small red spots (lesions) on the tongue, on the inside of the mouth, and at the back of the throat (on the pharynx). The mouth-and-throat lesions grow, releasing billions of virus particles into the saliva that may then be transmitted to other people. The lesions in the throat trigger coughing, which tends to spread the disease. About 24 hours after the appearance of the mouth-and-throat rash, a rash appears on the skin, first on the face and limbs and then on the trunk. The rashes become lumpier and fill with fluid. In about a week the lumps, now filled with pus and called pustules, have become round, raised, and hard to the touch, like beads under the skin. Generally, the more severe the rash, the greater the chance that the patient will die. In

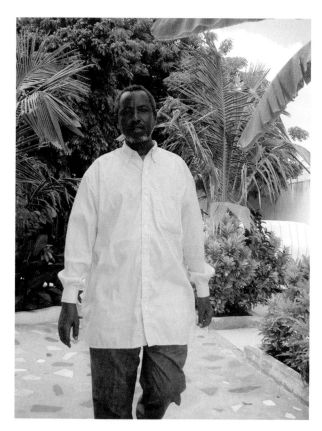

Ali Maow Maalim, the last known smallpox victim, was photographed in Mogadishu in late 2002. He still bears scars from the disease, which he caught in 1977 while vaccinating people against smallpox in a Somali hospital. *AP Images.*

another week the fluid in the pustules has been absorbed and a crust or scab begins to form over them. Finally, a week later, the crusts fall off, leaving bleached skin and indented scars. At this point the patient has ceased to be infectious.

Modified Smallpox

Modified smallpox is a milder form of the disease that sometimes occurs in persons who have been vaccinated. The fever does not return after the prodromal phase and the rash appears more quickly but produces fewer and smaller lesions. This form of the disease is almost never fatal.

Flat Smallpox

In flat smallpox, the raised lesions or pustules of ordinary smallpox do not develop on the skin. This form of the disease has been observed in a study in India to occur about 5–10% of the time, usually in children. The prodromic stage is more severe in flat smallpox, and so is the rash on the tongue and at the back of the throat. The skin lesions appear slowly and are flatter than in ordinary smallpox. This form of the disease is usually fatal.

Hemorrhagic Smallpox

Hemorrhagic smallpox occurs about 2% of the time in India. It is called "hemorrhagic" because to hemorrhage means to bleed; patients with this form of smallpox begin to bleed—sometimes only a few days into the course of the disease—in the eyes, gums, mouth, and skin lesions. Death usually occurs about a week after the onset of symptoms, before the skin rash has had a chance to develop much.

Transmission

Variola virus is quite virulent, that is, easy to spread from one person to another. Only a small number of virus particles need be taken into the body to cause the disease. Virus concentrations in the saliva and mucus are highest during the first week of symptomatic illness (after the prodromic stage), and it is during this time that the patient is most infectious. However, the patient remains infectious until all crusts have separated from the healing pustules on the skin. Virus particles can be transmitted through the air or by direct contact with the patient or materials they have touched. They do not enter through the skin, but may be transferred to the mucous membranes of the mouth, eyes, or nose by hand contact.

■ Scope and Distribution

Smallpox infection no longer occurs naturally. As of 2007, the only stocks of the virus known to exist are held by the governments of Russia and the United States.

■ Treatment and Prevention

Since smallpox is caused by a virus, it cannot be treated using antibiotics (which kill only bacteria). Nor, as of 2006, had any antiviral drug had been approved by the U.S. Food and Drug Administration for the treatment of smallpox. The Centers for Disease Control and Prevention suggested that the antiviral drug cidofovir might be used for smallpox under the supervision of an infectious diseases specialist, but warns that the drug can injure the kidneys. The usual treatment is strictly supportive: the patient is kept clean, sheltered, and hydrated, while their own immune system fights the infection.

The main method of preventing transmission of smallpox is to avoid having other people ingest the virus. To this end, all persons having contact with a smallpox patient should wear fitted breathing masks and disposable gloves, gowns, and shoes. Breathing masks prevent the inhalation of virus particles.

Where high-technology medical settings are available, a smallpox patient should be isolated in a room with negative pressure, that is, one where the air-circulation system draws air into the room and filters it before pumping it out rather than allowing it to escape. This is because smallpox transmission can be caused by virus particles conveyed in tiny, airborne particles. Air that has contacted a

---

WORDS TO KNOW

ERADICATION: The process of destroying or eliminating a microorganism or disease.

PRODROME: A prodrome of a disease is a symptom indicating the disease's onset; it may also be called a prodroma. For example, painful swallowing is often a prodrome of infection with a cold virus.

VARIOLATION: Variolation was the pre-modern practice of deliberately infecting a person with smallpox in order to make them immune to a more serious form of the disease. It was dangerous, but did confer immunity on survivors.

---

smallpox patient must be assumed to be potentially carrying the disease.

The primary method of preventing smallpox infection is the smallpox vaccine. It is not made using smallpox virus, but a live vaccinia virus strain. The standard vaccine available today was developed in the early 1980s and is supplied as a freeze-dried powder in 100-dose units. The dry vaccine mixture contains several antibiotics and is mixed with a special liquid consisting of water, glycerin, and phenol as a preservative. The vaccine is guaranteed to confer immunity for at least 10 years, but there is evidence that it may confer immunity for far longer. About 15 million doses of this vaccine are stockpiled in the United States as of 2007; this number could be increased in an emergency by diluting the vaccine to increase its volume by a factor as great as 5.

Smallpox vaccine causes a number of medical complications, but death is rare. It should not be taken by pregnant women, because the vaccinia virus can cause fetal vaccinia, an infection of the fetus with the vaccinia virus. This usually causes stillbirth or death of the child soon after birth.

■ Impacts and Issues

The eradication of smallpox was one of the major public health success stories of the twentieth century. This effort demonstrated that international cooperation on important health issues could be achieved. Moreover, it also demonstrated that it is possible to eradicate an infectious disease with an effective vaccination program, and that vaccination is a useful preventative method in the fight against infectious diseases. Smallpox stocks still exist, however, and if released into the environment, could cause an epidemic in an unvaccinated population. As of 2007, a large but unknown percentage of Americans were not immune to smallpox. This uncertainty arises because nobody is sure how much immunity is still conferred by immunizations received before 1972.

Smallpox has long been considered as a biological weapon of war or terror. In the mid–1700s, British army commanders in what is now Canada gave smallpox-infested blankets to Indians who were collaborating with the French (the enemies of the British at that time). Systematic bioweapons research by the U.S., Japan, the Soviet Union, and other countries began during World War II but concentrated on bacteria (e.g., anthrax) rather than viruses for some years. In the 1950s, American bioweapon developers, concerned that the Soviet Union might be developing smallpox and other viruses as well, began studying techniques for producing freeze-dried smallpox powder that could be efficiently spread over a wide area. In the mid-1960s, Army planners approached the U.S. bioweapons labs at Fort Detrick, Maryland, to see whether biological weapons could be used to attack military traffic between North and South Vietnam. Smallpox was considered the best candidate, but the idea was abandoned because U.S. use of biological warfare might be exposed, North Vietnam might retaliate in kind, and the disease might spread to friendly forces. At about this time, Soviet agents secretly sampled highly virulent smallpox strains in India for use in the large Soviet bioweapons program. In 1969, President Richard Nixon abolished the U.S. biological warfare program and supported an international ban on biological weapons. This was formalized as the 1972 Biological and Toxic Weapons Convention Treaty, which was eventually signed by the Soviet Union and most of the rest of the countries of the world.

After biological attacks using anthrax occurred in the United States in 2001, the issue of smallpox as a potential agent of biological terror again surfaced. In the United States, researchers, members of the military, key health personnel, and first responders in the community were vaccinated against smallpox so that response to any future threat by the smallpox virus can be prompt. Large reserves of smallpox vaccine are maintained by many countries in the developed world and the World Health Organization.

Today, the smallpox virus is only known to exist in two secure repositories, both authorized by WHO: one is at the Centers for Disease Control and Prevention in the United States and the other is at the State Research Center of Virology and Biotechnology of the Russian Federation in Siberia. Debate continues on whether the last remaining stocks of smallpox virus should be used for research or destroyed.

■ Primary Source Connection

Disease outbreaks are reported by World Health Organization (WHO, Epidemic and Pandemic Alert and Response (EPR), Disease Outbreak News.

WHO maintains the EPR as a "major pillar of global health security aimed at the detection, verification and containment of epidemics. In the event of the intentional release of a biological agent these activities would be vital to effective international containment efforts."

As the bulletin below indicates, the system is also used to clarify information and allay fear concerning infectious agents that could be used as biological weapons.

ACCIDENTAL EXPOSURE TO SMALLPOX VACCINE IN THE RUSSIAN FEDERATION

20 JUNE 2000

DISEASE OUTBREAK REPORTED

The recent report of illness amongst 8 young children in Vladivostock who had played with discarded ampoules of smallpox vaccine has now been confirmed by the Ministry of Health of the Russian Federation. Laboratory confirmation of the illness in the children is being sought. The report has evoked much public concern. In some of the reports, there were misconceptions about the components of the vaccine used to prevent smallpox, and about why any country might still be retaining stocks of smallpox vaccine. This note aims to clarify these issues.

1. Smallpox vaccine is not made from smallpox virus. The vaccine which was used for centuries to vaccinate against smallpox was not made from smallpox, but from vaccinia virus. Vaccinia is a different virus from the virus which causes smallpox. However, it is a member of the same family of viruses to which the smallpox virus belongs. The smallpox virus is also known as variola virus. Mass vaccinations with smallpox vaccine made from vaccinia virus led to the eradication of smallpox announced by WHO in 1980. People vaccinated with smallpox vaccine (vaccinia) develop reactions to it which range from mild and transient to severe, and very rarely, fatal.

2. Two countries still keep smallpox virus (variola) stocks. Although smallpox disease has been

eradicated, two laboratories still hold stocks of smallpox virus (variola). These are the WHO Collaborating Centres in Atlanta, USA and Koltsovo, Russian Federation.

3. Many countries still hold smallpox vaccine (vaccinia) stocks. WHO recommends that countries which still have stocks of smallpox vaccine (vaccinia) maintain these stocks. This recommendation has been made for two reasons. Firstly, small amounts of vaccine are still needed to vaccinate laboratory personnel handling vaccinia virus and other members of this virus family. Some of these viruses are found in nature and cause illness among animals, and some are used in research to make new, safer vaccines against a variety of infectious diseases. Secondly, smallpox vaccine (vaccinia) will also be needed in case of a deliberate or accidental release of smallpox virus (variola), which is a very unlikely event but currently of great concern to some countries. For further information on this topic, see the summary of the recent meeting of the WHO Advisory Committee on Variola Virus Research, published in the Weekly Epidemiological Record.

4. Disposal of biological materials and pharmaceuticals. All biological materials and pharmaceuticals such as vaccines, drugs and diagnostic specimens should be disposed of safely. Some may require inactivation before disposal. This can be accomplished by autoclaving or incineration.

World Health Organization

WORLD HEALTH ORGANIZATION, EPIDEMIC AND PANDEMIC ALERT AND RESPONSE (EPR), DISEASE OUTBREAK NEWS "ACCIDENTAL EXPOSURE TO SMALLPOX VACCINE IN THE RUSSIAN FEDERATION: 20 JUNE, 2000." <HTTP:// WWW.WHO.INT/CSR/DON/2000_06_20E/EN/INDEX.HTML> (ACCESSED APRIL 12, 2007)

SEE ALSO *Smallpox Eradication and Storage; Viral Disease; World Health Organization (WHO).*

BIBLIOGRAPHY

Books

Ian, Glynn, and Jennifer Glynn. *Life and Death of Smallpox.* London: Profile Books, 2005.

Miller, Judith, et al. *Germs: Biological Weapons and America's Secret War.* New York: Simon & Schuster, 2002.

Rodriguez, Ana Maria. *Edward Jenner: Conqueror of Smallpox.* Springfield, NJ: Enslow, 2006.

Periodicals

Cohen, Jon. "Leaks Produce a Torrent of Denials." *Science* 298 (2002): 1313–1314.

Esposito, Joseph J., et al. "Genome Sequence Diversity and Clues to the Evolution of Variola (Smallpox) Virus." *Science* 313 (2006): 807–812.

Koopman, Jim. "Controlling Smallpox." *Science* 298 (2002): 1342–1344.

Web Sites

Centers for Disease Control and Prevention. "Emergency Preparedness and Response: Smallpox." <http:// www.bt.cdc.gov/agent/smallpox/> (accessed February 21, 2007).

Journal of Young Investigators. "Smallpox: Historical Review of a Potential Bioterrorist Tool." September 2002. <http://www.jyi.org/volumes/volume6/ issue3/features/bourzac.html> (accessed February 21, 2007).

World Health. "Smallpox." <http://www.who.int/ mediacentre/factsheets/smallpox/en/> (accessed February 20, 2007).

Larry Gilman

Smallpox Eradication and Storage

■ Introduction

Smallpox is a disease caused by the smallpox virus, also called the variola virus or simply variola. The World Health Organization (WHO) of the United Nations declared smallpox eradicated in 1980 after a decades-long program of global vaccination. However, specimens of smallpox virus are still held in the United States, Russia, and possibly other countries. Samples of variola DNA may also be recoverable from old medical samples, such as the century-old smallpox scabs discovered in an envelope tucked in a nineteenth-century medical textbook in a New Mexico library in 2004. Since the 1990s, there has been ongoing debate about whether or not remaining stocks of smallpox should be destroyed. Issues include the morality of deliberately causing the extinction of a species; whether continued possession of the virus might someday result in its escape, potentially causing millions of deaths; whether the virus might be used to develop biological weapons; and whether keeping the virus intact is necessary as a precaution against the possible use of smallpox as a biowar or bioterror weapon or its accidental or natural re-release into human populations. The WHO has authorized some research with existing variola stocks, but faces continued controversy over the continued existence of the smallpox virus.

■ History and Scientific Foundations

The eradication of smallpox began with the discovery in 1796 by English physician Edward Jenner (1749–1823) that inoculating a person with pus from a cowpox lesion could prevent smallpox. This fact had been noticed before by a number of people, as had the possibility of inoculation using scabs or pus from people with milder cases of smallpox (variola minor). However, Jenner was the first person with professional standing to discover inoculation with the harmless cowpox virus, and so he

was able to publish his findings and make them a standard part of medical knowledge.

Widespread vaccination led to the disappearance of smallpox from industrialized countries. In the United States, for example, the last case was reported in Texas in 1949. From 1967 to 1980, the World Health Organization oversaw a global campaign, the WHO Intensified Smallpox Eradication Program, to eliminate

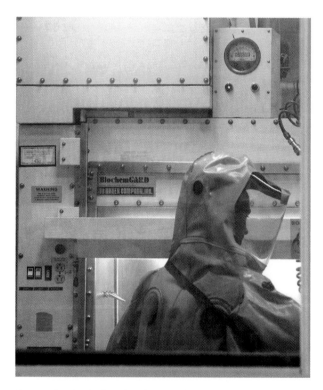

A researcher in the Poxvirus Section of the Centers for Disease Control and Prevention (CDC) in Atlanta shows the use of a biohazard suit. In an effort to modernize defenses against smallpox, the CDC has dedicated a maximum-containment laboratory to smallpox-only research. *AP Images.*

smallpox entirely. The program was declared an official success in May 1980, almost three years after the last case of natural smallpox on Earth was seen in 1977 in Somalia.

The eradication strategy had two basic features. First came mass vaccination campaigns in each target country, coordinated with that country's government. The goal was to vaccinate at least 80% of the population of each target country. Smallpox vaccination is a simple procedure involving multiple skin punctures in the side of the arm with a two-pronged metal tool resembling a lobster fork. The tool, termed a bifurcated needle, is dipped once into a vial containing liquid smallpox vaccine and then repeatedly stuck into the skin over a small area. Earlier, less-convenient methods were displaced by the bifurcated-needle procedure during the global eradication campaign.

The smallpox vaccine does not contain smallpox virus, but live vaccinia virus. Vaccinia virus almost never causes fatal disease; the reported death rate from smallpox vaccination is approximately one death per one million vaccinations. An immune system that has learned to recognize and attack the vaccinia virus will also recognize and attack the variola virus at its first appearance. Smallpox virus may enter the body of an immunized person, but is destroyed by the immune system before it can gain a foothold.

The second aspect of the eradication strategy was termed "surveillance and containment." Since some percentage of the population in most countries remained unvaccinated even at the height of the eradication campaign, smallpox still occurred. Surveillance and containment involved keeping a lookout for outbreaks of smallpox and then selectively, intensively vaccinating people in the vicinity of the outbreak.

This two-part strategy was successful. Smallpox was eliminated in Brazil in 1971 and in Indonesia in 1972. A few outbreaks in Europe were caused by travelers, but were rapidly contained. The last case of the more severe form of smallpox, variola major, occurred in Bangladesh in 1975. The last case of natural smallpox occurred in Somalia in 1977. After several years with no reported cases of the disease, the World Health Organization declared smallpox eradicated in 1980. As of 2007, no cases had been reported worldwide in 30 years.

Following eradication, the World Health Organization requested that all laboratories in the world either destroy their smallpox virus stocks or transfer them to one of two reference laboratories, the Institute of Viral Preparations in Moscow or the United States Centers for Disease Control and Prevention in Atlanta, Georgia. The stocks of the Institute of Viral Preparations were transferred in 1994 to the State Research Center of Virology and Biotechnology of the Russian Federation in Siberia, now the WHO Collaborating Centre for Orthopoxvirus Diagnostics.

WORDS TO KNOW

BIFURCATED NEEDLE: A bifurcated needle is a needle that has two prongs with a wire suspended between them. The wire is designed to hold a certain amount of vaccine. Development of the bifurcated needle was a major advance in vaccination against smallpox.

BIOSAFETY LEVEL 4 FACILITY: A specially equipped, secured laboratory where scientists study the most dangerous known microbes. These labs are designed to contain infectious agents and disease-causing microbes, prevent their dissemination, and protect researchers from exposure.

COWPOX: Cowpox refers to a disease that is caused by the cowpox or catpox virus. The virus is a member of the orthopoxvirus family. Other viruses in this family include the smallpox and vaccinia viruses. Cowpox is a rare disease, and is mostly noteworthy as the basis of the formulation, over 200 years ago, of an injection by Edward Jenner that proved successful in curing smallpox.

VACCINATION: Vaccination is the inoculation, or use of vaccines, to prevent specific diseases within humans and animals by producing immunity to such diseases. The introduction of weakened or dead viruses or microorganisms into the body to create immunity by the production of specific antibodies.

VACCINIA VIRUS: The vaccinia virus is a usually harmless virus that is closely related to the virus that causes smallpox, a dangerous disease. Infection with the vaccinia virus confers immunity against smallpox, so vaccinia virus has been used as a vaccine against smallpox.

VARIOLA VIRUS: Variola virus (or variola major virus) is the virus that causes smallpox. The virus is one of the members of the poxvirus group (Family Poxviridae). The virus particle is brick shaped and contains a double strand of deoxyribonucleic acid. The variola virus is among the most dangerous of all the potential biological weapons.

By United States law, smallpox virus can be stored and handled only at Biosafety Level 4 (BSL-4) facilities. Such a facility consists of a separate building or architecturally isolated section of a building specially equipped for biological isolation. Persons entering and leaving the facility must take sterilizing showers; air and sewage leaving the building must pass through special filters to remove any possible disease-carrying particles, and separate air supply and exhaust must be arranged for workers inside the laboratory space. The building must be ventilated so that air flows into the building and toward the part of the building where the most hazardous materials are kept. The building must also remain sealed in the event of a power failure. There are approximately 10 BSL-4 facilities in the United States as of 2007.

■ Applications and Research

Following eradication, the World Health Organization set 1999 as the deadline for the destruction of all variola virus stocks. However, both the United States and Russia failed to carry out this directive, citing the need for further research on the virus. The World Health Assembly (WHA), the governing body of WHO, accepted the continuing existence of the virus and established a Variola Advisory Committee to oversee variola virus research until the end of 2002. After that time, the virus stocks were to finally be destroyed. Some ethicists have raised the question of whether it is permissible to deliberately cause the extinction of any species, even a malignant virus, but this has not been a major concern in WHO or governmental debates on the fate of the variola virus. In 2002 the WHA decided, under combined United States and Russian pressure, that not enough research had been accomplished and that the deadline for variola destruction would be extended indefinitely.

The goals of variola virus research are said by workers in the field to be a better understanding of the genome of the virus, the proteins produced by the virus, and the precise means by which the virus infects cells in order to prepare for accidental, natural, or deliberate re-release of the virus in human populations. The genomes of several dozen varieties of variola virus were completely sequenced by 2007.

In 2004, the Variola Advisory Committee decided to allow the creation of genetically modified varieties of the variola virus, in particular, some containing reporter genes (genes that make it easy to identify the presence of the virus, such as a protein that glows green when exposed to blue light). In 2005, the advisory committee also voted to allow the transfer of variola DNA fragments up to 55 base pairs long between laboratories, the manufacture of gene chips containing smallpox DNA, and the splicing of smallpox genes into other orthopoxviruses.

■ Impacts and Issues

Research using the surviving smallpox virus stocks has been controversial for decades. The World Health Organization's Director-General opposed WHO's decision in 2005 to allow the transfer of smallpox genes to other viruses, a move also opposed by South Africa, China, the Netherlands, and a number of other countries. Developing countries, which would be more vulnerable to a new smallpox outbreak, are particularly keen on final destruction of virus stocks. Two groups, the Third World Network and the Sunshine Project, mounted campaigns in the early 2000s against continuing smallpox research of this type.

Also in 2005, a bill passed by the United States Congress made it illegal to "produce, engineer, [or] synthesize" the variola virus from scratch. The possibility of from-scratch (also called de novo) manufacture of smallpox virus is not farfetched. Poliovirus was first synthesized from scratch in 2001, starting solely with a record of its genome and without the aid of preexisting RNA, DNA, or living cells. In 2006, Sandia National Laboratory, an arm of the U.S. government, began experiments that involved inserting synthetic (de novo) variola genes into other organisms. Some critics of the continued existence of variola stocks say that since Sandia's historical mission has been the production of nuclear weapons and the laboratory has no biomedical mission, its research with variola virus genes is inappropriate and signifies deteriorating WHO control over smallpox research.

In January 2007, the WHO Executive Board adopted a draft smallpox resolution to be sent to the WHA in May 2007. The resolution asks the Director-General of the WHO to forbid genetic engineering of the variola virus and calls for the topic of setting a definite date for the destruction of variola virus stocks to be placed on the agenda of the WHA's 63rd or 64th session in 2010 or 2011.

SEE ALSO *Smallpox; Viral Disease; World Health Organization (WHO).*

BIBLIOGRAPHY

Books

Carrell, Jennifer Lee. *The Speckled Monster: A Historical Tale of Battling the Smallpox Epidemic.* New York: Dutton, 2003.

Koplow, David. *Smallpox: The Fight to Eradicate a Global Scourge.* Berkeley, CA: University of California Press, 2004.

Periodicals

Cohen, Jon. "Leaks Produce a Torrent of Denials." *Science* 298 (November 15, 2002): 1313–1315.

Enserink, Martin. "WHA Gives Yellow Light for Variola Studies." *Science* 308 (May 27, 2005): 1235.

Halloran, M. Elizabeth, et al. "Containing Bioterrorist Smallpox." *Science* 298 (November 15, 2002): 1428–1432.

Normile, Dennis. "WHO Gives a Cautious Green Light to Smallpox Experiments." *Science* 306 (November 19, 2004): 1270–1271.

Web Sites

Centers for Disease Control and Prevention. "The Pink Book: Smallpox." November 15, 2006. <http://www.cdc.gov/nip/publications/pink/smallpox.pdf> (accessed February 22, 2007).

World Health Organization. "Smallpox." <http://www.who.int/mediacentre/factsheets/smallpox/en/> (accessed February 20, 2007).

Larry Gilman

Sporotrichosis

Introduction

Sporotrichosis, also known as rose gardener's disease, is a mycotic (fungal) infection that is caused by the fungus *Sporothrix schenckii*. Humans most often become infected when they are pricked or scratched by plants that harbor the fungus. The resulting infection is usually a cutaneous (skin) infection involving the formation of ulcerous lesions. However, other forms of sporotrichosis can occur when the fungus is inhaled, and include pulmonary sporotrichosis, in which the lungs are infected, and disseminated sporotrichosis, in which the joints, gastrointestinal system, or central nervous system are infected.

Sporotrichosis infection occurs worldwide. Gardeners, florists, or children playing in hay bales who regularly come in contact with plants harboring the fungus are most at risk of becoming infected.

Sporotrichosis is most commonly treated with antifungal medication. Treatment may be required for months, and in cases left untreated, severe skin ulceration can occur. Development of the less common forms of the disease, that is pulmonary and disseminated sporotrichosis, can lead to serious complications such as tuberculosis, bone diseases, or swelling of the brain and may potentially be fatal. People with weakened immune systems are most at risk of these potentially fatal complications of sporotrichosis.

Disease History, Characteristics, and Transmission

The fungus was first identified as the causative agent of sporotrichosis by the American physician Benjamin Robinson Schenck (1873–1920) in 1896. For this reason, sporotrichosis is also sometimes known as Schenck's disease. After the French physician Charles Lucien de Beurmann (1851–1923) further explained the role of *S. schenckii* in causing disease in 1903, some scientists renamed the organism *Sporotrichum beurmanni*.

After an incubation period of about 1–12 weeks from exposure to the fungus, infection with *S. schenckii* causes a small painless nodule (bump), similar to an insect bite, to develop on the skin. This nodule can be red, pink, or purple, and tends to be located on the finger, hand, or arm. Eventually, a number of similar lesions form, spreading to other regions of the body.

Most sporotrichosis infections are limited to the skin. However, rarely, the fungus may spread through the lymphatic system after it is inhaled to infect the lungs, joints, or central nervous system. Serious complications can arise in these cases, particularly when the fungus spreads to the central nervous system. In this case, the disease is known as sporotrichosis meningitis, and can cause death. When the joints are affected, the disease is known as osteoarticular sporotrichosis. This condition can cause symptoms such as weight loss, bursitis, and weak, stiff joints. Pulmonary sporotrichosis is more common in middle aged men who have underlying risk factors such as alcoholism and existing pulmonary diseases like emphysema. People with pulmonary sporotrichosis often develop pneumonia.

The fungus is transmitted from plant material such as roses, hay, and sphagnum moss into humans via broken skin. Defensive mechanisms on these plants such as thorns, barbs, and pine needles can cause punctures or cuts in the skin, creating an entry route for transmission of the fungi. Sporotrichosis is not spread from person to person.

Scope and Distribution

Sporotrichosis occurs worldwide. The fungus *S. schenckii* occurs naturally on thorny plants such as roses, on sphagnum moss, and in hay. Therefore, people who come in contact with these plants are at the greatest risk of becoming infected. This includes gardeners, nursery workers, farmers, and greenhouse workers. In addition, children who often play on baled hay are at risk of contracting the disease.

Treatment and Prevention

The most common form of treatment for sporotrichosis is administration of the anti-fungal drug itraconazole. Oral administration of a saturated potassium iodide solution is sometimes given, and this treatment is given over a period of usually 3–6 months. Other anti-fungal drugs such as fluconazole may also be used. When the lesions have become large and filled with fluid, it is sometimes necessary to drain and remove the lesions surgically.

Other forms of sporotrichosis, such as in the lungs, joints, or central nervous system, may also require itraconazole or surgery. An additional treatment sometimes administered in complicated cases involves amphotericin B.

Wearing protective clothing, such as gloves and long sleeves while handling plants may provide protection against infection by *S. schenckii*. In particular, the Centers for Disease Control and Prevention (CDC) recommends that workers wear gloves when coming into contact with sphagnum moss due to a number of outbreaks of sporotrichosis associated with this plant.

Impacts and Issues

Sporotrichosis also occurs in other mammals such as cats and dogs, and pet owners, especially those living on a farm, are advised to seek treatment for pets showing nodules. Humans can become infected by coming in contact with the open sores present on animals. Therefore, veterinarians responsible for treating animals infected with sporotrichosis are also at risk of contracting this infection.

While disseminated variations of sporotrichosis rarely occur, they occur most commonly in people with compromised immune systems such as people living with diseased or weakened organs, cancer, diabetes, or AIDS. Therefore, these persons are at a greater risk of developing potentially fatal forms of sporotrichosis.

SEE ALSO *AIDS (Acquired Immunodeficiency Syndrome); Immune Response to Infection; Mycotic Disease; Pneumonia; Tuberculosis.*

WORDS TO KNOW

CUTANEOUS: Pertaining to the skin.

DISSEMINATED: Disseminated refers to the previous distribution of a disease-causing microorganism over a larger area.

INCUBATION PERIOD: Incubation period refers to the time between exposure to disease causing virus or bacteria and the appearance of symptoms of the infection. Depending on the microorganism, the incubation time can range from a few hours (an example is food poisoning due to *Salmonella*) to a decade or more (an example is acquired immunodeficiency syndrome, or AIDS).

MYCOTIC: Mycotic means having to do with or caused by a fungus. Any medical condition caused by a fungus is a mycotic condition, also called a mycosis.

BIBLIOGRAPHY

Periodicals

Coles FB, et al. "A Multistate Outbreak of Sporotrichosis Associated with Sphagnum Moss." *American Journal of Epidemiology* (1992): 136, 475–487.

Web Sites

Centers for Disease Control and Prevention (CDC). "Sporotrichosis." October 13, 2005 <http://www.cdc.gov/ncidod/dbmd/diseaseinfo/sporotrichosis_g.htm#How%20is%20sporotrichosis%20treated> (accessed March 12, 2007).

Department of Health, New York State. "Sporotrichosis." June 2004 <http://www.health.state.ny.us/diseases/communicable/sporotrichosis/fact_sheet.htm> (accessed March 12, 2007).

Standard Precautions

■ Introduction

Standard precautions are precautions that have been put into effect by the U.S. Centers for Disease Control and Prevention (CDC) aimed at reducing the risk of transfer of disease-causing viruses or bacteria (generally called pathogens) from the blood or other moist regions of the body—such as mucous membranes and damaged skin—that can harbor pathogens. Essentially, standard precautions involve good hygiene. This includes proper handwashing and, in a hospital, other practices, such as the proper use of protective equipment, environmental controls, and handling of used linen.

■ History and Scientific Foundations

The standard precaution criteria established by the CDC in January 1996 are an extension of guidelines that were known as universal precautions. Universal precautions were recommended in 1987 following the recognition that acquired immunodeficiency syndrome (AIDS, also cited as acquired immune deficiency syndrome) could be contracted by the transfer of blood that was contaminated with the human immunodeficiency virus (HIV).

Universal precautions applied to people known or suspected of having a blood-borne infection. Standard precautions are wider in their scope, and apply to all body fluids (except sweat) of all patients whether or not they are recognized as having an infection.

■ Applications and Research

Handwashing

One of the fundamental standard precautions is handwashing. Hands must be washed after direct contact with blood or other body fluids of a patient, or after contact with items, such as fluid-soaked linen, whether or not gloves have been worn. This ensures that pathogens that may have contacted the skin through tiny tears or an imperfection in a glove are killed.

Handwashing should be done immediately after contact with a patient and before moving on to another patient. Handwashing may also need to be done during the time with one patient, if different tasks are performed, for example, after probing inside the mouth and before examining other parts of the body.

For routine handwashing, use of ordinary household soap is acceptable, since the soap's ingredients and the friction from rubbing the hands together for a sufficient length of time (at least 30 seconds) will produce the desired antimicrobial effect. But, increasingly in hospital wards, an alcohol solution is being used. This is because the alcohol solution is effective more quickly, an important consideration in the time-constrained day of healthcare providers. In addition, washing the hands with soap many times every day can be harsh on skin, even to the point of causing breaks in the skin that can become infected.

Gloves

Healthcare providers should wear gloves when coming into contact with blood and other body fluids. Fresh gloves must be worn for each patient, otherwise the gloves can become a route of patient-to-patient transfer of microbes. Similar to handwashing, gloves should be worn and removed immediately before and after contact with a patient, and need to be disposed of in a designated container.

Gown

A hospital gown worn over clothing protects against splashing or spraying of blood and other body fluids. The choice of a gown depends to a large extent on the infection that a person might be exposed to. For example, a gown made out of plastic or other water-repellent material should be used when dealing with an infection suspected of being severe such as Ebola. A gown that became soaked with Ebola virus-laden blood could result in transfer of the virus to the healthcare provider. In contrast, cotton gowns can be appropriate in other cases.

A gown should be removed as soon as possible after seeing a patient and always before moving to another patient. Since the removal of a gown involves the hands, handwashing should be done only after a gown is removed and put in a designated container.

Patient-Care Equipment

Equipment that becomes contaminated with blood or other body fluid must be decontaminated before re-use. Equipment that is meant for one-time use must be disposed of properly after that use and should never be re-used. Needles and other sharp object must be disposed of after use in rigid containers to minimize the chances of accidental injury during their disposal.

Environmental Control

Microorganisms can stick to surfaces and, in some cases, can remain capable of causing an infection for hours. If a contaminated surface is touched by someone, the infectious microbes can be transferred to that person or someone else that person contacts. Thus, an important standard precaution is the disinfection of surfaces such as beds, bedrails, toilets and toilet assist rails, and equipment near a patient's bed. The disinfection needs to be done at regular intervals with an approved disinfectant, and all disinfections should be recorded on paper or electronically.

Linen

Soiled bedding needs to be cleaned to completely remove blood and body fluids. It should be washed in hot water to kill living bacteria that may have clung to the fabric. Another standard precaution involving linen relates to the transport of the linen from the bedside to the hospital laundry. Soiled linen should be transport in a closed and waterproof container to lessen the chances that microbes could leak out or become airborne.

■ Impacts and Issues

Standard precautions are an efficient way of minimizing the chances of the transfer of infectious microorganisms from patient to patient, and from patients to healthcare providers. However, diligence is required.

Unfortunately, diligence is not always practiced. A number of studies from the United States and Europe conducted since 2000 have revealed a dismal record of compliance with handwashing among healthcare providers. Even though the benefits of handwashing are well-established, fewer than 50% of healthcare providers regularly wash their hands after finishing with one patient and before seeing another patient. The common explanation is a lack of time. In an effort to increase compliance with handwashing, some hospitals have

---

WORDS TO KNOW

AUTOCLAVE: An autoclave is a device that is designed to kill microorganisms on solid items and in liquids by exposure to steam at a high pressure.

HYGIENE: Hygiene refers to the health practices that minimize the spread of infectious microorganisms between people or between other living things and people. Inanimate objects and surfaces such as contaminated cutlery or a cutting board may be a secondary part of this process.

PATHOGEN: A disease causing agent, such as a bacteria, virus, fungus, etc.

UNIVERSAL PRECAUTION: Universal precaution refers to an infection control strategy in which all human blood and other material is assumed to be potentially infectious, specifically with organisms such as Human Immunodeficiency Virus (HIV) and Hepatitis B Virus. The precautions are aimed at preventing contact with blood or the other materials.

---

installed alcohol-based handwashing stations at patient's bedsides. The pressure of being caught in noncompliance with handwashing precautions can be a powerful incentive to practice proper hygiene.

The need for standard precautions pertaining to equipment is highlighted by the observation that prions—proteins whose abnormal folding causes a severe, progressive damage to brain cells that is the basis of transmissible spongiform encephalopathies, such as Creutzfeldt-Jakob disease—can remain capable of causing disease even when surgical instruments have been sterilized using the combination of chemicals and the high pressure and high heat that is known as autoclaving. The World Health Organization has recommended that surgery on patients suspected of having a prion-related disease should be done using disposable instruments, or instruments should be incinerated before being used again.

A real-world example of this danger occurred in 2003 in New Brunswick, Canada, where seven patients likely contracted Creutzfeldt-Jakob disease (CJD) from surgical equipment that was contaminated with prions. An investigation revealed that the instruments had originally been used in neurosurgery on a patient who subsequently developed CJD. While the instruments were treated according to the required protocol, this was not sufficient to decontaminate them.

SEE ALSO *Airborne Precautions; Handwashing; Isolation and Quarantine; Personal Protective Equipment.*

BIBLIOGRAPHY

Books

DiClaudio, Dennis. *The Hypochondriac's Pocket Guide to Horrible Diseases You Probably Already Have.* New York: Bloomsbury, 2005.

Lawrence, Jean, and Dee May. *Infection Control in the Community.* New York: Churchill Livingstone, 2003.

Tierno, Philip M. *The Secret Life of Germs: What They Are, Why We Need Them, and How We Can Protect Ourselves Against Them.* New York: Atria, 2004.

Brian Hoyle

Staphylococcus aureus Infections

■ Introduction

Staphylococcus aureus is a bacterium that colonizes, or normally inhabitants the surface of the skin and, in about 25% of humans, the inside of the nose. In a healthy person, the bacterium is usually not a health concern. But, if a person's skin is damaged by a cut or a burn, or if *S. aureus* gains access to areas inside the body, infection can result.

S. *aureus* is the most common cause of the so-called staph infections. (Other species of *Staphylococcus* can also cause infections.) *S. aureus* can cause a number of life threatening infections, including toxic shock syndrome. While uncommon now, the marketing of super absorbent tampons in the 1970s caused illness and death of a large number of women. The tampon design encouraged the growth of the bacteria, which subsequently produced a poison (toxin) that entered the blood stream.

Other life-threatening infections can occur in susceptible people. These infections are described as being opportunistic infections, since they normally do not occur in healthy people.

■ Disease History, Characteristics, and Transmission

S. aureus is a spherical-shaped bacterium. It is a Gram-positive bacterium, meaning that it consists of a membrane layer made up mainly of lipids and proteins, and a thick, strong network called peptidoglycan. (Gram-negative bacteria have two membrane layers and a thin peptidoglycan.) The design of the bacterium makes it quite environmentally hardy, which enables it to live in microscopic depressions on the surface of the skin. The bacterium also thrives in the warm and moist atmosphere inside the nose.

S. *aureus* typically grows and divides to form microscopic clusters that appear grapelike. When grown on a solid food source that contains blood, the visible mounds of bacteria (colonies) that develop tend to be golden in color; *aureus* means "gold" in Latin. These characteristics aid in the identification of the organism. Other tests of biochemical activity, such the ability of the bacterium to clot blood, also are used in identification.

If the normal barrier of the skin's surface is breached, by a cut or a burn for example, or if a person is immuno-compromised (their immune system is not functioning properly) and so is less capable of fighting off invading microorganisms, *S. aureus* can rapidly cause infections. These range from skin infections that are relatively minor, such as boils and pimples, to life-threatening infections of the skin in infants (scalded skin syndrome), of the lungs (pneumonia), of the lining of certain nerves (meningitis), of the heart valves (endocarditis), and, in the case of toxic shock syndrome, of the blood (septicemia). Heart-related

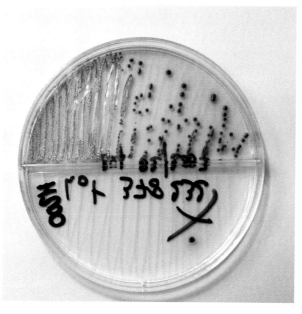

A culture of the *Staphylococcus aureus* bacterium (red) is shown growing in a petri dish. *CC Studio/Photo Researchers, Inc.*

WORDS TO KNOW

ANTIBIOTIC RESISTANCE: The ability of bacteria to resist the actions of antibiotic drugs.

COLONIZE: Colonize refers to the process where a microorganism is able to persist and grow at a given location.

IMMUNOCOMPROMISED: A reduction of the ability of the immune system to recognize and respond to the presence of foreign material.

OPPORTUNISTIC INFECTION: An opportunistic infection is so named because it occurs in people whose immune systems are diminished or are not functioning normally; such infections are opportunistic insofar as the infectious agents take advantage of their hosts' compromised immune systems and invade to cause disease.

RESISTANT ORGANISM: Resistant organisms are bacteria, viruses, parasites, or other disease-causing agents that have stopped responding to drugs that once killed them.

infections are associated with the implantation of devices designed to assist proper heart function. The devices can become contaminated before being implanted, if they are handled by bare hands that have not been washed properly. This transfers *S. aureus* from the skin to the plastic surface of the device, where the bacteria can adhere and grow.

The association of *S. aureus* and infections has been known since 1880, when the bacterium was isolated from wounds. The environmental hardiness of the bacterium is one important factor in its ability to cause infection. If present on a moist surface, such as a towel, the bacteria can remain alive and capable of causing infection for hours. Even more importantly, skin-to-skin contact can easily spread *S. aureus* from one person to another. The ability of the bacterium to invade host tissue is one cause of infection. Toxins can also be produced when *S. aureus* gets into a wound or other niche away from the skin's surface, or when the bacterium contaminates food.

■ Scope and Distribution

S. aureus infections occur virtually anywhere in the world and are very common. For example, even in a developed country like the United States with high-quality medical care, more than 500,000 people are hospitalized with *S. aureus* infections every year. The bacterium is one of the important causes of what are termed nosocomial (hospital-acquired) infections.

The bacterium is also a concern in agriculture, since it is the cause of a disease in cattle called mastitis.

■ Treatment and Prevention

Despite the antibiotic resistance of some types of *S. aureus*, infections still usually respond to treatment with antibiotics. Completing the full course of antibiotic treatment is very important. Some patients may stop taking antibiotics before the course of treatment is completed because they begin to feel better. This is very unwise, since the infection may not yet be eliminated. Surviving *S. aureus* can cause the illness to recur, and these survivors may even become resistant to the antibiotic(s) being used in the treatment.

■ Impacts and Issues

The impacts of *S. aureus* infections are enormous, both in terms of the number of serious illnesses and deaths caused, and also in terms of the financial cost of caring for these patients. In a nationwide analysis of hospitalized patients in 2001, patients with *S. aureus* were found to average three times the length of hospital stay, three times the total charges, and three times the risk of death while in the hospital than hospitalized patients without *S. aureus* infection.

Furthermore, the development of antibiotic resistance by the bacterium (strains that are resistant to almost all antibiotics exist) is ominous. At the time of the commercial introduction of the first antibiotic, penicillin, in 1943, antibiotic resistance among *S. aureus* isolated from infections was unknown. Only seven years later, approximately 40% of all isolates were resistant to penicillin. By 1960, 80% of hospital isolates of *S. aureus* were penicillin-resistant.

In addition, resistance to a variety of other antibiotics has developed. As of 2007, disease outbreaks due to *S. aureus* that are almost completely resistant to antibiotics are becoming much more common. The challenge now is to quickly discover new antibiotics and/or methods of infection control that protect hospitalized patients, who are the most susceptible to grave illness and death from these infections.

SEE ALSO *Antibiotic Resistance; Bacterial Disease; MRSA; Toxic Shock.*

BIBLIOGRAPHY

Books

Freeman-Cook, Lisa, and Kevin D. Freeman-Cook. *Staphylococcus aureus Infections.* London: Chelsea House, 2005.

Prescott, Lansing M., John P. Harley, and Donald A. Klein. *Microbiology*. New York: McGraw Hill, 2004.

Tortora, Gerard J., Berell R. Funke, and Christine L. Case. *Microbiology: An Introduction*. New York: Benjamin Cummings, 2006.

Brian Hoyle

Sterilization

■ Introduction

Sterilization refers to processes that eliminate microorganisms from surfaces, the interior of equipment, foods, and liquids. A catheter is one example of a device whose surface must be completely sterilized before it is inserted in a person to deliver food or medicine. A cardiac pacemaker is another example of a device whose surface must be sterilized before it is implanted inside the body to control the heart rate. A common example of a liquid requiring sterilization is the liquid-based nutrient medium used to grow bacteria in the laboratory.

Sterilization is intended to eliminate living microorganisms such as bacteria, fungi, and protozoa, along with nonliving microbes such as viruses that, given the appropriate host, can cause disease.

There are various methods of sterilization depending on the aim of the procedure. For example, surgical instruments are sterilized to guarantee the absence of pathogens (disease-causing organisms), while most laboratory growth media used for experimentation is sterilized to guarantee the absence of bacteria. Pharmaceutical medications also need to be free of all potential disease-causing agents.

WORDS TO KNOW

AUTOCLAVE: An autoclave is a device that is designed to kill microorganisms on solid items and in liquids by exposure to steam at a high pressure.

PATHOGEN: A disease causing agent, such as a bacteria, virus, fungus, etc.

■ History and Scientific Foundations

Heat has been used to sterilize objects for millennia. Until a few centuries ago, the flame of a fire was used. Today, the most common method of heat sterilization employs high temperature and pressure above atmospheric pressure. The combination of temperature and pressure most efficiently heats an object or a volume of liquid; exposure of the samples for a certain period of time has proved sufficient to kill even hardy microorganisms.

An autoclave is the most common instrument used for heat sterilization. Autoclaves range in size from small units that easily fit on the bench-top of a laboratory to large units that have the volume of an average kitchen refrigerator. An autoclave uses steam to sterilize the objects place inside it. Most typically, the steam is pumped into the autoclave chamber at a temperature of 250°F (121°C) and a pressure that is 15 pounds per square inch above atmospheric pressure. These conditions of temperature and pressure are maintained for at least 15 minutes (larger loads or greater volumes of liquid can be held longer). Then, the steam is released from the chamber in a controlled and safe manner. The chamber can be opened when it has returned to atmospheric pressure.

As a control over the process, indicator tape can be applied to the objects being autoclaved. Bands form on the tape when the proper conditions of temperature, pressure, and time have been attained. This helps the operator judge whether sterilization has been successful. To be even more certain, solutions that contain bacterial spores of *Bacillus stearothermophilus* can be included with the load being sterilized. Bacterial spores are very resistant to the killing action of heat. If the liquid containing the spores is incubated in a suitable liquid growth source and the medium remains clear, it indicates that sterilization was successful. In addition to the use of this so-called bio-indicator, many autoclaves record the temperature profile of each sterilization cycle, allowing the user to visually monitor whether the appropriate conditions were achieved.

Monitoring of autoclave performance is important. If, for example, too many items are autoclaved at once, the overcrowded conditions may not allow the steam to effectively penetrate the entire load, which can result in inadequate sterilization.

Although autoclaving is an effective method of sterilization with many applications, it is not foolproof. For example, it has been shown that prions—proteins whose abnormal folding stimulates damage of brain cells causing several similar diseases termed transmissible spongiform encephalopathies (an example is Creutzfeld-Jacob disease)—can remain potent following autoclaving of surgical instruments. Even the combination of autoclaving with chemicals has proven ineffective against prion contamination. The World Health Organization has recommended that surgery on patients suspected of having a prion-related disease be performed with disposable instruments, or that the instruments used be incinerated after the surgery is completed.

There are other methods of sterilization. Some metal objects can be surface-sterilized by holding them in an open flame. This is a common way of sterilizing a loop of metal called an inoculating loop that is used to transfer microorganisms from one place to another during experiments. Burning trash that contains medical waste is another way of sterilizing the residual ash. This ash can then be safety disposed of. Medical incinerators must be specially designed to retain the vapor given off, since infectious material can potentially be carried into the air during incineration. A common method for sterilizing drinking water is boiling. Boiling kills most bacteria and inactivates most viruses. However, agents like prions and some spore-forming bacteria can survive boiling for 15 minutes. However, in most situations, boiling is better than not treating water at all before drinking it.

Objects such as plastic, optical equipment, and electrical circuits that cannot stand heat can be sterilized using a chemical called ethylene oxide. This chemical is applied as a gas in a specialized machine. Another spore-forming bacterium, *Bacillus subtilus*, is used to monitor the success of ethylene oxide sterilization.

Ozone is another chemical sterilizer. Drinking water can be sterilized using ozone. A diluted solution of bleach (sodium hypochlorite) is an especially useful sterilizing agent for work surfaces. Other chemical sterilizers include glutaraldehyde and hydrogen peroxide.

Applications and Research

Sterilization is a necessity of everyday life in research, health care, and even the supermarket. Ongoing inves-

---

IN CONTEXT: BACTERIA SPORES SPUR STERILIZATION RESEARCH

The discovery of bacteria that are resistant to sterilization could potentially contaminate experiments and environments studied by NASA and other space agency probes. One species was tentatively named *B. odysseensis* after being isolated from the surfaces of the Mars *Odyssey* spacecraft following routine sterilization. The method of spore formation is suspected of having a role in resistance of spore-forming bacteria to sterilization.

Earth-bound benefits of such research offer hope of improved methods of sterilization and prevention of unintentional contamination.

SOURCE: *Jet Propulsion Laboratory, National Aeronautics and Space Administrations (NASA)*

---

tigations seek to develop chemicals that sterilize more efficiently and quickly, while being safe to use.

Impacts and Issues

Without the ability to sterilize growth media, many scientific experiments could not be accomplished, as it would be impossible to know if the results were due to the organism being studied or to a contaminant. In addition, surgeries would have a very poor survival rate, as was the case in the days before sterilization techniques were routinely employed.

In some instances, standard sterilization methods have not been sufficient to protect patients from developing disease as a result of contact with contaminated medical equipment. An example occurred in 2003 in the Canadian province of New Brunswick, where seven patients probably contracted Creutzfeld-Jacob disease from prion-contaminated instruments used during their neurosurgeries. The instruments became contaminated when used in an operation on a patient who was subsequently found to have the disease. The instruments were routinely sterilized, but it later became clear that this routine sterilization procedure did not remove the prions. It was this outbreak that resulted in the institution of hospital protocols mandating the use of disposable instruments during procedures on high-risk areas such as the brain and spinal cord involving patients suspected of having a prion-related disease.

Recently, scientists have found that prions can be digested by a particular enzyme. Enzymatic treatment of medical instruments has shown promise as

---

sterilization technique effective for prions, but it is not yet in general use.

While important, the quest for sterilization can go too far. One example is the marketing of surface sterilizing products designed for use in the kitchen and bathroom. Bacteria that are not killed by these products have the potential to become resistant to the particular chemical, which can make these bacteria a more serious concern than before they developed this resistance.

SEE ALSO *Disinfection; Infection Control and Asepsis; Sanitation.*

BIBLIOGRAPHY

Books

Gladwin, Mark, and Bill Trattler. *Clinical Microbiology Made Ridiculously Simple.* 3rd ed. Miami: Medmaster, 2003.

Prescott, Lansing M., John P. Harley, and Donald A. Klein. *Microbiology.* New York: McGraw-Hill, 2004.

Tortora, Gerard J., Berell R. Funke, and Christine L. Case. *Microbiology: An Introduction.* New York: Benjamin Cummings, 2006.

Brian Hoyle

Strep Throat

■ Introduction

A sore throat is one of the most common symptoms sending people to the doctor. It often precedes a cold, flu, or other respiratory infection. Most sore throats are caused by viral infection. Strep throat, or Streptococcal pharyngitis, is a bacterial throat infection with "strep" being a shortened for *Streptococcus pyogenes*, the causative agent. Most people carry *S. pyogenes* in their throat and on their skin and normally it causes no problems.

Strep throat is considered a mild infection, although it can be very painful. Left untreated, it can sometimes lead to serious complications, such as rheumatic fever. Strep throat responds promptly to antibiotic treatment, which will also stop the infection spreading to others. The majority of sore throats will not respond to anti-biotics, because they are caused by viruses. That is why strep throat should be properly diagnosed wherever possible, to prevent the unnecessary use of antibiotics.

■ Disease History, Characteristics, and Transmission

The *S. pyogenes* bacterium belongs to a large group of bacteria called the streptococci, which occur in characteristic long chains. They are subdivided according to the antigen proteins they bear on their surfaces. *S. pyogenes* is, therefore, sometimes called Group A streptococcus (GAS), since it carries the A antigen. A certain amount of GAS is found on the skin of most people

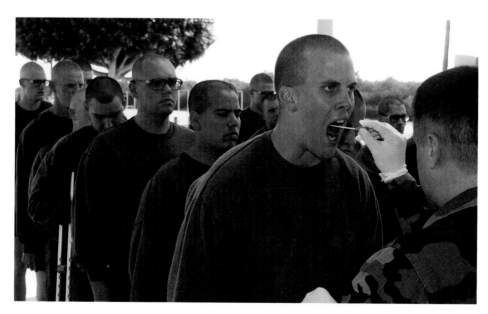

A U.S. Marine recruit receives a throat swab for a culture in 2002. During an outbreak of strep throat in San Diego, California, more than 300 recruits reported a sore throat and fever; 185 tested positive for the *Streptococcus* A bacteria, which causes strep throat. *Cpl. Anthony D. Pike/Getty Images.*

IN CONTEXT: SOCIAL AND PERSONAL RESPONSIBILITY

According to the Division of Bacterial and Mycotic Diseases at Centers for Disease Control and Prevention (CDC), "the spread of all types of GAS infection can be reduced by good hand-washing, especially after coughing and sneezing and before preparing foods or eating. Persons with sore throats should be seen by a doctor who can perform tests to find out whether the illness is strep throat. If the test result shows strep throat, the person should stay home from work, school, or day care until 24 hours after taking an antibiotic. All wounds should be kept clean and watched for possible signs of infection such as redness, swelling, drainage, and pain at the wound site. A person with signs of an infected wound, especially if fever occurs, should seek medical care. It is not necessary for all persons exposed to someone with an invasive group A strep infection (i.e., necrotizing fasciitis or strep toxic shock syndrome) to receive antibiotic therapy to prevent infection. However, in certain circumstances, antibiotic therapy may be appropriate. That decision should be made after consulting with your doctor."

SOURCE: *Centers for Disease Control and Prevention (CDC), Coordinating Center for Infectious Diseases, Division of Bacterial and Mycotic Diseases.*

without causing illness; this is known as colonization. However, besides strep throat, GAS can also cause impetigo (a skin infection) and scarlet fever. Some strains of GAS are also responsible for necrotizing fasciitis, which involves the soft tissue under the skin, and toxic shock syndrome, both of which are potentially fatal.

The symptoms of strep throat include throat pain and difficulty in swallowing, headache, fever, and swollen glands. The tonsils might be red and swollen with white patches and streaks of pus. Strep throat is distinguished from other conditions, such as tonsillitis or viral throat infection, by testing a throat swab for the presence of GAS.

Possible complications of strep throat include rheumatic fever and kidney inflammation. These may set in weeks after the first symptoms of the throat infection. Rheumatic fever may be indicated by joint pain or rash, while the urine may become dark if the kidneys are infected. Rheumatic fever is potentially serious, as it can lead to permanent damage of the heart valves with impairment of heart function. Other possible complications include tonsillitis, scarlet fever, sinus infection, and ear infection.

GAS is highly contagious and strep throat is spread through coughs, sneezes, and contact with objects, such as kitchen utensils and bathroom items, that have been used by an infected person (fomites). The infection often spreads rapidly through family members, schools and child care centers—anywhere, in fact, that people come into close contact.

■ Scope and Distribution

Strep throat is most common among children aged from 5 to 15, although it can affect people of any age. It is most often seen in late fall, winter, and spring. In the United States, the risk of complications from strep throat is low.

■ Treatment and Prevention

Strep throat is usually treated by an antibiotic, such as penicillin, amoxicillin, clarithromycin, or cephalosporin. The treatment reduces the severity and duration of symptoms, and stops the infection from passing to others. Symptoms will start to clear within a day or two of starting antibiotics. It is important to finish the whole course of prescribed antibiotics. Stopping medication early will increase the risk of complications and encourage the growth of resistant organisms.

Rest, plenty of water, and soothing foods will also help relieve the pain of strep throat, as will gargling with salt water. Acetaminophen and ibuprofen may be prescribed for pain and fever, although aspirin is not recommended for young children with strep throat because it can contribute to the development of Reye's syndrome, a potentially life-threatening illness.

As with many infections, the best way to prevent strep throat is by good personal hygiene, including covering the mouth and nose when coughing or sneezing and washing the hands frequently and thoroughly. For a child with recurrent strep throat, tonsillectomy (removal of the tonsils) may be helpful. A study carried out by the Mayo Clinic in 2006 showed that children with recurrent strep throat with intact tonsils are three times more likely to develop subsequent episodes compared to those who have their tonsils removed.

■ Impacts and Issues

Accurate diagnosis of the cause of a sore throat is important. Viral infections should not be treated with antibiotics. Not only will the infection not respond, but the inappropriate prescription of antibiotics has been linked to antibiotic resistance, which is a growing public health problem. Strep throat can be diagnosed with rapid tests for GAS antigen or DNA. Courses of antibiotics prescribed for strep throat should always be completed, because stopping early also encourages antibiotic resistance.

SEE ALSO *Antibiotic Resistance; Bacterial Disease; Impetigo; Necrotizing Fasciitis; Scarlet Fever; Toxic Shock.*

BIBLIOGRAPHY

Web Sites

Centers for Disease Control and Prevention. "Group A Streptococcal (GAS) Disease." October 11, 2005. <http://www.cdc.gov/ncidod/dbmd/diseaseinfo/groupastreptococcal_g.htm> (accessed May 1, 2007).

MayoClinic.com. "Strep throat." November 3, 2006. <http://www.mayoclinic.com/health/strep-throat/DS00260> (accessed May 1, 2007).

Streptococcal Infections, Group A

■ Introduction

Group A *Streptococcus* bacteria (also called group A streptococci or GAS for short) can cause many diseases. The species *Streptococcus pyogenes* (pronounced pie-AHJ-uh-neez) is the group A *Streptococcus* that causes most disease in humans and is often treated as synonymous with GAS, though there are also non-*S. pyogenes* group A streptococci. Among the diseases caused by GAS are scarlet fever, strep throat, toxic shock syndrome, and impetigo. GAS were often life-threatening before the

discovery and mass-production of antibiotics. Untreated GAS infections also threaten health by triggering auto-immune diseases, including glomerulonephritis and rheumatic fever. Rheumatic fever is life-threatening, killing from 2% to 5% of patients.

Some invasive GAS infections that invade the lungs, blood, or deep muscle and fat tissue are life threatening. Most invasive GAS illnesses have a mortality rate of 10–15%. Necrotizing fasciitis (also called "flesh-eating disease") and streptococcal toxic shock syndrome (STSS) are two of the least common, but most severe and

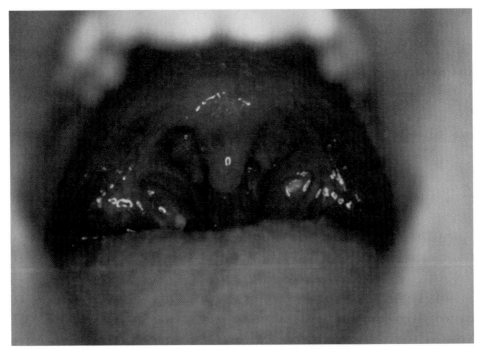

This close up of the mouth of a child shows severe streptococcal tonsillitis. The tonsils and pharynx appear deep red (center). Both tonsils are swollen and are narrowing the throat. A collection of whitish pus is visible on the patient's right tonsil (center left). A white coating covers the entire surface of the tongue. *Dr. P. Marazzi/Photo Researchers, Inc.*

aggressive forms of invasive GAS. Approximately 20% of patients with necrotizing fasciitis die, while STSS has a mortality rate of 60%.

Today, most routine GAS infections are routinely treated with antibiotics in industrialized countries, but resistance to earlier-developed antibiotics is an increasing problem. In the developing world, untreated GAS and its resultant autoimmune diseases are still a widespread problem.

■ Disease History, Characteristics, and Transmission

The streptococci bacteria were first described by German-Austrian physician Christian Theodor Billroth (1829–1894), who found *Streptococcus pyogenes* growing in infected wounds (the word "pyogenes" is from the Greek for "pus-forming"). *S. pyogenes* was actually named by German physician Michael Josef Rossbach (1842–94) in 1884, but was not termed a group A streptococcus until the 1930s, when American scientist Rebecca Lancefield (1895–1981) classed the streptococci into the alphabetically labeled groups that are still called Lancefield groups. Lancefield also established that a protein embedded in the cell wall of group A streptococci, M protein, is crucial to their power to cause disease. There are over 120 varieties of *S. pyogenes*, distinguished by their varying M proteins.

The streptococci are gram-positive bacteria that tend to grow in chains or pairs. They are classed into two basic groups based on their ability to break down blood cells under laboratory conditions, a process called hemolysis (hemo meaning blood, and lysis meaning breakup). The beta-hemolytic streptococci break up blood cells completely, creating clear areas around bacteria colonies growing on blood agar in petri dishes. (Petri dishes are small, round, shallow dishes used commonly in laboratories to grow microorganisms; agar is a form of jelly derived from seaweed or algae, chemically a sugar; and blood agar is agar mixed with blood cells, usually from horses or sheep.)

Further division of the beta-hemolytic streptococci into the Lancefield groups A to T is based on the chemical makeup of the cell wall. The group A streptococci, of which *S. pyogenes* is the most important, are globular and about 0.6 to 1 mm in diameter. These bacteria primarily invade human epithelial cells, which constitute the skin and line the respiratory and digestive tracts.

Strep throat is an infection of the throat with *S. pyogenes*. About 18 or 20 days after the end of a strep throat infection, acute rheumatic fever may occur. The primary symptom of rheumatic fever is pain in the joints. Inflammation of the heart may also occur, causing permanent damage to one or more heart valves. Post-streptococcal glomerulonephritis—inflammation of the

---

---

kidney—may also develop about 10 days after a GAS infection.

Transmission of *S. pyogenes* is via direct contact with mucus, saliva, and open sores, or through airborne saliva droplets released by sneezing or coughing.

Severe, invasive GAS infections are rare among otherwise healthy individuals. Invasive GAS infections are most likely to occur in persons with diabetes or weakened immune systems, persons who use steroids or some other medications, or in patients with recent trauma or surgical wounds.

■ Scope and Distribution

The only known reservoir for *S. pyogenes* is human beings. About 5% to 15% of health persons harbor *S. pyogenes*, usually in their upper respiratory tract, without any sign of infection. This bacterium is one of the most common causes of bacterial infection in human beings, and in many developed nations is the most common cause of bacterial infection of the upper respiratory tract for all age groups.

IN CONTEXT: TRENDS AND STATISTICS

Streptococcal pharyngitis (strep throat) is one of the most common childhood illnesses worldwide. In industrialized countries, thanks to antibiotic treatment of strep throat, rheumatic fever has an annual incidence of around 0.5 cases per 100,000 school-age children. In developing countries, however, the annual incidence of rheumatic fever ranges from 100 to 200 cases per 100,000 school-aged children—from 200 to 400 times higher than the developed-world rate. There are over 18 million cases of severe GAS disease such as rheumatic heart disease worldwide, with more than half a million deaths per year.

In the eighteenth and nineteenth centuries, scarlet fever was a major killer, and until antibiotics were available to treat GAS infections, rheumatic fever (usually following strep throat) was a widespread childhood disease. Moreover, puerperal fever was common in maternity wards, where sanitation was poor (the role of bacteria in causing infection was not yet known) and *S. pyogenes* was transmitted by doctors' unwashed hands. During childbirth, *S. pyogenes* would often infect the mother's bloodstream through tears in the vaginal wall or skin of the genital area. This commonly resulted in death rates in maternity wards of about 10% to 25%, with occasional epidemics leading to much higher death rates. Today, puerperal fever is rare in industrialized countries because of standardized medical hygiene and prevalent antibiotics.

■ Treatment and Prevention

For over a century, attempts have been made to develop a GAS vaccine. As of early 2007, one GAS vaccine was in phase 2 clinical human trials, with several others approaching the human trial phase. However, no GAS vaccine was yet available.

Prevention of GAS infections consists primarily of handwashing, sterilization in health-care environments, and avoiding contact with infected persons. According to the World Health Organization (WHO), the only effective and cost-effective large-scale control strategy for GAS diseases, apart from health education and medical hygiene, is treatment by antibiotics.

■ Impacts and Issues

WHO estimates that puerperal sepsis, infection of women giving birth, by GAS accounts for 15% of maternal deaths globally today. Most of these deaths occur in developing countries where sterile conditions and antibiotics are more rare.

Failure of penicillin to eradicate GAS from the throat has been reported with increasing frequency in recent years. Whether antibiotics other than penicillin should be added to standard treatment regimens for strep throat and other GAS infections is debated among physicians. Treating resistant infections requires more powerful and recently-developed antibiotics. However, many physicians worry that prescribing newer, more powerful antibiotics as a first course of treatment may encourage further antibiotic resistance in GAS infections.

SEE ALSO *Impetigo; Necrotizing Fasciitis; Puerperal Fever; Scarlet Fever; Streptococcal Infections, Group B.*

BIBLIOGRAPHY

Books

Smith, Tara and Edward Alcamo. *Streptococcus (Group A) (Deadly Diseases and Epidemics).* Philadelphia, PA: Chelsea House Publications, 2004.

Periodicals

Cunningham, Madeleine W. "Pathogenesis of Group A Streptococcal Infections." *Clinical Microbiology Reviews.* 13 (2000): 470-511.

Facklam, Richard. "What Happened to the Streptococci: Overview of Taxonomic and Nomenclature Changes." *Clinical Microbiology Reviews.* 15 (2002): 613-630.

Kaplan, Edward L., et al. "Reduced Ability of Penicillin to Eradicate Ingested Group A Streptococci from Epithelial Cells: Clinical and Pathogenic Implications." *Clinical Infectious Diseases.* 43 (2006): 1398–1406.

Web Sites

World Health Organization (United Nations). "A Review of the Technical Basis for the Control of Associated with Group A Streptococcal Infections." 2005 <http://www.who.int/ child-adolescent-health/New_Publications/ CHILD_HEALTH/DP/WHO_FCH_CAH_ 05.08.pdf> (accessed February 2, 2007).

Streptococcal Infections, Group B

■ Introduction

Group B *Streptococcus* bacteria, primarily the species *Streptococcus agalactiae*, are a major cause of sickness and death among newborns worldwide. Group B *Streptococcus* illnesses are also known as GBS, Beta strep, or group B *Streptococci*. GBS infection also increases risks to both the mother and the fetus before birth. In the newborn, infection can cause pneumonia (fluid in the lungs) and bacteremia (bacteria in the blood, which is normally sterile) within the first week after birth. The late-onset form of the disease occurs from 7 to 90 days after birth, usually causing meningitis, which is inflammation of the meninges (the tough membranes that surround the brain and spinal cord). Pneumonia, bacteremia, and meningitis can all be fatal. GBS infection can be treated with antibiotics, but no vaccine is currently available.

■ Disease History, Characteristics, and Transmission

Streptococci, which are Gram-positive bacteria that tend to grow in chains or pairs, were first described in 1874 by Christian Theodor Billroth (1829–1894). Around 1903, Hugo Shottmuller (1867–1936) distinguished between alpha-hemolytic and beta-hemolytic Streptococci. Beta-hemolytic Streptococci—which include almost all group A and many group B Streptococci—are distinguished by their ability to completely break up blood cells when grown in the laboratory, a process called hemolysis (hemo meaning blood, and lysis meaning breakup). Hemolysis creates clear areas around colonies of beta-hemolytic bacteria growing in petri dishes on the substance called blood agar, a jellylike substance derived from seaweed or algae mixed with (usually) sheep blood.

GBS is most often noted for causing pneumonia and meningitis in newborns, with a high fatality rate. GBS is also known to cause infections in adults with preexisting conditions such as breast cancer, cirrhosis of the liver, and diabetes. In adults, GBS can manifest as a soft-tissue infection, pneumonia, meningitis, or infections of the bones or joints. The elderly are at greatest risk from these invasive GBS infections.

GBS is usually transmitted by direct contact. Newborns may contract the bacteria during labor and delivery by mothers who are vaginally or anally colonized with the bacteria. Alternatively, fetuses may contract the bacteria from their mothers during development, before birth. This can lead to miscarriage or premature birth, and approximately triples the risk of cerebral palsy.

■ Scope and Distribution

Like group A streptococci, GBS are common in human populations. They are particularly important as a cause of infection in newborns, causing several thousand deaths per year in the United States alone. About 12% to 27% of women in North Africa, south-central Asia, Saudi Arabia, and the United States are colonized by GBS.

■ Treatment and Prevention

Although GBS can be treated with antibiotics, infection can spread quickly and symptoms can be difficult to diagnose in newborns. Administration of antibiotics—usually penicillin or ampicillin—to the mother during delivery can prevent infection in newborns.

Research is under way for the use of monoclonal antibodies as a vaccine for GBS, but, as of early 2007, had not yet reached the stage of clinical trials with human subjects. Strains of GBS causing bacteria can vary significantly in different parts of the world, challenging development of a single GBS vaccine that would be effective worldwide.

WORDS TO KNOW

BACTEREMIA: Bacteremia occurs when bacteria enter the bloodstream. This condition may occur through a wound or infection, or through a surgical procedure or injection. Bacteremia may cause no symptoms and resolve without treatment, or it may produce fever and other symptoms of infection. In some cases, bacteremia leads to septic shock, a potentially life-threatening condition.

COLONIZATION: Colonization is the process of occupation and increase in number of microorganisms at a specific site.

HEMOLYSIS: The destruction of blood cells, an abnormal rate of which may lead to lowered levels of these cells. For example, Hemolytic anemia is caused by destruction of red blood cells at a rate faster than which they can be produced.

MENINGITIS: Meningitis is an inflammation of the meninges—the three layers of protective membranes that line the spinal cord and the brain. Meningitis can occur when there is an infection near the brain or spinal cord, such as a respiratory infection in the sinuses, the mastoids, or the cavities around the ear. Disease organisms can also travel to the meninges through the bloodstream. The first signs may be a severe headache and neck stiffness followed by fever, vomiting, a rash, and, then, convulsions leading to loss of consciousness. Meningitis generally involves two types: non-bacterial meningitis, which is often called aseptic meningitis, and bacterial meningitis, which is referred to as purulent meningitis.

MONOCLONAL ANTIBODIES: Antibodies produced from a single cell line that are used in medical testing and, increasingly, in the treatment of some cancers.

■ Impacts and Issues

In the United States in the 1970s, there were 7,500 GBS infections in newborns per year. The death rate for GBS infection was as high as 50%. In the 1980s, it was found that giving antibiotics to women who tested positive for GBS and were therefore at risk for transmitting the bacteria to their babies greatly reduced the rate of early-onset (first week of life) disease. As a result, the U.S. Centers for Disease Control (CDC) issued guidelines in 1996 recommending vaginal and rectal screening between the 35th and 37th weeks of pregnancy to identify women with GBS; women who test positive are offered antibiotics during labor.

In developing countries, infection rates in newborns are surprisingly low; in a recent study of newborns in India, the Middle East, and elsewhere, only about 1% of newborns tested positive for GBS, even though their mothers were colonized by GBS at a rate of 12% to 27%. It is possible, according to the World Health Organization (WHO), that GBS causes infant death in developing countries primarily by causing miscarriage or premature birth, leading to an artificially low figure for GBS infant mortality.

SEE ALSO *Streptococcal Infections, Group A.*

BIBLIOGRAPHY

Periodicals

Osrin, David, et al. "Serious Bacterial Infections in Newborn Infants in Developing Countries." *Pediatric and Neonatal Infections.* 17 (2004): 217–224.

Benitz, Willem E., et al. "Risk Factors for Early-onset Group B Streptococcal Sepsis: Estimation of Odds Ratios by Critical Literature Review." *Pediatrics.* 103 (1999): 1–14.

Web Sites

Centers for Disease Control and Prevention. "Prevention of Perinatal Group B Streptococcal Disease." August 16, 2002 <http://www.cdc.gov/mmwr/preview/mmwrhtml/rr5111a1.htm> (accessed February 2, 2007).

Royal College of Obstetricians and Gynaecologists (United Kingdom). "Prevention of Early Onset Neonatal Group B Streptococcal Disease." November, 2003 <http://www.rcog.org.uk/index.asp?PageID=520> (accessed February 2, 2007).

Strongyloidiasis

■ Introduction

Strongyloidiasis is an infection with a parasitic round-worm known as *Strongyloides stercoralis*. It occurs in tropical and subtropical areas, as well as in the southern part of the United States. *S. stercoralis* has a complex life cycle involving infection through the skin by the larvae which travel to the intestine, where they reproduce causing chronic infection in the original host. They can also pass onto new hosts and cause further infections.

In persons with compromised immunity, such as organ transplant recipients, strongyloidiasis can cause a hyperinfection involving the intestines and the rest of the body. The condition can also be difficult to diagnose, since the symptoms are varied and non-specific. However, the parasitic worms can be eliminated by drug treatment. All patients at risk of hyperinfection should be treated and those about to undergo an organ transplant ought to be screened for the infection.

■ Disease History, Characteristics, and Transmission

S. stercoralis has a more complicated life cycle than other parasitic worms, which means it can set up a high burden of persistent infection in a human host, especially one who has weakened immunity. Where the burden of parasites is low, the individual may have no, or merely intermittent, symptoms.

The parasites enter the skin and pass through the blood and lungs to the intestines. Therefore, those with a significant burden of parasites will develop symptoms relating to these areas. Skin symptoms include dermatitis and irritation, while the lung stage may involve dry cough, wheezing, fever, shortness of breath, and maybe coughing up blood. Parasites in the intestine will cause bloating, swelling, flatulence, indigestion, and diarrhea.

Hyperinfection—sometimes called disseminated stronglyoidiasis—may cause blood poisoning, peritonitis (inflammation of the lining of the abdominal cavity), neurological complications, and liver problems. The symptoms of strongyloidiasis are easily confused with other medical conditions, such as irritable bowel syndrome. Diagnosis depends upon identifying the *S. stercoralis* larvae within either a stool or a duodenal fluid sample.

Transmission of stronglyoidiasis starts when larvae in contaminated soil penetrate the skin of the human host and are transported through blood to the lungs. Here they first penetrate the alveoli, the tiny air sacs through which gases are exchanged between the lung surface and the blood. From here, the larvae travel up to the throat area and are swallowed, reaching the small intestine.

In the small intestine, the larvae become female adult worms. These lay eggs, by parthenogenesis—that is, without involvement of a male worm. The resulting larvae may pass through the stool, returning to the environment to repeat the cycle and infect other hosts. They can also cause so-called autoinfection in which the larvae continue to develop and penetrate the mucosal surface of the intestine, or the skin of the anal area. They then repeat the previous infection cycle—skin, lungs, and intestine—thereby massively increasing the parasitic burden on the host. Alternatively, the larvae may spread throughout the body, causing the complications described above.

■ Scope and Distribution

S. stercoralis infection is found in humid tropical and subtropical areas where the larvae can survive in the soil. Cases have also been found in temperate areas, including the southeastern part of the United States. The infection is more frequently found in rural areas, institutional settings, and among immigrants from the developing world. Those with reduced immunity, including patients with leukemia, organ transplant recipients, or those

WORDS TO KNOW

AUTOINFECTION: Re-infection of the body by a disease organism already in the body, such as eggs left by a parasitic worm, is autoinfection.

HOST: Organism that serves as the habitat for a parasite, or possibly for a symbiont. A host may provide nutrition to the parasite or symbiont, or simply a place in which to live.

HYPERINFECTION: A hyperinfection is an infection that is caused by very high number of disease causing microorganisms. The infection results from an abnormality in the immune system that allows the infecting cells to grow and divide more easily than would normally be the case.

IMMUNOCOMPROMISED: A reduction of the ability of the immune system to recognize and respond to the presence of foreign material.

ROUNDWORM: Also known as nematodes; a type of helminth characterized by long, cylindrical bodies. Roundworm infections are diseases of the digestive tract and other organ systems that are caused by roundworms. Roundworm infections are widespread throughout the world, and humans acquire most types of roundworm infection from contaminated food or by touching the mouth with unwashed hands that have come into contact with the parasite larva. The severity of infection varies considerably from person to person. Children are more likely to have heavy infestations and are also more likely to suffer from malabsorption and malnutrition than adults.

receiving steroids, seem to be at higher risk of strongyloidiasis. However, HIV/AIDS does not seem to be a risk factor, despite the patient's immunocompromised status. In the Caribbean and Japan, an association between strongyloidiasis and human T-cell leukemia has been found.

■ Treatment and Prevention

S. stercoralis infection can be treated successfully by ivermectin. People being assessed for an organ transplant ought to be screened for infection and treated before the operation is performed. Travelers should avoid contamination with soil in areas of the world where *S. stercoralis* is endemic.

■ Impacts and Issues

Although infection with *S. sterocoralis* may not cause any symptoms, the nature of the parasite's life cycle means that some patients may be at risk of life-threatening complications. The path the larvae take through the body mean that there are many and varied symptoms, which cause confusion with other conditions. Careful diagnosis of the condition is essential, so the parasite can be eradicated before the infection spreads throughout the body in those whose immunity is compromised.

SEE ALSO *Parasitic Diseases; Tropical Infectious Diseases.*

BIBLIOGRAPHY

Books

Peters, Wallace, and Geoffrey Pasvol. *Tropical Medicine and Parasitology.* 5th ed. London: Mosby, 2002.

Wilson, Walter R., and Merle A. Sande. *Current Diagnosis & Treatment in Infectious Diseases.* New York: McGraw Hill, 2001.

Web Sites

Centers for Disease Control and Prevention. "Parasites and Health: Strongyloidiasis." September 26, 2005. <http://www.dpd.cdc.gov/dpdx/HTML/Strongyloidiasis.htm> (accessed May 1, 2007).

Swimmer's Ear and Swimmer's Itch (Cercarial Dermatitis)

■ Introduction

Swimmer's ear (otitis externa) is an infection of the ear canal and swimmer's itch (cercarial dermatitis) is an allergic reaction to various types of microscopic water-borne parasites infecting human skin.

Many different types of fungi or bacteria can infect the ear canal—the hollow cylindrical-like opening that allows sounds to enter the eardrum. Swimmer's ear often results.

Swimmer's itch—sometimes also called duck itch and clam digger's itch in the United States and various other names around the world—is a distinctly different infection caused by parasitic schistosomes (small flukes that live in blood) that infect snails and vertebrates. Most schistosomes infect waterfowl. The parasites are discharged from infected snails and vertebrates into fresh waters (often slow-moving ponds and lakes). The para-sites then burrow into the skin of swimming humans. They cause an allergic reaction, itch, and rash.

These schistosomes cannot become long-term para-sites in humans. They only cause mild itchy spots, which later can become raised bumps that are much itchier. The parasites die within a few hours, and the symptoms disappear.

■ Disease History, Characteristics, and Transmission

Swimmer's ear occurs frequently in children because they usually spend more time swimming. It can also occur in environments with high humidity. The infec-tion can also arise any time a break in the skin occurs within the ear canal. Thus, any extended exposure to moisture in the ear often irritates the ear canal, which

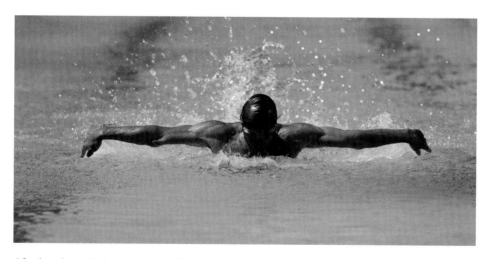

After long hours in the pool, competitive swimmers can be susceptible to swimmer's ear. When too much moisture is in the ear, it can become irritated and infected as the skin in the canal breaks down, allowing bacteria or fungi to invade. © Stefan Schuetz/zefa/Corbis.

WORDS TO KNOW

MALIGNANT: A general term for cells that can dislodge from the original tumor, invade and destroy other tissues and organs.

PARASITE: An organism that lives in or on a host organism and that gets its nourishment from that host. The parasite usually gains all the benefits of this relationship, while the host may suffer from various diseases and discomforts, or show no signs of the infection. The life cycle of a typical parasite usually includes several developmental stages and morphological changes as the parasite lives and moves through the environment and one or more hosts. Parasites that remain on a host's body surface to feed are called ectoparasites, while those that live inside a host's body are called endoparasites. Parasitism is a highly successful biological adaptation. There are more known parasitic species than nonparasitic ones, and parasites affect just about every form of life, including most all animals, plants, and even bacteria.

SCHISTOSOMES: Blood flukes that infect an estimated 200 million people.

allows fungi or bacteria to enter. People often get swimmer's ear when they have dry skin or eczema, frequently or aggressively scratch or clean the ear canal, or insert objects into the ear canal, such as cotton swabs, pencil tips, or paper clips.

Trichobilharzia and *Gigantobilharzia* are two genera of schistosome that commonly cause swimmer's itch. These schistosomes infect waterfowl, such as ducks and geese, and aquatic mammals, such as beavers. The parasites lay eggs that are transferred in the feces of infected birds or mammals. The eggs, if dropped into water, hatch and release larvae that can infect humans.

Schistosomatium douthitti is a species of schistosome that infects snails. It first infects a non-human vertebrate, such as a waterfowl or mammal, and completes its life-cycle within these hosts. However, humans can become indirectly infected when coming into contact with infected waters or shorelines.

Symptoms of swimmer's ear include fever, skin inflammation inside the ear canal, temporarily reduced hearing (caused by swollen tissue), and itchiness. More severe symptoms include reddening and swelling of the outer ear, enlarged and tender lymph nodes around the ear, and yellowish drainage. Sharp pain often affects the earlobe or other external parts. In severe cases, the skin infection spreads to the face and salivary gland in the cheek. Eating can become painful. According to the Nemours Foundation, swimmer's ear is not contagious.

Swimmer's itch has symptoms that occur from minutes to days after contact. Common symptoms include mild itchy areas on the skin, which can become more itchy and redder after a few hours. There is also a tingling or burning sensation in the infected areas. Later, small blisters can appear. Itching usually stops within a week and other symptoms gradually disappear. Children are more likely to become infected due to the simple fact that they spend more time around water. According to the U.S. Centers for Disease Control and Prevention, swimmer's itch cannot be spread from person to person.

■ Scope and Distribution

Swimmer's ear is found is all temperate climates of the world where water is available for swimming. It is considered an infection that frequently occurs.

Swimmer's itch occurs throughout the world. The parasites causing the infection are more frequently found around lakes or other such bodies of slow-moving fresh and salt water. Inshore waters, rather than open waters, are more likely to contain schistosomes. They commonly infect humans during the hotter months of the year, and often infect humans that wade or swim close to shore or in shallow water.

■ Treatment and Prevention

Treatment of swimmer's ear includes using over-the-counter drops of a dilute solution—usually about 2%—of acetic acid or alcohol. Such ear drops are usually used several times a day for a maximum of ten days. Care should be taken because improper use can irritate or damage membranes located past the ear canal. Ear drops containing quinolone antibiotics are useful for stopping fluid discharge and combating bacterial infection. A corticosteroid is used to prevent inflammation, itching, and swelling. Treatment usually will cure the problem within seven to ten days.

Swimmer's ear can be prevented by drying a child's ears with a towel. Battery powered ear dryers can also be used. The child's head also can be tilted to the side so that excess water runs out. Doctors may recommend earplugs while swimming; however, the earplugs should be professionally fitted because they can irritate the ear canal if improperly used. Until the infection has cleared up, doctors recommend that a child should not swim or wash his or her hair. To prevent damage to the ear canal, children should not be allowed to place objects in their ears or to clean their ears themselves.

The American Osteopathic College of Dermatology recommends that swimmer's itch be treated with an antihistamine cream or a mild corticosteroid cream. Both can be purchased as over-the-counter medicines. However, if symptoms, such as scratching, continue longer than three days, the AOCD recommends a visit to a dermatologist.

Prevention of swimmer's itch usually involves the long-term removal of the schistosome hosts. For instance, various control agents such as copper sulfate have been used to eliminate snail populations around lakes. The application of the insect repellant DEET (N, N-diethyl-m-toluamide) to the body can help to repel schistosomes.

■ Impacts and Issues

People with diabetes or immune system disorders should get medical assistance immediately when affected with swimmer's ear. They are more likely to suffer severe symptoms including malignant otitis externa, which is a rare form of otitis externa. Rather than staying on the surface of the outer ear, this disease can move into the bony structures of the ear and may permanently destroy them.

Because marine pollution is increasing around the world, especially in developed and developing countries, more incidents of swimmer's itch are occurring. In addition, global warming is creating conditions favorable to expanded populations of water-borne parasites. Many people have more leisure time and may choose to spend this time around water. More people are also moving to areas containing slow-moving bodies of water, such as lakes and estuaries. The rate of swimmer's itch increases both with the amount of time spent in infected waters and with the level of pollution in waters where swimming is done.

SEE ALSO *Ear infections (Otitis Media); Water-borne Disease.*

BIBLIOGRAPHY

Books

Bluestone, Charles D. *Targeting Therapies in Otitis Media and Otitis Externa*. Hamilton, Ontario, Canada: Decker DTC, 2004.

Zhai, Hongho, and Howard I. Maibach. *Dermatotoxicology*. New York: CRC Press, 2004.

Periodicals

Beers, S., and T. Abramo. "Otitis Externa Review." *Pediatric Emergency Care* 20 (April 2004): 250–256.

Verbrugge, L. M., et al. "Prospective Study of Swimmer's Itch Incidence and Severity." *Journal of Parasitology* 90 (2004): 697–704.

Web Sites

Centers for Disease Control and Prevention. "Cercarial Dermatitis." September 17, 2004. <http://www.cdc.gov/ncidod/dpd/parasites/cercarialdermatitis/factsht_cercarialdermatitis.htm> (accessed March 24, 2007).

Health Canada. "Material Safety Data Sheet—Infectious Substances: Ascaris lumbricoides." January 23, 2001. <http://www.phac-aspc.gc.ca/msds-ftss/msds9e.html> (accessed March 23, 2007).

KidsHealth for Parents. "Infections: Swimmer's Ear." March 2006. <http://www.kidshealth.org/parent/infections/ear/swimmer_ear.html> (accessed March 27, 2007).

THE EXTERNAL EAR

The external ear consists of the flesh and cartilage structure on either side of the head, known as the auricle or pinna, and of the hole into the head. The auricle helps focus the incoming sound waves. The hole leads into the auditory canal, a roughly cylinder-shaped, small diameter canal that is about 2.5 cm long. Towards the inner end, the canal widens slightly and ends at the eardrum. The ear canal can be thought of as a shaped tube with a resonating column of air inside it, having open and closed ends, similar to the construction of an organ pipe.

This analogy is apt, for the ear canal enhances the sound vibrations that have traveled in from the outside. The canal can resonate, or vibrate, typically at frequencies that the ear hears most sharply. The vibration increases the wavelength of the sound waves traveling down the canal. The amplified waves eventually contact the ear drum, which is positioned at the inner end of the canal, and marks the boundary between the outer ear and the middle ear.

The ear drum is a membrane. It is capable of vibration, which occurs when the sound waves contact it. The vibrational energy of the ear drum is converted to mechanical vibrations in the solid materials of the middle ear. These solid materials are three bones: the malleus, incus and stapes. The bones form a system of levers that are linked together and are driven by the eardrum. The outer malleus pushes on the incus, which in turn pushes on the stapes. This further amplifies the sound vibrations, typically 2–3 fold. Muscles are positioned around the bones, the smallest muscles in the body, and 'dampen down' the mechanical vibrations if they become too pronounced. They are a form of safety device, restricting movement of one or more of the bones. This protects against the creation of too great a vibration from a very loud sound.

Syphilis

■ Introduction

Syphilis is one of the most significant of the sexually transmitted diseases (STDs) with an estimated 12 million new infections occurring each year worldwide. It is a deceptive condition, starting with a single, painless sore which may not even be detected but which may progress over a period of years to potentially fatal complications such as heart damage, dementia, and paralysis. Syphilis is very infectious, and most cases are caused by sexual contact with people who may not even be aware that they have themselves contracted the disease.

Syphilis is caused by the bacterium *Treponema pallidum* and the advent of penicillin in the late 1940s led to a dramatic decrease in the number of cases. However, syphilis has been on the increase again in recent years in the United States and in other countries, so there is a great need to treat the disease at an early stage and to educate people about the risks.

■ Disease History, Characteristics, and Transmission

Syphilis is caused by *T. pallidum*, which belongs to the spirochaete class of fine, spiral, highly motile bacteria. Its incubation time is from nine to 90 days and the disease

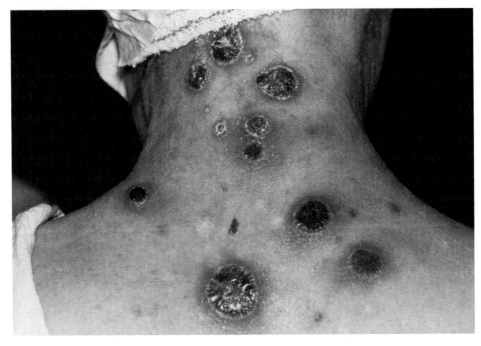

A person displays the signs of secondary syphilis rash and inflammation on the back.   *CNRI/Photo Researchers, Inc.*

progresses through an infectious and a non-infectious stage. The infectious stage lasts for a few months, during which time symptoms may cause little, or no, illness. The non-infectious stage, which follows if syphilis is not treated early on, may also be without symptoms—or it may be accompanied by major heart or neurological damage.

Infectious syphilis is divided into two stages. The primary stage is characterized by the appearance of a single sore, known as a chancre, either on or inside the genitals or elsewhere on the body, such as on the eyelid or lip. Typically, the chancre is firm, round, small and painless. It appears at the site of entry of *T. pallidum* into the body. The chancre, which those affected may be completely unaware of, lasts for three to six weeks and heals without treatment. However, if treatment is not administered, the infection will progress to the secondary stage.

A skin rash and mucous membrane lesions are the prime symptoms of the secondary stage. A non-itching rash develops, either while the chancre is healing or several weeks afterwards. This might appear as rough red or reddish-brown spots on the palms of the hands and the soles of the feet. However, a rash might appear on some other part of the body and resemble that from some other disease—especially if the primary stage has not been identified.

Sometimes the rash from secondary syphilis is so faint as to be unnoticeable. There may be other symptoms such as fever, swollen glands, weight loss, headaches, loss of appetite, and fatigue. However, this stage also resolves within a few weeks without any treatment.

Latent syphilis is untreated disease past the primary and secondary stage. It has no obvious symptoms and is known as early or late, depending on whether it develops earlier or later than two years after the first infection. This is an arbitrary cut-off time that refers to whether or not the disease is likely to still be infectious.

Late latent syphilis may lead to complications of the nervous system. Ten percent of people with latent syphilis will develop neurosyphilis, of which there are various types, depending on which part of the brain and nervous system is affected. Neurosyphilis produces early symptoms such as personality change, tremor, and impaired memory, often followed by paralysis, delusions and seizures. Another form of neurosyphilis, tabes doralis, is accompanied by sharp pains in the legs and an absence of normal reflexes. The meningovascular type of neurosyphilis is an inflammation of the covering of the brain, and headache is usually a major symptom. Neurosyphilis may not have any symptoms at all, but evidence of infection can still be found in the cerebrospinal fluid.

Another ten percent of those with late disease will develop cardiovascular syphilis, which affects the aorta—the main vessel leaving the heart to supply the rest of the body with oxygenated blood. The disease leads to aneur-

---

WORDS TO KNOW

ANTIBIOTIC: A drug, such as penicillin, used to fight infections caused by bacteria. Antibiotics act only on bacteria and are not effective against viruses.

SEXUALLY TRANSMITTED DISEASE (STD): Sexually transmitted diseases (STDs) vary in their susceptibility to treatment, their signs and symptoms, and the consequences if they are left untreated. Some are caused by bacteria. These usually can be treated and cured. Others are caused by viruses and can typically be treated but not cured. More than 15 million new cases of STD are diagnosed annually in the United States.

VENEREAL DISEASE: Venereal diseases are diseases that are transmitted by sexual contact. They are named after Venus, the Roman goddess of female sexuality.

---

ysm, which is a weakness in the artery, which may lead to a potentially fatal rupture. Finally, gummatous syphilis affects 15 percent of those with later disease and leads to the presence of sores on the skin and mucous membranes, many years after the primary infection.

A pregnant woman with syphilis might pass the disease on to her unborn child. Congenital syphilis leads to stillbirth, death shortly after birth, physical deformity, or neurological problems. Increasing awareness of the dangers of syphilis can decrease the risk of all these complications, by treating cases at the earliest possible stage with antibiotics.

Transmission of syphilis is by direct contact with a chancre, which usually occurs through sexual contact. Since the sore may be inside the body—on the cervix, for instance—it is possible that neither person will realize the danger of infection. It is also possible to become re-infected with syphilis at some later stage—unlike with some other infectious diseases, one infection does not confer lifelong immunity.

■ Scope and Distribution

According to the World Health Organization, there are around 12 million new syphilis infections each year. South and Southeast Asia account for about four million, sub-Saharan Africa for another four million. Other areas where syphilis is a significant health problem include Eastern Europe and the United States.

IN CONTEXT: SCIENTIFIC, POLITICAL, AND ETHICAL ISSUES

In 1932, the U.S. Public Health Service (USPHS). Venereal Disease Division began an experiment in Macon County, Alabama, to determine the natural course of untreated, latent syphilis in African American men. The experiment, known as the Tuskegee Syphilis Study, involved 400 men with syphilis, as well as 200 uninfected men who served as controls. The men were told that they were ill with "bad blood," a rural Southern colloquialism for syphilis and anemia, but were never informed that they were participants in a study. The USPHS was investigating the possibility that anti-syphilitic treatment was unnecessary.

Despite the fact that major medical textbooks in 1932 advocated treating syphilis at the latent stage, the USPHS actively prevented the men enrolled in the study from receiving treatment. They were never given a clear diagnosis. In 1934, the USPHS advised local black hospitals not to treat the study subjects, and when the Alabama Health Department took a mobile venereal disease unit into Macon County in the early 1940s, the USPHS advised the health officials to deny treatment to the test subjects. At the start of World War II (1941–1945), several of the men were drafted for military service and were told by the Army to begin anti-syphilitic treatment. Concerned about the continuation of the experiment, the USPHS gave the names of 256 study members to the Alabama state draft board and asked that they not be drafted and, thus, receive treatment in the military. The draft board complied with the request. When penicillin became widely available by the early 1950s as a cure for syphilis, the men enrolled in the study did not receive treatment.

No effort was made by the USPHS to protect the wives and families of the diseased men from syphilis. The officials in charge of the experiment presumed that syphilis existed naturally in the black community, presumed that African American men were promiscuous, and presumed they would not seek or continue treatment even if given the choice.

The first published report of the Tuskegee Syphilis Study appeared in 1936, with subsequent papers issued every four to six years throughout the 1960s. Each report noted the ravages of untreated syphilis. In 1969, a committee from the Centers for Disease Control decided that the study should be continued. However, by this time, some of the test subjects had received antibiotics for other illnesses, thereby compromising the syphilis study. Only in July 1972, when the Associated Press reported the story, did the Department of Health, Education, and Welfare (HEW) halt the experiment amid great public outrage. At that time, 74 of the test subjects were still alive. Many of the subjects had died from untreated syphilis with estimates of the dead ranging from twenty-eight to one hundred men. In August 1972, HEW appointed an investigatory panel, which subsequently found the study to be "ethically unjustified." HEW declared that penicillin should have been provided to the men. None of the physicians who participated in the study were ever prosecuted for any crimes, although the United States did settle a lawsuit brought by the survivors and their families for $10 million.

The Tuskegee Syphilis Study led to new standards for experiments that employ human subjects. In U.S. Senate hearings on human experimentation held in the wake of publicity about the study, physicians were reminded that the goal of human experimentation must always be to advance the human condition and to improve the situation of the subjects of the study. Institutional review boards were established to guarantee that studies are grounded in scientific principles and that the rights of study participants are protected.

In May 1997, President Bill Clinton issued a formal apology for the Tuskegee Syphilis Study on behalf of the United States government.

According to the Centers for Disease Control and Prevention (CDC), where data on syphilis infection is collected, the disease fell to an all-time low in 2000 but has been increasing since then. Accordingly, there were 7,940 reported cases of primary and secondary syphilis in 2004 and 8,724 in 2005. But there has been a decrease in congenital syphilis during that time period from 9.1 to 8.0 per 100,000 births.

■ Treatment and Prevention

Penicillin is still the mainstay of treatment for syphilis. Doxycycline and erythromycin are alternatives for those who are allergic to penicillin. Early cases can be treated by a single injection of penicillin but the more the disease progresses, the longer the duration of treatment must be. Treatment is effective and it halts progression to the later stages of syphilis and its progression.

Prevention of the disease includes the tracing of the sexual contacts of those in the infectious stages of syphilis. If they are found to be infected, they should be treated promptly. Sexual abstinence, or having monogamous sexual contact with a partner known not to be infected, are the most effective way of avoiding infection with syphilis.

■ Impacts and Issues

During World War I (1914–1918), many involved nations launched public campaigns to combat the spread of sexually transmitted diseases (then commonly called venereal disease or VD) that often rose dramatically during and immediately after wartime. Posters and pamphlets warned soldiers of contracting venereal disease from prostitutes and transmitting venereal disease to wives back home. Syphilis was the focus of most anti-VD campaigns since it then was the most devastating and difficult to treat venereal disease. Anti-VD, and especially anti-syphilis campaigns were again launched during World War II (1939–1945), but the advent of antibiotics shifted their focus to one of wartime rationing and conservation—saving precious antibiotics for those most in need by reducing the risk of exposure to venereal disease.

The Tuskegee Syphilis Study (1932–1972) documented the effects of untreated syphilis in approximately 400 African-Americans living near Tuskegee, Alabama. Most of the subjects of the study were poor and had scant access to health care. Many were illiterate, or had little formal education. The study was kept secret for almost four decades, with minimal concern for the welfare of participants. Individuals who volunteered for the study were told they would receive free meals and medical care for their "bad blood." The families of participants who died were eligible to receive $35 for funeral expenses. When the Tuskegee Syphilis Study began in 1932, antibiotic penicillin had been discovered but was not yet commonly available for medical use. Standard treatments for syphilis were neither effective of safe, many involved toxic substances that damaged the liver, kidneys, and nervous system.

The originators of the Tuskegee Syphilis Study claimed that it might be more beneficial for patients to receive no treatment at all than to be subjected to the syphilis remedies then available. However, the Study continued long after penicillin became commonly available after World War II (1939–1945), and patients were denied antibiotics or information about antibiotic treatments. Participants were never fully informed that they had syphilis or that treatment was available. Throughout the course of the study, participants were subjected to repeated injections of non-medicinal solution, routine examinations, and medical testing. Many participants suffered painful symptoms for many years; many died from complications related to untreated syphilis. The experiment terminated abruptly in 1972 after information about the Tuskegee Study was leaked to the press.

While incidence of syphilis in the United States, especially in young adults, reached a new low in the 1990s, an isolated outbreak in 1996 garnered national media attention when public health officials documented 17 cases of syphilis in teenagers in a suburban county near Atlanta, Georgia. Health officials asserted that as many as 250 teens may have been exposed to syphilis. Testing and disease tracking found that many of the teens routinely engaged in high-risk sexual behaviors including having multiple partners, group sex, and unprotected sex.

Much of the increase in syphilis cases in recent years has occurred among men who have sex with men who now account for nearly half of all cases. There has also been an increase in syphilis cases among women, for the first time in more than ten years, and among African-Americans.

Syphilis infection is a major risk for those who already have HIV infection. The presence of the chancre makes it easier for the virus to enter the body. Studies have shown that the risk of HIV transmission is two to five times higher among those who already have syphilis. The symptoms of HIV and syphilis tend to overlap one another, which may confuse the diagnosis. Also, people who are HIV positive might progress quicker to the complications of syphilis. For these reasons, those who are diagnosed with syphilis are recommended to have an HIV test and those who are HIV positive should be tested for syphilis, so treatment can be given as soon as possible.

Primary Source Connection

In the aftermath of the Tuskegee Experiment revelations, calls for government investigations, reparations, and apologies were met with Congressional hearings. The Henderson Act of 1943 had required that all forms of venereal disease be documented and treated; the U.S. Surgeon General had sent letters of commendation to men enrolled in the study on its twenty-fifth anniversary in 1957; and the study violated the 1964 World Health Organization's Declaration of Helsinki, in which informed consent is required. All of these events pointed to a level of government involvement and neglect that led the National Association for the Advancement of Colored People (NAACP) to file a 1973 class-action lawsuit that resulted in a financial settlement.

President William Jefferson Clinton's apology was part of an effort on the part of the Clinton administration to further correct the omission of an apology from the federal government. In 1997, when President Clinton issued his apology, only 8 of the 399 study participants who had syphilis were still alive.

President William Jefferson Clinton's apology on behalf of the United States of America

The East Room.

2:26 P.M. EDT.

THE PRESIDENT: Ladies and gentlemen, on Sunday, Mr. Shaw will celebrate his 95th birthday. I would like to recognize the other survivors who are here today and their families: Mr. Charlie Pollard is here. Mr. Carter Howard. Mr. Fred Simmons. Mr. Simmons just took his first airplane ride, and he reckons he's about 110 years old, so I think it's time for him to take a chance or two. I'm glad he did. And Mr. Frederick Moss, thank you, sir.

I would also like to ask three family representatives who are here—Sam Doner is represented by his daughter, Gwendolyn Cox. Thank you, Gwendolyn. Ernest Hendon, who is watching in Tuskegee, is represented by his brother, North Hendon. Thank you, sir, for being here. And George Key is represented by his grandson, Christopher Monroe. Thank you, Chris.

I also acknowledge the families, community leaders, teachers and students watching today by satellite from Tuskegee. The White House is the people's house; we are glad to have all of you here today. I thank Dr. David Satcher for his role in this. I thank Congresswoman Waters and Congressman Hilliard, Congressman Stokes, the entire Congressional Black Caucus. Dr. Satcher, members of the Cabinet who are here, Secretary Herman, Secretary Slater, members of the Cabinet who are here, Secretary Herman, Secretary Slater. A great friend of freedom, Fred Gray, thank you for fighting this long battle all these long years.

The eight men who are survivors of the syphilis study at Tuskegee are a living link to a time not so very long ago that many Americans would prefer not to remember, but we dare not forget. It was a time when our nation failed to live up to its ideals, when our nation broke the trust with our people that is the very foundation of our democracy. It is not only in remembering that shameful past that we can make amends and repair our nation, but it is in remembering that past that we can build a better present and a better future. And without remembering it, we cannot make amends and we cannot go forward.

So today America does remember the hundreds of men used in research without their knowledge and consent. We remember them and their family members. Men who were poor and African American, without resources and with few alternatives, they belived they had found hope when they were offered free medical care by the United States Public Health Service.

They were betrayed.

Medical people are supposed to help when we need care but even once a cure was discovered, they were denied help, and they were lied to by their government. Our government is supposed to protect the rights of its citizens; their rights were trampled upon. Forty years, hundreds of men betrayed, along with their wives and children, along with the community in Macon County, Alabama, the City of Tuskegee, the fine university there, and the larger African American community.

The United States government did something that was wrong—deeply, profoundly, morally wrong. It was an outrage to our commitment to integrity and equality for all our citizens.

To the survivors, to the wives and family members, the children and the grandchildren, I say what you know: No power on Earth can give you back the lives lost, the pain suffered, the years of internal torment and anguish. What was done cannot be undone. But we can end the silence. We can stop turning our heads away. We can look at you in the eye and finally say on behalf of the American people, what the United States government did was shameful, and I am sorry.

The American people are sorry—for the loss, for the years of hurt. You did nothing wrong, but you were grievously wronged. I apologize and I am sorry that this apology has been so long in coming.

To Macon County, to Tuskegee, to the doctors who have been wrongly associated with the events there, you have our apology, as well. To our African American citizens, I am sorry that your federal government orchestrated a study so clearly racist. That can never be allowed to happen again. It is against everything our country stands for and what we must stand against is what it was.

So let us resolve to hold forever in our hearts and minds the memory of a time not long ago in Macon County, Alabama, so that we can always see how adrift we can become when the rights of any citizens are neglected, ignored and betrayed. And let us resolve here and now to move forward together.

The legacy of the study at Tuskegee has reached far and deep, in ways that hurt our progress and divide our nation. We cannot be one America when a whole segment of our nation has no trust in America. An apology is the first step, and we take it with a commitment to rebuild that broken trust. We can begin by making sure there is never again another episode like this one. We need to do more to ensure that medical research practices are sound and ethical, and that researchers work more closely with communities.

Today I would like to announce several steps to help us achieve these goals. First, we will help to build that lasting memorial at Tuskegee. (Applause.) The school founded by Booker T. Washington, distinguished by the renowned scientist George Washington Carver and so many others who advanced the health and well-being of African Americans and all Americans, is a fitting site. The Department of Health and Human Services will award a planning grant so the school can pursue establishing a center for bioethics in research and health care. The center will serve as a museum of the study and support efforts to address its legacy and strengthen bioethics training.

Second, we commit to increase our community involvement so that we may begin restoring lost trust. The study at Tuskegee served to sow distrust of our medical institutions, especially where research is involved. Since the study was halted, abuses have been checked by making informed consent and local review mandatory in federally-funded and mandated research.

Still, 25 years later, many medical studies have little African American participation and African American organ donors are few. This impedes efforts to conduct promising research and to provide the best health care to all our people, including African Americans. So today, I'm directing the Secretary of Health and Human Services, Donna Shalala, to issue a report in 180 days about how we can best involve communities, especially minority communities, in research and health care. You must—every American group must be involved in medical research in ways that are positive. We have put the curse behind us; now we must bring the benefits to all Americans.

Third, we commit to strengthen researchers' training in bioethics. We are constantly working on making breakthroughs in protecting the health of our people and in vanquishing diseases. But all our people must be assured that their rights and dignity will be respected as new drugs, treatments and therapies are tested and used. So I am directing Secretary Shalala to work in partnership with higher education to prepare training materials for medical researchers. They will be available in a year. They will help researchers build on core ethical principles of respect for individuals, justice and informed consent, and advise them on how to use these principles effectively in diverse populations.

Fourth, to increase and broaden our understanding of ethical issues and clinical research, we commit to providing postgraduate fellowships to train bioethicists especially among African Americans and other minority groups. HHS will offer these fellowships beginning in September of 1998 to promising students enrolled in bioethics graduate programs.

And, finally, by executive order I am also today extending the charter of the National Bioethics Advisory Commission to October of 1999. The need for this commission is clear. We must be able to call on the thoughtful, collective wisdom of experts and community representatives to find ways to further strengthen our protections for subjects in human research.

We face a challenge in our time. Science and technology are rapidly changing our lives with the promise of making us much healthier, much more productive and more prosperous. But with these changes we must work harder to see that as we advance we don't leave behind our conscience. No ground is gained and, indeed, much

is lost if we lose our moral bearings in the name of progress.

The people who ran the study at Tuskegee diminished the stature of man by abandoning the most basic ethical precepts. They forgot their pledge to heal and repair. They had the power to heal the survivors and all the others and they did not. Today, all we can do is apologize. But you have the power, for only you—Mr. Shaw, the others who are here, the family members who are with us in Tuskegee—only you have the power to forgive. Your presence here shows us that you have chosen a better path than your government did so long ago. You have not withheld the power to forgive. I hope today and tomorrow every American will remember your lesson and live by it.

Thank you, and God bless you.

CLINTON, WILLIAM J. *APOLOGY FOR STUDY DONE IN TUSKEGEE.* WHITE HOUSE OFFICE OF PRESS SECRETARY, 1997.

SEE ALSO *Sexually Transmitted Diseases.*

BIBLIOGRAPHY

Books

Adler, Michael, et al. *ABC of Sexually Transmitted Diseases.* London: BMJ, 2004.

Web Sites

Centers for Disease Control and Prevention (CDC). "Trends in reportable sexually transmitted diseases in the United States, 2005." December 2006 <http://www.cdc.gov/std/stats/trends2005.htm#trendssyphilis> (accessed May 1, 2007).
World Health Organization. "Sexually Transmitted Infections." <http://www.who.int/reproductive-health/stis/docs/sti_factsheet_2004.pdf> (accessed May 1, 2007).

Susan Aldridge

Taeniasis (*Taenia* Infection)

■ Introduction

Taenia infection, or taeniasis, is an infection of the digestive tract caused by parasitic flatworms generally called cestodes, or tapeworms. It is specifically caused by only the species within the *Taenia* genus, those that infect carnivores (flesh eating animals). Taeniasis is acquired when humans (definitive hosts) eat raw or undercooked meat from infected animals (intermediate hosts).

For instance, cows (and other ruminants) carry the tapeworm species *Taenia saginata* and pigs (and dogs, cats, and sheep) harbor the species *Taenia solium*. When humans acquire taeniasis from cows the tapeworm is commonly called beef tapeworm and when it is from pigs the tapeworm is called pig tapeworm. In addition, *Taenia multiceps* infect hares, rabbits, and squirrels, while only rarely infecting humans.

■ Disease History, Characteristics, and Transmission

When humans eat infected meat from an intermediate host, tapeworm larvae hatch and develop inside the intestines. *T. saginata* matures to a length of 13 to 26 feet (4 to 8 meters). *T. solium* reaches adulthood at a length of 3 to 7 feet (1 to 2 meters). Both tapeworms can be found as an adult in the human intestines and as larvae in muscles and other tissues of cattle (and other ruminants) and pigs (and dogs, cats, and sheep), respectively. Adult tapeworms can stay inside their hosts for many years. The eggs are passed into the soil from human feces where they are eaten by intermediate hosts. Then, the eggs hatch and larvae enter tissues of the animal host where they enclose themselves in cysts (this is called encysts). When humans eat infected animal flesh, they also eat the cysts.

Tapeworms are long, segmented worms with each segment able to produce eggs. Each segment can detach from the worm and pass out through the feces or they can also crawl on their own through the anus. The worms do not have an intestinal tract, so must obtain their nourishment through their outer covering (integument). The structure of an adult consists of a head, neck, and segmented body that contain both male and female reproductive features. The head attaches to the mucous lining of the intestine.

Humans infected with *T. solium* can become infected again when eggs are ingested from human hands after coming in contact with the anal area. These infected individuals can infect other humans through improper food handling and other unsanitary means. These humans are considered intermediate hosts. The larvae will travel to various tissues of organs within the human host. Thus, *T. solium* are tapeworms that can infect humans as intermediate and definitive hosts.

Taenia infection does not usually cause any symptoms. However, sometimes there can be minor gastrointestinal pain, weight loss, and persistent ill feelings. The infection is usually recognized when the infected person passes tapeworm segments in the stool, especially if the segment is moving.

■ Scope and Distribution

Taenia infection is found worldwide, but only rarely in the United States. In the United States, *T. saginata*it is found in less than 1% of cattle because cattle are thoroughly treated for tapeworms. *T. solium* is also rare in the United States, but it is becoming more frequent as immigrants come in increasing numbers from areas infected with the parasite.

*T. saginata*it is found most often in Latin America, central Asia, Africa, and the Middle East. It is also found somewhat in Europe, southern Asia, Japan, and the Philippines. *T. solium* is found mostly in Latin America, Africa, the Slavic countries of central and southern Europe, southeast Asia, India, and China.

According to the Division of Parasitic Diseases (DPD), of the U.S. Centers for Disease Control and

WORDS TO KNOW

CHEMOTHERAPY: Chemotherapy is the treatment of a disease, infection, or condition with chemicals that have a specific effect on its cause, such as a microorganism or cancer cell. The first modern therapeutic chemical was derived from a synthetic dye. The sulfonamide drugs developed in the 1930s, penicillin and other antibiotics of the 1940s, hormones in the 1950s, and more recent drugs that interfere with cancer cell metabolism and reproduction have all been part of the chemotherapeutic arsenal.

ERADICATION: The process of destroying or eliminating a microorganism or disease.

HOST: Organism that serves as the habitat for a parasite, or possibly for a symbiont. A host may provide nutrition to the parasite or symbiont, or simply a place in which to live.

PARASITE: An organism that lives in or on a host organism and that gets its nourishment from that host. The parasite usually gains all the benefits of this relationship, while the host may suffer from various diseases and discomforts, or show no signs of the infection. The life cycle of a typical parasite usually includes several developmental stages and morphological changes as the parasite lives and moves through the environment and one or more hosts. Parasites that remain on a host's body surface to feed are called ectoparasites, while those that live

inside a host's body are called endoparasites. Parasitism is a highly successful biological adaptation. There are more known parasitic species than nonparasitic ones, and parasites affect just about every form of life, including most all animals, plants, and even bacteria.

RUMINANTS: Cud-chewing animals with a four-chambered stomachs and even-toed hooves.

SEIZURE: A seizure is a sudden disruption of the brain's normal electrical activity accompanied by altered consciousness and/or other neurological and behavioral abnormalities. Epilepsy is a condition characterized by recurrent seizures that may include repetitive muscle jerking called convulsions. Seizures are traditionally divided into two major categories: generalized seizures and focal seizures. Within each major category, however, there are many different types of seizures. Generalized seizures come about due to abnormal neuronal activity on both sides of the brain, while focal seizures, also named partial seizures, occur in only one part of the brain.

TAPEWORM: Tapeworms are parasitic flatworms of class *Cestoidea*, phylum *Platyhelminthes*, that live inside the intestine. Tapeworms have no digestive system, but absorb predigested nutrients directly from their surroundings.

Prevention (CDC), *T. solium* is found more than *T. saginatait* in underdeveloped areas because people live very close to pigs and often eat undercooked pork.

■ Treatment and Prevention

Taenia infection is diagnosed with a stool sample. Tapeworm eggs can be found with a medical examination. Segments of worms can also be readily seen in feces after they are passed from the body. An infected person is treated with oral anti-parasitic worm medications. Usually one dose of niclosamide (Niclocide®) is used, and sometimes either praziquantel (Biltricide®) or albendazole (Albenza®, Eskazole®, or Zentel®) is given. After the treatment is complete, tapeworm infection is normally eliminated, but reinfection is possible if more cysts are ingested.

Any complications are usually from an infected person re-infecting themselves with tapeworm eggs. In rare

cases, worms may cause blockage of the intestines and obstruct the bowels, resulting in a medical emergency.

Taenia infection is prevented in the United States and other industrial countries with strict federal law governing the feeding and inspection of domesticated animals slaughtered for food. According to the CDC's Division of Parasitic Diseases, taeniasis has been largely eliminated in the United States. In addition, fully cooking meat destroys any tapeworm larvae that may be present and any infection they may carry. Anyone infected with tapeworms can prevent infecting oneself again by practicing good hygiene, especially by thoroughly washing one's hands after using the toilet.

■ Impacts and Issues

T. saginatait infection can cause obstruction of the appendix (small outgrowth of intestines), pancreatic duct (carrier of pancreatic juices), and biliary duct (transporter of bile).

Infections involving *T. solium* can cause debilitating complications with regards to the central nervous system and the skeletal muscles. Under many conditions, a neurologic examination comes back normal, making it very difficult to diagnosis the infection. Other complications that can set in include meningitis (inflammation of the meninges), dementia (deterioration of memory functions), and hydrocephalus (increased fluid around the brain).

Larvae can also migrate from the intestines to other tissues of the body. If larvae migrate to the brain, they can cause neurological problems that are generally called cysticercosis. Seizure can occur when the brain is affected, along with earlier signs of vomiting, confusion, visual changes, and headaches.

Several international health organizations, including the World Health Organization (WHO), have identified taeniasis as potentially eradicable, meaning that health officials hope to eliminate the disease in humans. As of 2007, current efforts to eradicate taeniasis focus on hygiene education, improved sanitation, and preventative vaccinations for carrier animals. In South America and parts of Asia and Africa, efforts to control *Taenia solium* employ aggressive chemotherapy (using drugs or chemicals that are toxic to sources of diseases within the body) campaigns to reduce the number of human carriers.

SEE ALSO *Helminth Disease; Parasitic Diseases; Tapeworm Infections.*

BIBLIOGRAPHY

Books

Maule, Aaron G., and Nikki J. Marks, eds. *Parasitic Flatworms: Molecular Biology, Biochemistry, Immunology and Physiology.* Wallingford, UK: CABI Publishing, 2006.

Singh G., and S. Prabhakar, eds. *Taenia Solium Cysticercosis: From Basic to Clinical Science.* Chandigarh, India: CABI Publishing, 2002.

Periodicals

Beers, S., and T. Abramo. "Otitis externa review." *Pediatric Emergency Care.* 20(4) (2004): 250–256.

Verbrugge, L.M., et al. "Prospective study of swimmer's itch incidence and severity." *Journal of Parasitology.* 90 (2004): 697–704.

Web Sites

Division of Parasitic Diseases, U.S. Centers for Disease Control and Prevention. "Taeniasis." November 29, 2006 <http://www.dpd.cdc.gov/dpdx/Default.htm> (accessed March 27, 2007).

Tapeworm Infections

■ Introduction

Tapeworms are parasitic animals also known as cest-odes. The life cycle of the tapeworm involves humans as either a primary or intermediate host. Both of these situations cause infection in humans. Humans become infected with tapeworms when they either ingest meat containing encysted tapeworms or when they ingest tapeworm eggs. In the first case, humans act as primary hosts. In the second case, humans act as intermediate hosts.

While tapeworm infections tend to be asympto-matic, some symptoms may appear, including abdominal pain, nausea, diarrhea, stools containing mucus, and the passing of tapeworm segments, or proglottids. How-ever, if a human is infected with eggs, more serious complications can arise. The cysts formed by the larvae in tissues can cause damage, including damage to vital organs, such as the brain.

Tapeworm infections occur worldwide, but are more prevalent in countries with low hygiene and sani-tation conditions or in areas where humans live close to

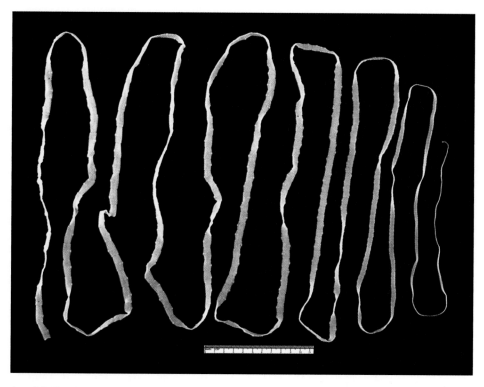

An adult *Taenia saginata* tapeworm is shown. Humans become infected with tapeworms by ingesting raw or undercooked infected meat. *Science Source.*

WORDS TO KNOW

CESTODE: A class of worms characterized by flat, segmented bodies, commonly known as tapeworms.

INTERMEDIATE HOST: An organism infected by a parasite while the parasite is in a developmental form, not sexually mature.

PRIMARY HOST: The primary host is an organism that provides food and shelter for a parasite while allowing it to become sexually mature, while a secondary host is one occupied by a parasite during the larval or asexual stages of its life cycle.

livestock. Tapeworms are passed on predominantly through ingesting meat containing encysted tapeworms or ingesting food and water contaminated with infected human feces. Treatment involves anti-parasitic medications, such as praziquantel, and is usually effective.

■ Disease History, Characteristics, and Transmission

Tapeworms are parasitic flatworms belonging to the class Cestoda. The life cycle of a tapeworm generally involves a primary host and an intermediate host. The life cycle begins when a tapeworm egg is passed from a primary host into soil or water. An intermediate host ingests the egg and the larvae hatch, enter tissues, and form cysts. A primary host then ingests cysts when they consume the flesh of the intermediate host. These cysts develop into adults, which sexually reproduce in the host's intestines.

In most cases, humans become infected with tapeworms after eating undercooked or raw animal flesh containing tapeworm cysts. These worms migrate to the intestines where they reproduce. The fecal matter of these infected individuals is infectious, since it contains tapeworm eggs. The most common tapeworms that infect humans in this manner are: *Taenia solium*, which is present in pigs; *Taenia saginata*, which is present in cattle; *Diphyllobothrium* species, which are present in freshwater fishes; *Hymenolepis* species, which are found in rodents and insects; and *Diphyllobothrium caninum*, which is present in cat and dog fleas.

In some cases, humans are intermediate hosts. In these cases, humans ingest the tapeworm eggs. These hatch, and the larvae migrate to tissues within the body and form cysts. This occurs with *Taenia solium* if humans swallow food or water that contains contami-

nated human fecal matter. It also occurs when humans accidentally swallow insects containing the larvae of *Hymenolepis* species.

Tapeworm infections tend to be asymptomatic. However, possible symptoms include abdominal pain, nausea, diarrhea, stools containing mucus, and the passing of tapeworm segments, or proglottids. A serious risk associated with an infestation of *T. solium* is the risk of developing cysticercosis. This occurs when the eggs are ingested and the larvae form cysts within tissues. The most serious form of this infection involves cysts that form in the central nervous system—a condition known as neurocysticercosis. This can cause neurological problems and seizures. In severe cases, permanent brain damage or death may occur.

■ Scope and Distribution

Tapeworm infections occur worldwide. However, certain species are only present, or are more prevalent, in certain regions. In the United States, only a few tapeworms commonly cause infection. Infection by *T. saginata* and *T. solium* is rare in the United States, with less than a 1% infection rate for *T. saginata*. This is a result of the almost complete absence of these parasites from the livestock industry. However, infection by *Diphyllobothrium* species, which is caused by ingesting raw or undercooked fish, occurs more commonly.

Elsewhere in the world, *T. saginata* and *T. solium* are more prevalent. *T. saginata* is endemic in Latin America, Africa, the Middle East, and central Asia. It also occurs in Europe, south Asia, Japan, and the Philippines. *T. solium* is common in Latin America, the Slavic countries, Africa, Southeast Asia, India, and China. It also occurs in Europe, but with lower prevalence. Cysticercosis, which occurs when humans are infected by the larval form of tapeworms, is endemic in almost all Latin American countries.

Infection from *Diphyllobothrium* species also commonly occurs in Europe, Canada, Africa, some Asian countries, South America, and Australia. However, the most common tapeworm infection in humans is caused by *Hymenolepis nana*. Infection arises when humans accidentally ingest infected insects, or ingest food or water contaminated by infected insects. In addition, the eggs are transmissible from human to human through contaminated feces. Children, the developmentally disabled, and psychiatric patients are most commonly infected. In addition, these parasites are commonly found in regions with poor hygiene and sanitation methods.

■ Treatment and Prevention

Tapeworm infections are usually treated with anti-parasitic drugs. One of the most common and effective medications is praziquantel. This drug effectively kills adult tapeworms. There are a few mild side effects of praziquantel, but these are generally short-lived. Albendazole is an alternative to praziquantel, with similar effects. Another alternative to praziquantal is niclosamide, which is used to treat infections by *Taenia* and *Diphyllobothrium* tapeworms. The side effects of this drug include nausea, abdominal pain, vomiting, diarrhea, light-headedness, and skin rash. In the case of neurocysticercosis, in which tapeworm larvae form cysts in the central nervous system, early treatment of this infection can minimize damage to the system, and thus decrease the risk of neurological complications.

These treatments kill the adult tapeworms, not the eggs, so it is possible for a patient to remain infected following treatment. Therefore, a visit to the doctor three months after treatment is necessary to check for continued infection and to determine whether further treatment is needed.

There are no vaccinations to prevent tapeworm infections. Therefore, the best method of prevention is to avoid becoming contaminated. For tapeworms found in meats, cooking the meat above a temperature of 150°F (65.5°C) or freezing it for 12–24 hours kills the tapeworms. In addition, ensuring that livestock are dewormed decreases the risk that they are infected and likely to pass on an infection to humans.

Food and water may be contaminated with infected fecal matter, particularly in regions with poor hygiene and sanitation. Therefore, washing raw food or thoroughly cooking it helps to ensure parasites are removed. In addition, boiling or filtering drinking water decreases the chance of ingesting parasites from the water. Good personal hygiene, such as washing hands with soap and water prior to handling food, and rigorous sanitation practices, especially where human waste is involved, also decrease the likelihood that parasites will be transmitted among a human population.

■ Impacts and Issues

Tapeworms are a major health issue for a number of countries. Since tapeworms are usually originate in livestock or contaminated human feces, regions in which humans live near their livestock and areas with poor hygiene and sanitation standards have a higher prevalence of tapeworm infections. Tapeworm infections tend to be endemic in developing countries, where sanitation is poor due to a lack of funding and medical treatment is often unavailable.

Tapeworm infections do still occur in developed countries for a number of reasons. Travel and immigration have become a source of tapeworm infection as infected people interact with non-infected people, potentially spreading the tapeworms. In addition, since tapeworm infections are usually asymptomatic, the tapeworm may go undetected for years before treatment is given and the tapeworm is removed from the body.

Since tapeworms form cysts in animal flesh, eating raw or undercooked meats increases the likelihood of becoming infected. This is not a significant problem for countries such as the United States in which livestock are almost totally free of tapeworm infestations due to deworming practices. However, for countries where the practices associated with livestock farming are more relaxed, there is a higher chance that eating meat may cause infection.

Although many cases of tapeworm infection go undetected for years due to the asymptomatic nature of infection, the most severe form of infection—cysticercosis—can cause serious health issues. If a human ingests tapeworm eggs, they hatch and the larvae form cysts in tissues within the body. This can cause damage to vital body organs, and, in the worst-case scenario, can damage the nervous system. This may result in death or permanent brain injury.

SEE ALSO *Endemicity; Food-borne Disease and Food Safety; Handwashing; Parasitic Diseases; Sanitation; Taeniasis* (Taenia *Infection*).

BIBLIOGRAPHY

Books

Beers, M. H. *The Merck Manual of Medical Information.* New York: Pocket Books, 2003.

Bush, A.O., et al. *Parasitism: The Diversity and Ecology of Animal Parasites.* New York: Cambridge University Press, 2001.

Mandell, G.L., J.E. Bennett, and R. Dolin. *Principles and Practice of Infectious Diseases.* 6th ed. Philadelphia: Elsevier, 2004.

Web Sites

Centers for Disease Control and Prevention. "Hymenolepis Infection." September 21, 2004. <http://www.cdc.gov/ncidod/dpd/parasites/hymenolepis/factsht_hymenolepis.htm> (accessed March 9, 2007).

WebMD. "Tapeworm Infestation." August 8, 2005. <http://www.emedicine.com/emerg/topic567.htm> (accessed March 9, 2007).

Tetanus

■ Introduction

Tetanus is a serious but easily prevented acute neurological disease that affects the muscles and nerves of the human body. The bacterium *Clostridium tetani* causes the disease, typically through any injury to the skin, such as a burn, crushing injury, cut, gangrene, or wound, that becomes contaminated. Tetanus can also come about from the use of non-sterile needles in drug use, body piercing, and tattooing. Tetanus can be classified as local tetanus (muscle contraction in one local area) and cephalic tetanus (found in the middle ear). Newborn babies can also get neonatal tetanus, a special type of tetanus, when they are born in unsanitary conditions.

However, most tetanus is generalized tetanus, which descends from the head down through the body. Once in the human body, the bacteria produce a neurotoxin (a poisonous protein that acts on the nervous system) called tetanospasmin. The neurotoxin causes contraction and rigidity of the skeletal muscles. According to the U.S. Centers for Disease Control and Prevention (CDC), tetanus cannot be spread from human to human. Thus, it is not contagious.

■ Disease History, Characteristics, and Transmission

Tetanus has been medically reported as far back as the fifth century BC. According to the CDC, the first passively transferred antitoxin (an antibody that is able to neutralize a toxin) was developed in 1897. In 1924, the first tetanus toxoid was developed. A toxoid is a toxin that has been treated to destroy toxicity, but the toxoid is still capable of inducing the formation of antibodies when injected into the human body.

C. tetani is widely found in soil and in the intestines and feces of such animals as cattle, chickens, cats and dogs, guinea pigs, horses, rats, and sheep. Manure-treated soils also may contain large amounts of the bacteria. Cases of tetanus in the United States are usually from a cut or deep wound that has been contaminated with feces, saliva, or soil.

The puncture of the skin with a rusty nail, for instance, is typically seen as the source of possible tetanus. However, rust does not cause tetanus, but the nail itself causes the puncture into the skin and the rust may only harbor *C. tetani* on its surface.

The first sign of tetanus is usually in the nerves that control the muscles near the wound, which first allowed the bacterium to enter the body. Later, as the bacteria have had time to travel through the bloodstream and lymph system, other nerves become adversely affected. The widely spreading bacteria soon produce general muscle spasms. Without treatment, tetanus can cause death to humans.

The incubation period for tetanus is 2–21 days. Symptoms often begin around the seventh or eighth day. Initial symptoms include muscle spasms in the jaw (what is called trismus and what gives tetanus its commonly used name—lockjaw). Later, swallowing may become difficult and stiffness or pain may occur in the muscles of the shoulders, neck, and back. Still later, additional spasms may spread throughout the muscles of the upper arms, thighs, and abdomen. Other symptoms include fever, sweating, high blood pressure, and rapid heart rate. Symptoms generally begin to subside after about 17 days. Spasms may continue for three to four weeks. A complete recovery may take months.

■ Scope and Distribution

Tetanus is relatively rare in the United States and other countries with comprehensive tetanus vaccination programs to prevent and immunize their citizens when compared to countries without such programs. Most cases of tetanus occur in densely populated areas with hot, humid climates and rich organic soils. Around five cases are reported in the United States in an average

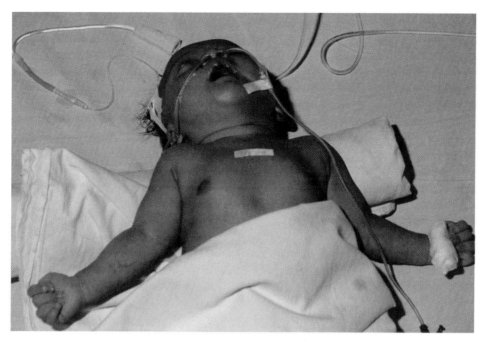

A hospitalized infant shows the characteristic muscle contractions of tetanus, such as lockjaw. Contamination of the umbilical stump can cause tetanus in newborns. *Sue Ford/Photo Researchers, Inc.*

year. Over two million cases are reported worldwide each year. According to the CDC, about 11% of all reported cases of tetanus around the world are fatal, totaling over 225,000 people. People most susceptible to death from tetanus are unvaccinated persons and those people over the age of 60 years.

■ Treatment and Prevention

Tetanus is diagnosed only by clinical signs and symptoms. There is no laboratory confirmation for the bacteria. It is treated with a tetanus booster (for children still receiving their series of tetanus shots) or an injection of tetanus antitoxin, such as tetanus immune globulin (TIG), to neutralize any toxin released by the bacteria. Intravenous immune globulin (IVIG) can be given if TIG is unavailable. Metronidazole can be given to control bacteria. The wound should be cleaned and all dead or infected skin should be removed. Severe cases of tetanus should be treated in the intensive care unit of a hospital. Medicines to control breathing and prevent muscle spasms are usually given.

Tetanus is prevented with a routine tetanus immunization. Children in the United States and other such countries usually receive an injection that combines diphtheria and tetanus toxoids with pertussis vaccine. This immunization protects children from diphtheria (throat and respiratory infection), tetanus, and pertussis (whooping cough). According to the Mayo Clinic, the latest version is called the diphtheria and tetanus toxoids

and acellular pertussis (DTaP) vaccine. The DTaP vaccine generally consists of a series of five shots in the arm or thigh given to children at two months, four months, eight months, 15–18 months, and 4–6 years of age. The Mayo Clinic recommends that adolescents get a booster shot between the ages of 11 and 18 years. Thereafter, a vaccination should be given every 10 years. A medical professional should be consulted for each particular situation.

■ Impacts and Issues

Although tetanus is rare, it is still a serious illness. Tetanus is considered an international health problem because so many people around the world are still unvaccinated or inadequately vaccinated. It is especially serious in children. As a result, children are often treated in intensive care units of hospitals after contracting tetanus. The child being treated in such situations will usually be given antibiotics to kill bacteria and TIG to neutralize the toxins. Medicines may be given to control muscle spasms. Other medicines may need to be given to support life functions for cases involving pneumonia and other respiratory problems.

Adults may also have complications including spasms of the vocal cords, spasms of the muscles of respiration, and fractures of the spine and longer bones of the body. Various treatment methods have been tried in such serious cases. However, no medical consensus has yet been reached as to the best method to use.

WORDS TO KNOW

ANTITOXIN: An antidote to a toxin that neutralizes its poisonous effects.

INCUBATION PERIOD: Incubation period refers to the time between exposure to disease causing virus or bacteria and the appearance of symptoms of the infection. Depending on the microorganism, the incubation time can range from a few hours (an example is food poisoning due to *Salmonella*) to a decade or more (an example is acquired immunodeficiency syndrome, or AIDS).

TOXIN: A poison that is produced by a living organism.

TOXOID: A toxoid is a bacterial toxin that has been altered chemically to make it incapable of causing damage, but still capable of stimulating an immune response. Toxoids are used to stimulate antibody production, which is protective in the event of exposure to the active toxin.

TRISMUS: Trismus the medical term for lockjaw, a condition often associated with tetanus, infection by the *Clostridium tetani* bacillus. In trismus or lockjaw, the major muscles of the jaw contract involuntarily.

Even though tetanus can be prevented and treated, many countries still do not immunize their citizens against tetanus. For example, in India about 90% of the population is inadequately protected against tetanus. Many underdeveloped and developing countries continue to ignore the problem. Newborn babies are especially at risk in such countries, since their umbilical cords are likely to become infected due to unhygienic conditions during and following birth.

SEE ALSO *Bacterial Disease; CDC (Centers for Disease Control and Prevention); Diphtheria.*

BIBLIOGRAPHY

Books

Atkinson, William, et al., eds. *Epidemiology and Prevention of Vaccine-preventable Diseases.* Atlanta: U.S. Centers for Disease Control and Prevention, 2002.

Bellenir, Karen, ed. *Infectious Diseases Sourcebook.* Detroit, MI: Omnigraphics, 2004.

Periodicals

Centers for Disease Control and Prevention. Advisory Committee on Immunization Practices. "Preventing Tetanus, Diphtheria, and Pertussis Among Adolescents: Use of Tetanus Toxoid, Reduced Diphtheria Toxoid and Acellular Pertussis Vaccines." *Morbidity and Mortality Weekly Report* 55 (February 23, 2006): 1–34. Also available online at: <http://www.cdc.gov/mmwr/preview/mmwrhtml/rr55e223a1.htm> (accessed May 11, 2007).

Centers for Disease Control and Prevention. Advisory Committee on Immunization Practices. "Preventing Tetanus, Diphtheria, and Pertussis Among Adults: Use of Tetanus Toxoid, Reduced Diphtheria Toxoid and Acellular Pertussis Vaccines." *Morbidity and Mortality Weekly Report* 55 (December 15, 2006): 1–33. Also available online at: <http://www.cdc.gov/mmwr/preview/mmwrhtml/rr5517a1.htm> (accessed May 11, 2007).

Web Sites

Centers for Disease Control and Prevention. "Tetanus." <http://www.cdc.gov/niP/publications/pink/tetanus.pdf> (accessed March 27, 2007).

MayoClinic.com. "Tetanus." December 29, 2006. <http://www.mayoclinic.com/health/tetanus/DS00227/DSECTION=7> (accessed March 27, 2007).

Toxic Shock

■ Introduction

Toxic shock syndrome (TSS) is a potentially fatal form of blood poisoning that is usually associated with a toxin-producing strain of the bacterium *Staphylococcus aureus*. It has been associated with the use of high-absorbency tampons during menstruation, but may also arise after surgery and as a consequence of severe burns.

In any form of shock, the circulation is impaired, blood pressure falls dramatically, and body organs begin to fail. Burns, severe blood loss, traumatic injury, and infections can cause shock, but in toxic shock the bacterial toxin is the underlying cause. Intensive care with rehydration and monitoring of vital functions such as respiration and blood pressure are necessary to treat a patient in shock. Toxic shock syndrome is a rare condition, and in its early stages may be confused with other illnesses. Prompt and accurate diagnosis of TSS is essential.

■ Disease History, Characteristics, and Transmission

Most cases of toxic shock are caused by exposure to a toxin-producing strain of *S. aureus*, a normally harmless bacterium. *S. aureus* is normally present on the skin and in the nose, but some strains produce toxins that can cause toxic shock. The most common of these is known as toxic shock syndrome toxin, but others have been identified. The toxin invades the blood through some kind of 'focus' of infection, such as a post-operative wound, an intrauterine contraceptive device or a tampon used during menstruation. A few cases of toxic shock have been linked to Group A streptococcus or *Streptococcus pyogenes*, which also causes scarlet fever and necrotizing fasciitis, a deep tissue infection.

Symptoms of toxic shock come on very suddenly and include high fever, a sunburnlike rash, diarrhea, vomiting, fainting, dizziness, and confusion. There is a dramatic fall in blood pressure, which can lead to multi-organ failure affecting the liver, kidneys, heart, and brain. The fatality rate of toxic shock is between three and five percent. It can mimic other conditions, such as severe flu, in its earlier stages. One or two weeks after the illness, the skin on the palms and soles may start to peel off. Long-term complications of toxic shock include memory loss, decreased ability to concentrate, and emotional instability.

■ Scope and Distribution

Toxic shock is rare, but the risk of TSS is greater among young people.

About half of all cases of toxic shock are associated with women using tampons, and the rest result from localized infections, usually following burns, boils, insect bites, or surgery. The presence of intrauterine contraceptive devices (IUDs) is also a risk factor for toxic shock.

■ Treatment and Prevention

Antibiotics can reduce the risk of recurrence of toxic shock but cannot always modify the course of the illness. Clindamycin, usually in combination with another antibiotic, is often recommended, as it reduces the rate of production of toxin from *S. aureus*. Foreign bodies associated with the infection, such as a tampon, must be removed and infected wounds cleaned up.

Intensive care is generally needed to treat shock. The circulation and supply of oxygen to affected organs must be restored with rehydration therapy. Blood pressure, respiration, and other vital functions must be monitored constantly.

Women can avoid TSS associated with tampons by always using a tampon with the lowest possible absorbency and changing them regularly. It is never advisable to insert more than one tampon at a time, and the hands

WORDS TO KNOW

SHOCK: Shock is a medical emergency in which the organs and tissues of the body are not receiving an adequate flow of blood. This condition deprives the organs and tissues of oxygen (carried in the blood) and allows the buildup of waste products. Shock can result in serious damage or even death.

TOXIC: Something that is poisonous and that can cause illness or death.

TOXIN: A poison that is produced by a living organism.

IN CONTEXT: TRENDS AND STATISTICS

According to the Division of Bacterial and Mycotic Diseases at Centers for Disease Control and Prevention (CDC): the "annual incidence (in the United States) is 1 in 2/100,000 women 15–44 years of age" and that "5% of all cases are fatal." However the last active surveillance was performed in 1987.

SOURCE: *Centers for Disease Control and Prevention (CDC), Coordinating Center for Infectious Diseases, Division of Bacterial and Mycotic Diseases.*

should be washed thoroughly before and after inserting a tampon. Women should also be sure to remove the final tampon when their period is over and not use tampons between periods.

■ Impacts and Issues

Toxic shock is a rare condition and may not be readily recognized. The symptoms accompanying TSS, such as fever or rash, occur in many other illnesses. However, multi-organ failure can occur rapidly once the *S. aureus* toxin has entered the bloodstream; then, the patient's life may be in danger. Therefore, prompt medical attention is needed whenever there is a rapid onset of fever and other symptoms.

In 1980, an outbreak of TSS occurred among women who used a certain brand of tampon. Researchers traced most cases to use of the Rely superabsorbent tampon designed to be used over several hours or even days, though there were cases in women who used other superabsorbent brands. From March 1980 to March 1981, almost 1,000 U.S. women were diagnosed with TSS. Forty women died. When Rely and similar superabsorbent tampons were taken off the market, incidence of TSS dropped dramatically the following year. However, researchers noted that fewer women used any tampons immediately following the TSS outbreak. Today, tampons are designed to be changed more frequently, and women are encouraged to used tampons of varying absorbencies to match their menstrual flow. Tampons are now packaged and sold with informative literature about TSS and TSS prevention.

SEE ALSO *Streptococcal Infections, Group A;* Staphylococcus aureus *Infections.*

BIBLIOGRAPHY

Books

Wilson, Walter R., and Merle A. Sande. *Current Diagnosis & Treatment in Infectious Diseases.* New York: McGraw Hill, 2001.

Wilks, David, Mark Farrington, and David Rubenstein. *The Infectious Disease Manual.* Malden: Blackwell, 2003.

Web Sites

Centers for Disease Control and Prevention (CDC). "Toxic Shock Syndrome." October 24, 2005. <http://www.cdc.gov/ncidod/dbmd/diseaseinfo/toxicshock_t.htm> (accessed May 2, 2007).

The Toxic Shock Information Service. "Toxic Shock Syndrome: The Facts." <http://www.toxicshock.com> (accessed May 2, 2007).

Toxoplasmosis (*Toxoplasma* Infection)

■ Introduction

Toxoplasmosis (TOX-o-plaz-MO-sis) refers to an infection caused by a type of microorganisms known as a protozoan. The particular protozoan responsible for the infection is *Toxoplasma gondii*. The infection is part of a parasitic association between *T. gondii* and a human host—the microbe benefits from the association, but the host does not. In the case of toxoplasmosis, the infection enables the protozoan to complete its life cycle.

Toxoplasmosis (sometimes called "toxo") is a serious concern in people whose immune systems are not functioning properly, such as those with acquired immunodeficiency syndrome (AIDS, also cited as acquired immune deficiency syndrome). For those with AIDS, toxoplasmosis can be lethal.

■ Disease History, Characteristics, and Transmission

Toxoplasmosis is an example of a zoonotic disease—a disease that is passed from animals to humans. The animal that is most important in the spread of toxoplasmosis is the cat. The United States Centers for Disease Control and Prevention has estimated that approximately 30% of domestic cats in the United States harbor *T. gondii*. Cats can acquire the protozoan by eating an infected rodent. Other animals can also carry the protozoan, in particular cattle, sheep, or other livestock, which poses an increased risk to farmers, ranchers, and others who come in contact with farm animals.

T. gondii has a life cycle that involves two forms of the organism. The actively growing and dividing form actually causes the disease. But, typically this is not the form of the organism that first enters the body. Rather, a person ingests the form that is called an oocyst. An oocyst is a smaller and hardier form of *T. gondii* that is analogous to a bacterial spore—an oocyst is designed to survive environmental conditions that would otherwise kill the growing protozoan. When ingested, the oocyst can convert to the growing form in the less hostile conditions of the intestinal tract.

Oocysts are shed in the feces of cats and the other animals. People can ingest the oocysts after stroking a cat's fur (on which oocysts can stick, although this route is rare), by handling a cat's litter box and not properly washing their hands before hand-to-mouth contact, by eating produce that was irrigated with oocyst-contaminated water, or by eating undercooked

WORDS TO KNOW

OOCYST: An oocyst is a spore phase of certain infectious organisms that can survive for a long time outside the organism and so continue to cause infection and resist treatment.

PROTOZOA: Single-celled animal-like microscopic organisms that live by taking in food rather than making it by photosynthesis and must live in the presence of water. (Singular: protozoan.) Protozoa are a diverse group of single-celled organisms, with more than 50,000 different types represented. The vast majority are microscopic, many measuring less than 5 one-thousandth of an inch (or 0.005 millimeters), but some, such as the freshwater Spirostomun, may reach 0.17 inches (3 millimeters) in length, large enough to enable it to be seen with the naked eye.

ZOONOSES: Zoonoses are diseases of microbiological origin that can be transmitted from animals to people. The causes of the diseases can be bacteria, viruses, parasites, and fungi.

IN CONTEXT: PERSONAL RESPONSIBILITY AND PROTECTION

The Centers for Disease Control and Prevention (CDC), Division of Parasitic Diseases recommends the following to reduce chances of becoming infected with *Toxoplasma*:

- Wear gloves when you garden or do anything outdoors that involves handling soil. Cats, which may pass the parasite in their feces, often use gardens and sandboxes as litter boxes. Wash your hands well with soap and water after outdoor activities, especially before you eat or prepare any food.
- When preparing raw meat, wash any cutting boards, sinks, knives, and other utensils that might have touched the raw meat thoroughly with soap and hot water to avoid cross-contaminating other foods. Wash your hands well with soap and water after handling raw meat.
- Cook all meat thoroughly; that is, to an internal temperature of 160° F (71° C) and until it is no longer pink in the center or until the juices become colorless. Do not taste meat before it is fully cooked.

SOURCE: *Division of Parasitic Diseases. The Centers for Disease Control and Prevention (CDC)*

meat that contains the protozoan. Eating undercooked meat is the most common route of infection.

Following the regeneration of the *T. gondii* oocysts into the growing form, the symptoms of toxoplasmosis are produced. These include a fever that comes and goes, swollen lymph nodes, generalized muscle pain, and fatigue. For those who recover fairly rapidly, protection from a future infection is guaranteed for life. For others, toxoplasmosis can persist—this is generally referred to as a chronic infection. Chronic toxoplasmosis can cause retinochoroiditis, which is an inflammation of the eyes. This condition can cause a yellowing of the skin and the whites of the eyes that is called jaundice. More seriously, inflammation of the brain, which is called encephalitis, can produce numbness, severe headaches, impaired vision or even blindness, and convulsions.

Toxoplasmosis is not readily spread from person to person. An exception is the spread from mother to fetus that can occur during pregnancy. Approximately six of every 1,000 pregnant women acquire the infection; about half of these women pass the infection on to the fetus. In the United States, over 3,000 cases of congenital toxoplasmosis occur each year. In newborns, toxoplasmosis can be rapidly lethal. Other newborns will retain the infection and display symptoms months or years later.

■ Scope and Distribution

Toxoplasmosis is global in distribution and its incidence is common. Up to 60% of the world's population may carry the protozoan. In the United States alone, over 60 million people are thought to be infected with *T. gondii*.

■ Treatment and Prevention

As for many other microbial diseases, good personal hygiene including handwashing is an important preventative measure. Pregnant women should not handle cat litter. Common sense food handling precautions including washing cutting boards after use help minimize the risk of transferring meat-borne *T. gondii*.

Medication can be prescribed for pregnant women and those with AIDS to kill the protozoan, even those residing in the brain. Other medications prevent the protozoan from acquiring vitamin B, which is vital for its survival.

■ Impacts and Issues

For most people who become infected with *T. gondii*, there is little concern, as they have the immune system capability to fight off the infection. But, for people with a malfunctioning immune system, toxoplamosis is a serious, even lethal, disease. The millions of people with AIDS, infants, the elderly, and those whose immune system has been deliberately impaired to avoid rejection of a transplant are at risk.

Toxoplasmosis is also becoming an indicator of how human activity can affect other forms of life. Along the coast of California, deaths of sea lions and sea otters due to toxoplasmosis has been increasing from the 1990s to the present. The cause is thought to be the disposal of cat litter in municipal waste; *T. gondii* oocysts survive the journey to the ocean water, where they can infect the sea lions and sea otters.

SEE ALSO *Parasitic Diseases; Zoonoses.*

BIBLIOGRAPHY

Books

Fields, Denise, and Ari Brown. *Toddler 411: Clear Answers and Smart Advice for Your Toddler.* Boulder: Windsor Peak Press, 2006.

Joynson, David H.M., and Tim G. Wreghitt. *Toxoplasmosis.* Cambridge: Cambridge University Press, 2005.

Lindsay, David S., and Louis M. Weiss. *Opportunistic Infections: Toxoplasma, Sarcocystis, and Microsporidia (World Class Parasites).* New York: Springer, 2004.

Web Sites

Centers for Disease Control and Prevention.
"Toxoplasmosis: An Important Message for Cat Owners." <http://www.cdc.gov/ncidod/dpd/parasites/toxoplasmosis/toxoplasmosis_brochure_8.2004.pdf> (accessed on April 2, 2007).

Brian Hoyle

IN CONTEXT: EFFECTIVE RULES AND REGULATIONS FOR KEEPING A CAT

Some people living in public housing or special care centers are forced to give up beloved pets due to illness or fear of *Toxoplasma*. However, the Centers for Disease Control & Prevention, National Center for HIV, STD, and TB Prevention, Divisions of HIV/AIDS Prevention state that even persons at risk for a severe infection (e.g., you have a weakened immune system or are pregnant) may still keep cats as pets (often offering love, comfort, and other emotional benefits) if at risk persons follow safety precautions as shown below to avoid being exposed to *Toxoplasma*. Persons at risk should consult with their personal health care provider for full details.

- Have someone who is healthy and not pregnant change your cat's litter box daily. If this is not possible, wear gloves and clean the litter box every day, because the parasite found in cat feces needs one or more days after being passed to become infectious. Wash your hands well with soap and water afterward.
- Keep your cat indoors to prevent it from hunting. Feed your cat dry or canned cat food rather than allowing it to have access to wild birds and rodents or to eat food scraps. A cat can become infected by eating infected prey or by eating raw or undercooked meat infected with the parasite. Do not bring a new cat into your house that might have spent time out of doors or might have been fed raw meat.
- Feed your cat only cat food or cook all meat thoroughly before giving it to your cat.
- Do not give your cat raw or undercooked meat.
- If you adopt or buy a cat, get one that is healthy and at least 1 year old.
- Avoid stray cats and kittens. They are more likely than other cats to be infected.
- Your veterinarian can answer any other questions you may have regarding your cat and risk for toxoplasmosis.

SOURCE: *Centers for Disease Control & Prevention,, National Center for HIV, STD, and TB Prevention, Divisions of HIV/AIDS Prevention*

Trachoma

■ Introduction

Trachoma, also called granular conjunctivitis and Egyptian ophthalmia, is a contagious bacterial disease of the eye caused by the bacterium *Chlamydia trachomatis*. Flies become infected when they lay eggs on human feces lying in soil. The infection occurs when a host fly, infected with the bacterium, bites a human. A fly can also become a host and harbor the bacteria when it makes direct contact with eye, nose, or throat secretions from an infected person. The bacterium can also be carried directly to humans from contaminated hands by fomites (objects contaminated with infective material) such as clothing. The disease is reported as one of the leading infectious causes of blindness.

■ Disease History, Characteristics, and Transmission

The International Trachoma Initiate (ITI) states that trachoma is one of the oldest infectious diseases known to humankind, and was reported as far back as ancient Egypt. General improvements in public health and sanitation have eliminated trachoma from most industrialized nations such as those in North America and Europe. However, it continues to infect people at high rates in underdeveloped and developing countries, especially in the poorest areas of Africa, Asia, Australia, Latin America, and the Middle East.

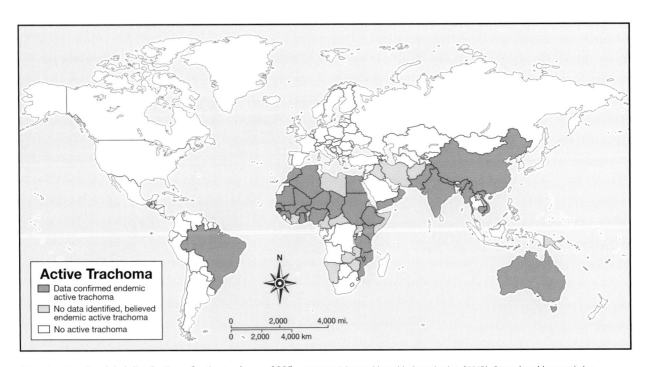

Active Trachoma
- Data confirmed endemic active trachoma
- No data identified, believed endemic active trachoma
- No active trachoma

Map showing the global distribution of active trachoma, 2005. © *Copyright World Health Organization (WHO). Reproduced by permission.*

An incubation period of about five to 12 days occurs before the eye becomes inflamed. Then, additional symptoms occur, including pus discharge, eyelid swelling, eye tearing, and light sensitivity. Within a few weeks, more symptoms begin to appear including chronic swelling (such as swelling of lymph nodes in front of the ears), eye blisters, cornea clouding, and cornea scarring. Extensive damage to the cornea can eventually lead to blindness.

■ Scope and Distribution

The ITI estimates that about eight million people are visually impaired due to trachoma and about 84 million people in 55 endemic countries suffer active symptoms. The World Health Organization (WHO) states that about 3.6 million people are blind from trachoma.

Trachoma occurs most commonly among populations living in overcrowded conditions and with limited contact to clean water and health care facilities such as in undeveloped villages in northern Africa. Children and women who take care of children are most susceptible to trachoma. Children between the ages of three and five years, according to the WHO, are most at risk of all groups of children. When infected early in life, the person may not notice the degradation in sight until adulthood.

Because close personal contact allows easier transmission of the disease, the ITI states that in many crowded African communities it is so prevalent that trachoma is considered a regular part of life. In the United States and other technologically advanced countries, trachoma is rare, but can occur in populations living in extreme poverty and crowdedness, and with poor hygienic conditions.

■ Treatment and Prevention

According to the National Library of Medicine (NLM), of the National Institutes of Health (NIH), symptoms start as an apparent irritation near the eye, what is sometimes called conjunctivitis (commonly called pink eye). Soon, hard pimples or granular outgrowths appear on the inner surface of the eyelids and inflammation occurs on its membrane.

If left untreated, scar tissue develops on the inside of the eyelid. Such scarring in children is usually not noticeable until later in the adult years. Formation of scarring eventually forces the eyelid to curve inward and the eyelashes to scrape the eye. Severe infection of the cornea can later occur. This activity can cause eye ulcers, which further cause scarring and vision problems. Eventually, slow and painful blindness develops over many years.

In the early stage of the infection, trachoma responds well to oral or topical antibiotics such as azithromycin, doxycycline, and erythromycin. Officials from NLM/NIH report that people who receive early treatment

WORDS TO KNOW

FOMITE: A fomite is an object or a surface to which an infectious microorganism such as bacteria or viruses can adhere and be transmitted. Transmission is often by touch.

HOST: Organism that serves as the habitat for a parasite, or possibly for a symbiont. A host may provide nutrition to the parasite or symbiont, or simply a place in which to live.

MORBIDITY: The term "morbidity" comes from the Latin word "morbus," which means sick. In medicine it refers not just to the state of being ill, but also to the severity of the illness. A serious disease is said to have a high morbidity.

for trachoma before scarring and lid deformities occur have excellent chances to be cured. WHO recommends using oral eye ointments such as azithromycin and tetracycline to control trachoma.

According to WHO, relief from trachoma can be attained by following the SAFE strategy: surgery, antibiotics, facial cleanliness, and environmental improvement. Thus, surgery can be performed to correct advanced problems related to the disease. Early treatment with antibiotics can prevent long-term complications. Good hygiene should be consistently and thoroughly practiced such as washing of the face in order to reduce transmission. Access to clean water and improved sanitation facilities (especially the safe disposal of human and animal feces) also greatly help to reduce the occurrence and severity of the disease.

In addition, regular eye examinations can pinpoint abnormal redness on the white areas of the eyes, scarring on the inside of the upper eyelid, and improper blood vessel growth on the corneas. Laboratory tests, especially the polymerase chain reaction (PCR) technique, are used to identify the bacterium that causes trachoma. Such tests, however, are usually too costly for use in the poorest areas of the world where trachoma occurs the most.

■ Impacts and Issues

The infection often results in significant morbidity (ill effects arising from a state of disease), striking people during their productive working years. According to WHO, women are two to four times more likely to become blind after becoming infected with trachoma than men. Often they cannot take care of themselves and their children when infected by the disease,

IN CONTEXT: DISEASE IN DEVELOPING NATIONS

The CDC assists the World Health Organization in reducing the occurrence of trachoma, and asserts that major declines are now found in those countries associated with multifaceted control programs. The CDC reports that "WHO has initiated a global campaign for the elimination of blindness due to trachoma, that recommends a strategy including antibiotics, improved personal and community hygiene and sanitation, and surgery to correct trichiasis. Campaign challenges include: establishing surveillance for endemic trachoma, determining when mass treatment with antibiotics is necessary (i.e., retreatment), determining the effectiveness of improved hygiene and sanitation at preventing a resurgence of endemic disease, monitoring for adverse effects of mass treatment with antibiotics..."

SOURCE: *Centers for Disease Control and Prevention (CDC), Coordinating Center for Infectious Diseases, Division of Bacterial and Mycotic Diseases.*

Common complications of trachoma include scarring of the conjunctiva (membrane under the eyes) and cornea, eye lid abnormalities, turned-in eyelashes, vision reductions, and, in severe cases, blindness. The prognosis for each individual person depends on the severity of the disease, the treatment used to combat it, and the number of times the eyes are re-infected. Persons with trachoma who are treated with the proper drugs and in the early stage of the infection are much more likely to fully recover. Severe symptoms can be often eliminated but eyesight, once lost, cannot be regained.

SEE ALSO *Antibacterial Drugs; Bacterial Disease; Chlamydia Infection; Handwashing.*

BIBLIOGRAPHY

Books

Bellenir, Karen, ed. *Infectious Diseases Sourcebook.* Detroit, MI: Omnigraphics, 2004.

Parker, James N. *The Official Patient's Sourcebook on Trachoma.* San Diego, CA: Icon Health Publications, 2002.

Periodicals

Mabey, D.C., A. Foster, and A.W. Solomon. "Trachoma." *Lancet.* 362 (9379) (July 2003): 223–229.

Web Sites

International Trachoma Initiative. "Trachoma is a hidden disease." 2005 <http http://www.trachoma.org/trachoma.php> (accessed April 2, 2007).

National Library of Medicine, National Institutes of Health. "Trachoma." September 22, 2006 <http://www.nlm.nih.gov/medlineplus/ency/article/001486.htm> (accessed April 2, 2007).

especially when they are blinded. It is often the case that the oldest daughter, or another child, is taken out of school to tend to family needs. Because of the child's incomplete education, she/he is then unable to earn a living outside the family unit, and is restricted to providing care to the family. This vicious cycle continues in the future by keeping families, and sometimes entire villages, in poverty. Consequently, ITI reports that about $2.9 billion (in U.S. currency) is lost worldwide annually in human productivity because of trachoma.

Travel and Infectious Disease

■ Introduction

The global movement of infection is as old as the wanderings of mankind itself. A vast variety of bacteria, viruses, fungi, and parasites move on or in the bodies of humans, their clothing, belongings, pets, food, water, fleas, lice, and other fellow travelers. In fact, the widespread global presence of most infectious diseases reflects human travel dating to the earliest years of mankind itself.

■ History and Scientific Foundations

Travel-related infection has clearly changed world history for hundreds of years. The Black Death (plague) which began in Europe during the fourteenth century was caused by bacteria which infected rat-fleas introduced into Italy by ships. The "great pox" which affected Europe during the sixteenth century was caused by a new disease introduced by travelers from Africa, or possibly South America. The disease eventually evolved into modern day syphilis. Another pox disease that traveled in the opposite direction was instrumental in decimating Indian tribes in the New World during later years. In similar fashion, liver fluke and river blindness were introduced into Latin America as disease of slaves, but went on to adopt themselves to the local ecology, residing in insects or snails.

Although major diseases have crossed geographical borders for centuries, such events have only become commonplace in the twentieth century—as a result of widespread immigration, world conflict, and air travel. In earlier times, a disease characterized by an incubation period measured in days would appear, run its course (or kill the infected person) long before the human host could arrive to a far-off country by horse or schooner. Many will recall an outbreak of Ebola in Africa during 1995, when moviegoers and the world media debated a scenario in which an infected person travels to the United States and infects an unsuspecting population. The Ebola virus can remain in the human host for up to 21 days before onset of symptoms. The flight from Africa takes less than 12 hours.

Many infectious diseases are limited to specific regions, or even specific countries because of a requirement for specific plants, animals, insects, or climatic factors necessary for their propagation and survival. Others diseases are quite capable of adapting to new countries if introduced by man or his activities. Examples in recent years have included West Nile fever, which arrived to the United States in 1999, and quickly entered a favorable ecological environment consisting of compatible insects (mosquitoes) and birds (primarily crows). AIDS, which scientists suspect evolved into a human disease in Africa during the 1950s, exploded onto the world stage because largely because of universal air travel, injecting drug use, and sexual practices. More recently, SARS broke out of China when an infected physician visited Hong Kong, and when others went on to spread the disease to Canada, the Philippines, and other countries.

Impacts and Issues

As of 2000, many people would associate the word malaria with exotic jungles in far off lands. In fact, until the early twentieth century, malaria was quite common in North America and Europe. The mosquitoes that serve as vectors (transmitters) of this disease are still found in most developed countries, and an increasing number of small outbreaks in the United States and other malaria-free countries have followed introduction of the disease by an infected traveler. In fact, many cases of "airport malaria" infecting airport personnel and surrounding communities have been related to the presence of infected mosquitoes in the cargo holds of arriving aircraft.

Each year, billions of travelers cross international boundaries. The vast majority will not seek medical advice and will remain well. The most common medical problem will be traveler's diarrhea, affecting as many as 40 percent of tourists to some countries. Many medical problems are unrelated to infectious disease—automobile accidents, exposure to sun and high altitude, jet lag, petty crime, political instability. The chance of contracting malaria during a one-month tour varies from less than 1 per 1,000 (in southeast Asia) to over one percent (in sub-Saharan Africa). Many will be exposed to venereal disease, and a few will acquire AIDS. Rare instances of exotic and even life-threatening diseases such as yellow fever and African sleeping sickness are also acquired by tourists.

Since 1990, specialists expert in travel medicine have increasingly been involved in the prevention of all such problems. The pre-travel consultation consists of vaccination, prescription of prophylactic medications, and most importantly advice regarding medical risks and prevention. The informed tourist is a healthy tourist.

SEE ALSO *AIDS: Origin of the Modern Pandemic; Dysentery; Globalization and Infectious Disease; Plague, Early History; Plague, Modern History; Tropical Infectious Diseases.*

BIBLIOGRAPHY

Books

Berger, Stephen A., Charles A. Calisher, J.S. Keystone. *Exotic Viral Diseases: A Global Guide.* Hamilton, ON: BC Decker, 2003.

Centers for Disease Control and Prevention. *Health Information for International Travel.* Atlanta: CDC, 2005.

Web Sites

Centers for Disease Control and Prevention. "Traveler' Health." <http://www.cdc.gov/travel/> (accessed May 28, 2007).

Stephen A. Berger

Trichinellosis

■ Introduction

Trichinellosis (TRICK-a-NELL-o-sis), also known as trichinosis or trichiniasis, is an infection caused by a roundworm of the genus *Trichinella*, usually the species *Trichinella spiralis*. The infection is contracted by eating meat (usually pork, but also the meat of wild game) that contains live helminth (parasitic worm) cysts. These cysts are the larvae or young of the worm, which are curled up inside tiny protective capsules. The cysts hatch in the small intestine and breed a new generation of larval worms, which then infect various body tissues. Thorough cooking destroys the larvae and renders infected meat safe to eat. Trichinellosis is rare in most of the world, but is fairly common in Eastern Europe and is increasing in frequency in other areas. Eating undercooked pork is the most common path of trichinellosis infection worldwide; in North American, eating wild game is the most common path of infection. Death from the infection is rare.

■ Disease History, Characteristics, and Transmission

History

British physician James Paget (1814–1899) discovered the worm that causes trichinellosis in 1835 while still a medical student. However, he did not know how humans became infected with the worm. In 1846, American parasitologist Joseph Leidy (1823–1891) discovered the parasite in pork. His early results were misreported in 1851 in Europe, the other region where trichinellosis is common, as being descriptions of *Trichinella affinis*, which does not infect humans. In 1853 and 1856 Leidy again published accounts of finding *Trichinella spiralis* in pork and reported that thorough cooking destroyed the parasite and made the meat safe to eat. Despite these later publications, European appli-

cation of his results was delayed for decades by the original error.

Today, some experts consider that trichinellosis should be categorized as a reemerging disease because it is increasingly being reported in previously unaffected areas.

Characteristics and Transmission

When meat containing encysted larvae is eaten, the larvae are liberated by the digestive process. They develop into adults in the small intestine, then mate and produce offspring. These adult worms are eventually excreted. The new larvae drill through the wall of the intestine and enter the bloodstream, which conveys them to destinations throughout the body, including the muscles, eyes, lungs, and brain. The larvae encyst themselves in muscle and become dormant. Since humans with the disease are usually not eaten by other animals or people, that is usually the end of the disease cycle in human beings. If the encysted larvae are in the muscle of any animal that might be eaten by human beings or other carnivores, the life cycle can continue.

Abdominal symptoms appear a day or two after infection and include nausea, diarrhea, vomiting, and abdominal pain. Other symptoms may appear two to four weeks after infection and include headaches, fevers and chills, muscle and joint pain, itching, diarrhea, rash, and swelling of the eyes. The later-stage symptoms are caused by the larvae encysting in the muscles and the body's immune response to their presence. Not all cases of infection, even in humans, produce noticeable symptoms.

■ Scope and Distribution

Trichinellosis occurs worldwide today but is found mostly in North America, Europe, and China. From 1991 to 1992, there were more than 20,000 cases in Europe. In Eastern Europe and parts of China, some swine herds have a trichinellosis prevalence of about 50%.

WORDS TO KNOW

DORMANT: Inactive, but still alive. A resting non-active state.

ENCYSTED LARVAE: Encysted larvae are larvae that are not actively growing and dividing, and which are more resistant to environmental conditions.

HELMINTH: A representative of various phyla of worm-like animals.

IN CONTEXT: PERSONAL RESPONSIBILITY AND PROTECTION

To prevent trichinellosis the Centers for Disease Control and Prevention (CDC), National Center for Infectious Diseases, Division of Parasitic Diseases, recommends the following:

- Cook meat products until the juices run clear or to an internal temperature of 170°F (76.6°C).
- Freeze pork less than 6 inches thick for 20 days at 5°F (15°C) to kill any worms.
- Cook wild game meat thoroughly. Freezing wild game meats, unlike freezing pork products, even for long periods of time, may not effectively kill all worms.
- Cook all meat fed to pigs or other wild animals.
- Do not allow hogs to eat uncooked carcasses of other animals, including rats, which may be infected with trichinellosis.
- Clean meat grinders thoroughly if you prepare your own ground meats.

SOURCE: *Centers for Disease Control and Prevention, National Center for Infectious Diseases, Division of Parasitic Diseases*

In North America, the primary source of trichinellosis infection is wild game, with only about 12 cases per year being reported in the United States. Outbreaks of trichinellosis have occurred among Eskimos eating undercooked walrus. Almost all mammals can be infected by one or more species of Trichinella, but humans are more likely than most other species to develop symptoms.

Pork and bear meat are primary sources of *Trichinella spiralis* infection in humans. Beaver, opossums,

rats, walruses, and whales can also carry the parasite. Infected animals remain asymptomatic; however, symptoms in humans—which can begin as soon as five or a late as 45 days after exposure—can range from asymptomatic to, rarely, death. Severity depends upon the number of parasites ingested. Although trichinosis is found in some grain-fed pigs, swine fed on garbage containing infected meat scraps are the primary source of human trichinosis.

■ Treatment and Prevention

Diagnosis is confirmed by observing the adult worms in a stool sample or through finding larvae in a muscle biopsy (a small piece of muscle tissue removed for laboratory testing). Treatment is supportive, except during the intestinal phase of the infection when several drugs can be given to kill the worms in the intestine. These anti-helminthic drugs include mebendazole and thiabendazole. No drug exists that can kill the encysted larvae, which may persist alive in the tissue—though inactive—for many years.

Trichinellosis can be prevented by eating only thoroughly cooked meats. Laws have been passed in both the United States and Europe forbidding feeding garbage-containing raw meat to hogs. To prevent trichinellosis, the U.S. Centers for Disease Control (CDC) recommends cooking pork to a temperature of 160 degrees Fahrenheit (71°C) before eating or freezing pork less than six inches thick for 20 days at 5°F (−15°C). Microwaving does not reliably kill larvae in meat.

■ Impacts and Issues

The economic impact of trichinellosis is high, because the measures taken to reduce its presence in the food supply can be so expensive. In the European Union, the domestic pig control program designed to minimize trichinellosis costs $500 million per year. In China, large herds of infected pigs are occasionally destroyed, which can be a severe hardship for uninsured farmers.

In recent years, an increase in trichinellosis cases related to travel prompted many countries to adopt stricter bans on the importation of pork and game products by travelers to some regions. Many popular tourist destinations, such as Argentina, Croatia, Mexico, Romania, Serbia, and Laos, have endemic problems with trichinellosis. In 2005, nearly two-thirds of the reported cases of trichinellosis in the United Kingdom and France were in people who had contracted the infection while traveling abroad or who had consumed infected products—such as sausages—that had been imported by travelers. Many nations now include trichinellosis in traveler health warnings.

SEE ALSO *Parasitic Diseases; Zoonoses.*

BIBLIOGRAPHY

Books

Despommier, Dickson D., et al. *Parasitic Diseases*, 5th ed. New York: Apple Trees Productions, 2005.

Periodicals

Bruschi, F., and K.D. Murrel. "New Aspects of Human Trichinellosis: The Impact of New Trichinella Species." *Postgraduate Medical Journal.* 78 (2002): 15–23.

Moorhead, Andrew. "Trichinellosis in the United States, 1991–1996: Declining but not Gone." *Journal of the American Medical Association.* 281 (1999): 1472.

Web Sites

Centers for Disease Control (U.S. Government). "Trichinellosis Fact Sheet." February 6, 2007. <http://www.cdc.gov/ncidod/dpd/parasites/trichinosis/factsht_trichinosis.htm> (accessed April 12, 2007).

IN CONTEXT: EFFECTIVE RULES AND REGULATIONS

The Centers for Disease Control and Prevention, National Center for Infectious Diseases, Division of Parasitic Diseases, states that trichinellosis "infection is now relatively rare. During 1997–2001, an average of 12 cases per year were reported." The CDC further asserts that "the number of cases has decreased because of legislation prohibiting the feeding of raw-meat garbage to hogs, commercial and home freezing of pork, and the public awareness of the danger of eating raw or undercooked pork products. Cases are less commonly associated with pork products and more often associated with eating raw or undercooked wild game meats."

SOURCE: *Centers for Disease Control and Prevention, National Center for Infectious Diseases, Division of Parasitic Diseases*

Trichomonas Infection

■ Introduction

Trichomonas infection, also called trichomoniasis, is a sexually transmitted disease of the urogenital system (relating to urinary and reproductive organs) of humans. It is caused one-celled parasitic microbes of the species *Trichomonas vaginalis.* The *T. vaginalis* parasite has a round body with four flagella (tail) that gives it a distinctive appearance that is easily identifiable under a microscope by medical professionals. The species, sometimes commonly called trich, is classified within the order Trichomonadida, and genus *Trichomonas.*

The World Health Organization (WHO) estimates that 180 million people around the world are infected annually with *Trichomonas.* The highest incidence of trichomoniasis occurs within sexually active women who have multiple partners. WHO and the U.S. Centers for Disease Control and Prevention (CDC) consider it to be the most common pathogenic (disease-causing) protozoan infection of humans in the industrialized world, with over 175 million infections annually occurring each year. The CDC Division of Parasitic Diseases (DPD) estimates that over eight million people become infected annually in North America. *Trichomonas* infection is considered a sexually transmitted disease or sexually transmitted infection (STD/STI).

■ Disease History, Characteristics, and Transmission

Trichomonas infection is transmitted by sexual intercourse. It occurs more often in females than males. In females it is commonly found in the vagina, where it frequently causes burning and itching and an irritating discharge. It can also occur in the urinary tract, fallopian tubes, and pelvis of women. In males, it may occur in the prostate gland and urethra; and in both sexes it may irritate the bladder.

The parasite cannot survive in the human mouth or rectum or on dry objects such as toilet seats. It can live for up to 24 hours on moist surfaces such as bathing suits and hot tubs. However, such environments rarely contribute to transmission of the infection. It is, instead, almost always transmitted between humans through sexual intercourse or genital-to-genital contact.

Most symptoms do not show up until four to 28 days after being infected. General symptoms in women include abdominal soreness; discomfort with sexual intercourse; vaginal itching; oral lesions; vagina inflammation with gray, greenish-white, or greenish-yellow secretions that are often foul-smelling; labial swelling; vulvar itching; inner thigh itching; and the urge to urinate. Symptoms in pregnant females can often include preterm labor and birth of babies, low birth weight babies, and increased mortality of babies.

Other conditions more likely to occur are pneumonia, bronchitis, infertility, cervicitis (inflammation of the cervix), ectopic pregnancy, non-gonoccal urethritis (urethral inflammation), pelvic inflammatory disease, and reactive arthritis. Infected women are more likely to contract human immunodeficiency virus (HIV) infection and cervical cancer.

There are usually no symptoms in men. If symptoms occur they are usually described as itching of the genital area, burning feeling while urinating or ejaculating, and fluid discharge from urethra. In men, this infection stops on its own within several weeks. However, in rare cases men can develop epididymitis or prostatitis (inflammation of the epididymis or prostate).

■ Scope and Distribution

Trichomoniasis occurs worldwide. Women between the ages of 16 to 35 years of age, according to the National Library of Medicine (NLM), of the National Institutes of Health (NIH), contract the disease more often than any other U.S. group. The frequency in the United

States and Europe are similar, but its rate of incidence is much higher in Africa.

■ Treatment and Prevention

The infection can be diagnosed in women by studying fluid discharge from the vagina with a Pap smear. Such an examination under a microscope reveals the parasites causing the infection. In addition, a visual examination of the pelvis area will locate red blotches on the vaginal wall or cervix of infected women.

The infection is more difficult to diagnosis in men. More often than not, it is first diagnosed in their female sexual partner. However, men can be diagnosed through continued symptoms of burning or itching in the genital area even with treatment for Chlamydia or gonorrhea, two other sexually transmitted diseases. Specimens for examination under a microscope are often collected from the urethra (the tube that urine flows through).

Antibiotic medicines such as metronidazole are usually taken orally, intravenously, or as an intravaginal suppository gel. Sometimes tinidazole is given orally. Antibiotic medicines should be prescribed to the sexual partner, too.

The disease can be prevented either with total abstinence from sexual activities or can be minimized with the proper use of latex condoms during sex and with having a minimal number of sexual partners. The prognosis for *Trichomonas* infection is excellent if treated properly. Complications can happen, however, if proper treatment is not given in a timely basis. Extended infection in women can cause degradation in the tissues on the cervical surface.

■ Impacts and Issues

Trichomonas infection is a sexually transmitted disease (often called STD, or SDI for sexually transmitted infection) that is normally not serious when antibiotics are used to treat the disease. However, its symptoms can be unpleasant, and an untreated infection can lead to pelvic inflammatory disease and resulting infertility. It causes an increased risk of contracting HIV. Although rare, pregnant women who are infected can give the infection to their baby during the delivery process.

Infection in young children can be an indication of sexual abuse. These children are treated for the infection and, if sexual abuse suspected, additional investigations are conducted.

SEE ALSO *Antibiotic Resistance; Gonorrhea; HIV; Parasitic Diseases; Sexually Transmitted Diseases.*

WORDS TO KNOW

PATHOGEN: A disease causing agent, such as a bacteria, virus, fungus, etc.

PROTOZOA: Single-celled animal-like microscopic organisms that live by taking in food rather than making it by photosynthesis and must live in the presence of water. (Singular: protozoan.) Protozoa are a diverse group of single-celled organisms, with more than 50,000 different types represented. The vast majority are microscopic, many measuring less than 5 one-thousandth of an inch (or 0.005 millimeters), but some, such as the freshwater Spirostomun, may reach 0.17 inches (3 millimeters) in length, large enough to enable it to be seen with the naked eye.

SEXUALLY TRANSMITTED: Sexually transmitted diseases (STDs) and infections vary in their susceptibility to treatment, their signs and symptoms, and the consequences if they are left untreated. Some are caused by bacteria. These usually can be treated and cured. Others are caused by viruses and can typically be treated but not cured. More than 15 million new cases of STD are diagnosed annually in the United States.

BIBLIOGRAPHY

Books

Cohen, Jonathan, and William G. Powderly, eds. *Infectious Diseases.* New York: Mosby, 2004.

Ryan, Kenneth J., and C. George Ray, eds. *Sherris Medical Microbiology: An Introduction to Infectious Diseases.* New York: McGraw Hill, 2004.

Periodicals

Schwebke, J.R., and D. Burgess. "Trichomoniasis Is a Common Infection Whose Prevention Has Not Been a Priority." *Clinical Microbiology Review* 17 (2004): 794–803.

Web Sites

Centers of Disease Control and Prevention. "Trichomonas." <http://www.dpd.cdc.gov/dpdx/HTML/Trichomoniasis.htm> (accessed April 7, 2007).

Tropical Infectious Diseases

■ Introduction

The warm humid climate of the tropics can, in itself, encourage diseases that are rare or unknown in the West, such as those borne by mosquitoes. Conditions of poverty and poor sanitation are also common in tropical regions, such as sub-Saharan Africa, which encourages the spread of these diseases, even when there is a known cure for them.

Compared to heart disease, cancer, and even malaria or AIDS, many tropical diseases are neglected in terms of research and efforts to get medicines and vaccines to all affected. The World Health Organization (WHO) estimates that one in six of the world's population suffers from a neglected tropical disease, including leprosy, sleeping sickness or elephantiasis. Control of some tropical diseases has been successful in the past. The WHO and its collaborators now seek to fight tropical infectious disease by improving both surveillance and drug delivery.

■ Disease History, Characteristics, and Transmission

Malaria is perhaps the best known of the tropical infectious diseases, not least because it can affect returning travelers, sometimes with fatal consequences. Another significant mosquito-borne disease is yellow fever, whose causative agent is a flavivirus spread by certain *Aedes* and *Haemogogus* mosquito species. The name comes from the jaundice that often accompanies the late or toxic form of the disease, which has a 50% fatality rate. Lymphatic filariasis—or elephantiasis—is also spread by mosquitoes, the infective agent being microscopic parasitic worms of the *Wuchereria bancrofti* and *Brugia malayi* species. These lodge in the lymphatic system, causing immense and disfiguring swelling of the arms, legs, genitals, vulva, and breast, which may be accompanied by internal damage to the kidneys and lymphatic system.

Leishmaniasis is spread by the bite of sandflies infected with parasites of various *Leishmania* species; there are two types of leishmaniasis, visceral and cutaneous. Untreated, visceral leishmaniasis is fatal in 95% of cases. It typically causes extensive internal organ damage after an initial phase of fever, night sweats, and weight loss. The cutaneous form causes a long-term rash which sometimes leads to internal tissue damage and accompanying secondary bacterial infection, which is potentially fatal.

Meanwhile, African trypanosomiasis, or sleeping sickness, is spread by tsetse flies that carry protozoa of the *trypanosome* genus. More than 90% of cases are caused by *T. brucei gambiense*, the rest by *T. brucei rhodesiense*, with the former being of slower onset than the latter. At first, the trypanosomes multiply in subcutaneous tissues, blood and lymph, then they cross the blood-brain barrier to infect the central nervous system. Left untreated, sleeping sickness will prove fatal.

There are many tropical infectious diseases which do require an insect vector. Leprosy has been a feared and stigmatizing disease since antiquity. Today, however, leprosy is easily treatable and need not be debilitating. Untreated, it may lead to permanent damage and disfigurement to skin, nerves, limbs, and eyes. Leprosy is caused by the bacillus *Mycobacterium leprae* which is related to the bacterium that causes tuberculosis (TB). It is spread by droplets from the nose and mouth from untreated cases, although it is not highly infectious.

Yaws is one of the more neglected of the infectious tropical diseases. It is a chronic infection that affects mainly skin, bone, and cartilage, whose cause is the bacterium *Treponema pertenue*. Another less known condition is buruli ulcer disease, which is caused by the bacterium *Mycobacterium ulcerans*, which is also related to the TB bacterium. The infection leads to destruction of the skin and soft tissue, with the formation of large ulcers on the arms and legs. The disease is not only disfiguring, but can also cause disability through restriction in joint movement.

There are many other tropical infectious diseases, varying widely in their cause, symptoms, and health consequences. Tropical diseases remain a serious health threat because many people in tropical disease-prone areas do not have access to existing treatment. Furthermore, medical research has not yet discovered effective therapies for all tropical diseases.

Scope and Distribution

Malaria is known to affect up to 900 million people worldwide and causes an estimated 2.7 million deaths a year, mainly among children in Africa. The WHO also collects data on many other infectious tropical diseases, but warns that such diseases are underreported and their effects likely underestimated. For example, there are an estimated 200,000 cases of yellow fever each year, causing 30,000 deaths. Only a fraction of the occurrences is officially reported.

Yellow fever is present in 33 African countries, and in nine South American countries. Meanwhile, millions of people in 36 different countries in sub-Saharan Africa are at risk of sleeping sickness, although only a small proportion of the countries are under constant surveillance and medical monitoring. Leishmaniasis is widely distributed around the Mediterranean, tropical Africa, South America, and in East and Central Asia with an estimated two million new cases per year.

More than one billion people in more than 80 countries are at risk of lymphatic filariasis with 120 million already being affected; one third are in India, another third in Africa and the rest in South East Asia, the Pacific, and the Americas. Leprosy is still a public health problem in nine remaining countries in Africa, Asia, and South America but the global toll of the disease has fallen dramatically in recent years, from 5.2 million in 1985 to 286,000 cases at the end of 1999. Incidences of leprosy have continued to decrease. Since the mid-1980s, 116 of 122 countries once endemic for leprosy have eliminated the disease as a public health problem.

The trend has been the opposite for yaws. There had been some success in controlling the disease up to 1970s. However, as some anti-yaws campaigns were scaled down, the disease incidence once again increased. By the 1990s, there were thought to be 2.5 million cases, of which nearly half a million were new.

Finally, Buruli ulcer is found in 30 countries in Africa, the Americas, Asia, and the Western Pacific. Surveillance is patchy, but there have been 24,000 cases reported in Côte d'Ivoire (Ivory Coast) between 1989 and 2006. More than 11,000 cases have been reported in Ghana since 1993.

Treatment and Prevention

There is an effective vaccine, but no treatment for yellow fever. Sleeping sickness is treatable by a regime of differ-

WORDS TO KNOW

NEGLECTED TROPICAL DISEASE: Many tropical diseases are considered to be neglected because despite their prevalence in less-developed areas, new vaccines and treatments are not being developed for them. Malaria was once considered to be a neglected tropical disease, but recently a great deal of research and money have been devoted to its treatment and cure.

PARASITE: An organism that lives in or on a host organism and that gets its nourishment from that host. The parasite usually gains all the benefits of this relationship, while the host may suffer from various diseases and discomforts, or show no signs of the infection. The life cycle of a typical parasite usually includes several developmental stages and morphological changes as the parasite lives and moves through the environment and one or more hosts. Parasites that remain on a host's body surface to feed are called ectoparasites, while those that live inside a host's body are called endoparasites. Parasitism is a highly successful biological adaptation. There are more known parasitic species than nonparasitic ones, and parasites affect just about every form of life, including most all animals, plants, and even bacteria.

VECTOR: Any agent, living or otherwise, that carries and transmits parasites and diseases. Also, an organism or chemical used to transport a gene into a new host cell.

ent drugs, depending on the stage of the disease. Lymphatic filariasis can be cured by treatment with the antiparasitic drugs albendazole or ivermectin and the World Health Organization is working with the assistance of the drugs' manufacturers in a bid to eliminate the disease, in programs similar to those used to tackle river blindness. There are a number of drugs which can treat leishmaniasis, but many of these have severe side effects.

Leprosy usually responds to treatment with a combination therapy consisting of rifampicin, clofazimine and dapsone. The World Health Organization aims to eliminate this disease, with assistance from participating pharmaceutical companies and nongovernment organizations. It may also be possible to eliminate yaws. The disease is curable with just a single injection of penicillin, but more global coordination is needed to get the drug to those at risk. Buruli ulcer can be also be effectively treated by antibiotics and global efforts are underway to eliminate this tropical disease also.

■ Impacts and Issues

Tropical infectious diseases have an impact upon many millions of people, particularly in Africa, causing death, disability, loss of economic productivity, and impaired quality of life. There are many approaches to keeping these diseases under control or eliminating them. Where the disease is well understood and a cure or vaccine is available, then surveillance, monitoring, and effective distribution are key to targeting supplies where they are needed. Public-private partnerships—between the World Health Organization and drug companies, for instance—can be very valuable.

Tropical infectious diseases should also be higher up the agenda when it comes to basic and applied research. There is still an urgent need, for instance, to understand the life cycle of the malaria parasite better in the search for a vaccine. Meanwhile, genomics may prove a powerful tool for understanding tropical diseases—the genome of *M.ulcerans* was published in February 2007, potentially speeding development of new treatments and simpler and more rapid diagnostic tests.

Though tropical infectious diseases have received increased attention in recent years, they remain a significant global health threat. Over one billion people are affected by neglected tropical diseases. These diseases are called "neglected" because they have been essentially eliminated from developed nations, but are endemic to some of the world's most underdeveloped nations and marginalized communities. Neglected tropical diseases (NTDs) flourish in tropical and subtropical regions, especially those with poor sanitation systems, contaminated drinking water, lack of adequate healthcare, and endemic disease-carrying insect problems. The World Health Organization considers the following neglected tropical diseases (NTDs): African sleeping sickness, Buruli ulcer, Chagas disease, cholera, dengue fever, endemic syphilis, epidemic diarrhoeal diseases, guinea-worm, leishmaniasis, leprosy, lymphatic filariasis, onchocerciais, pinta, schistosomiasis, soil-transmitted helminthiasis, trachoma, and yaws.

Neglected tropical diseases bring significant impact to local societies and economies. Since NTDs often strike subsistence cultures, the ability to work and grow food is vitally important to survival. Endemic threat of NTDs such as sleeping sickness has forced many people to flee productive—and sometimes scarce—farm and grazing lands in river valleys. Farming less-productive soils has contributed to food scarcity in some regions. Migration and increased local population density has exacerbated malnutrition and fueled incidence of disease. Some survivors of NTDs experience life-long pain or physical disability, curtailing their ability to work. Despite the significant social and economic effects of NTDs, less than 1% of all new drugs registered between 1975–2000 were indicated to treat or prevent tropical diseases.

The World Health Organization and other organizations have reenergized international research on tropical diseases. Several NTDs can be treated with drugs that cost as little as two United States cents per dose. International health organizations have focused on educating health officials and training community volunteers to administer and distribute therapeutic drugs. Improved sanitation and hygiene programs, increased access to clean drinking water, and use of anti-insect pesticides, traps, and mosquito netting have helped to reduce incidence of NTDs. However, treatments for some NTDs remain expensive, outdated, and toxic or dangerous if administered incorrectly. Development of vaccines and cheaper, more effective, and safer drugs are vital to combating these NTDs.

Some scientists predict that global climate change may increase the incidence of tropical diseases. Warmer temperatures and increased surface water may increase the habitat of disease vectors such as insects. Some assert that tropical diseases will become more common, more widespread, and increasingly virulent.

SEE ALSO *African Sleeping Sickness (Trypanosomiasis); Buruli (Bairnsdale) Ulcer; Climate Change and Infectious Disease; Developing Nations and Drug Delivery; Filariasis; Leishmaniasis; Leprosy (Hansen's Disease); Malaria; Mosquito-borne Diseases; River Blindness (Onchocerciasis); Yellow Fever.*

BIBLIOGRAPHY

Books

Peters, W., and G. Pasvol. *Tropical Medicine and Parasitology.* 5th ed. London: Mosby, 2002.

Wilks, D., M. Farrington, and D. Rubenstein. *The Infectious Diseases Manual.* 2nd ed. Malden: Blackwell, 2003.

Web Sites

World Health Organization. "Neglected Tropical Diseases." <http://www.who.int/neglected_diseases/en/> (accessed May 17, 2007).

Susan Aldridge

Tuberculosis

Introduction

Tuberculosis, often known as TB, is a disease caused by infection with the bacterium called *Mycobacterium tuberculosis*. A few other types of mycobacterium are capable of causing a tuberculosislike illness, but are only rarely encountered. Most commonly, the infection affects the lungs. However, along with the pulmonary form of tuberculosis, the infection can become extrapulmonary, affecting other parts of the body, including the central nervous system, kidneys, joints, spine, and skin.

In a tuberculosis infection, symptoms may be absent initially. Sometime later, in about 10% of those who are infected, this so-called latent tuberculosis, which cannot be spread from person to person, becomes active and more serious, killing up to 50% of those who are infected. The presence of the latent form of tuberculosis is especially dangerous in people whose immune systems are not functioning properly, such as those with acquired immunodeficiency syndrome (AIDS, also cited as acquired immune deficiency syndrome).

Disease History, Characteristics, and Transmission

Tuberculosis is an ancient disease. In about 400 BC, the Greek physician Hippocrates (460–377 BC) described a disease that is thought to have been tuberculosis. Then the disease was called phthisis, a name derived from the

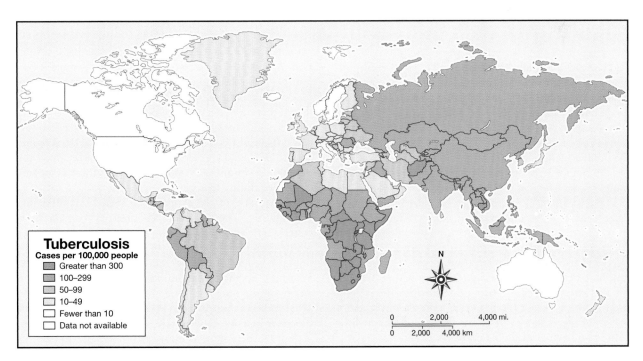

Map depicting estimated tuberculosis cases, 2001.   © Copyright World Health Organization (WHO). Reproduced by permission.

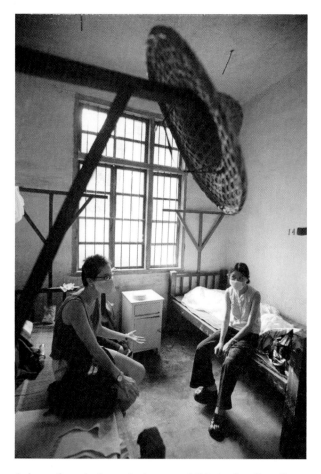

A doctor from the humanitarian group Médecins Sans Frontières (Doctors Without Borders) explains treatment details to a new patient who suffers from tuberculosis at a hospital in China's southern Guangxi province. *AP Images.*

Greek word meaning "to waste away". This description was apt, since, then, as now, a hallmark feature of tuberculosis is weight loss and physical deterioration that occurs over the often considerable length of time that the infection persists. In more recent times, the characteristic physical wasting associated with the disease led to its popular name—consumption.

A fragment of *M. tuberculosis* DNA was found in lung tissue from an Egyptian mummy approximately 3,000 years old. It has been argued that diseases like tuberculosis were unknown in South America until being introduced by European explorers hundreds of years ago. However, this may not be true, since preserved remains of people with tuberculosislike lung damage have been dated to hundreds of years before the time of Columbus. (There is no evidence that the Viking explorations, which pre-date Columbus, took them south of the equator.) It seems likely that tuberculosis may have been globally common even centuries ago.

The name tuberculosis was coined in 1839 by Johann Schönlein. At that time, the pathogen responsi-

ble for the disease had not been discovered. *M. tuberculosis* was finally identified in 1882 by Robert Koch (1843–1910), one of the pioneers of the study of bacteria (bacteriology). In 1890, Koch reported on the extraction of a bacterial protein from dead bacteria recovered from tuberculosis infections. The protein, which he called tuberculin, is still important as a means of detecting the presence of the bacteria. With the discovery and use of x rays at the end of the nineteenth century, the presence of the lung infection that is a consequence of the growth of *M. tuberculosis* was revealed. On x-ray images, the masses of bacteria that develop are seen as more opaque regions in the lungs.

Lung infection with *M. tuberculosis* results from inhaling droplets of moisture that contain the bacteria. Most commonly this occurs when someone who has the infection expels droplets from their lungs by coughing. The droplets, which tend to be 0.5–5 microns in diameter (a micron is a millionth of a meter) can contain more than 40,000 living *M. tuberculosis* bacteria. *M. tuberculosis* also can be transmitted in milk that has not been pasteurized to kill the bacteria. Symptoms of this form of tuberculosis, which is called active tuberculosis, include a feeling of tiredness, loss of weight, a fever that tends to occur during sleep, chills, and a cough that persists for weeks. The coughing can dislodge and expel sputum, which may be tinged with blood, as the infection can damage cells lining the lungs. In some people, the infection can spread beyond the lungs to other parts of the body. If not treated, this extrapulmonary tuberculosis is fatal in up to 50% of the cases. The extrapulmonary form cannot be spread from person to person.

■ Scope and Distribution

Tuberculosis is a common disease with a global distribution. About 30% of the world's population—some 2 billion people—have tuberculosis, according to the World Health Organization (WHO). The organization has estimated that new infections are occurring at the rate of one every second. In 2004, almost 15 million people had the active form of tuberculosis, according to the WHO, and about 1.7 million people died of the disease, most in developing countries. Nearly 9 million of these cases had developed during that year.

Some people are at increased risk for contracting tuberculosis. These include children, whose immune systems are not fully developed, and elderly people, whose immune function may have deteriorated. The immune system can also deteriorate due to diseases (for example, acquired immunodeficiency syndrome, or AIDS), poor nutrition, and the physical consequences of chronic alcohol or drug abuse. In addition, immune function may be deliberately suppressed in transplant patients to help minimize the chance of rejection of the transplanted organ. Health care providers may also be at risk of contracting tuberculosis, since they are exposed

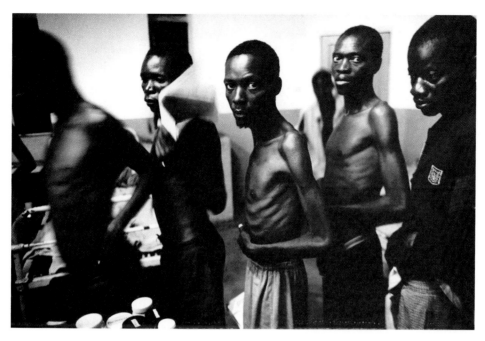

Patients in the TB ward at a hospital in Malawi line up for their medication. In 2000, 76 percent of tuberculosis cases in the hospital were found to be HIV related. © *Gideon Mendel/Corbis.*

more frequently to people with the infection. Other risk factors include diabetes, various cancers, kidney disease, and abnormally low body weight.

While present in every country, tuberculosis can be especially prevalent in regions where health care is substandard and poverty affects the overall health of the inhabitants. Traditionally, this has been a more significant problem in underdeveloped and developing countries. However, even in the United States, increasing poverty has contributed to a resurgence of tuberculosis. More than 14,000 cases of tuberculosis were reported in the United States in 2004, according to the CDC.

■ Treatment and Prevention

The diagnosis of tuberculosis relies of the recognition of the symptoms and the detection of the infection. The presence of the lung infection can be visualized using a chest x ray. *M. tuberculosis* also can be detected, either by obtaining sputum samples and growing the organism or by isolating protein components of the bacterium. The latter test can be faster, since the bacterium can be difficult to grow in laboratory conditions. For example, the length of time for *M. tuberculosis* to grow and divide in the nutritionally rich conditions of a laboratory culture dish can be 16–20 hours, which is far longer than the 15–20 minutes required by the common intestinal bacterium *Escherichia coli*. Thus, identification of the tuberculosis bacterium by laboratory culturing can take days.

A well-known test for tuberculosis is called a skin test. In this test, the tuberculin protein from *M. tuberculosis* is injected just under the skin of the forearm. The development of redness and swelling at the injection site within several days indicates that the person has at least been exposed to the infection. The test does not necessarily show that the infection is active, and so is valuable in the detection of the latent form of tuberculosis.

In May 2005, the U.S. Food and Drug Administration approved the QuantiFERON®-TB Gold test for use in the diagnosis of *M. tuberculosis* infection in the United States. The test detects the release of a compound called interferon-gamma from blood cells in those who have tuberculosis. The test has been approved as a replacement for the skin test, and to confirm the results of the skin test. As of 2007, the test is not widely available, and can still be beyond the budget of smaller health care centers.

In the past, the treatment of tuberculosis was associated with images of hospital wards filled with bedridden patients or images of people slowly recovering from the infection while at sanatoriums located in the countryside. Even into the 1960s, sanatoriums that were located in areas with clean, dry air were a popular part of treatment for tuberculosis.

Sanatoriums did aid recovery, but their usefulness was supplanted during the 1960s by the introduction of antibiotics that were effective against *M. tuberculosis*. The antibiotic treatment needs to be carried out for up to six months to be effective, in part because of the slow growth of the bacteria (many antibiotics are effective

IN CONTEXT: EXTENSIVELY DRUG-RESISTANT TUBERCULOSIS (XDR TB)

In May 2007 a Centers for Disease Control and Prevention (CDC) investigation of a suspected case of Extensively Drug-Resistant Tuberculosis (XDR TB) made news headlines around the world and heightened public awareness of XDR TB. The case involved a U.S. citizen that the CDC publicly asserted had a "potentially infectious XDR TB who traveled to and from Europe on commercial flights between May 12 and May 24, (2007) and then re-entered the United States at the Canada-U.S. border via automobile."

Because of the international travel implications, for the first time in more than 40 years, CDC issued a Federal isolation order under authority of the U.S. Public Health Service Act. Such are orders are rare because state and local health departments usually order isolation (in fact, in early June 2007, the Denver Health Authority Public Health Department issued an order that the patient be detained for treatment at the Denver area hospital where the patient had ultimately been transferred for treatment and so the federal order was lifted).

Although the patient was asymptomatic and physicians later stated that he did not appear to be highly infectious, the case came under intense media scrutiny. At the time of the printing of this book, many issues existed concerning the facts and timeline of events related to the case, including the investigation of how the patient may have initially contracted the disease and the events surrounding the response by a number of health and security agencies to his infection and subsequent travel. Intense media coverage was also fueled by initial disinformation about the nature of transmission, with reports failing to specify that transmission of the bacterium responsible usually takes prolonged contact.

The CDC states that Extensively drug-resistant tuberculosis (XDR TB) is "a relatively rare type of multidrug-resistant tuberculosis (MDR TB). It is resistant to almost all drugs used to treat TB, including the two best first-line drugs: isoniazid and rifampin. XDR TB is also resistant to the best second-line medications: fluoroquinolones and at least one of three injectable drugs (i.e., amikacin, kanamycin, or capreomycin)."

"Because XDR TB is resistant to the most powerful first-line and second-line drugs, patients are left with treatment options that are much less effective and often have worse treatment outcomes."

"XDR TB is of special concern for persons with HIV infection or other conditions that can weaken the immune system. These persons are more likely to develop TB disease once they are infected, and also have a higher risk of death once they develop TB disease."

"The risk of acquiring XDR TB in the United States appears to be relatively low. However, it is important to acknowledge the ease at which TB can spread. As long as XDR TB exists, the United States is at risk and must address the threat."

SOURCE: *Centers for Disease Control and Prevention, Division of Tuberculosis Elimination National Center for HIV/AIDS, Viral Hepatitis, STD, and TB Prevention*

---

only on bacteria that are growing). It can be tempting to stop taking the antibiotics before the end of the prescribed period of treatment, since the patient begins to feel better after only a few weeks. But, as with other bacterial infections, discontinuing treatment prematurely is dangerous, since it can allow surviving bacteria to re-establish the infection. In fact, the surviving bacteria may be resistant to the antibiotics used, making treatment more difficult and more expensive.

The first few decades of the antibiotic therapy were resoundingly successful. Over 90% of tuberculosis infections were cured. However, in the early years of the twenty-first century, resistance to the antibiotics emerged and became more prevalent.

A tuberculosis vaccine does exist. It was developed during World War I (1914–1918) by French scientists Albert Calmette (1863–1933) and Camille Guérin, (1872–1961) and was first used in 1921. The vaccine uses a live, but weakened, strain of the bacterium *Mycobacterium bovis*. BCG (for Bacillus-Calmette-Guérin) is still the only vaccine for tuberculosis, although researchers are continuing to investigate new vaccine candidates.

The vaccine is not recommended for use in the United States by the CDC. This is due to a combination of factors—the relatively low number of cases of the disease in the United States, the vaccine's 80% success rate, and the risks associated with the use of live bacteria in a vaccine. Health care providers and others at higher risk to acquire the infection are vaccinated, however, as are people who have the multidrug-resistant form of tuberculosis. People who come to the United States from areas of the world where tuberculosis is prevalent are required to be examined for the presence of the active and latent forms of the infection and to be treated if necessary.

Efforts to develop new tuberculosis vaccines are ongoing. Several vaccine candidates have been developed using recombinant genetic techniques. These techniques involve splicing genetic material into an organism that can then ferry the recombined genetic material into animals or humans to generate antibodies to combat the infection. As of 2007, the U.S. National Institute of Allergy and Infectious Diseases and other agencies around the world continue to sponsor trials to evaluate the effectiveness and safety of the recombinant vaccines.

■ Impacts and Issues

Throughout history, tuberculosis has been a threat to health and life. For example, in the mid-nineteenth century, about 25% of all deaths were due to tuberculosis. The devastation caused to families and the economic consequences of the loss of so many wage-earners were immense. At that time, the disease was especially prevalent in children, adolescents, and young adults; whole generations of people were affected.

This situation changed during the 1940s with the introduction of antibiotics that were effective against *M. tuberculosis*. There was a steep drop in the number of cases of tuberculosis worldwide. This fueled optimism that the disease had been controlled. But, as with other bacterial diseases that were initially suppressed by antibiotic therapy, this optimism was premature. Several factors have fueled the return of tuberculosis, including the increasing incidence of immunosuppressive diseases (primarily AIDS), the impact of growing gap in health care between the richer and poorer nations, and the emergence of a type of tuberculosis infection that is resistant to multiple antibiotics.

Currently, the impact of tuberculosis is most severe in the poorest regions of the world. For example, South Africa had the highest incidence of tuberculosis in the world in 2004, according to the WHO, and India had the most infections. WHO statistics show that more than 80% of the new cases of tuberculosis in 2004 were found among people living in Africa, Southeast Asia (including India), and the Western Pacific.

In other countries, including the United States, tuberculosis is less common and is mainly found in cities among the poor and homeless. In the United States, a program called Directly Observed Therapy (DOT) is being used by some states to help deal with the rising prevalence of tuberculosis. The program, which focuses on the poor and homeless in cities such as New York, involves direct meetings between the patient and a health care provider and the delivery of every scheduled dose of tuberculosis medication by that health care provider. DOT has been successful in reducing the number of reported cases of the disease.

DOT is also used in 182 other nations. It is estimated that this surveillance program, which relies on the microscopic detection of *M. tuberculosis* in blood samples, detected over 60% of the cases of tuberculosis worldwide in 2005.

In 1990, there were 7,537,000 tuberculosis cases worldwide, according to the WHO, with approximately 30,000 of those cases reported in the United States. The 14,097 reported cases in the United States in 2005 represent a 47% decline from 1990. However, in some states and among certain ethnic groups in the country, the prevalence of tuberculosis is still increasing. Furthermore, the situation elsewhere in the world is bleak. During the decade from 2000–2009, the WHO projects that 30 million people will die of tuberculosis. Since many cases are never reported, the actual death toll likely will be much higher.

In 2004, there were almost 9 million new cases of tuberculosis around the world, according to the WHO. Of these, 740,000 infections arose in people already infected with the human immunodeficiency virus (HIV). The immunocompromised condition of these patients makes it more likely that their cases of tuberculosis will be more serious, life threatening, and costly to treat.

IN CONTEXT: SCIENTIFIC, POLITICAL, AND ETHICAL ISSUES

The interplay of complex ethical and social considerations is also evident when considering the general rise of infectious diseases that sometimes occurs as an unintended side effect of the otherwise beneficial use of medications. Nearly half the world's population, for example, is infected with the bacterium causing TB (although for most people the infection is inactive) yet the organism causing some new cases of TB is evolving toward a greater resistance to the antibiotics that were once effective in treating TB. Such statistics also take on added social dimension when considering that TB disproportionately impacts certain social groups (the elderly, minority groups, and people infected with HIV).

The resurgence of tuberculosis has resulted in part from the increasing prevalence of immunodeficiency diseases, but also from a lack of attention to the control of tuberculosis. As with diseases such as polio, the early success in combating the disease led to complacency regarding control programs, with the result that the disease rebounded.

The emergence of antibiotic-resistant forms of *M. tuberculosis* is especially troubling. From 2000–2004, according to the CDC, 20% of tuberculosis cases in the United States were resistant to commonly used antibiotics and approximately 2% were resistant to the more potent and more expensive drugs employed as a next step. MDR-TB (multidrug-resistant TB) includes strains of tuberculosis that are resistant to at least two first-line drugs—isoniazid and rifampicin—used to treat TB.

Extremely drug-resistant tuberculosis (XDR-TB) is another emerging threat, according to the WHO. The disease is initially latent; when the symptoms appear and treatment is initiated, the resistance of the infection to virtually all antibiotics makes XDR-TB extremely difficult to treat.

As of 2007, identified XDR-TB is rare. Yet, the WHO estimates that in 2004 there were over 500,000 cases worldwide and that this number will rise in the coming years. The increased expense of treating XDR-TB will become a significant issue for poorer nations. By 2015, according to the WHO, the treatment of tuberculosis will cost $650 million each year, in part due to elaborate airborne precautions in hospitals that include isolation rooms with specialized air exchanges and N-95 masks that can serve as a barrier for the extra-small bacteria that cause tuberculosis. More than $600 million will also be needed for programs aimed at curbing the spread of the multidrug-resistant bacteria. As of 2007, the funds budgeted by various governments around the world to battle tuberculosis total $250 million—$400 million less than the projected $650 million needed. In 2006, the WHO spearheaded the Stop TB Partnership, an initiative that aims to save 14 million lives by 2015, partly by encouraging nations worldwide to commit the needed money. The campaign also seeks to increase access to treatment for nations most in need, and to reduce the economic burden associated with the costs of tuberculosis health care and the work force losses due to the disease.

■ Primary Source Connection

The World Care Council (WCC), based in France, is a non-governmental organization (NGO) dedicated to mobilizing public and private forces together worldwide in the fight against AIDS, malaria, and tuberculosis. The Patients Charter for Tuberculosis Care, developed by the WCC, aims to empower people with tuberculosis by describing their rights and responsibilities regarding the disease. WCC intends for the charter to become the catalyst for effective collaboration between health providers, authorities, and persons with TB. The charter is the first global patient-powered standard for care.

The Patients' Charter for Tuberculosis Care

The Patients' Charter outlines the Rights and Responsibilities of People with Tuberculosis. It empowers people with the disease and their communities through this knowledge. Initiated and developed by patients from around the world, the Charter makes the relationship with health care providers a mutually beneficial one.

The Charter sets out the ways in which patients, the community, health providers, both private and public, and governments can work as partners in a positive and open relationship with a view to improving tuberculosis care and enhancing the effectiveness of the health care process. It allows for all parties to be held more accountable to each other, fostering mutual interaction and a 'positive partnership'.

Developed in tandem with the **International Standards for Tuberculosis Care** to promote a 'patient-centered' approach, the Charter bears in mind the principles on health and human rights of the United Nations, UNESCO, WHO, Council of Europe, as well as other local and national charters and conventions.

The Patients Charter for Tuberculosis Care practices the principle of Greater Involvement of People with TB. This affirms that the empowerment of people with the disease is the catalyst for effective collaboration with health providers and authorities, and is essential to vic-

tory in the fight to stop TB. The Patients' Charter, the first global 'patient-powered' standard for care, is a cooperative tool, forged from common cause, for the entire TB Community.

PATIENTS' RIGHTS

You have the right to:

Care

- The right to free and equitable access to tuberculosis care, from diagnosis through treatment completion, regardless of resources, race, gender, age, language, legal status, religious beliefs, sexual orientation, culture or having another illness.

- The right to receive medical advice and treatment which fully meets the new International Standards for Tuberculosis Care, centering on patient needs, including those with MDR-TB or TB-HIV coinfections, and preventative treatment for young children and others considered to be at high risk.

- The right to benefit from proactive health sector community outreach, education and prevention campaigns as part of comprehensive care programs.

Dignity

- The right to be treated with respect and dignity, including the delivery of services without stigma, prejudice or discrimination by health providers and authorities.

- The right to quality health care in a dignified environment, with moral support from family, friends and the community.

Information

- The right to information about what health care services are available for tuberculosis, and what responsibilities, engagements, and direct or indirect costs, are involved.

- The right to receive a timely, concise and clear description of the medical condition, with diagnosis, prognosis (an opinion as to the likely future course of the illness), and treatment proposed, with communication of common risks and appropriate alternatives.

- The right to know the names and dosages of any medication or intervention to be prescribed, its normal actions and potential side-effects, and its possible impact on other conditions or treatments.

- The right of access to medical information which relates to the patient's condition and treatment, and a copy of the medical record if requested by the patient or a person authorized by the patient.

- The right to meet, share experiences with peers and other patients, and to voluntary counseling at any time from diagnosis through treatment completion.

Choice

- The right to a second medical opinion, with access to previous medical records.
- The right to accept or refuse surgical interventions if chemotherapy is possible, and to be informed of the likely medical and statutory consequences within the context of a communicable disease.
- The right to choose whether or not to take part in research programs without compromising care.

Confidence

- The right to have personal privacy, dignity, religious beliefs and culture respected.
- The right to have information relating to the medical condition kept confidential, and released to other authorities contingent upon the patient's consent.

Justice

- The right to make a complaint through channels provided for this purpose by the health authority, and to have any complaint dealt with promptly and fairly.
- The right to appeal to a higher authority if the above is not respected, and to be informed in writing of the outcome.

Organization

- The right to join, or to establish, organizations of people with or affected by tuberculosis, and to seek support for the development of these clubs and community based associations through the health providers, authorities, and civil society.
- The right to participate as 'stakeholders' in the development, implementation, monitoring and evaluation of TB policies and programs with local, national and international health authorities.

Security

- The right to job security after diagnosis or appropriate rehabilitation upon completion of treatment.
- The right to nutritional security or food supplements if needed to meet treatment requirements.

PATIENTS' RESPONSIBILITIES

You have the responsibility to:

Share Information

- The responsibility to provide the health care giver as much information as possible about present health, past illnesses, any allergies and any other relevant details.

> ## WORDS TO KNOW
>
> **ACTIVE INFECTION:** An active infection is one which is currently producing symptoms or in which the infective agent is multiplying rapidly. In contrast, a latent infection is one in which the infective agent is present, but not causing symptoms or damage to the body, nor reproducing at a significant rate.
>
> **AIRBORNE PRECAUTIONS:** Airborne precautions are procedures that are designed to reduce the chance that certain disease-causing (pathogenic) microorganisms will be transmitted through the air.
>
> **AIRBORNE TRANSMISSION:** Airborne transmission refers to the ability of a disease-causing (pathogenic) microorganism to be spread through the air by droplets expelled during sneezing or coughing.
>
> **ANTIBIOTIC RESISTANCE:** The ability of bacteria to resist the actions of antibiotic drugs.
>
> **LATENT INFECTION:** An infection already established in the body but not yet causing symptoms, or having ceased to cause symptoms after an active period, is a latent infection.

- The responsibility to provide information to the health provider about contacts with immediate family, friends and others who may be vulnerable to tuberculosis or may have been infected by contact.

Follow Treatment

- The responsibility to follow the prescribed and agreed treatment plan, and to conscientiously comply with the instructions given to protect the patient's health, and that of others.
- The responsibility to inform the health provider of any difficulties or problems with following treatment, or if any part of the treatment is not clearly understood.

Contribute to Community Health

- The responsibility to contribute to community well being by encouraging others to seek medical advice if they exhibit the symptoms of tuberculosis.
- The responsibility to show consideration for the rights of other patients and health care providers, understanding that this is the dignified

basis and respectful foundation of the TB Community.

Show Solidarity

- The moral responsibility of showing solidarity with other patients, marching together towards cure.

- The moral responsibility to share information and knowledge gained during treatment, and to pass this expertise to others in the community, making empowerment contagious.

- The moral responsibility to join in efforts to make the community TB Free.

World Care Council

WORLD CARE COUNCIL. "THE PATIENTS' CHARTER FOR TUBERCULOSIS CARE." 2006. AVAILABLE ONLINE AT <HTTP://WWW.WHO.INT/TB/PUBLICATIONS/2006/ISTC_CHARTER.PDF> (ACCESSED APRIL 10, 2007).

SEE ALSO *Airborne Precautions; Antibiotic Resistance; Developing Nations and Drug Delivery; Re-emerging Infectious Diseases; Resistant Organisms.*

BIBLIOGRAPHY

Books

Daniel Thomas M. *Captain of Death: The Story of Tuberculosis.* Rochester, NY: University of Rochester Press, 2005.

Gandy, Matthew, and Alimuddin Zumla. *The Return of the White Plague: Global Poverty and the 'New' Tuberculosis.* New York: Verso, 2003.

Mayho, Paul, and Richard Coker. *The Tuberculosis Survival Handbook.* West Palm Beach, FL: Merit Publishing International, 2006.

Periodicals

Hoffman, Michelle. "New Medicine for Old Mummies: Diagnosing Disease in Some Very Old 'Patients'." *American Scientist* 86 (May–June 1998).

Web Sites

World Health Organization. "World TB Day—March 24th." <http://www.stoptb.org/events/world_tb_day/> (accessed April 10, 2007).

Brian Hoyle

Tularemia

■ Introduction

Tularemia, also known as rabbit fever, deerfly fever, and lemming fever, is a highly infectious bacterial zoonotic (acquired from animals) disease that is endemic (occurs naturally) throughout the United States. The highly infectious nature of the bacterium poses a significant threat to humans and *Francisella tularensis,* the bacteria that causes tularemia, has also been considered a potential bioterrorism agent.

Francisella tularensis, is a highly infectious bacterium that naturally colonizes (lives at population levels below that which cause disease) many species of small animals. Transmission of the disease to humans is via vectors such as ticks and mosquitoes, contact with infected animals, or ingestion of contaminated soil, water, or food. Symptoms present after a short incubation and may include fever, nausea, headache, diarrhea, and joint and muscle pain. The infection can spread to the lungs, liver, and lymphatic system. In around two percent of cases, tularemia is fatal.

Treatment with antibiotics is usually effective and readily available. Prevention may be achieved through the use of insect repellents, avoidance of contact with infected animals, and the maintenance of uncontaminated food and water sources.

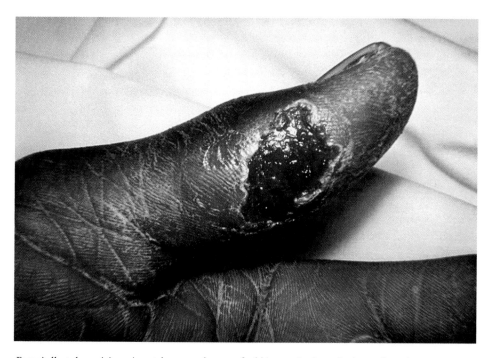

Francisella tularensis is an insect-borne pathogen of rabbits, squirrels, and other rodents in many countries, including Russia and the western United States. Ticks, fleas, and flies may transmit the organism to humans. *Science Source.*

WORDS TO KNOW

AEROSOL: Particles of liquid or solid dispersed as a suspension in gas.

ARTHROPOD: A member of the largest single animal phylum, consisting of organisms with segmented bodies, jointed legs or wings, and exoskeletons.

COLONIZE: Colonize refers to the process where a microorganism is able to persist and grow at a given location.

ENDEMIC: Present in a particular area or among a particular group of people.

FULMINATE: In medicine, a disease that appears suddenly and follows a severe, intense course is said to fulminate. In chemistry, a fulminate is fulminic acid, HONC, or any other compound containing the -ONC group.

HOST: Organism that serves as the habitat for a parasite, or possibly for a symbiont. A host may provide nutrition to the parasite or symbiont, or simply a place in which to live.

INOCULUM: An inoculum is a substance such as virus, bacterial toxin, or a viral or bacterial component that is added to the body to stimulate the immune system, which provides protection from an infection by the particular microorganism.

RESERVOIR: The animal or organism in which the virus or parasite normally resides.

VECTOR: Any agent, living or otherwise, that carries and transmits parasites and diseases. Also, an organism or chemical used to transport a gene into a new host cell.

VIRULENCE: Virulence is the ability of a disease organism to cause disease: a more virulent organism is more infective and liable to produce more serious disease.

ZOONOSES: Zoonoses are diseases of microbiological origin that can be transmitted from animals to people. The causes of the diseases can be bacteria, viruses, parasites, and fungi.

■ Disease History, Characteristics, and Transmission

Tularemia was first described in Japan in 1837, but gained its name from Tulare County, California, where a plague-like illness arose among squirrels in 1911. The causative agent, *Francisella tularensis,* is considered to be among the most infectious bacteria known, and, if left untreated, infection may prove fatal.

Symptoms of tularemia usually appear within three to five days of exposure, but can take up to 14 days in some cases. Presentation includes a sudden fever, chills, headache, diarrhea, muscle aches, joint pain, dry cough, and progressive weakness. Disease caused by tularemia can vary in severity and presentation according to virulence (pathogenicity, or the ability to cause disease) of the infecting organism, dose, and site of inoculums (where the bacteria enters the body). Symptoms can include ulcers on the skin or mouth, swollen painful lymph glands, and a sore throat. Some persons with tularemia also become susceptible to pneumonia and develop chest pain, bloody sputum (mucus from the lungs), and have breathing complications.

Only a small number of the bacteria are required for tularemia disease to fulminate (appear suddenly and intensely); the infection is established when particles invade white blood cells and subsequently attack the immune system following multiplication. The major target organs are the lymph nodes, lungs, spleen, liver, and kidneys. While the inoculation may be focal, the disease will often become disseminated and cause problems throughout the body. The disease is fatal in around two percent of cases, with the most common cause of death being failure of the respiratory system or multiple organs.

Many small animals, including rodents, rabbits, and hares, provide natural reservoirs for the bacteria. Transmission of the infection to humans may occur through vectors such as ticks, biting flies, and mosquitoes. Humans may also contract the disease by handling infected animals or by ingesting contaminated water, soil, or food. Inhalation is also a significant form of transmission, but person-to-person transmission has not been established.

■ Scope and Distribution

The *F. tularenisis* bacterium is endemic throughout North America and in parts of Europe and Asia. Cases of tularemia have been reported in every state of America except Hawaii, with the majority occurring in south-central and western states. The widely present nature of the bacteria may be attributed to the fact that *F. tularensis* is found in diverse hosts and habitats, and it can survive for weeks at low temperatures in water, moist soil, hay, straw, and decaying animal carcasses.

People at a higher risk of contracting tularemia include hunters and trappers engaging in the skinning of potentially infected animals. Activities that lead to the aerosolization (dispersion into the air) of the bacteria can also increase the likelihood of infection, with lawn mowing the most common example of such an activity.

Currently in the United States, cases of tularemia occur most commonly between May and August when they are largely attributed to transmission by arthropod (a group of invertebrate animals including insects) vectors. This is in contrast to the historical incidence of tularemia, which was previously considered a winter disease contracted mostly from infected rabbits.

The incidence of tularemia has dropped significantly in the United States, from several thousand cases per year in the 1950s to around 200 per year in the 1990s. The fatality rate in the United States has also declined and is relatively low, at 1.4%. This is most likely due to the current availability of antimicrobial therapies. The exact prevalence of tularemia, however, is unknown, as it is assumed that the disease is greatly under-recognized and therefore, underreported. Tularemia occurs more often among males than females; it is also more prevalent among children between the ages of five and nine and adults between the ages of 75–84.

■ Treatment and Prevention

Treatment of tularemia is generally effective with antibiotics, usually streptomycin or gentamicin. Due to the nature of the infection, treatment should be continued for at least 10 days to ensure complete recovery. Long-term immunity will usually follow recovery from tularemia, but re-infection is possible, and repeated cases have been reported.

Although not yet available to the market, a vaccine was developed using a live attenuated strain of the disease. As of 2007, the vaccine is under review by the Food and Drug Administration. Post-exposure vaccination is not considered a viable public health strategy due to the three-to-five day incubation period of the disease, as well as the time necessary for immunity to develop.

Preventative measures should be adopted by people working in endemic areas. These should include the use of insect repellent on skin and clothing to minimize chance of insect bites and effective handwashing using antibacterial soap for people handling animal carcasses. The general public can also minimize infection by thoroughly cooking animal meat and ensuring the safety of water sources.

■ Impacts and Issues

Tularemia is identified as a Category A agent by the Centers for Disease Control (CDC), meaning that it is considered a high risk to society poses a potential threat

IN CONTEXT: TERRORISM AND BIOLOGICAL WARFARE

The Division of Vector-Borne Infectious Diseases at Centers for Disease Control and Prevention (CDC) states that "Francisella tularensis is very infectious. A small number (10-50 or so organisms) can cause disease. If F. tularensis were used as a weapon, the bacteria would likely be made airborne for exposure by inhalation. People who inhale an infectious aerosol would generally experience severe respiratory illness, including life-threatening pneumonia and systemic infection, if they are not treated. The bacteria that cause tularemia occur widely in nature and could be isolated and grown in quantity in a laboratory, although manufacturing an effective aerosol weapon would require considerable sophistication."

A part of the CDC program for bioterrorism preparedness and response the CDC states that as part of its preparations the CDC (or partners in the preparedness program) is:

- Stockpiling antibiotics to treat infected people
- Coordinating a nation-wide program where states share information about tularemia
- Creating new education tools and programs for health professionals, the public, and the media.

SOURCE: *Centers for Disease Control and Prevention, National Center for Infectious Diseases, Division of Vector-Borne Infectious Diseases*

to national security. The extremely low infectious dose required by the *F. tularensis* bacteria, in addition to the possible aerosol nature of transmission, makes tularemia potentially hazardous in large populations.

It is for these reasons that tularemia has been previously considered a viable option as a biological warfare agent. During World War II (1939–1945), Japanese researchers investigated this avenue. In the 1950s and 1960s, the United States developed weapons to deliver aerosolized *F. tularensis* organisms. These were destroyed in 1973. The World Health Organization (WHO) released a statement in 1969 that estimated that the successful release of 50 kilograms of the virulent bacteria over a metropolitan area housing five million people in a developed country would result in 250,000 cases of illness, including 19,000 fatalities. Although it was removed from the list of nationally notifiable diseases in 1994, it was reinstated in 2000 due to its potential for use as a biological weapon. As of 2007, this impact is still recognized and the CDC acts to ensure the rapid availability of substantial amounts of available antibiotics effective against the bacteria that causes tularemia.

SEE ALSO *Antibacterial Drugs; Bacterial Disease; Bioterrorism; CDC (Centers for Disease Control and Prevention); Vaccines and Vaccine Development; World Health Organization (WHO); Zoonoses.*

BIBLIOGRAPHY

Books

Mandell, G.L., J.E. Bennett, and R. Dolin. *Principles and Practice of Infectious Diseases,* Vol. 2. Philadelphia, PA: Elsevier, 2005.

Fong, I.W., and K. Alibek. *Bioterrorism and Infectious Agents: A New Dilemma for the 21st Century.* New York: Springer Science, 2005.

Mims, C., H. Dockrell, R. Goering, I. Roitt, D. Wakelin, and M. Zuckerman. *Medical Microbiology.* St. Louis, MO: Mosby, 2004.

Web Sites

Centers for Disease Control (CDC). "Consensus Statement: Tularemia as a Biological Weapon: Medical and Public Health Management." June 6, 2001. <http://www.bt.cdc.gov/agent/tularemia/tularemia-biological-weapon-abstract.asp#2> (accessed April 5, 2007).

Centers for Disease Control (CDC). "Tularemia." February 21, 2005. <http://www.cdc.gov/ncidod/dvbid/tularemia.htm> (accessed April 5, 2007).

Infectious Diseases Society of America. "Tularemia: Current, Comprehensive Information on Pathogenesis, Microbiology, Epidemiology, Diagnosis, Treatment, and Prophylaxis." March 5, 2007. <http://www.cidrap.umn.edu/idsa/bt/tularemia/biofacts/tularemiafactsheet.html#_Agent> (accessed April 5, 2007).

Tony Hawas

Typhoid Fever

Introduction

Typhoid fever, sometimes also known as enteric fever, is a potentially life-threatening infection caused by the bacterium *Salmonella typhi*. It is rare in the United States and other Western countries, and most cases in these areas have been acquired when traveling abroad. The disease is spread by contaminated food and water.

People who have had typhoid fever may be infectious for many months after they have recovered. One of the most famous carriers of typhoid fever was Mary Mallon, a cook for a family in New York City between 1901 and 1915. She infected 53 people with typhoid, and three of those she infected died. Typhoid is treatable with antibiotics, but can have a fatality rate of up to 30% if it goes untreated. There is also a vaccine that travelers can use to protect themselves in areas where typhoid is endemic. However, protection afforded by the vaccine is not lifelong and those who may be exposed may need to have a booster dose.

Disease History, Characteristics, and Transmission

Typhoid fever is caused by the bacterium *Salmonella typhi*, which infects the blood and the intestines. Paratyphoid fever is a milder condition caused by related species of *Salmonella*. The two are sometimes referred to as enteric fever, because of the site of infection. *Salmonella* species also cause food poisoning and only infect humans—there is no animal reservoir. At one time, typhoid was confused with typhus, because of the similarity between the symptoms. However, it is now known that the causes and pathology of the two diseases are very different.

The symptoms of typhoid include high fever, chills, cough, muscle pain, weakness, stomach pain, headache, and a rash made up of flat, rose-colored spots. Diarrhea is a less common symptom of typhoid fever, even though it is a gastrointestinal disease. Sometimes there are mental changes, known as "typhoid psychosis." A characteristic feature of typhoid psychosis is plucking at the bedclothes, if the patient is confined to bed.

Typhoid fever is diagnosed by identification of *S. typhi* in blood or in stool samples. Left untreated, fever may persist for many months, leading to potentially fatal complications. For instance, the mucosal walls of the

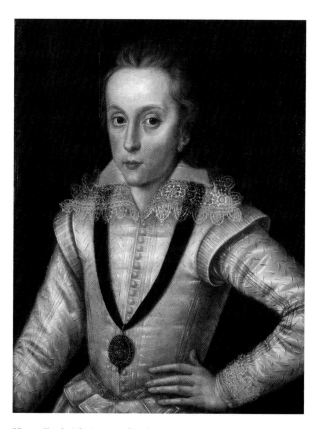

Henry Frederick, Prince of Wales (1594–1612), died of typhoid fever at the age of 18. He was the eldest son of King James I of England (1566–1625). *HIP/Art Resource, NY.*

intestine may weaken, allowing the infection to spread into the bowel. Typhoid fever has a 1% fatality rate in the United States, assuming prompt treatment with antibiotics. Without treatment, the death rate rises to about 10%. In parts of Africa and Asia, where the disease is far more common, mortality rates from typhoid may approach 30%.

Typhoid fever is spread through food and water contaminated by people with typhoid shedding *S. typhi*. About 1–4% of typhoid cases become chronic carriers—that is, they continue to shed *S. typhi* in their urine and feces for more than a year after recovery. Typhoid is also transmitted by water into which contaminated sewage has been discharged.

■ Scope and Distribution

Typhoid has long been a feared human disease. According to the World Health Organization (WHO), there are around 17 million cases of typhoid fever each year, of which 600,000 prove fatal. This is considered to be a conservative estimate of the scale of the problem. Typhoid fever is endemic in the Indian subcontinent and in parts of Asia, Africa, and Central and South America. In some of these places, typhoid is one of the top five causes of death. The peak age for contracting typhoid in countries where it is endemic is between five and 19 years, although it can affect people of either sex at any age.

In the United States, around 400 cases of typhoid fever are reported each year, of which 70% are contracted during travel to areas where it is endemic. In England and Wales, there are 150–200 cases of typhoid annually, again mainly in returning travelers. People have been known to develop typhoid after less than one week's stay in an endemic country. The disease has been all but eliminated from developed nations, although sporadic cases such as those mentioned above still arise.

■ Treatment and Prevention

Typhoid fever is treated with antibiotics, with ampicillin, trimethoprim-sulfamethoxazole, and ciprofloxacin being the preferred choices. However, a major concern is the emergence of multi-drug resistant strains of *S. typhi* in parts of Asia and South America. Therefore, the choice of antibiotic should be guided by local knowledge of which drugs will be effective against the strain of *S. typhi* involved in the infection.

There are two vaccines against typhoid—oral and injectable—and they are about 75% effective. Travelers should consult their national public health authority as to whether they need to be vaccinated against typhoid, if they are going to a country where the disease is endemic. Even if they have been previously vaccinated, a booster dose may be necessary.

Taking care to avoid risky food or drink is as important as being vaccinated in protecting against typhoid fever. All drinking water should either be bottled or boiled rapidly for one minute. Ice should be avoided, since it could have been made from contaminated water. Travelers in countries where there is typhoid should only eat food that is thoroughly cooked and is still hot and steaming. Raw vegetables and fruits should be avoided—unless they can be peeled, in which case hands should be carefully washed first. Many travelers get sick with typhoid—and other gastrointestinal illnesses—by eating food they bought from street vendors. It is impossible to observe a high standard of cooking hygiene under street conditions.

People who have had typhoid fever ought to assume they have carrier status, unless a series of stool samples analyses for *S. typhi* proves negative for the bacterium. Therefore, they should not prepare or serve food, and should take extra care with personal hygiene.

■ Impacts and Issues

Typhoid continues to be a problem worldwide because of poor sanitation, which forces people into frequent contact with contaminated water and food. Inadequate sewage disposal continues to be an issue in too many places, placing the populations at risk of many diseases, including typhoid fever.

The higher mortality rates from typhoid fever seen in many developing countries can be attributed to a weak—or non-existent—healthcare infrastructure, which does not provide ready access to the antibiotics that could cure the disease. War and natural disasters, such as earthquakes, disrupt clean water supplies, which is why typhoid has often accompanied such disasters, both today and throughout the course of history.

For example, the WHO reported a significant outbreak of typhoid fever in Kinshasa in the Democratic Republic of the Congo involving a total of 13,400 cases by mid-December 2004. The fatality rate from the outbreak was 22% (134 deaths), mainly due to peritonitis, a severe inflammation of the lining of the abdominal cavity. Very poor sanitation and lack of access to clean drinking water had been reported in the affected areas. The number of cases increased to over 42,000 through the early months of 2005, while the death toll mounted to 214. The medical charity Médicins sans Frontières Belgium helped to provide clean water which, along with other control measures including health education, began to bring the outbreak under control.

SEE ALSO *Travel and Infectious Disease; War and Infectious Disease.*

BIBLIOGRAPHY

Books

Wilks, David, Mark Farrington, and David Rubenstein. *The Infectious Diseases Manual.* 2nd ed. Malden, UK: Blackwell, 2003.

Wilson, Walter R., and Merle A. Sande. *Current Diagnosis & Treatment in Infectious Diseases.* New York: McGraw Hill, 2001.

Web Sites

Centers for Disease Control and Prevention. "Typhoid Fever." January 10, 2005. <http://www.cdc.gov/ncidod/dbmd/diseaseinfo/typhoidfever_g.htm> (accessed May 2, 2007).

World Health Organization. Initiative for Vaccine Research. "Typhoid." <http://www.who.int/vaccine_research/diseases/typhoid/en/index.html> (accessed May 2, 2007).

Susan Aldridge

IN CONTEXT: TYPHOID MARY

Mary Mallon, a known carrier of typhoid, refused to stop behaving in ways that risked spreading the disease and forced the government to jail her to protect the public health. The first person in North America to be identified as a healthy typhoid carrier, Mallon was an Irish-born cook who worked for wealthy New Yorkers. In 1906, she was employed in the rented summer home of banker Charles Henry Warren in Oyster Bay, Long Island, when typhoid fever struck six people in the household of eleven. The owners of the rental house hired investigators to determine the source of the epidemic. The detectives traced forty-seven cases of typhoid and three deaths to Mallon.

A contagious bacterial disease, typhoid had a fatality rate of ten percent, although milder cases also occurred. Typhoid bacteria remain in the intestine, liver, and bile ducts until they are transmitted via urine and feces. Victims suffer fever, chills, headaches, malaise, severe cramping, and diarrhea or constipation. The symptoms often continue for over a month. While sick, persons with typhoid weaken and became susceptible to complications such as dehydration or intestinal bleeding.

As a single, working class woman, Mallon needed to work in order to support herself. She was reputedly an excellent cook, but was unaware of the germ theory of disease and of the simple measures (such as handwashing) necessary to prevent spreading disease. Investigators discovered that thirty percent of the bacteria excreted by Mallon in her urine were the bacteria that cause typhoid.

In March 1907, New York City health officials literally dragged Mallon kicking and screaming into a city ambulance. They deposited her in a small cottage on North Brother Island that formed part of the grounds of an isolation hospital. Although she was released for brief periods, Mallon died in captivity in 1938 at the age of sixty-nine, after spending twenty-six years in her island prison.

Typhus

Introduction

Typhus is a group of diseases caused by bacteria belonging to the *Rickettsiae* genus. They are spread by ticks and small insects and are found in specific geographical locations around the world. Typhus has caused millions of deaths over the course of human history, being particularly common under conditions of war, famine, and mass migration.

There are four main types of typhus. Epidemic typhus is spread by lice and tends to occur in conditions of overcrowding and poor hygiene. The spotted fevers (sometimes also known as tick-borne typhus), like Rocky Mountain spotted fever, are a group of tick and mite-borne rickettsial diseases found in parts of the United States, Africa, India, Australia, and parts of the Mediterranean. Endemic flea-borne typhus is spread by rats and occurs in rodent-infested environments such as garbage dumps and markets. Scrub typhus is spread by mites and is found in parts of South East Asia. Typhus is a potentially fatal disease, with prevention depending on control of its insect vectors (transmitters from one host to another).

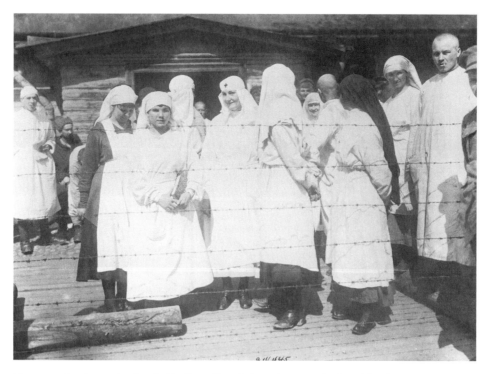

Nurses on duty in a typhus hospital in Narva, Estonia (now known as the Republic of Estonia) are shown during an outbreak in 1920. The nurses received ten cents a day; half of the staff died of typhus during the outbreak.   © *Bettmann/Corbis.*

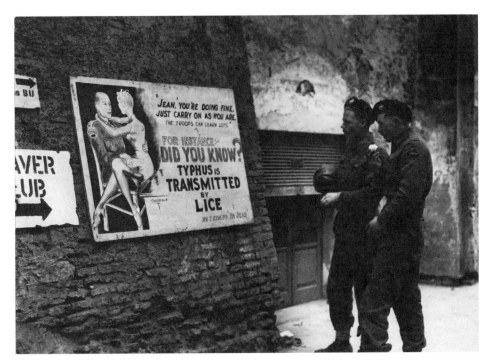

Allied soldiers read a poster warning of the dangers of catching typhus from lice in Italy, 1943.
© *Hulton-Deutsch Collection/Corbis.*

■ Disease History, Characteristics, and Transmission

Typhus was confused with typhoid fever until the 1830s, when it was shown to be a separate disease, although the similarity between the two names persists. The *Rickettsiae*, which are the causative agents of the various forms of typhus, get their name from Howard Taylor Ricketts (1871–1910), the American pathologist who discovered them, and who also died from typhus. They are Gram-negative cocci or bacilli, having an oval shape or existing as chains. Gram-negative refers to the way in which the bacteria react with Gram's stain, which is used to prepare samples for microscopy.

The specific *Rickettsiae* associated with the different types of typhus have been identified. Therefore, *R. prowazekii* is the agent of epidemic louse-born typhus, and *R. rickettsii, R. conorii, R. africae, R. japonica R. australis* and several other species are involved in tick-borne typhus, each organism being found in a different geographical area. Endemic flea-borne typhus is associated with *R. mooseri*, and *R. tsutugamusi* is the agent of scrub typhus.

The incubation time of typhus is 12–15 days. The bacteria enter the bloodstream and can spread throughout the body. They invade the endothelial cells, which line the inner walls of the small veins, arteries and capillaries and make them swell up. This can cause thrombosis, or blood clotting, and in addition, small characteristic nodules made up of white blood cells and platelets may develop in the blood.

The early symptoms of all kinds of typhus are nonspecific and may range from mild to severe, consisting of fever, headache, an extensive rash, and perhaps mental confusion. Symptoms persist for about two weeks, but several months may pass before complete recovery occurs. A characteristic eschar, or thick blackened scab, is seen at the site of the vector bite in scrub typhus and some of the spotted fevers. It is not uncommon for typhus to be improperly diagnosed.

Epidemic typhus may cause a high fever, headache, chills, confusion, and limb pain, progressing to agitation, coma, and many other complications. Photophobia, which is an aversion to light, vomiting, and a rash that starts on the trunk can also occur. Epidemic typhus is a far more severe condition than endemic typhus, whose symptoms are milder, but similar.

Rocky Mountain spotted fever causes headache, fever, abdominal pain, and a rash that begins on the hands and feet and spreads to the rest of the body. The other spotted fevers cause similar symptoms, but with some regional variations. So, for example, African tick-bite fever is not usually associated with a rash, and its symptoms are very similar to those of North Asian tick typhus. Scrub typhus causes breathing difficulties, cough, fever, headache, sweating, swollen glands, a swelling at the site of the bite, and a rash starting on the trunk.

WORDS TO KNOW

ARTHROPOD: A member of the largest single animal phylum, consisting of organisms with segmented bodies, jointed legs or wings, and exoskeletons.

ENDEMIC: Present in a particular area or among a particular group of people.

ESCHAR: Any scab or crust forming on the skin as a result of a burn or disease is an eschar. Scabs from cuts or scrapes are not eschars.

HOST: Organism that serves as the habitat for a parasite, or possibly for a symbiont. A host may provide nutrition to the parasite or symbiont, or simply a place in which to live.

MACULOPAPULAR: A macule is any discolored skin spot that is flush or level with the surrounding skin surface: a papule is a small, solid bump on the skin. A maculopapular skin disturbance is one that combines macules and papules.

PROPHYLAXIS: Treatment to prevent the onset or recurrence of disease.

RESERVOIR: The animal or organism in which the virus or parasite normally resides.

VECTOR: Any agent, living or otherwise, that carries and transmits parasites and diseases. Also, an organism or chemical used to transport a gene into a new host cell.

Rickettsiae may damage blood vessels, causing clotting and even gangrene, the death of tissue at the extremities of the body because of oxygen deprivation. This can lead to the loss of limbs or digits (fingers and toes). The infection can also lead to organ failure. Other complications may occur, depending upon the type of typhus involved. For instance, tick-borne typhus may result in liver and kidney failure, while brain damage and coma can occur with scrub typhus.

Typhus is usually more severe in adults than in children. The introduction of antibiotics has reduced overall mortality (death) rates to between three to four percent. Untreated, the mortality rate of epidemic typhus, which is the most serious form of the disease, ranges from five to 40 percent; in healthy individuals, the mortality rate is around 20 percent, but can be as high as 60 percent in elderly, malnourished, or debilitated individuals. Mortality from treated murine typhus

is about one to four percent, and is less than one percent for scrub typhus.

Those who survive endemic typhus generally have lifelong immunity to another attack, but may relapse many years later with a milder form called Brill-Zinsser disease. This occurs because the *Rickettsiae* may linger even after antibiotic treatment, especially if this has been incomplete or the person is malnourished. People surviving other forms of typhus generally have long-term or lifelong immunity from further attacks.

Transmission of typhus is from an animal or human host infected with *Rickettsiae* through an arthropod (flea, tick, mite) vector. In epidemic, louse-borne typhus, the bacteria pass—usually under crowded, unhygienic conditions—from one person to another via the body (clothing) louse, which thrives on worn, unwashed clothing. Head and pubic lice do not usually acts as vectors for *Rickettsiae*.

The *Rickettsiae* live in the digestive tract of the louse and are shed in its feces. Transmission usually occurs when the louse bites a human for a blood meal, defecating as it eats. The bite itches and scratching it crushes the louse and releases the bacteria from contaminated louse feces into the bloodstream. *Rickettsia* can survive for many months in dust containing dried louse feces and may be transmitted in this form through the eyes or mouth.

Endemic typhus, sometimes called murine typhus, is carried by the flea *Xenopsylla cheopis*, with rats, mice, opossums, raccoons, and skunks acting as the animal reservoirs. In tick-borne typhus, including the spotted fevers, rodents, dogs, cats, opossums, and hares act as animal reservoirs in various locations, with the vectors usually being ticks. However, Rickettsiael pox, which occurs in Russia, South Africa, and Korea, is carried by mites and *R. felis* infection, which is similar to endemic typhus, is spread by cat and dog fleas in parts of Europe and South America. Finally, scrub typhus is spread by mite bites.

■ Scope and Distribution

Typhus is a disease that has killed millions over the course of human history and is particularly prevalent under conditions of war, famine, and natural disaster where hygiene is poor and overcrowding and malnutrition are common. First described in the fifteenth century, typhus has been known as famine fever, ship fever, camp fever, and gaol (jail) fever, names that reflect the conditions under which it is most commonly found. It arrived in Europe in 1489 with soldiers who had been fighting in Cyprus. An outbreak between 1557–1559 killed around ten percent of the English population.

In the nineteenth century, typhus ravaged Napoleon's troops on their Moscow campaign, typhus hit Ireland between 1816–1819, and again during the famine of the 1840s. London experienced a serious typhus epidemic in the 1840s during a time of railway construction and building trade strikes that led to dislocation and deprivation in the city, and the disease began to claim more lives than smallpox.

During World War I (1914–1918), typhus caused 150,000 deaths in Serbia in 1915, and this epidemic was eventually brought under control by a British sanitary team. In the four years from 1918, epidemic louse-borne typhus caused 30 million cases and three million deaths in Eastern Europe and Russia. This epidemic was triggered by war and revolution, food and fuel shortages, and economic collapse, and was spread by the railways that enabled mass movement of people.

A famous victim of typhus was the teenage diarist of the second World War (1939–1945), Anne Frank, who died of typhus in the Bergen-Belsen concentration camp in 1945. Frank was just one victim in an epidemic which had a mortality of around 50 percent, killing almost 35,000 of the inhabitants of the camp.

More recently, in 1997, the World Health Organization (WHO) reported an outbreak of nearly 24,000 cases of epidemic typhus in Burundi, the largest outbreak in 50 years. The epidemic began with 216 cases occurring in a prison in N'Gozi, ideal conditions for contracting the disease, and then spread to the malnourished residents of refugee camps in the central highlands. WHO joined local teams in investigating the focal points of the outbreak, handing out doses of antibiotics to get the epidemic under control.

Epidemic typhus now occurs mainly in northeastern and central Africa. It is rare in most developed countries and would generally only be seen in communities and populations where body louse infestations are common, such as in refugee and prisoner populations during wars or famine.

In the eastern and central United States, around 15 cases of epidemic typhus have been reported among people with no history of lice infestation, but all described contact with flying squirrels and their nests. Therefore, campers and wildlife workers could be at risk of typhus if they come into contact with the squirrels or their nests, which are typically made in houses or in tree holes. The insect vector in such cases is the flying squirrel louse or flea.

Epidemic typhus today occurs sporadically outside the United States in cool mountainous regions of Africa, Asia, and Central and South America, especially during the colder months when louse-infested clothing may not be washed frequently. Travelers who do not come into contact with either lice or people with lice are not at risk in areas where epidemic typhus occurs. However, healthcare workers and military personnel who do have such contact may be at risk of contracting typhus.

Tick-borne typhus occurs in many places throughout the world, including the eastern United States, Brazil, the Mediterranean basin, the African veldt, India, and Australia. For instance, Rocky Mountain spotted fever occurs in Mexico, Central America, and South America, while tick-borne disease caused by *R. slovaca* is found in Europe. The spring and summer months are the peak times for transmission of tick-borne typhus. Travelers taking part in outdoor activities such as camping or hiking, could be at risk of acquiring tick-borne typhus if they do not take adequate precautions against tick bites.

Endemic flea-borne typhus causes sporadic cases in locations worldwide where humans and rodents live close together, such as in markets and garbage dumps. Flea infested rats are found all year round in humid tropical climates, and are more common in the warmer winter months in temperate regions. In the United States, cases have occurred in southern California and southern Texas, more commonly among adults. Travelers to places where there are rat-infested buildings and homes, especially by rivers and coastal port regions, could be at risk of contracting endemic typhus. Other animals, such as feral cats and opossums may carry the flea vectors of the disease, and contact with them should be avoided in endemic countries.

Scrub typhus is acquired from the bite of larval mites living on waist high Imperata grass that grows in previously cleared jungle around villages and in plantations. It occurs in South East Asia, the Indian subcontinent, Sri Lanka, and the other Indian Ocean islands, Papua New Guinea, and North Queensland in Australia. No cases have occurred in the United States except among travelers coming back from endemic areas. The incidence of scrub typhus worldwide is unknown, because its rather non-specific symptoms make it difficult to diagnose and there is a lack of diagnostic lab facilities in many parts of the world where it is endemic.

■ Treatment and Prevention

In 1948, the antibiotic chloramphenicol was introduced for the treatment of scrub typhus. Tetracycline became an alternative drug but, these days, doxycycline is the recommended treatment. Some antibiotic-resistant cases of scrub typhus have been reported. In areas where this is so, first-line treatment with rifampicin or ciprofloxacin might be recommended. The type of antibiotic treatment for all forms of typhus is similar.

Lab tests are important to determine the cause of the disease, but treatment is usually begun before the results of these are available to prevent complications. Treatment usually continues for up to three days after the fever has cleared.

There is no vaccine against typhus. Where there is epidemic typhus, mass prophylaxis with doxycycline is often necessary, as was accomplished in the Burundi outbreak. Long-term prevention efforts depend upon controlling the insect vector and the animal reservoirs of *Rickettsia*. Therefore, for louse-borne typhus, clean clothes, dusted with one percent malathion or one percent permethrin insecticide helps protect against the disease.

Prevention of endemic typhus depends upon controlling the local rodent population, while those at risk should use insect repellent to keep the fleas away. Tick-borne typhus can be prevented by the use of DEET (diethyltoluamide) or permethrin. Finally, prevention of scrub typhus is aided by clearing jungle grass within or near affected villages. Travelers should protect themselves with jungle boots, long trousers, and impregnate their clothing with DEET or permethrin. Prophylactic doxycycline may also be useful for those who must travel through high-risk areas.

Travelers are generally not at high risk of developing typhus via exposure to an infected person, except in cases of epidemic typhus. However, people traveling to any of the many countries where typhus is endemic seek advice from their healthcare provider about precautions. In general, covering the body to avoid tick and fleabites, and frequent washing and changing of clothes will help prevent typhus. Insecticides also have an important role to play in keeping the vectors under control.

■ Impacts and Issues

Typhus has long been one of the great human killers. It remains a threat in many parts of the world where the relevant animal reservoirs and disease vectors are not adequately controlled, and where sanitation and the health infrastructure are poor. War, famine, and mass migration have created epidemics of typhus in the past and will continue to do so, especially in the absence of an effective vaccine against the disease.

The advent of antibiotic treatment has greatly reduced the death toll from typhus, where it is available. However, in Thailand there have been reports of strains of *Rickettsiae* that are becoming resistant to the drug of choice, doxycycline, Small clinical trials conducted in areas of drug resistance have suggested that rifampicin and azithromycin may be effective alternative treatments. But in case resistance against these drugs also emerges, researchers are focusing on developing a wider range of treatments for all types of typhus.

■ Primary Source Connection

Ludwick Gross (1904–1999) was a physician and medical researcher who pioneered the study of viruses as a possible cause of human cancers. After earning his medical degree in 1929 in his native Poland, Gross began a long association with the Pasteur Institute in Paris, where he met Charles Nicolle (1866–1936), the scientists who unraveled the mystery of how epidemic typhus is transmitted. Gross recounts Nicolle and the significance of his typhus research in the following excerpted memoir.

How Charles Nicolle of the Pasteur Institute Discovered that Epidemic Typhus Is Transmitted by Lice: Reminiscences from My Years at the Pasteur Institute in Paris

Until the first decade of this century, our information about epidemic, i.e., exanthematic typhus was rather scarce. We knew only that there existed a very dangerous, easily communicable disease, which decimated populations during wars, hunger, or flood, spreading with great speed and affecting large numbers of people. After World War I, 20–30 million people died in Eastern Europe from this disease, and an additional several million died during and after World War II. Crowding, the scarcity of clean clothes, and dirt were the principal factors enabling the spread of typhus. The disease causes high fever and maculo-papular [small, red, raised] eruptions of the skin. Typhus is similar to a disease that occurs in the Rocky Mountains in the United States and is transmitted by ticks.

The fact that epidemic typhus is transmitted by lice was discovered by Dr. Charles Nicolle; a discovery for which he received the Nobel Prize in 1928. I met Dr. Nicolle in 1934 at the Pasteur Institute in Paris during my years as a guest investigator. I spoke to him several times in the corridor adjoining my laboratory. At my invitation he came to visit. He was a tall man, distinguished looking, impeccably dressed, lean, and slightly stooped, with dry skin and sparkling eyes. He was 68 years old at that time. It was difficult to talk with him because he was hard of hearing. In spite of his listening device, with its batteries and wires, which he was carrying, one had to almost shout to be understood. He was, like many Frenchmen, very polite and attentive. He agreed, at my request, to spend some time in my laboratory at the Pasteur Institute, and talk about his discovery.

Before long, still a few years before World War II, he came to my laboratory. He arrived wearing a shirt with a starched collar and starched cuffs, and sat himself comfortably in a large chair. He told the following story.

"I was delegated, some 30 years ago," recalled Dr. Nicolle, "to become director of the Pasteur Institute in Tunis, and decided to do something about typhus, which was decimating the local population. The first step was to try to transmit the disease to experimental animals. I injected guinea pigs with blood from patients with typhus and observed that, at least in some of these animals, the injection produced only high temperature. I realized, nevertheless, that even though some of them did not develop fever, they still carried the causative agent. This way we learned that typhus could exist, at least in some species, without any symptoms, except now and then, only fever. The most important point, however, was to discover how it was transmitted from man to man under natural life conditions. I learned this by accident. Tunis was full of typhus patients; the hospital was full and the number of new patients increased every day. Not only was every bed occupied and waiting rooms filled, but patients were waiting in front of the hospital, on the streets, to be admitted. At that point I made the crucial observation," said Dr. Nicolle, "that patients infected others out on the street, and also that their clothing was infectious; service personnel at the hospital and also in the laundry room became infected. The moment the patients were admitted to the hospital, however, after they had a hot bath and were dressed in hospital clothing, they ceased to be infectious. There was no longer fear of disease transmission in a hospital room full of patients. This observation was so simple and uncomplicated that it could have been made not necessarily by a physician, but by an administrator without professional medical training. I determined that there must therefore exist a transmitting vector, in the clothing and underwear of the patients. I anticipated," said Dr. Nicolle, "that most probably lice could be responsible for the transmission of typhus from man to man."

Dr. Nicolle continued his story.

"At the end of June, 1909, I asked Dr. Emile Roux, who was at that time Director of the Pasteur Institute in Paris, for a few chimpanzees. My request was granted, and the chimpanzees arrived promptly. I injected one chimpanzee with blood from a patient suffering from typhus. After several days, I collected from the injected chimpanzee a few lice, and transferred them to another chimpanzee; before long, after about 10 days, this animal developed typhus. I repeated this experiment, with similar results. It was now obvious that typhus was transmitted by lice. That was in September 1909. The first step in the search for typhus control was accomplished. Lice were demonstrated to be the transmitting vectors. The Tunisian government now began intensive measures to limit the typhus epidemic with attempts to combat infestation by lice.

The initial step had been accomplished, but great difficulties were ahead. Typhus is very infectious and many laboratory workers engaged in research on the typhus epidemic became infected accidentally, in the course of their laboratory work, and some of them died of the disease."

Ludwik Gross, M.D.

GROSS, LUDWICK. "HOW CHARLES NICOLLE OF THE PASTEUR INSTITUTE DISCOVERED THAT EPIDEMIC TYPHUS IS TRANSMITTED BY LICE: REMINISCENCES FROM MY YEARS AT THE PASTEUR INSTITUTE IN PARIS." *PROCEEDINGS OF THE NATIONAL ACADEMY OF SCIENCES OF THE UNITED STATES OF AMERICA.* (OCTOBER 1996): VOL. 93, 10539–10540.

SEE ALSO *Arthropod-borne Disease; Lice Infestation (Pediculosis); Rickettsial Disease; Rocky Mountain Spotted Fever.*

BIBLIOGRAPHY

Books

Pelis, Kim.*Charles Nicolle, Pasteur's Imperial Missionary: Typhus and Tunisia*. Rochester: University of Rochester, 2006.

Periodicals

Cowan, George. "Rickettsial Diseases: the Typhus Group of Fevers - a Review." *Postgraduate Medical Journal.* 76 (2000): 269–272.

Web Sites

Centers for Disease Control and Prevention (CDC). "Traveler's Health: Rickettsial Infections." 2005–2006 <http://www2.ncid.cdc.gov/travel/yb/utils/ybGet.asp?section=dis&obj=rickettsial.htm> (accessed May 5, 2007).

Susan Aldridge

UNICEF

◼ Introduction

Founded by the United Nations (UN), the United Nations Children's Fund (UNICEF, retained from its original name United Nations International Children's Emergency Fund) is an organization responsible for providing humanitarian assistance to children in developing countries. Its services promote the development of community groups for the well-being of local children.

As of 2006, UNICEF, headquartered in New York City, participates in efforts to improve children's rights in 191 developing and transitional countries. It is actively established within 156 developing countries. UNICEF works with organizations around the world to counter the devastating effects that abuse, disease, discrimination, exploitation, neglect, poverty, and violence have on children.

◼ History and Scientific Foundations

UNICEF was founded in December 11, 1946, to furnish clothing, food, health care, and other necessities to European children adversely affected by World War II (1939–1945). The U.N. expanded its charter in 1950, making it responsible for children's welfare in over 150 developing countries.

In 1953, UNICEF became a permanent part of the United Nations. Its first major activity was a global campaign to eliminate the infectious disease yaws that, at the time, affected millions of children. The disfiguring tropical disease of the bones, joints, and skin is caused by the bacterium *Treponema pertenue*. The incidence of yaws was reduced among children with the use of penicillin.

In 1959, UNICEF became guided by the U.N.'s Declaration of the Rights of the Child, which made it easier to establish international standards for children's rights in education, health care, nutrition, protection, and shelter.

The Nobel Peace Prize was awarded to UNICEF in 1965 for "the promotion of brotherhood among nations." UNICEF highlighted the rights of children in 1979— naming it the U.N. International Year of the Child.

During the 1980s, UNICEF adopted the International Code of Marketing of Breast-milk Substitutes (to promote breast milk use); launched Child Survival and Development Revolution (founded on low-cost techniques applied to breastfeeding, child development, and immunization); and adopted the Convention on the Rights of the Child (which became a global human rights treaty).

In the decade of the 1990s, UNICEF sponsored the World Summit for Children, whose goal is to improve children's education, health, and nutrition. UNICEF also emphasized the harmful influence that armed conflicts have on children. In the 2000s, UNICEF sponsors the Global Movement for Children and organized a historic Special Session of the UN General Assembly that was dedicated to children's rights.

◼ Applications and Research

The United Nations Economic and Social Council (ECO-SOC) is the parent organization to UNICEF. The five primary goals of UNICEF are: (1) establish international rights for children and create an international ethical standard of behavior toward children; (2) provide survival and developmental opportunities for children; (3) ensure that children are provided basic care, education, gender equality, health, nutrition, and nurturing; (4) protect children from abuse, exploitation, and violence; and (5) counter infectious diseases, especially HIV/AIDS, which has spread among children.

UNICEF upholds the United Nation's Convention on the Rights of the Child (CRC). The CRC is an international convention that establishes the cultural, economic, political, and social rights of children. UNICEF also participates in the Global Movement for Children, an international effort dedicated to building a better world for children by assuring that violations of their rights do not occur.

In some countries, such as the United States and Canada, fundraising for UNICEF is especially popular at Halloween when its "Trick-Or-Treat for UNICEF" program takes place, where children go from house to house collecting donations for UNICEF.

■ Impacts and Issues

UNICEF works to counter diseases within children around the world. Its Immunization Plus program has made significant improvements in children's health with respect to infectious diseases over the last three decades. UNICEF provides information, services, and products to fight childhood diseases such as educational programs, immunizations, and nutritional supplements. However, UNICEF estimates that two million children still die from diseases that are preventable with inexpensive vaccines.

UNICEF is especially concerned with children who are targets of abuse, exploitation, and violence. Its child protection programs include the countering of such practices as childhood marriages, child labor, female genital mutilation, sexual exploitation, slave trafficking, and other crimes.

In September 2000, the Millennium Declaration was established at the U.N. Millennium Summit in New York City. Among the global statistics held at the time of the Summit concerning children, hunger, poverty, and diseases are: nearly 600 million children live on less than one dollar (U.S. equivalence) a day; over 500 million do not have access to sanitation facilities; around 15 million have seen one or both parents die from HIV/AIDS (human immunodeficiency virus/acquired immunodeficiency syndrome); and over ten million die of hunger and preventable diseases each year.

UNICEF personnel work to break the connection between poverty, hunger, and diseases among children. Poverty contributes to hunger and malnutrition in children, which, leads to increased incidences in diseases, which, in turn, is a leading factor that causes over one-half of all children's deaths under five years of age in developing countries.

The goals of the Millennium Declaration state that by the year 2015: it will reduce by 50% the proportion of people living on less than one dollar per day and the proportion of people who suffer from hunger. Consequently, UNICEF is dedicated to reducing hunger and poverty in children throughout developing countries. Immunization for infectious diseases is the critical factor in UNICEF's work. As a result, UNICEF has become an international leader in providing vaccines to children. UNICEF purchases and distributes vaccines to over 40% of children located in developing countries. It also works to create and maintain local health systems and to improve at-home child care.

SEE ALSO *Childhood Infectious Diseases, Immunization Impacts; Tropical Infectious Diseases; United Nations*

WORDS TO KNOW

IMMUNODEFICIENCY DISORDER: In immunodeficiency disorders, part of the body's immune system is missing or defective, thus impairing the body's ability to fight infections. As a result, the person with an immunodeficiency disorder will have frequent infections that are generally more severe and last longer than usual.

NUTRITIONAL SUPPLEMENTS: Nutritional supplements are substances necessary to health, such as calcium or protein, that are taken in concentrated form to compensate for dietary insufficiency, poor absorption, unusually high demand for that nutrient, or other reasons.

SANITATION: Sanitation is the use of hygienic recycling and disposal measures that prevent disease and promote health through sewage disposal, solid waste disposal, waste material recycling, and food processing and preparation.

Millennium Goals and Infectious Disease; Vaccines and Vaccine Development.

BIBLIOGRAPHY

Books

Maddocks, Steven. *UNICEF.* Chicago, IL: Raintree, 2004.
UNICEF. *1946–2006: Sixty Years for Children.* New York: UNICEF, 2006.

Web Sites

NobelPrize.org, Nobel Foundation. "The Nobel Peace Price 1965." <http://nobelprize.org/nobel_prizes/peace/laureates/1965/> (accessed June 17, 2007).
UNICEF. "Home website of UNICEF." <http://www.unicef.org/> (accessed June 17, 2007).
UNICEF. "A Promise to Children." <http://www.unicef.org/wsc/> (accessed June 17, 2007).
United Nations. "Millennium Campaign." <http://www.millenniumcampaign.org/> (accessed June 17, 2007).
United Nations Cyber School Bus. "Declaration of the Rights of the Child (1959)." <http://www0.un.org/cyberschoolbus/humanrights/resources/child.asp> (accessed June 17, 2007).
United Nations Economic and Social Council (ECOSOC). "Home website of ECOSOC." <http://www.un.org/ecosoc/> (accessed June 17, 2007).

William Arthur Atkins

United Nations Millennium Goals and Infectious Disease

■ Introduction

In 2000, the United Nations (UN) adopted a series of goals designed to improve the lives of people throughout the world by reducing poverty, hunger, disease, maternal and infant mortality, by providing better education for children, equal opportunities for women, and moving toward a healthier environment. According to the UN, these eight Millennium Development Goals (MDGs) are providing "a framework for countries around the world for development, as well as time-bound targets by which progress can be measured." Several of these goals are aimed specifically at reducing the incidence and prevalence of infectious disease, most notably HIV, malaria, and tuberculosis, as well as the prevention of infectious disease, especially measles, among children.

Data subsequently collected by the UN suggests that several countries in sub-Saharan Africa are successfully lowering HIV infection rates and expanding treatment, thus demonstrating that the war against AIDS is not a hopeless endeavor. In addition, the resurgence of tuberculosis and malaria in Africa have been linked to the HIV/AIDS epidemic due to the increased vulnerability of immunocompromised persons (those with weakened immune systems) who are co-infected with both HIV and either malaria or tuberculosis. However, the resurgence of malaria and tuberculosis is also independent of HIV/AIDS, and combating these diseases is addressed separately in the Millennium goals.

The Millennium Goals pertaining to the global control of infectious disease include 1) "Reduce child mortality," a major part of which is the reduction of childhood deaths from measles through vaccination programs, and 2) "Combat HIV/AIDS, malaria and other diseases," which will be achieved mainly by international aid to poor nations to help implement prevention and treatment measures that are known to be effective.

■ History and Policy Response

HIV/AIDS

Over the past 25 years, more than 25 million people have died from AIDS. This death toll among adults in their sexual and occupational prime has resulted in the orphaning of 15 million children and economic devastation, which has in turn, exacerbated poverty and hunger. HIV/AIDS has become the leading cause of death among adults ages 15–59, and has afflicted both genders equally worldwide. It has taken most of these 25 years for the world community to mount a strong and concerted response to the epidemic, signified by the adoption of the Declaration of Commitment on HIV/AIDS in June 2001. A major component of this response has been the establishment of The Global Fund to Fight AIDS, Tuberculosis, and Malaria in 2002 to provide low- and middle-income nations with financial aid to help control the epidemic. In addition, the prices of some AIDS medicines have been significantly reduced. Groups such as the World Health Organization (WHO) and The Joint United Nations Program on HIV/AIDS (UNAIDS) have launched the "Three by Five Initiative," which has helped to substantially increase the number of people receiving antiretroviral treatment.

Despite these efforts, the overall growth of the HIV epidemic worldwide continues to overwhelm the effect of current efforts. Several countries report success in reducing HIV infection rates through programs that promote behavior changes such as reducing the number of sexual partners, using condoms, and avoiding sharing needles. However, infection rates overall are still growing. Approximately 39 million people globally were infected with HIV in 2005, while some 4.1 million people became infected with HIV and an estimated 2.8 million died from AIDS. The *Human Development Report 2005* of the United Nations Development Program (UNDP) concluded that the HIV/AIDS pandemic had done more to reverse human development than any other single factor. Sub-Saharan Africa remains the center of the epidemic. With just over 10% of the world population, 64% of HIV-positive people and in some areas, up to 90% of children under age 15 are infected with the virus. Twelve million sub-Saharan African children are orphans. Women comprise 59% of HIV-positive adults in sub-Saharan Africa (13.2 million people). HIV prevalence among people aged 15–49 in sub-Saharan Africa appears to be leveling off, although at an extremely high rate. However, this apparent stabilization reflects the fact that as new people acquire the virus, nearly the same number die from AIDS.

Malaria

A greater awareness of the heavy toll exacted by malaria has been matched in recent years with greater commitment to contain the disease. Increased funding coming from the World Bank's Global Fund to Fight AIDS, Tuberculosis, and Malaria, along with the United States President's Malaria Initiative and the Bill and Melinda Gates Foundation, among others, are expected to encourage important malaria control interventions, particularly insecticide-treated net use and access to effective anti-malarial drugs. The sale of insecticide-treated mosquito nets has increased ten-fold, but mostly among urban-dwellers. Poor rural communities in endemic areas remain extremely vulnerable to malaria.

Tuberculosis

The number of new tuberculosis cases grow by about 1% annually, with the most rapid increases occurring in sub-Saharan Africa. In the Commonwealth of Independent States (the nations comprising the former Soviet Union), tuberculosis incidence increased during the 1990s, but peaked around 2001, and has since fallen. Worldwide, tuberculosis kills about 1.7 million people per year. Of the nearly nine million new cases in 2004, almost 9% were among people infected with HIV.

Measles

One major aspect of the MDGs concerning child mortality includes reducing measles deaths through immunization. Measles vaccination of children is one of the most cost-effective public health interventions on record. However, the disease killed nearly a half-million children in 2004, and left many others blind or deaf. A majority of unvaccinated children live in China, Congo, India, Indonesia, Nigeria, and Pakistan. On the other hand, considerable progress in measles immunization has been achieved in Latin America, the Caribbean, and sub-Saharan Africa. According to the MDG report, sub-Saharan Africa achieved the largest reduction in measles deaths of any region, with a decrease of nearly 60% between 1999 and 2004.

WORDS TO KNOW

ENDEMIC: Present in a particular area or among a particular group of people.

IMMUNOCOMPROMISED: A reduction of the ability of the immune system to recognize and respond to the presence of foreign material.

INCIDENCE: The number of new cases of a disease or injury that occur in a population during a specified period of time.

PANDEMIC: Pandemic, which means all the people, describes an epidemic that occurs in more than one country or population simultaneously.

IN CONTEXT: DISEASE IN DEVELOPING NATIONS

Three out of the eight Millennium Development Goals and 18 quantitative of the 48 total quantitative indicators monitor progress relate directly to health issues. In May 2005 the United Nations stated that "some developing countries have made impressive gains in achieving the health-related Millennium Development Goals, targets and indicators. However, many more are falling behind. Progress is particularly slow in sub-Saharan Africa."

With regard to reducing child mortality, the U.N. states, "Some progress has taken place in specific countries. However, nearly 11 million children under the age of five die every year globally. In 16 countries, 14 of which are in Africa, levels of under-five mortality are higher than in 1990."

With regard to combating the spread of HIV/AIDS, malaria, and other diseases, the United Nations states "There have been successes in selected countries where they have made progress on reversing the spread of HIV/AIDS. However, the story is bleak in many countries. With three million deaths from HIV/AIDS alone each year, the worsening global pandemic has reversed life expectancy and economic gains in several African countries."

SOURCE: *World Health Organization, Fact Sheet 290, May, 2005*

■ Impacts and Issues

Of the four diseases mentioned in the Millennium Goals report; HIV/AIDS, malaria, tuberculosis, and measles, HIV/AIDS presents the greatest long-term challenge from both technical and policy standpoints. To a large extent, malaria, tuberculosis, and measles require more assiduous application of existing therapies and prevention

WHO AND THE MILLENNIUM DEVELOPMENT GOALS (MDG)

In May 2005 (Fact Sheet 290), the United Nations estimated that "the global estimate of what is required is a doubling of aid from US$ 50 to US$ 100 billion each year to achieve all of the Millennium Development Goals which would require a fivefold increase in donor spending on health (The Zedillo Commission: Monterey Conference)."

Moreover, to reach millennium goals, "the economic and health policies in developing countries must reflect the needs: current health spending in most low-income countries is insufficient for the achievement of the health MDGs. African leaders pledged to raise public spending on health to 15% of GNP at the African summit in 2001."

SOURCE: *World Health Organization*

methods as well as the prevention of resistant strains. While the fight against HIV/AIDS will also require all of these measures, it will additionally require the development of new treatments and vaccines. The AIDS pandemic has helped fuel current malaria and tuberculosis epidemics due to co-infection. Therefore, containing the HIV/AIDS epidemic is the paramount public health challenge worldwide.

The world community has agreed to redouble efforts to control HIV/AIDS, and at the 2005 World Summit Outcome, national political leaders pledged a massive increase in HIV prevention, treatment, and care programs with the aim of approaching the goal of universal access to treatment by the year 2010. These programs have begun to reduce some trends in national HIV prevalence, with recent declines noted in Cambodia, Thailand, Kenya, and Zimbabwe, in urban areas of Burkina Faso and Haiti, and in four states in India. The numbers of people receiving antiretroviral therapy for HIV infection in low- and middle-income countries by December 2005 increased to 1.3 million people, including an eightfold increase from 100,000 to 810,000 treated persons in sub-Saharan Africa between 2003 and 2005 (more than doubling in 2005 alone). The number of people receiving antiretroviral therapy in Asia nearly tripled to 180,000, in 2005.

In response to the call from the UN General Assembly to increase efforts against the AIDS pandemic, UNAIDS and its co-sponsors developed a program to help countries move towards universal access to anti-retroviral treatment and issued a report on these efforts entitled *Towards Universal Access,* which includes practical recommendations on setting and supporting national priorities, including

- ensuring predictable and sustainable financing

- strengthening human resources and systems

- removing the barriers to ensure affordable commodities

- protecting the AIDS-related human rights of people living with HIV, women, and children, and people in vulnerable groups

- setting targets and accountability mechanisms.

In June 2006, five years after the issuance of the Declaration of Commitment on HIV/AIDS, UN member states

- committed to specific actions to achieve the goal of universal access to HIV prevention, treatment, care and support by 2010

- recognized the UNAIDS estimate that $20 billion to $23 billion would be required annually by 2010 to fund sufficient responses

- committed to setting up ambitious national targets and estimated the cost of national plans

- agreed to focus on the key factors of the epidemic such as gender disparity, social and behavioral challenges for young people and stigma and discrimination against AIDS victims.

Political leaders of every persuasion worldwide now agree that the HIV/AIDS epidemic requires an extraordinary response. In order to bring the pandemic under control, among the main challenges in the future will be the need to work more closely and openly with populations impacted most by HIV/AIDS, including men who have sex with men, sex workers, and injecting drug users. Moving from short-term emergency responses to a longer-term response that recognizes the uniqueness of AIDS and is incorporated into national development planning and execution is envisioned. Strategies that are rational and ambitious, striking a balance between prevention and treatment based on adequate urgent funding have been called for to achieve the UN Millennium Development Goals as they relate to infectious disease. With such an urgent approach, progress made to date indicates that a considerable impact on even the HIV/AIDS epidemic could be made in a short period of time.

SEE ALSO *AIDS (Acquired Immunodeficiency Syndrome); Antiviral Drugs; Developing Nations and Drug Delivery; Malaria; Médecins Sans Frontières (Doctors Without Borders); Measles (Rubeola); Mosquito-borne Disease; Puerperal Fever; Re-emerging Infectious Diseases; Tuberculosis; Vector-borne Disease; War and Infectious Disease.*

BIBLIOGRAPHY

Web Sites

United Nations. "Millennium Development Goals Report 2006." Sections 2.10–11 (Child Mortality from Infectious Disease), Sections 2.14–15 (Malaria and AIDS Goals) <http://unstats.un.org/unsd/mdg/

Resources/Static/Products/Progress2006/MDG Report2006.pdf> (accessed March 11, 2007).

United Nations. "Progress towards the Millennium Development Goals, 1990–2005." <http://mdgs. un.org/unsd/mdg/Host.aspx?Content=Products/ Progress2005.htm> (accessed March 11, 2007).

United Nations. "Secretary General's Report on the Work of the Organization." <http://mdgs. un.org/unsd/mdg/Resources/Static/Products/ SGReports/61_1/a_61_1_e.pdf> (accessed March 11, 2007).

United Nations. "UN Development Group National Monitoring Reports." <http://www.undg.org/ index.cfm?P=87> (accessed March 11, 2007).

Kenneth T. LaPensee

Urinary Tract Infection

■ Introduction

The urinary tract is the system that produces, stores, and excretes urine. Its purpose is to remove undesirable compounds and some of the waste products of body processes. The human urinary tract is comprised of a pair of kidneys that filter waste from blood, two tubes (ureters) that connect the kidneys to a storage bag called the urinary bladder, a pair of sphincter muscles that help control urine flow, and the exit channel (urethra).

An infection of involving all or a portion of the urinary system is a urinary tract infection (UTI). The infection may remained confined to the urinary system—common sites of infection are the urethra and the bladder, but the kidney(s) can also become infected. Alternatively, a UTI can infrequently spread elsewhere in the body via the circulatory system. Infections of the urinary tract are the second most common type of infection in the human body.

■ Disease History, Characteristics, and Transmission

Although some people with a UTI do not display symptoms (asymptomatic), most men and women with a UTI display a range of characteristic symptoms, including urgent and frequent urination, a burning feeling when urinating, frequent urination but only in small amounts, urine that is cloudy and strong-smelling instead of clear yellow and relatively odorless, and blood in the urine (a condition called hematuria).

Pyelonephritis is an infection of the kidney. This usually occurs after the bladder has been infected, and the infection grows up the inner wall of the ureters that connect the bladder with each kidney. A kidney infection is accompanied by a high fever and flank pain. An infection of the bladder is known as cystitis. This infection is associated with abdominal discomfort, frequent and painful urination, and strong-smelling urine. Urethritis,

an infection of the urethra, is associated with the buring sensation upon urination.

UTIs begin when bacteria enter the urethra from the outside world. This can occur if the external region around the urethra is touched by hands that have not been properly washed, or it can occur accidently during a bowel movement. Females are more prone to this accidental contact, since their anus is nearer to the urethra than in males. The typical contaminating bacterium is *Escherichia coli*, which is a normal resident of the gastrointestinal tract and so is present in feces.

Another way of contracting an infection is through sexual activity. In women, the pathogens typically involved are the herpes simplex virus and the bacterium *Chlamydia trachomatis*, which are normal causes of sexually transmitted disease. In men, *C. trachomatis* and *Neisseria gonorrhoeae*, (the bacterium that causes gonorrhea) are typically involved.

■ Scope and Distribution

While they occur both in males and females, UTIs are almost a fact of life for some women. The chances that a woman will have a bladder infection during her liftime is about 50%. Physicians are not sure why women have more urinary infections than men, but one factor may be anatomical—a woman's urethra is short, allowing bacteria to access the bladder quickly. Also, a woman's urethra opens near sources of bacteria from the anus and vagina. In addition, post-menopausal women tend to be more infection-prone, since hormonal change makes the urinary tract walls thinner and more susceptible to infection. Both men and women who are sexually active with multiple partners also tend to have more urinary tract infections.

Another factor that contributes to the development of a UTI is the presence of an obstruction in the urinary tract; in men this can be an enlarged prostate. Other conditions that can predispose a person to UTIs include kidney stones, diabetes, and diseases or drugs that impair the function of the immune system. In addition, extended use of a catheter (tube) to help drain the bladder can increase the risk of a UTI. Epidemiologists estimate that a catheterized patient in a hospital has a 10% greater chance of developing a UTI for each day that the same catheter is in place. This is because bacteria readily adhere to catheter material and form biofilms, which can then migrate upwards towards the bladder.

■ Treatment and Prevention

UTIs are often treated using antibiotics, especially if they cause troublesome symptoms. These infections can be minimized by drinking plenty of water, which prevents urine from stagnating. Cranberry juice is also beneficial for some people, since a compound in the juice can outcompete bacteria for a specific attachment site on the bladder wall. In addition, wiping from front to back after a bowel movement lessens the chance that bacteria in feces will be accidentally deposited at the end of the urethra.

■ Impacts and Issues

The majority of urinary tract infections can be treated successfully and the patient suffers no lasting ill effects. However, kidney infections can be a serious complication of an untreated UTI. In addition, a chronic or complicated UTI in a pregnant woman increases the risk of premature birth or lower than average birth weight, which can pose risks for the newborn.

Urinary tract infections are a special concern for persons who have spinal cord injuries or who are immobile. If the muscles responsible for emptying the urinary bladder are paralyzed, repeated catheterizations or the placement of indwelling catheters are necessary to empty the bladder of urine and recurrent UTIs often develop. Pyelonephritis and sepsis (infection in the blood) are more common complications of UTI in this group, and these persons sometimes receive prolonged antibiotic therapy.

Even if a UTI is asymptomatic, it is important to finish the entire course of the prescribed antibiotic. Failure to do this can contribute to specific and overall antibiotic resistance. UTIs are sometimes caused by bacteria that grow as biofilms—colonies of bacteria that adhere to tissue. When enclosed in a biofilm, bacteria can be very resistant to antibiotics and may not be all killed if antibiotic use is stopped prematurely. Moreover, the surviving bacteria, which may have been exposed to a sublethal dose of an antibiotic, may develop resistance to the drug. When the UTI recurs as the bacterial numbers subsequently rebound, the antibiotic may no longer be effective against the pathogen.

WORDS TO KNOW

BIOFILM: Biofilms are populations of microorganisms that form following the adhesion of bacteria, algae, yeast, or fungi to a surface. These surface growths can be found in natural settings such as on rocks in streams, and in infections such as can occur on catheters. Microorganisms can colonize living and inert natural and synthetic surfaces.

PYELONEPHRITIS: Inflammation caused by bacteria infection of the kidney and associated blood vessels is termed pyelonephritis.

RESISTANT ORGANISM: An organism that has developed the ability to counter something trying to harm it. Within infectious diseases, the organism, such as a bacterium, has developed a resistance to drugs, such as antibiotics.

IN CONTEXT: REAL-WORLD RISKS

Urinary tract infections (UTIs) are any type of communicable diseases that occur along the urinary tract—which include the kidneys, ureters, bladder, and urethra. There are several kinds of UTIs. Cystitis is defined as inflammation of the urinary bladder. Urethritis is an inflammation of the urethra, which is the passageway that connects the bladder with the exterior of the body. Sometimes cystitis and urethritis are referred to collectively as a lower urinary tract infection, or UTI. Infection of the upper urinary tract involves the spread of bacteria to the kidney and is called pyelonephritis.

SEE ALSO *Bacterial Disease; Chlamydia Infection; Resistant Organisms.*

BIBLIOGRAPHY

Books

Iannini, Paul B. *Contemporary Diagnosis and Management of Urinary Tract Infections.* Newtown, PA: Handbooks in Health Care, 2003.

Kavaler, Elizabeth. *A Seat on the Aisle, Please! The Essential Guide to Urinary Tract Problems in Women.* New York: Springer, 2006.

OPERATION SEA SPRAY

The US Army conducted a study in 1951-52 called "Operation Sea Spray" to study wind currents that might carry biological weapons. As part of the project design, balloons were filled with *Serratia marcescens* (then thought to be harmless) and exploded over San Francisco. Shortly thereafter, there was a corresponding dramatic increase in reported pneumonia and urinary tract infections.

Prescott, Lansing M., John P. Harley, and Donald A. Klein. *Microbiology.* New York: McGraw-Hill, 2004.

Tortora, Gerard J., Berell R. Funke, and Christine L. Case. *Microbiology: An Introduction.* New York: Benjamin Cummings, 2006.

Web Sites

Medline Plus. "Urinary Tract Infection." <http://www.nlm.nih.gov/medlineplus/ency/article/000521.htm> (accessed March 20, 2007).

Brian Hoyle

USAMRIID (United States Army Medical Research Institute of Infectious Diseases)

■ Introduction

USAMRIID is an acronym for the United States Army Medical Research Institute of Infectious Diseases. The facility is operated by the Department of Defense and serves as the country's principal laboratory for research into the medical aspects of biological warfare. Specifically, the facility aims to develop vaccines for infectious diseases, other treatments such as drugs, and tests to detect and identify disease-causing microorganisms.

■ History and Scientific Foundations

The Office of the Surgeon General of the Army established USAMRIID on January 27, 1969. The facility replaced the U.S. Army Medical Unit (USAMU), which had been operating at the Fort Detrick, Maryland, location since 1956. The USAMU had a mandate to conduct research into the offensive use of biological and chemical weapons. This research was stopped by U.S. President Richard Nixon in 1969. In 1971 and 1972, the stockpiled biological weapons were ordered destroyed.

The defensive research that USAMU had been conducting, such as vaccine development, was continued by USAMRIID. In 1971, the facility was reassigned to the U.S. Army Medical Research and Development Command.

USAMRIID has a Biosafety Level 4 facility (the highest level of safety and security controls) and a Biosafety Level 3 area and is one of the largest high-level containment facilities in the United States.

The USAMRIID Biosafety Level 4 patient ward can house people who have been infected during a disease outbreak or researchers who have been accidentally exposed to an infectious microbe. This ward was used in 1982 to care for two researchers from the Centers for Disease Control and Prevention who were exposed to rat blood contaminated with the virus that causes Lassa fever. The two researchers, along with three others

thought to have been exposed to the virus, remained in the containment ward until they were determined to be free of infection.

Equipment is also available that allows the Biosafety Level 4 conditions to be mimicked in the field. Thus, an infected person can be isolated at the site of an outbreak and transported back to Fort Detrick for medical treatment and study of the infection.

■ Applications and Research

The research staff at USAMRIID numbers over 500 people and includes physicians, microbiologists, molecular biologists, virologists, pathologists, and veterinarians. Among the support staff who assist the researchers are laboratory technicians who have volunteered to be test subjects during clinical trials of vaccines and drugs.

USAMRIID scientists have the ability to rapidly identify infectious microorganisms. Vaccines are in various stages of development for several microbes including the anthrax bacterium and the Ebola and Marburg viruses.

Researchers and support staff can also respond to disease outbreaks. On short notice, teams can journey to the site of the infection to begin an investigation. This response is often conducted in conjunction with personnel from the Centers for Disease Control and Prevention. USAMRIID teams can also respond to combat. A portable laboratory to treat biological warfare casualties can be quickly set up near a battlefield.

One well-known USAMRIID response occurred in 1989, when an outbreak of an Ebola virus occurred at a primate holding facility in nearby Reston, Virginia. Some personnel even became infected with the virus, which was later determined to be a different variety from that which causes hemorrhagic Ebola fever in humans. The response of the USAMRIID personnel was subsequently detailed in best-selling books and popular movies.

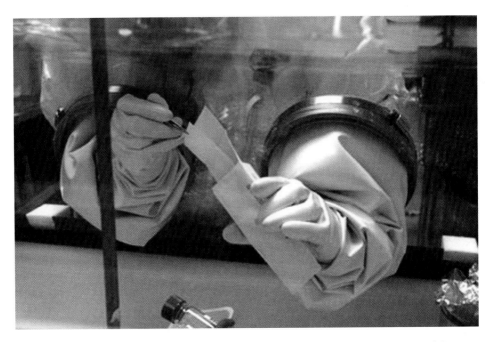

An anthrax-laden letter sent to Senator Patrick Leahy (D-VT) in 2001 is shown being removed from its envelope with tweezers at the Army's biomedical research laboratory at Fort Detrick in Maryland. © *Reuters/Corbis.*

The facility has played an important role in several military campaigns where it served as the medical support staging area for vaccines, drugs, and medical equipment.

In the aftermath of the September 11, 2001, terrorist attacks on targets in the United States, several letters containing anthrax spores were sent to various locations in the eastern United States via the United States Postal Service. The culprits have not been identified or apprehended as of May 2007. Sequencing of the genetic material from the spores determined that the source of the anthrax was a strain of the microbe that had been developed in the USAMRIID labs in the 1980s. Whether the bacteria actually used in the incidents came from USAMRIID or from another lab that acquired the bacteria from USAMRIID has not been established.

IN CONTEXT: LABORATORY SAFETY

Laboratories have a rating system with respect to the types of microbes that can safely be studied. There are four levels possible. A typical university research lab with no specialized safety features (i.e., fume hood, biological safety cabinet, filtering of exhausted air) is a Biosafety Level 1. Progression to a higher level requires more stringent safety and biological controls. A Biosafety Level 4 laboratory is the only laboratory that can safely handle microbes such as the Ebola virus, *Bacillus anthracis* (the cause of anthrax), the Marburg virus, and hantavirus.

Entry to the Level 4 area requires passage through several checkpoints and the keying in of a security code that is issued only after the person has been successfully vaccinated against the microorganism under study. All work in the level 4 lab is conducted in a pressurized and ventilated suit. Air for breathing is passed into the suit through a hose and is filtered so as to be free of microorganisms.

■ Impacts and Issues

While some of the research conducted at USAMRIID is classified, other research findings of the resident civilian and military scientists are used to benefit the larger public community. USAMRIID and its counterpart USAMRICD (U.S. Army Medical Research Institute of Chemical Diseases) train military medical personnel each year on biological and chemical defense measures. Furthermore, military and civilian medical professionals attend annual courses and seminars on such topics as "The Medical Management of Biological Casualties."

USAMRIID is mandated to explore the use of the treatments and tests in the battlefield environment. According to the law, the research conducted at USAMRIID is defensive in nature. Infectious microbes are to be investigated only to develop means of protecting soldiers from the use of the microbes by opposition forces during a conflict.

The infectious disease research expertise at USAMRIID is also utilized to develop strategies and training programs to do with medical defense against infectious microorganisms. For example, the agency regularly updates and publishes a handbook that details the various medical defenses against biological warfare or terrorism. This handbook is available to the public.

SEE ALSO *Biological Weapons Convention; Bioterrorism; War and Infectious Disease.*

BIBLIOGRAPHY

Books

USAMRIID. *USAMRIID's Medical Management of Biological Casualties Handbook,* 6th ed. Fort Detrick, MD: U.S. Army Medical research Institute of Infectious Diseases, 2005.

Web Sites

USAMRIID. "Welcome to USAMRIID." The U.S. Army Medical Research Institute of Infectious Diseases. Fort Detrick, MD. <http://www.usamriid.army.mil/> (accessed May 25, 2007)

Paul Davies

WORDS TO KNOW

HEMORRHAGIC FEVER: A hemorrhagic fever is caused by viral infection and features a high fever and a high volume of (copious) bleeding. The bleeding is caused by the formation of tiny blood clots throughout the bloodstream. These blood clots—also called microthrombi—deplete platelets and fibrinogen in the bloodstream. When bleeding begins, the factors needed for the clotting of the blood are scarce. Thus, uncontrolled bleeding (hemorrhage) ensues.

MIMICKED: In biology, mimicry is the imitation of another organism, often for evolutionary advantage. A disease that resembles another (for whatever reason) is sometimes said to have mimicked the other. Pathomimicry is the faking of symptoms by a patient, also called malingering.

OUTBREAK: The appearance of new cases of a disease in numbers greater than the established incidence rate, or the appearance of even one case of an emergent or rare disease in an area.

SEQUENCING: Finding the order of chemical bases in a section of DNA.

STRAIN: A subclass or a specific genetic variation of an organism.

Vaccines and Vaccine Development

■ Introduction

Vaccines, the introduction of a substance to create an immune response against a pathogen (disease-causing organism), have been responsible for great advances in public health since their advent in the late 1700s. Vaccines have greatly decreased the incidence of once-common diseases that caused innumerable deaths and huge public-health expenditures, not to mention terrible human suffering. Even diseases that were once universally fatal, such as rabies, are now averted with vaccines.

■ History and Research

Smallpox was a very serious disease in humans from its first recorded appearances in Europe and China in the third century AD until its eradication in the 1970s. The smallpox virus produced fever and headache, followed by a rash of pustules (small, pus-filled swellings), which gave the disease its name. In about 30% of cases, such severe damage was done to the skin or internal organs that death occurred. Even when the victims survived, they would often be badly scarred or even blinded by the ordeal.

Efforts to avoid infection with smallpox were early and widespread. Variolation, or intentional infection with smallpox, was prevalent because it was thought to produce a less virulent infection. This method was eventually recognized to be ineffective and even dangerous, leading to serious disease and deaths. At the end of the eighteenth century, Edward Jenner noticed that many milkmaids who had been infected with the cowpox virus did not contract smallpox. Jenner proved his theory by vaccinating a young boy with cowpox virus and then exposing him to smallpox. The vaccine was further developed into a stable and convenient dehydrated form in the 1950s.

The work of Louis Pasteur led to the germ theory of disease and the first vaccine for rabies. Later, the 1920s saw an increased number of inoculations for diseases such as diphtheria, pertussis (whooping cough), and tuberculosis, followed later by tetanus, yellow fever, polio, measles, mumps, and rubella. These familiar vaccinations, routinely given to children in the western world, markedly reduced incidences of these diseases. Expanded vaccination programs led to the goal of disease eradication, though to date only smallpox has been eliminated in natural settings.

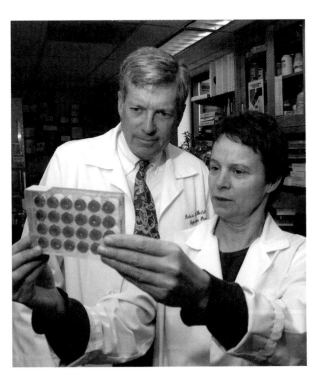

Doctors examine cultures at St. Louis University Hospital in Missouri in April 2002. The doctors discovered a way to successfully dilute up to five times the U.S. supply of 15.4 million doses of smallpox vaccine and retain its potency. This effectively expanded the number of individuals that can be protected from the contagious disease. *Bill Greenblatt/Getty Images.*

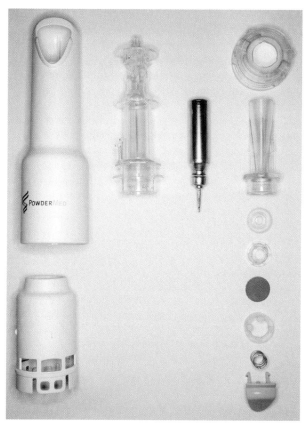

PowderMed, based in the United Kingdom, developed a vaccine for the H5N1 strain of bird flu as well as a means of delivery called PMED (Particle Mediated Epidermal Delivery). The delivery system fires the vaccine into the skin without the use of needles, stimulating rapid immunity. *Bruno Vincent/Getty Images.*

■ Impacts and Issues

Despite the great advances in human health due to vaccines, controversy has arisen over their possible unintended effects, with the result of some parents choosing not to vaccinate their young children against disease. Indeed, different groups have opposed vaccination since the technique was developed. Early arguments were religious in nature, stating that God sent smallpox afflictions as punishment and thus to circumvent the disease was to thwart God's will. More recent objections have focused on a purported link between vaccines and serious conditions such as autism.

In 1998, Andrew Wakefield published a study in the journal *Lancet* that purported to link the MMR (measles, mumps, and rubella) vaccine with the development of bowel disease and autism. His appearance at a press conference fed a media frenzy that caused many concerned parents to reject the MMR vaccine specifically and sometimes vaccines in general. Subsequent reassurances by the medical establishment and politicians were disbelieved by so many United Kingdom parents that

vaccination rates fell and outbreaks of disease were recorded. Though this hypothesis has not found support in many subsequent studies, distrust of the MMR vaccine has persisted; the United States Center for Disease Control and Prevention has recommended the removal of the mercury-containing vaccine preservative Thimerosal, identified by anti-vaccinationists as a possible source of vaccine contamination, as a cautionary measure.

Vaccines are not, and have never been, without risk. Localized reactions, such as itching, swelling, pain, or discomfort are quite common, while systemic reactions, such as fever, headache, and malaise are less so. More seriously, illnesses such as encephalitis, dangerous seizures, unintentional infection with the target pathogen, and even death have occurred. The smallpox vaccine in particular, despite its long history, has been known to be comparatively more dangerous than other vaccines in use today. For this reason, only a small number of persons with specific occupations have been recommended for pre-exposure vaccination against smallpox, despite the concern about potential bio-terrorism attacks in the post-September-11th environment.

Regardless of these concerns, vaccines are still considered an important foundation of public health efforts around the world. The Center for Disease Control prudently considers it better to prevent a disease than to treat its symptoms. Though many once-fatal diseases can be successfully treated with today's advanced supportive care and antibiotics, the costs of vaccination are much lower than those of treating infection. Indeed, the National Institute of Allergy and Infectious Diseases cites a study stating that for each dollar spent on vaccinating against rubella, eight dollars are saved in costs that would have been spent treating the infection.

Two infectious disease outbreaks have created public interest in the quick development of therapeutic vaccines: the 2004 outbreak of SARS (Severe Acute Respiratory Syndrome) and the ongoing, low-intensity occurrences of H5N1 avian influenza, particularly in Asia. In the face of epidemics, however, mass vaccination is not always feasible and may present hazards to public health. Ring vaccination, or administering vaccine to populations within and immediately surrounding the outbreak, is an alternative measure used in many outbreaks of infectious disease. Similarly, development of vaccines is a long and complex process that requires great amounts of research and testing before vaccines become available.

Many different types of vaccines exist, some of which are easier to produce than others. Different types of vaccines produce varying degrees of resistance to disease, some requiring multiple doses or "booster shots" to remain effective. A great deal of study and preparation is required before work on a vaccine can begin. The life cycle of the pathogen, the way it functions and causes harm in the body, and the response of the immune

WORDS TO KNOW

ATTENUATED STRAIN: A bacterium or virus that has been weakened, often used as the basis of a vaccine against the specific disease caused by the bacterium or virus.

RING VACCINATION: Ring vaccination is the vaccination of all susceptible people in an area surrounding a case of an infectious disease. Since vaccination makes people immune to the disease, the hope is that the disease will not spread from the known case to other people. Ring vaccination was used in eliminating the smallpox virus.

VARIOLATION: Variolation was the pre-modern practice of deliberately infecting a person with smallpox in order to make them immune to a more serious form of the disease. It was dangerous, but did confer immunity on survivors.

VACCINE TYPES

Vaccines with living, but weakened, viruses are termed attenuated vaccines. The attenuated virus does not cause a severe infection, but does present the body with sufficient challenge to mount and thus "learn" an immune response. MMR vaccines (the common abbreviation for the measles, mumps, and rubella vaccine) is an example of an attenuated vaccine.

Vaccination can also involve the use of dead viruses and bacteria. The antigen, usually a specific molecule that resides on the surface of the cell, is sufficient alone to provoke an immune response that subsequently provides protection against live bacteria or virus carrying the same surface molecule.

The third type of vaccination uses toxin produced by the living bacterium, but not the bacteria themselves. Diphtheria and tetanus vaccines are examples of toxoid vaccines promoted by the poster.

The fourth class of vaccine is engineered, or uses a chemical compound formed from the fusion of portions of two antigens. The Hib vaccine is such a biosynthetic vaccine.

system must all be examined before the most appropriate course of action can be determined.

Some types of vaccines are well understood, produce reliable immune responses, and are easy to produce. Many of these use attenuated (weakened but live) pathogens while others use dead organisms or portions of their proteins or antigens. Vaccines containing live, attenuated pathogens are not always appropriate for patients with weakened immune systems; likewise, vaccines containing dead pathogens often produce a weak or short-lived immune response. Newer, possibly more effective types of vaccines are being explored, including those that use parts of the pathogen's DNA to cause the body to produce "natural vaccine" on its own. Once a vaccine is developed, it must undergo the usual three phases of clinical trials to establish safety, dosage, and effectiveness, as well as a stringent licensing process and continued monitoring for safety and contamination. The length of this process means that new vaccines cannot always be quickly developed to meet an immediate need.

The risk of an epidemic must also be balanced with the real likelihood of adverse events associated with vaccinating large numbers of people in short periods of time. If mass vaccinations are required, the timing of the campaign can help the healthcare system deal with adverse events more successfully. By increasing the length of a vaccination campaign from two to ten days, fewer people will experience adverse events at the same time, reducing strain on doctors and hospitals. In cases of extreme shortage, vaccines such as smallpox can be diluted to much weaker solutions than their intended strength and still produce immunity in a portion of those vaccinated.

As a public health tool, vaccines are an inexpensive way to prevent serious disease before it develops and spreads. Health officials, individuals, and parents must maintain high levels of compliance to ensure protection against disease outbreak. At the same time, one must responsibly evaluate the risks of vaccines when faced with the outbreak of dangerous disease.

■ Primary Source Connection

The following newspaper article appeared in the *The New York Times* in 2004. It explains the economics of vaccine development from the drug manufacturers' point of view. Mentioned in the article is a vaccine under development for shingles, a chickenpox-related virus, and the overall trend for more vaccines for adolescents and adults rather than children. In an update to the article, the vaccine for shingles was approved in May 2006 and is recommended by the Centers for Disease Control and Prevention for all adults over age sixty.

Vaccines Are Good Business for Drug Makers

As the nation tries to comprehend this year's shortage of flu vaccine, many experts have explained that the vaccines business holds little allure for drug companies, because of low prices, strict regulations and uncertain demand.

But try telling that to Nabi Biopharmaceuticals, a small company in Boca Raton, Fla., which is testing one vaccine to protect patients in hospitals and kidney dialysis centers from potentially fatal bacterial infections and another to help people quit smoking.

Or tell it to Vical, a San Diego company trying to develop an arsenal of bioengineered vaccines for viruses like those that cause Ebola, West Nile, and SARS.

Or tell it to Wyeth, a big drug maker whose vaccine Prevnar, used against the pneumococcal bacteria that can cause pneumonia, meningitis and ear infections, costs more than $250 for the four-dose treatment given to infants. Despite the price, the government has recommended that all infants get the vaccine, and insurers generally pay for it—as does the federal Vaccines for Children program for low-income families. Prevnar, with sales expected to top $1 billion this year, would be the world's first "blockbuster" vaccine.

Vaccines, it turns out, can make for pretty good business.

Even flu vaccines, despite challenges that include the need to reformulate the medicine each season, are potentially more lucrative than they used to be, with wholesale prices up fourfold since the late 90's.

"I am not one of those who think this is an industry plagued by low prices, because it's not true," said Anthony F. Holler, chief executive of ID Biomedical, a Canadian company whose excess inventory of flu shots might help augment the American supply this winter. "I just think that people are thinking of the business that occurred 10, 15 years ago."

The current shortage has more to do with past government and industry decisions, which reduced the nation's suppliers to two: Chiron and the vaccine unit of Sanofi-Aventis. That occurred in part because the business requires a heavy investment, which, economists say, tends to favor having fewer, big suppliers rather than many smaller ones.

Now, to help prevent shortages, the government is considering steps that include expanding the amount of flu vaccine it puts into an emergency stockpile for childhood vaccines. This was the first year the government decided to add flu vaccine to that stockpile. Another possibility is guaranteeing the purchase of a certain number of flu shots each year, possibly beyond what the industry is contemplating manufacturing. That might attract more companies to the business or induce existing ones to produce more than needed, providing some cushion in case one supplier runs into problems.

As those proposals indicate, the vaccine business is as complex as the market dynamics that drive it. That is why the medicines receiving the biggest push from the industry are likely to be ones with a perceived market in the United States, which spends more than half the world's drug dollars.

With American free-market forces so heavily in play, vaccines for malaria or other diseases that mainly afflict developing countries are not likely to be pursued except through philanthropic efforts. But with diseases that affect Americans, the combination of new technologies, higher prices and new target populations—adults, not children, for instance—are opening new vistas for the business, even as the older childhood vaccines generally remain lower-priced commodities.

"It's a tough business for older products," said R. Gordon Douglas, an industry consultant who ran the vaccine business for 10 years at Merck & Company. "It's a good business for new products."

The role played by government can be crucial to determining what vaccines get produced, at what prices and in what quantities.

For older vaccines used to prevent childhood diseases like mumps, measles and diphtheria, for example, more than half the doses are purchased by the federal Vaccines for Children program. Prices are capped so they rise no faster than inflation. At $10 to $30 a dose, such vaccines are not a growth market, which helps explain why there is only a single supplier for five of the eight recommended childhood vaccines and why periodic shortages still occur.

Like many of the older childhood immunizations, flu vaccines are considered commodities. But because most are sold through the private sector, there are no caps on prices.

In the late 1990's four companies supplied flu vaccines but two—Wyeth and King Pharmaceuticals—dropped out, citing low profits and heavy expenditures to meet increasingly stringent regulatory requirements to prevent contamination.

In the same period, however, demand for flu shots was on the rise as government health officials expanded the categories of people recommended to receive the vaccine. As a result of that demand and the reduction in the number of suppliers, flu vaccine prices have quadrupled since the late 1990's, to around $8 a dose wholesale.

That trend appeared to be attracting more companies to the field even before the recent shortage. Chiron, for instance, acquired a British flu vaccine company last year largely to enter the American market; it was problems at the British plant, not a lack of profit motive, that created Chiron's shortage.

And ID Biomedical of Canada had been planning to enter the American market in a few years, though the shortage might now speed its entry. Others, like Baxter International, have been weighing entering the market within a few years.

Various economic arguments can be made for why the government should play a role in promoting the use of vaccines. One is that they are among the most cost-effective modes of medicine. Preventing a disease—often, the inoculation lasts a lifetime—can be far less expensive than treating it once it develops and spreads. Economists have estimated that every dollar spent on some of the inexpensive childhood vaccines has yielded benefits as high as $27. But left to their own devices, individuals may not highly value vaccines because of the uncertainty that they themselves will ever get the disease.

Whatever the government's role, there are business obstacles for vaccines, including a much smaller market than with drugs. Total sales of all vaccines worldwide are around $8 billion, less than sales of Pfizer's Lipitor cholesterol-lowering pill alone.

And because vaccines are given to healthy people, safety and liability concerns can be greater than with drugs, which are given to sick people, who are willing to bear some risk of side effects to get better. Liability concerns drove many companies out of the vaccine business before Congress enacted a law in 1986 providing some protection to makers of childhood vaccines. Companies say they are still vulnerable on adult vaccines and are still being sued for the use of thimerosal, a mercury-containing preservative that has been largely removed from pediatric vaccines.

Potential liability is also on the mind of Merck, which hopes to get approval for a vaccine aimed at rotavirus, a cause of life-threatening diarrhea. The company is testing it on 70,000 children—an enormous number for a clinical trial—because the company wants to rule out a rare side effect that caused a rotavirus vaccine by Wyeth to be pulled from the market in 1999.

Merck, which recently withdrew its painkiller Vioxx from the market and has had several drugs fail in clinical trials, is counting three vaccines among the most important products it expects to bring to market in the next few years. Besides the rotavirus vaccine, there is one for human papilloma virus, which is thought to cause cervical cancer. The third is for shingles, a disease of adults caused by the chickenpox virus.

As Merck's efforts indicate, many of the newer vaccines aim at adult diseases. "In the next 15 to 20 years we're going to move from pediatric vaccines to adolescent vaccines and adult vaccines," said Vijay B. Samant, chief executive of Vical.

If, as some economists argue, vaccines are underused relative to their value to public health, then the government could have several roles.

Urging vaccination, as is done for childhood diseases, assures manufacturers of a market. And the government can buy vaccines for a stockpile, as it is now doing for vaccines for anthrax and smallpox.

But industry officials, like Wayne Pisano of Aventis Pasteur, the vaccine unit of Sanofi-Aventis, say the most important factor for a healthy vaccine business is higher prices. "You can't have high investment, high regulatory requirements and low prices," Mr. Pisano said.

Andrew Pollack

POLLACK, ANDREW. "VACCINES ARE GOOD BUSINESS FOR DRUG MAKERS." *THE NEW YORK TIMES.* OCTOBER 29, 2004.

S‌ee Also *Childhood Infectious Diseases, Immunization Impacts; Influenza, Tracking Seasonal Influences and Virus Mutation; Polio Eradication Campaign; Smallpox; Smallpox Eradication And Storage.*

BIBLIOGRAPHY

Periodicals

Belongia, Edward A., and Allison L. Naleway. "Smallpox Vaccine: The Good, the Bad, and the Ugly." *Clinical Medicine and Research* 1, 2 (2003): 87-92.

Web Sites

Centers for Disease Control and Prevention. "Mercury and Vaccines (Thimerosal)." <http://www.cdc.gov/od/science/iso/concerns/thimerosal.htm> (accessed June 14, 2007).

McCulloch, J. Huston, and James R. Meginniss. *Ohio State University.* "A Statistical Model of Smallpox Vaccine Dilution." May 17, 2002. <http://www.econ.ohio-state.edu/jhm/smallpox.htm> (accessed June 14, 2007).

National Institutes of Health, National Institute of Allergy and Infectious Diseases. "Understanding Vaccines." July 2003. <http://www.niaid.nih.gov/publications/vaccine/pdf/undvacc.pdf> (accessed June 14, 2007).

White, Andrew Dickinson. *A History of the Warfare of Science with Theology in Christendom.* "Chapter X: Theological Opposition to Inoculation, Vaccination, and the Use of Anaesthetics." <http://abob.libs.uga.edu/bobk/whitem10.html> (accessed June 14, 2007).

World Health Organization. "Vaccines" <http://www.who.int/topics/vaccines/en> (accessed June 14, 2007).

Kenneth LaPensee

Vancomycin-Resistant Enterococci

◼ Introduction

The World Health Organization (WHO) reports that drug-resistant germs infect more than two million people in the United States every year and that 14,000 die as a result. The rise of drug resistance among microorganisms is tied to the widespread use of antibiotics in humans and animals. Vancomycin-resistant enterococcus (VRE) is one of a group of drug resistant bacteria that were first reported in 1986, almost 30 years after the antibiotic vancomycin was introduced. Vancomycin has been a mainstay of hospital infection control since the emergence of microorganisms that are resistant to

the original antibiotics developed in the early and mid-twentieth century, such as penicillin, methicillin, and ampicillin.

◼ History and Scientific Foundations

When large amounts of oral vancomycin are taken for an infection, some of the drug's proteins are not absorbed and remain in the gastrointestinal tract. This environment leads to colonization (the presence of microorganisms that normally do not cause disease) with vancomycin-

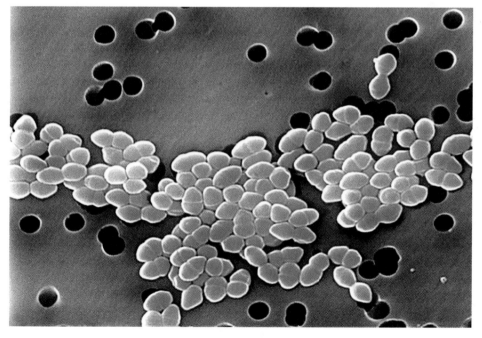

A color enhanced scanning electron micrograph (SEM) shows Vancomycin-resistant Enterococci (VRE). *Science Source.*

WORDS TO KNOW

COLONIZATION: Colonization is the process of occupation and increase in number of micro-organisms at a specific site.

ISOLATION: Isolation, within the health community, refers to the precautions that are taken in the hospital to prevent the spread of an infectious agent from an infected or colonized patient to susceptible persons. Isolation practices are designed to minimize the transmission of infection.

PATHOGEN: A disease causing agent, such as a bacteria, virus, fungus, etc.

PREVALENCE: The actual number of cases of disease (or injury) that exist in a population.

RESISTANT ORGANISM: Resistant organisms are bacteria, viruses, parasites, or other disease-causing agents that have stopped responding to drugs that once killed them.

resistant organisms when the antibiotic concentrations in the intestines are high enough to encourage resistant enterococci bacteria to grow, but not sufficiently high to kill these organisms.

For decades, vancomycin was the only effective therapy for potentially life-threatening infections with resistant bacteria such as methicillin-resistant *Staphylococcus aureus* (MRSA). Throughout the 1990s, there were few if any antimicrobial agents to treat VRE infections. In recent years, newly developed antibiotics have been effective against VRE and other multi-drug resistant organisms, but strains (types) of microorganisms that are resistant to these new agents have already emerged. Many of these strains are resistant not only to vancomycin, but are also to other antibiotics that have been widely used against infections with similar bacteria in hospital settings, a condition called cross-resistance.

The connection between VRE and MRSA is particularly alarming. In one study, almost 25% of hospitalized persons who were co-colonized with both bacteria (had growing populations of both bacteria present on their bodies) died. Another nearly 35% were discharged to other facilities and took with them significant risk of further transmitting the infection to other patients.

Most of the VRE recovered in the United States are one of two species of enterococcus bacteria *E. faecium* or *E. faecalis*. These enterococci occur naturally in the intestinal tract of all people and are not generally harm-

ful, whether or not they are vancomycin-resistant, and most infections resolve without treatment. Nevertheless, infections with these microbes, especially with *E. faecalis* can be dangerous to immunocompromised persons (those receiving chemotherapy for cancer, organ transplantation, or who have weakened immune systems due to a variety of conditions such as AIDS).

From 1990 to 1997 the prevalence of VRE in hospitalized patients with infections arising from enterococci bacteria increased from less than one percent to about 15%. By 1999, VRE accounted for nearly a quarter of all enterococcus infections in hospital intensive care units (ICUs), as reported by the National Nosocomial Infection Surveillance System (NNIS). This figure rose to 28.5% in 2003.

■ Applications and Research

The Centers for Disease Control (CDC) publishes and revises guidelines for the management of VRE and other antibiotic resistant organisms in healthcare settings. Local advisories based on the CDC guidelines are now widely disseminated and public health agencies are attempting to increase public awareness of VRE. A notice on the website of the New York State Department of Health states, "Serious VRE infections usually occur in hospitalized patients with serious underlying illnesses such as cancer, blood disorders, kidney disease or immune deficiencies. People in good health are not at risk of infection, but health care workers may play a role in transmitting the organism, if careful handwashing and other infection control precautions are not practiced." The notice goes on to say that VRE is usually spread by "direct contact with hands, environmental surfaces or medical equipment that has been contaminated by the feces of an infected person."

■ Impacts and Issues

In the United States and around the world, VRE infections present a growing burden of illness with considerable economic impact. A recent analysis documented increased mortality (deaths), length of hospital stay, ICU admissions, surgical procedures, and costs for VRE patients compared to a matched hospital population. VRE prevalence in the United States has steadily increased over the past two decades.

During this time, public health officials as well as hospital-based infectious disease specialists and hospital pharmacists have become increasingly concerned with the spread of infection with VRE in hospitals, rehabilitation centers, and nursing homes. The CDC reports that concerted efforts involving the isolation of VRE-infected patients, active surveillance, use of a waterless hand disinfectant, and staff training have resulted in significant local decreases in VRE prevalence.

Hospitals are responding with strategies designed to limit the spread of VRE by limiting the use of vancomycin. Powerful new antibiotics such as piperacillin-tazobactam are often effective against VRE, but are expensive and require intravenous administration.

Such anti-VRE strategies can be highly effective across an entire health care system. Some hospitals in the Netherlands and Denmark, for example, pro-actively isolate all patients considered at risk for VRE until tests show them to be free of multi-drug resistant organisms. This step prevents carriers from passing infections to other patients and hospital workers. The strategy has significantly reduced VRE-related infections in these countries. Also in the European Union, the non-therapeutic use of antibiotics in animals was banned in 2006 in order to stop the transfer of resistant bacteria from farm animals to people. This prescription was on top of a pre-existing ban on the agricultural use of vancomycin-type drugs in animal feed.

The "tried and true" methods of infection control are not universally considered to be an adequate response to the antibiotic resistant infection crisis. Some observers are now advocating environmental strategies directed at farming practices such as restricting the use of antibiotics in farm animal feed that promote VRE and related cross resistant strains which multiply in dairy effluent lagoons. Such broad ranging strategies have a political and economic policy aspect, and have not yet been endorsed by the CDC, which continues to emphasize institutional infection control measures. However, as alarm spreads over the increase in antibiotic resistance, more comprehensive, environmentally based, and economy-wide measures may eventually be implemented in order to preserve the effectiveness of antibiotics as life-saving drugs.

SEE ALSO *Antibiotic Resistance; Contact Precautions; Microbial Evolution; Resistant Organisms.*

BIBLIOGRAPHY

Books

Shnayersen, Michael, and Mark J. Plotkin. *The Killers Within: the Deadly Rise of Drug-Resistant Bacteria.* Boston: Back Bay, 2003.

Periodicals

Rice, L.B. "Emergence of Vancomycin-resistant Enterococci." *Emerging Infectious Diseases,* (March-April 2001):7(2)183–87.

Web Sites

Healthcare Infection Control Practices Advisory Committee. *Centers for Disease Control and Prevention.*"Management of Multidrug-Resistant Organisms In Healthcare Settings- 2006." <http://www.cdc.gov/ncidod/dhqp/pdf/ar/mdroGuideline2006.pdf> (accessed May 21, 2007.)

New York State Department of Health. "Vancomycin Resistant Enterococcus (VRE)." <http://www.health.state.ny.us/diseases/communicable/vancomycin_resistant_enterococcus/fact_sheet.htm> (accessed may 21, 2007).

Kenneth T. LaPensee

Vector-borne Disease

Introduction

Vector-borne disease refers to the transmission of a disease that is caused by a microorganism from one organism (the host) to another organism via a third organism (the vector). Put another way, a vector is the means by which microbes can get from their normal place of residence, where they typically cause no harm, to a susceptible organism, in which an infection results.

There are numerous examples of vector-borne diseases that involve a variety of pathogens and vectors, including such well-known maladies as malaria, yellow fever, Lyme disease, plague, and West Nile disease.

Disease History, Characteristics, and Transmission

Vector-borne diseases are characterized by the vector-mediated movement of a microorganism (such as a bacterium, virus, or protozoa) from the host to a recipient. The host and recipient can belong to the same species. A well-known example of this is malaria, in which the protozoan that causes the infection is acquired from an infected person by a mosquito during a blood meal and transferred to another human that the mosquito subsequently feeds on. Alternatively, the host and recipient can belong to different species. An example is western equine encephalitis, in which the host is a bird that is infected by the disease-causing species of arbovirus and the recipient is a horse or a human. As with malaria, the vector is a mosquito.

Dengue hemorrhagic fever is another example of a vector-borne disease. Dengue is caused by a virus in the *Flavivirus* genus. The virus is transmitted from the host to the susceptible person by a species of mosquito called *Aedes aegypti*.

Lyme disease is also a vector-borne disease. The disease, which is transmitted from contaminated animals such as deer to humans by the bite of several species of

tick, is the most prevalent tick-borne ailment in North America. Lyme disease is caused by a bacterium called *Borrelia burgdorferi*. It is very debilitating if not treated promptly, and can cause severe fatigue, joint pain, and heart trouble that can persist for years even when the disease is diagnosed and treated.

Still another bacterial vector-borne disease is plague. The disease, which is caused by *Yersinia pestis*, is ancient. Passages found in the Old Testament of the Bible describe the ravages of epidemics of plague. Rodents harbor the

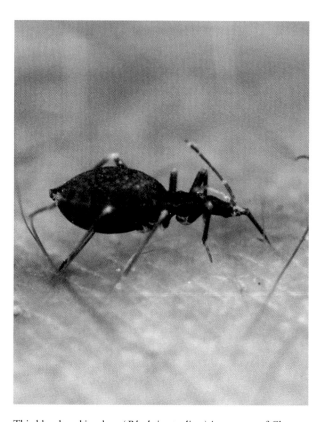

This blood-sucking bug (*Rhodnius prolixus*) is a vector of Chagas disease in humans. *Nigel Cattlin/Photo Researchers, Inc.*

bacterium. The vector that transmits the bacterium from rodents to humans is another rat or, more commonly, a flea. Both can feed on an infected rat and subsequently spread the infection to a human that they bite. There are several types of plague, depending on the site of the infection. Infection of the lungs (pneumonic plague) is almost always fatal within a week if not treated.

A final example of a vector-borne disease is yellow fever. Another viral disease caused by a member of the *Flavivirus* genus, the disease is transferred from the host (a type of monkey) to humans via a mosquito. In tropical regions, devastating outbreaks of yellow fever have occurred over the past several hundred years. A noteworthy outbreak occurred during the construction of the Panama Canal. Even today, several hundred thousand people are infected each year and about 30,000 die, according to the World Health Organization.

■ Scope and Distribution

Vector-borne diseases occur worldwide. While some diseases, such as malaria, are concentrated in tropical equatorial regions of the globe, other diseases can occur in more temperate climates. One example of a vector-borne disease found in more temperate regions is the mosquito-borne disease called West Nile disease. The West Nile virus that causes this disease has spread as far north as Canada, where it can be transmitted by mosquitoes during the warmer months of the year and even during the cooler days of spring by mosquitoes that have survived the winter.

■ Treatment and Prevention

Vector-borne diseases can be treated, and even prevented, by interrupting the vector-mediated transmission between the infected host and the susceptible person or animal. Treatment and prevention strategies for malaria focus on the mosquito vector. For example, spraying mosquito breeding grounds with insecticide can be an effective control. Indeed, the carefully controlled application of dichloro-diphenyl-trichloroethane (DDT), a powerful insecticide used in the 1960s that effectively reduced malaria vectors, but also resulted in significant loss of bird populations, is again beginning to be used as a means of mosquito control.

Another efficient and environmentally friendly way of controlling the mosquito-borne spread of malarial protozoa is draping beds with insecticide-treated mosquito netting to protect people during sleep. Organizations such as World Vision have campaigns to supply villages in Africa with bed netting. Similarly, protective clothing with overlapping upper and lower layers minimize the amount of skin that is exposed to a bite from the vector.

WORDS TO KNOW
HOST: Organism that serves as the habitat for a parasite, or possibly for a symbiont. A host may provide nutrition to the parasite or symbiont, or simply a place in which to live.
VECTOR: Any agent, living or otherwise, that carries and transmits parasites and diseases. Also, an organism or chemical used to transport a gene into a new host cell.

Another trial program aimed at preventing malaria involves releasing laboratory-bred infertile male mosquitoes. The program is based on the hypothesis that a greater population of infertile males will decrease the numbers of female mosquitoes due to reduced reproductive success. Since malaria is transmitted by female mosquitoes, fewer female mosquitoes should result in a reduction in the number of cases of malaria. There have been several successful small scale trials of this program, but the large number of sterile male mosquitoes needed is likely to make this approach impractical for larger scale implementation.

Other treatment and prevention strategies include vaccine development and the use of genetic material (known as morpholino antisense oligonucleotides) that can out-compete viral genetic material for binding onto cells of the host, blocking a crucial step in the formation of new virus particles.

■ Impacts and Issues

Vector-borne diseases exact a large toll worldwide. For example, more than 500 million cases of malaria occur each year, with approximately three million deaths attributed to the disease. One million of these deaths are children. The disease is particularly prevalent in Africa. The World Health Organization (WHO) estimates that more than 2.5 billion people are at risk for malaria. Yellow fever continues to infect hundreds of thousands of people in less developed tropical countries annually, despite the fact that a vaccine exists that can provide long-term protection. In Asia, a form of encephalitis puts about three billion people at risk each year.

The burden of these and other vector-borne diseases have a substantial economic and social impact on areas of the world that are already destitute. In malaria-prone areas, school attendance can be poor, as schoolchildren are either sick, tending for other sick family members, or have been pressed into work as parents and older siblings can no longer work due to illness.

IN CONTEXT: CHILDREN LESS THAN FIVE-YEARS-OLD SLEEPING UNDER INSECTICIDE-TREATED NETS

One means of preventing vector-borne disease is sleeping under treated nets. According to the U.S. Centers for Disease Control and Prevention (CDC), and more than one million people die from malaria (just one of many vector-transmitted diseases) per year. Young children are particularly at risk for many vector-borne disease. In some areas, bed nets are considered one of the most sustainable effective means to fight vector-borne disease.

Although disease risks vary, the list below reflects selected data from the World Health Organization that demonstrates the widest spectrum in results reported by WHO as of February 2007. Data was not available for all countries, including a lack of data for: Bangladesh, Brazil, China, Cuba, Egypt, Haiti, India, Mexico, Philippines, and not reported from some nations such as the United Kingdom and United States of America).

Lowest reported percentage of children under age 5 sleeping under insecticide-treated nets (with year data collected or reported):

- Indonesia 0.1% (2000)
- Swaziland 0.1% (2000)
- Madagascar 0.2% (2000)
- Uganda 0.2% (2000–01)
- Somalia 0.3% (1999)
- Sudan 0.4% (2000)
- Chad 0.6% (2000)
- Democratic Republic of the Congo 0.7% (2001)
- Equatorial Guinea 0.7% (2000)
- Cameroon 0.9% (2004)
- Niger 1% (2000)

Mid-range reported percentage of children under age 5 sleeping under insecticide-treated nets:

- Kenya 4.6% (2003)
- Rwanda 5% (2000)
- Zambia 6.5% (2001-02)

Highest percentage of children under age 5 sleeping under insecticide-treated nets:

- Viet Nam 15.8% (2000)
- Sao Tome and Principe 22.8% (2000)
- Malawi 35.5% (2004)

SOURCE: *World malaria report 2005. Geneva, World Health Organization and United Nations Children's Fund, 2005*

Through its Healthy Environments for Children Alliance, the WHO seeks to reduce environmental risks posed to children in under-developed countries; a major part of this program is directed at vector-borne diseases. Areas of concern include control of the spread of the vectors from their breeding grounds, the effect of increasing urbanization on the proximity of people to vector breeding grounds, and the poorer nutrition of under-developed regions (which can affect the efficiency of the immune system).

Vector-borne diseases are often difficult to treat. The vector is mobile and may be capable of movement over considerable distances. In addition, vectors can develop resistance to insecticides, as has occurred in some malaria prevention programs. Many vector insects, such as mosquitoes, have been around for millennia, and one reason for their persistence is their ability to adapt to changing environmental circumstances. Knowledge of a vector's habitat, life cycle, and migratory patterns is crucial in any effort to reduce the vector-borne spread of disease.

Global climate change is another factor in vector-borne disease. Some vectors, such as mosquitoes, thrive in warmer climates. The recent warming of the Earth's atmosphere could allow mosquitoes to inhabit more of the globe, which would undoubtedly increase the incidence of malaria and other diseases spread by these vectors.

The global nature of modern travel is an additional contributing factor to vector-borne disease transmission. Products and foods that harbor an insect vector can move virtually anywhere within hours. This increases the need for scrutiny of imported items at border crossings. In areas of the world where certain vector-borne diseases are endemic, aircraft are now routinely sprayed with insecticide after the hatches are closed and before takeoff to prevent any potential arthropod disease vectors aboard from reaching a new destination.

SEE ALSO *Arthropod-borne Disease; Bloodborne Pathogens; Host and Vector.*

BIBLIOGRAPHY

Books

Honigsbaum, Mark. *The Fever Trail: In Search of the Cure for Malaria.* New York: Picador, 2003.

Marquardt, William H. *Biology of Disease Vectors.* 2nd ed. New York: Academic Press, 2004.

Marqulies, Phillip. *West Nile Virus.* New York: Rosen Publishing Group, 2003.

Web Sites

Centers for Disease Control and Prevention. "Malaria: Vector Control." <http://www.cdc.gov/malaria/control_prevention/vector_control.htm> (accessed February 14, 2007).

Brian Hoyle

With a lack of education, hope for a more promising future can diminish, and the economy of a nation can be undermined by the illness of a sizable portion of the work force.

Viral Disease

Introduction

Viruses are microorganisms that do not have the ability to independently produce new copies of themselves. Instead, the intact virus or its payload of deoxyribonucleic acid (DNA) or ribonucleic acid (RNA) must get inside the host cell. Once inside, copies of the genetic material are made at the same time as the host's genetic material is being replicated, using the various constituents of the host's replication machinery.

Typically, the host cell eventually ruptures, releasing the newly made viruses, which in turn initiate another cycle by infecting other host cells. The host suffers, since cells are being destroyed.

There are many types of viruses that can cause infections in virtually every living thing, including humans.

Disease History, Characteristics, and Transmission

In general, viral diseases result from the attachment of a virus to the host cell and entry of either the virus particle or its genetic material into the cell. The attachment of a virion to a host involves the interaction of components of the viral and host cell outer surfaces. Often, these components are proteins, but carbohydrates and lipids can be involved. The host component is also known as the receptor. The receptor is not present specifically to allow viral infection. Rather, this host constituent has another function, and the infecting virus has evolved the capability of using this constituent to adhere to the cell surface. As one example, human immunodeficiency virus (HIV), which causes acquired immunodeficiency syndrome (AIDS, also cited as acquired immune deficiency syndrome), uses a host protein called CD4 as the receptor. HIV enters only cells, such as white blood cells, that have this receptor. The entry of the virus kills the white blood cell. Since white blood cells are important in the proper functioning of the host's immune system, their gradual destruction by HIV causes the immune system to break down, leaving the infected person vulnerable to a variety of opportunistic infections and maladies, including some types of cancer.

Following the fusion between the virion and the host cell surface, the virion or the viral genetic material enters the host cell. This fusion can happen in several different ways. An individual virion can enter the host cell in a process called endocytosis—the folding of a portion of the cell surface around the virion. The folding creates a spherical portion of the host cell's surface (a vesicle) that buds off inside the cell. The virion located inside the vesicle is degraded, releasing its genetic material. For other viruses, the viral surface layer melds with the host cell's outer surface, which releases the genetic material inside the host cell. Finally, the viral DNA or RNA can directly enter the host cell, leaving the viral particle stuck to the host cell's surface. An example of this process is the injection of DNA from a bacteriophage into the host cell that it specifically adheres to.

The viral DNA or RNA can then be replicated. In the case of DNA, this replication can occur directly, since the host's genetic material is also DNA. RNA-containing viruses, such as retroviruses (an example is HIV), require an additional step in which the viral RNA is used to make DNA. This is done using an virus-encoded enzyme called reverse transcriptase.

Depending on the virus, the replicated DNA, which is not recognized as foreign by the host's replication machinery, is used to manufacture the proteins that are encoded by the viral genes. The proteins assemble around the copies of replicated genetic material to form the new virus particles that are the hallmark of the viral disease. For other, so-called latent viruses, the replicated genetic material is incorporated into the host's DNA, where it can remain for years until certain conditions—as yet only partially understood—stimulate the viral DNA to excise and begin the production of virus particles. An active infection results. Examples of latent viral infections include AIDS, hepatitis B, Creutzfeld-Jacob disease, and herpes.

WORDS TO KNOW

BACTERIOPHAGE: A virus that infects bacteria. When a bacteriophage that carries the diphtheria toxin gene infects diphtheria bacteria, the bacteria produce diphtheria toxin.

DEGRADED: Any complex chemical that is broken down into less-complex molecules.

DEOXYRIBONUCLEIC ACID (DNA): Deoxyribonucleic acid (DNA) is a double-stranded, helical molecule that forms the molecular basis for heredity in most organisms.

ENDOCYTOSIS: Endocytosis is a process by which host cells allow the entry of outside substances, including viruses, through their cell membranes.

HOST: Organism that serves as the habitat for a parasite, or possibly for a symbiont. A host may provide nutrition to the parasite or symbiont, or simply a place in which to live.

LATENT VIRUS: Latent viruses are those viruses that can incorporate their genetic material into the genetic material of the infected host cell. Because the viral genetic material can then be replicated along with the host material, the virus becomes effectively "silent" with respect to detection by the host. Latent viruses usually contain the information necessary to reverse the latent state. The viral genetic material can leave the host genome to begin the manufacture of new virus particles.

RECEPTOR: Protein molecules on a cells surface that acts as a "signal receiver" and allow communication between cells.

REVERSE TRANSCRIPTASE: An enzyme that makes it possible for a retrovirus to produce DNA (deoxyribonucleic acid) from RNA (ribonucleic acid).

RIBONUCLEIC ACID (RNA): Any of a group of nucleic acids that carry out several important tasks in the synthesis of proteins. Unlike DNA (deoxyribonucleic acid), it has only a single strand. Nucleic acids are complex molecules that contain a cell's genetic information and the instructions for carrying out cellular processes. In eukaryotic cells, the two nucleic acids, ribonucleic acid (RNA) and deoxyribonucleic acid (DNA), work together to direct protein synthesis. Although it is DNA (deoxyribonucleic acid) that contains the instructions for directing the synthesis of specific structural and enzymatic proteins, several types of RNA actually carry out the processes required to produce these proteins. These include messenger RNA (mRNA), ribosomal RNA (rRNA), and transfer RNA (tRNA). Further processing of the various RNAs is carried out by another type of RNA called small nuclear RNA (snRNA). The structure of RNA is very similar to that of DNA, however, instead of the base thymine, RNA co

VIRION: A virion is a mature virus particle, consisting of a core of ribonucleic acid (RNA) or deoxyribonucleic acid (DNA) surrounded by a protein coat. This is the form in which a virus exists outside of its host cell.

■ Scope and Distribution

Viruses are classified into a number of families. The members of a given family share similarities in the type of genetic material and its arrangement (either as a double-strand of DNA or RNA or a single strand of the genetic material), chemistry, and physical properties, such as viral size and shape. Members of a given family differ in some characteristics from the members of another family, and different families of viruses cause different diseases.

Parvoviruses are members of the family Parvoviridae. These DNA-containing viruses are small. Their genetic material only codes for three of four proteins. Nonetheless, this small protein armada is sufficient to establish an infection. Diseases caused by parvoviruses include fifth disease, a mild illness characterized by a rash that usually occurs in children.

Papovaviruses are members of the family Papovaviridae. These DNA viruses also have a small genome that encodes five to eight proteins. Examples of papovavirus infections include warts, inflammation of the kidney (nephritis) and the urethra (urethritis), and progressive multifocal leukoencephalopathy. The latter is a disease that causes the loss of a brain component called myelin. The increasing damage to the transmission of nerve impulses is progressively disabling and can be fatal.

The 88 known adenoviruses are members of the family Adenoviridae. These viruses have a distinctive shape that consists of 20 triangular faces (an icosahedron) with long fibers protruding from 12 regions around the viral surface. Adenoviruses cause the common cold, and infections of the liver, bladder (cystitis), eye (keratoconjunctivitis), and gastrointestinal tract (gastroenteritis).

Herpesviruses are members of the family Herpesviridae. These viruses cause latent infections whose symptoms may not appear for years. The eight types of herpesvirus that can be recognized by the immune system cause a variety of infections. These infections include cell damage and the formation of ulcers in the mouth, lips (cold sores), skin, and genitals; keratoconjunctivitis, chickenpox, shingles, two forms of mononucleosis, three types of cancer (Burkitt's lymphoma, orophayngeal carcinoma, and, in AIDS patients, Kaposi's sarcoma), cytomegalovirus infection (which can be fatal in infants), and inflammation of the brain (encephalitis).

Poxviruses are members of the family Poxviridae. The name of the virus refers to the major characteristic of the diseases caused by poxviruses, namely a raised lesion on the skin (pox). Poxviruses are the largest viruses known and may be an intermediate between viruses and bacteria. However, they are still classified as viruses because they are not capable of independent replication. Diseases caused by poxviruses include smallpox, monkeypox, cowpox, and a type of skin infection. But, all poxviruses are not deadly. A poxvirus called vaccinia virus can bestow immunity to smallpox.

Viruses in the families Hepadnaviridae and Coronaviridae cause type B hepatitis and liver cancer, and the common cold, respectively.

Picornaviruses are RNA-containing viruses that are members of the family Picornaviridae. They are the smallest of the RNA viruses, coding for only six to nine genes. Infections caused by picornaviruses include polio, meningitis, the common cold, inflammation of the heart (myocarditis), and inflammation of the tissue surrounding the heart (pericarditis).

Calciviruses are members of the family Calciviridae. There are two members of note. The first is the Norwalk virus, which is notorious for causing disease outbreaks on cruise ships and in crowded communal areas, such as university residences. The virus causes a contagious form of gastroenteritis that is characterized by several days of intense diarrhea and vomiting. The second virus is hepatitis E, which is frequently fatal if contracted by pregnant women. In fact, Hepatitis E is fatal to the woman up to 20% of the time, especially during the third trimester.

Of the more than 150 known types of reovirus, two are significant to humans, causing encephalitis and, most commonly, diarrhea in infants. The latter infection, which is caused by rotavirus, produces dehydration that is fatal if not treated quickly.

Togaviruses are members of the family Togaviridae. Infections caused by togaviruses include rubella (also called German measles), various forms of encephalitis, inflammation of joints (arthritis), and skin inflammation.

Flaviviruses are members of the family Flaviviridae. These viruses cause a number of serious human infections that are transmitted by insects, such as mosquitoes. These infections include yellow fever, dengue, West Nile disease, and encephalitis.

Arenaviruses are members of the family Arenaviridae. The infections caused by arenaviruses are also serious and include hemorrhagic fever and inflammation of the brain and spinal cord or the membranes that cover these regions (lymphocytic choriomeningitis).

Retroviruses, which are members of the family Retroviridae, are given this name because they contain genetic information for the production of an enzyme called reverse transcriptase. The enzyme allows the viral RNA to be used to produce DNA. Retroviruses are important human pathogens, causing cancer of the blood (leukemia) and, most significantly, AIDS.

Orthomyxoviruses include several types of influenza virus, including influenza A (H5N1), which is the cause of avian influenza. Avian influenza is one example of an emerging disease. Other orthomyxoviruses can cause hemorrhagic fever and, along with bunyaviruses, encephalitis. Another viral class, paramyxovirus, includes the virus that causes measles.

Coronaviruses belongs to the family Coronaviridae. A coronavirus of particular significance causes severe acute respiratory syndrome (SARS), and is another example of an emerging disease.

Finally, filoviruses are members of the family Filoviridae. The two known filoviruses are Marburg and Ebola virus, which cause hemorrhagic fevers that can be severe and rapidly lethal. Relatively little is known about the infectious disease processes of these viruses or of their natural hosts because they are so dangerous to work with (a special containment facility called a biosafety level 4 laboratory is required for research on these microbes) and because illness outbreaks appear sporadically and end quickly.

■ Treatment and Prevention

Reflecting the diversity of viruses and viral diseases, treatment is variable. One common characteristic is the ineffectiveness of antibiotics, since antibiotics are effective against bacteria. Treatment strategies include blocking the attachment of the virus to host cells by occupying the host cell receptor with another molecule, use of a vaccine that has been developed for a particular virus or a similar target of different viruses, and taking medications that assist the immune system in responding to the presence of the infecting virus.

Likewise, prevention strategies vary. Wearing a protective mask to prevent inhalation of viral-contaminated droplets is mandated for healthcare providers when treating someone known or suspected of having SARS, for example. Protective gowns and gloves can be prudent measures when coming into contact with someone who has a hemorrhagic fever, since splashing or copious loss of blood can occur. Another viral barrier is the condom. Wearing a condom can lessen the risk of transmission of HIV during sexual intercourse. Complete abstinence from sex is the ultimate preventative strategy for sexually-transmitted viral disease, although this strategy can be difficult to follow in everyday life.

The incidence of viral diseases, such as West Nile disease, that are transmitted by insects can be reduced by eradicating insect breeding grounds and wearing clothing that protects the body from insect bites. Insect repellents are also a helpful preventative measure.

■ Impacts and Issues

The toll from viral diseases throughout history is incalculable. The death toll from viral gastroenteritis and measles exceeds 2 million each year, according to the World Health Organization (WHO). In the past 40 years, AIDS has grown in scope from a handful of cases to over 40 million cases and almost 3 million deaths in 2006.

The tragedy of many viral diseases is their concentration in poorer regions of the world, where access to health care and personal living conditions are not as good as in developed countries, such as the United States. AIDS, for example, exacts a huge toll in sub-Saharan Africa. It is common to find villages populated mainly by pre-adolescents and the elderly, with the generations from 20–60 having been decimated. Aside from the human tragedy, the massive loss of the majority of productive wage earners is economically devastating. Many African nations have been economically crippled and little relief is foreseen for generations.

One tragic aspect of the viral disease situation in under-developed and developing countries is that treatments, including vaccines, exist for some of these diseases, but they are not readily available or affordable in these countries. Distribution of the needed medical supplies has been and continues to be driven mainly by humanitarian initiatives of organizations such as the WHO, UNICEF, and the U.S. Centers for Disease Control and Prevention, rather than by commercial interests.

Finally, several of the highest profile emerging diseases are viral diseases. Ebola, avian influenza, and SARS are examples of diseases that have emerged as problems only relatively recently. Of these, avian influenza is a particular concern, since the virus that causes this disease may have developed the ability to spread directly from person to person, instead of only spreading from poultry to humans. This evolution combined with the expanding geographical range of the disease has raised concerns that this virus could cause a worldwide epidemic of a serious and frequently lethal form of influenza.

SEE ALSO *AIDS (Acquired Immunodeficiency Syndrome); Antiviral Drugs; Arthropod-borne Disease; Avian Influenza; B virus (Cercopithecine herpesvirus 1) Infection; CMV (Cytomegalovirus) Infection; Eastern Equine Encephalitis; Ebola; H5N1 Virus; Hepatitis A; Hepatitis B; Hepatitis C; Hepatitis D; Hepatitis E; Influenza Pandemic of 1918; Influenza Pandemic of 1957; Influenza, Tracking Seasonal Influences and Virus Mutation; Influenza; Measles (Rubeola); Monkeypox; Mononucleosis; Mosquito-borne diseases; Mumps; Nipah Virus Encephalitis; Norovirus Infection; Polio (Poliomyelitis); Polio Eradication Campaign; Rabies; Retroviruses; Rotavirus Infection; RSV (Respiratory Syncytial Virus) Infection; SARS (Severe Acute Respiratory Syndrome); St. Louis Encephalitis; West Nile.*

BIBLIOGRAPHY

Books

Collier, Leslie, and John Oxford. *Human Virology.* New York: Oxford University Press, 2006.

Tabor, Edward. *Emerging Viruses in Human Populations.* New York: Elsevier, 2007.

Periodicals

The Writing Committee of the World Health Organization Consultation on Human Influenza A/H5. "Avian Influenza A (H5N1) Infection in Humans." *New England Journal of Medicine* 353 (September 29, 2005): 1374–1385.

Brian Hoyle

Virus Hunters

The people of San Joaquim were dying—they were bleeding to death from a disease nobody had ever seen before. They called it "el tifo negro," the black typhus, later to become known as Bolivian hemorrhagic fever. In this little one-horse garrison town in the lowlands on the Amazonian side of the Bolivian Andes, close to the Brazil border, soldiers and citizens alike were sickening, and no one knew why.

Under the Alliance for Progress established by President John F. Kennedy (1917–1963) between the United States and Latin America, Bolivia asked for help from the United States, and a team was flown in from the National Institute of Health's Middle America Research Unit in the Panama Canal Zone. Heading it was physician Karl Johnson, one of the great virus hunters of the end of the twentieth century. I was greatly privileged to be working with his team, on a traveling fellowship from the Rockefeller Foundation, at the time he isolated the causative agent from a human case. It was a new virus, which he named Machupo virus, after a local place name.

Everybody knows that viruses are really nasty pieces of work. They are even smaller than bacteria, and untouched by antibiotics, so for many there is no cure, nor even a preventive vaccine. They are responsible for some of the deadliest diseases on the planet: Ebola,

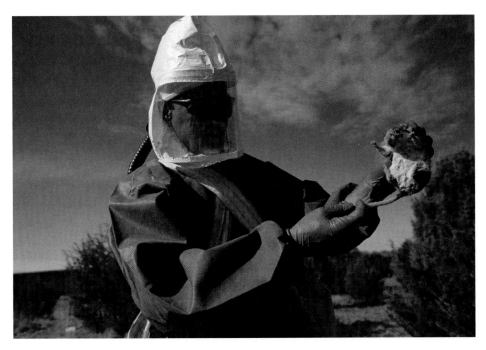

A researcher from the Centers for Disease Control and Prevention (CDC) inspects a deer mouse that was trapped for a study of hantaviruses in New Mexico in 2000. The deer mouse is a carrier of the Hantavirus, which can cause the often-deadly Hantavirus pulmonary syndrome in humans. © Karen Kasmauski/Corbis.

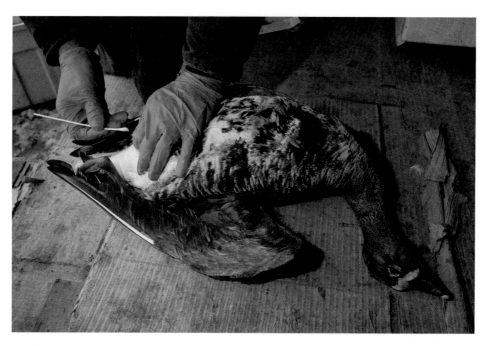

A wildlife biologist uses a cotton swab to sample fecal matter from a white-fronted goose in Alaska in June 2006. Officials from the USDA began testing migratory birds arriving from Asia and Russia for the avian influenza, also known as the bird flu. *Justin Sullivan/Getty Images.*

yellow fever, smallpox, AIDS, SARS (severe acute respiratory syndrome), polio, and influenza, both human and bird, to name only seven. The scientists who tackled them have gone down in history as the "virus hunters," and some of them paid for their research with their lives.

At the beginning of the twentieth century, the United States Army played a prominent role in the fight against yellow fever. A number of United States military physicians and volunteers died in early tests that proved that the virus was transmitted by mosquitoes. This discovery paved the way for control programs led by General William C. Gorgas, which resulted in the eradication of yellow fever from Havana, Cuba, and of the urban disease from Brazil. It also permitted the completion of the Panama Canal, work on which had been stalled by the huge toll exacted by yellow fever and malaria.

The Rockefeller Foundation's International Health Division set up laboratories in Africa and South America specifically to study yellow fever at its source. Six of their researchers died of the disease, but their work paid off with the isolation of the virus and the development of the 17D yellow fever vaccine, still one of the best vaccines ever invented.

The stories of these pioneer researchers are told in many books, but I want to tell you about two modern virus hunters with whom I had the good fortune to work myself. In San Joaquim, Karl Johnson had set up a breeding colony of hamsters and a separate infected animal room, well screened against mosquitoes and with the individual cages fitted with virus filters in their steel

mesh lids. A separate lab had a glove box, inside which the hamsters could be inoculated safely with specimens. The only problem with this was that there was only one glove box, and it had to be sterilized with a disinfectant spray and left for an hour between each litter of hamsters inoculated, which slowed down the work and meant working very late hours. There was also a thatched hut where the zoologist took the rodents he trapped in the town for processing and where the entomologist combed their fur for ectoparasites, such as ticks and mites, in case these were involved in the transmission of the disease (they weren't). There was an autopsy room for humans, but the dead cow that came in at night with a history of bleeding had to be necropsied on a wooden bullock cart in the open air by the light of hurricane lamps. The cow was negative for the virus.

The colonel in charge of the town's garrison invited us to take our meals with him in his quarters. There is a photo of him at the head of the table dining with the team. A week later he was dead from the black typhus. But shortly after that there was euphoria—hamsters inoculated with autopsy material from another victim came down with signs of infection, and a virus was isolated from their brains. Now reagents could be made to test for antibodies in the blood of survivors and wildlife.

The next step was to find out where the disease was coming from and how to stop its transmission. Karl suspected the wild rodents that seemed to have recently overrun the town. He set up a system to trap out all the rats in one half of the place. Lo and behold, after that,

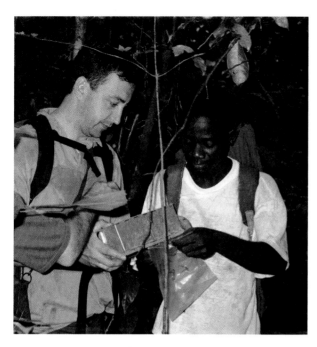

Dr. Pierre Formenty transfers a mouse from a trap into a plastic bag in the Tai Forest on the Ivory Coast in 1996. Formenty led a World Health Organization (WHO) team studying mice and other animals in the Tai Forest as they tried to locate the source of the deadly Ebola virus. *AP Images.*

WORDS TO KNOW

ANTIGEN: Antigens, which are usually proteins or polysaccharides, stimulate the immune system to produce antibodies. The antibodies inactivate the antigen and help to remove it from the body. While antigens can be the source of infections from pathogenic bacteria and viruses, organic molecules detrimental to the body from internal or environmental sources also act as antigens. Genetic engineering and the use of various mutational mechanisms allow the construction of a vast array of antibodies (each with a unique genetic sequence).

ANTIGENIC SHIFT: Antigenic shift describes an abrupt and major genetic change (e.g. in genes coding for surface proteins of a virus).

DROPLET TRANSMISSION: Droplet transmission is the spread of microorganisms from one space to another (including from person to person) via droplets that are larger than 5 microns in diameter. Droplets are typically expelled into the air by coughing and sneezing.

NECROPSY: A necropsy is a medical examination of a dead body: also called an autopsy.

PANDEMIC: Pandemic, which means all the people, describes an epidemic that occurs in more than one country or population simultaneously.

STRAIN: A subclass or a specific genetic variation of an organism.

no more cases occurred in that area. So the trapping was extended to the whole town, and the epidemic was stopped cold.

What eventually emerged was an extraordinary story. Apparently anti-malaria teams had deluged the town with DDT on a control visit. Cats are highly susceptible to DDT, and they get a fatal dose of it by preening their fur after being caught in the spraying or rubbing against surfaces that have been sprayed. All the cats in the town had died, so the wild rodents from the fields and forest around the town were able to infiltrate the houses in their quest for easy pickings. Some of them were infected with the virus, which they excreted in their urine and droppings inside houses. These dried out in the tropical heat and turned to dust, which, when stirred up by walking through or sweeping the rooms, was inhaled by the inhabitants, giving them the disease. So an intervention to control one fatal disease ended up causing another.

All this was in 1963. Thirteen years later, Karl was working for the United States Public Health Service as head of the Centers for Disease Control's Special Pathogens lab (the euphemism for the lab that handled the most dangerous disease agents known, needing Biosafety Level 4 containment, either in a chain of glove boxes or in negative pressure labs with the researchers wearing space suits). He found himself called out to investigate another hemorrhagic fever epidemic, this time in Yambuku, Zaire (now known as the Democratic Republic of the Congo). The American researchers found that the virus was transmitted by the inadequately sterilized, reused needles and syringes used for giving injections to the patients. The epidemic was being spread in the hospital. Worse, local burial custom demanded that the relatives remove by hand the viscera of the dead person, and of course this was done with out any concept of sterile precautions, so that the blood of the deceased infected the relatives. When these practices in the hospital and home were stopped, the epidemic ceased.

Karl's lab showed that the disease agent was a new member of a new family of viruses, the Filoviridae or "thread viruses" because they looked like partially coiled threads (some say more like shepherd's crooks) under the electron microscope. Karl named it Ebola virus, after a nearby river. He couldn't call it Congo virus because that name had already been taken by another, different virus isolated earlier in the same country, which was eventually named as the causative agent of Crimean-Congo hemorrhagic fever.

The labs run by Karl were dynamic places full of eager young researchers bubbling over with ideas about the viruses that cause disease and their epidemiology—where they hide in nature, how they are transmitted, and why they suddenly emerge to cause outbreaks. I would dearly have liked to have joined his lab, but instead I was hired by the Rockefeller Foundation to run their virus lab at the mouth of the Amazon, and so came to know well another modern virus hunter—Bob Shope.

I first met Bob on that same Rockefeller Foundation travel fellowship that took me to Bolivia. His family was away at the time and I was a guest in his home in Belem, Brazil, so we spent many happy hours both in the lab and in his house discussing the riddles of the viruses of the rain forest. His lab had a small mammal recapture program with a grid of traps in the forest at the edge of town, where wild rodents and marsupials were trapped daily, weighed and measured, and obliged to donate a blood sample so that their medical history could be followed. They were exposed to forest mosquitoes that transmitted all sorts of interesting viruses to them, which were then isolated from their blood samples in lab mice. Many of the viruses were new to science. Other mammals such as bats, sloths, and tree porcupines were also caught and studied, and a series of ingenious mosquito traps baited with monkeys or mice were run daily to provide pools of mosquitoes, sorted by species, which also yielded more such viruses. There were even lab workers who volunteered to go out into the forest at night to catch mosquitoes coming to bite them. Some of the human volunteers didn't manage to catch all the mosquitoes before the insects got their bites in, so they came down with jungle fevers. The viruses isolated from their blood provided proof that some of these new viruses could cause disease in people who went into the forest to hunt, collect timber, or clear plantations.

When Bob left Belem for the Yale Arbovirus Research Center (YARU), where he worked as researcher and then director for 30 years, I took over his lab and kept in close touch with him for many years. "Arbovirus" is short for "arthropod-borne virus," meaning viruses transmitted by fleas, ticks, and mites, as well as mosquitoes. YARU became a World Health Organization Collaborating Center and the world reference center for these and other viruses, because many viruses isolated from wildlife by field labs established around the world by the Rockefeller Foundation, France's Pasteur Institutes, and others turned out not to be transmitted by arthropods—notably Machupo and Ebola. Bob became a living encyclopedia of information on the origins and interrelationships of hundreds of viruses from around the world, including the many viruses from wildlife related to rabies. Some of these have become what we now call emerging diseases. He mentored students and post-docs from around the world, who worked in his lab on Rift Valley fever, Lassa fever, Argentinean, Brazilian, and Venezuelan hemorrhagic fevers, and other dangerous viruses. But he never forgot the lessons from his field experience in Brazil with exotically named viruses such as Caraparu, Oriboca, and Marituba. After his retirement, the YARU lab closed and he took the world reference collection of arboviruses to the University of Texas Medical Branch at Galveston, where he worked until his death in 2004.

So although it is all the rage now to go into molecular virology and sequencing, I hope that at least some of today's students will be inspired by the examples of Karl and Bob to go out into the field and get their hands dirty trapping wildlife and mosquitoes, finding out what viruses they are carrying and what makes those viruses tick. Because those viruses are the emerging diseases of the future, and we need to know as much as we can about them before they strike.

SEE ALSO *Arthropod-borne Disease; Ebola; Emerging Infectious Diseases; Epidemiology; Hemorrhagic Fevers; Tropical Infectious Diseases; Vector-borne Disease.*

BIBLIOGRAPHY

Books

Peters, C.J., and Mark Olshaker. *Virus Hunter: Thirty Years of Battling Hot Viruses around the World.* New York: Anchor, 1998.

Periodicals

Cowley, Geoffrey. "The Life of a Virus Hunter." *Newsweek* (May 15, 2006).

Glaser, Vicki. "A Career Path in Arbovirology—An Interview with Robert E. Shope, M.D." *Vector-bone and Zoonotic Diseases* 3, 1 (March 2003): 53-56.

Sheldon, Tony. "The Virus Hunter." *BMJ* 327 (October 25, 2003): 950.

Web Sites

Centers for Disease Control and Prevention. "Tracking a Mystery Disease: The Detailed Story of Hantavirus Pulmonary Syndrome." <http://www.cdc.gov/ncidod/diseases/hanta/hps/noframes/outbreak.htm> (accessed June 14, 2007).

Jack Woodall

War and Infectious Disease

■ Introduction

Throughout history, war epidemics have sapped and destroyed the ability of armies to fight, halted military operations, and brought death and disaster to the civilian populations of the warring factions as well as non-belligerent states. The historical occurrence and geographical spread of infectious diseases associated with wars raises the question of how the distribution of disease in epidemics is influenced by military operations. Historically, epidemics have been associated with military mobilization and the bringing together of tens and even hundreds of thousands of individuals into close quarters and contact in camps and garrisons. Deployment to parts of the world in which diseases are endemic, emerging, or re-emerging expose troops to diseases for which they have no immunity. Lastly, there is the age-old and familiar association of soldiers with prostitutes harboring sexually transmitted diseases. While the history of the impact of war on the emergence and spread of epidemics is long and tragic, this article will be focused on a few instances that bear on contemporary public health issues.

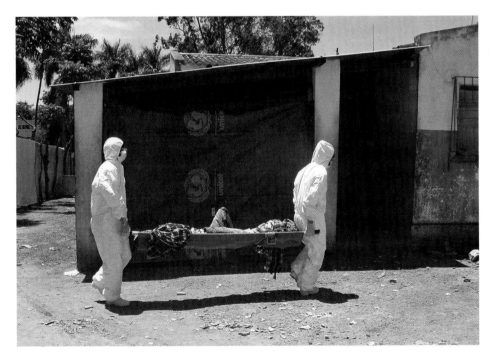

Medical workers carry a resident suffering from the deadly Marburg hemorrhagic fever in northern Angola in 2005. Battered by nearly three decades of civil war, hospitals in the country became a breeding ground for the Marburg virus, which has killed more than 200 people. © Reuters/Corbis.

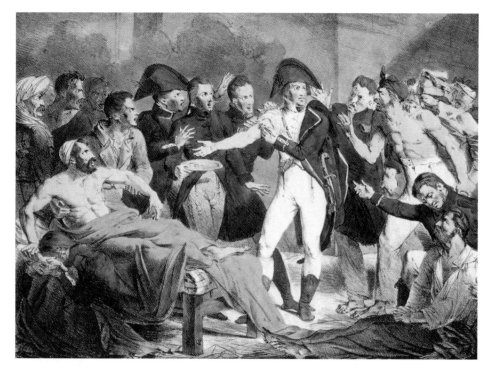

In this 19th-century engraving, the chief medical officer of the French army in Egypt, Baron René-Nicolas Dufriche Desgenettes (1762–1837), inoculates himself with the plague in the presence of sick soldiers. *Réunion des Musées Nationaux/Art Resource, NY.*

History and Scientific Foundations

The 1918 Influenza Pandemic and World War I

In view of contemporary concerns about the recurrence of a worldwide bird flu pandemic, the association of World War I with the first known avian influenza pandemic is of particular interest. With the possible exception of the ultimate death toll of the AIDS pandemic, which has unfolded over more than a quarter of a century, the 1918–1919 influenza pandemic killed more people than any other outbreak of disease in human history. Estimates of the death toll range from a low of 21 million to a more recent and well-supported estimate of 50 to 100 million dead. At the time of the epidemic, the world population was only 28% of what it is currently, and the majority of the deaths occurred during a sixteen-week period, from mid-September to mid-December of 1918.

The origin of the 1918 pandemic, sometimes called the "Spanish flu," is still a mystery. Except that the virus did not originate in Spain, the exact origin of the virus strain that caused the 1918 flu pandemic remains in dispute. One hypothesis recently advanced is based upon epidemiological research that suggests the most likely site of origin was Haskell County, Kansas, an isolated

and sparsely populated county in the southwest corner of the state, in January 1918. Some epidemiologists argue that competing hypotheses (that the pandemic originated in Asia, or that it began in British Army camps) are not as well supported as evidence that the flu might have spread between United States Army camps and might have been carried by American troops to Europe. The first known U.S. outbreak of epidemic influenza was identified in epidemiological studies and in lay accounts as having occurred at Camp Funston, now Fort Riley, in Kansas. However, a previously unknown epidemic of influenza occurred in Haskell County, Kansas, 300 mi (483 km) west of Funston.

In late January and early February of 1918, a local physician in the county faced an epidemic of influenza of extraordinary suddenness and lethality. Dozens of previously strong and healthy patients were struck down as suddenly "as if they had been shot." They then progressed to pneumonia and began to die. The local epidemic raged and worsened for several weeks and then disappeared as suddenly as it had emerged. Although influenza was not a reportable disease, the physician warned national public health officials, and this warning was published by the U.S. Public Health Service in "Public Health Reports" the Service's progenitor report to Morbidity and Mortality Weekly Report (MMWR). This report was the only reference in that journal to influenza anywhere in the world during the first six months of 1918. It was the first recorded instance in history of an influenza outbreak so violent that a physician warned public health officials, suggesting a new virus was adapting to humans with lethal effect.

During the Haskell County outbreak, local Army personnel reported to Funston for training. Also, friends and family visited them at Funston and soldiers came home on leave and then returned to Funston. The local press recorded several cases between February 26 and March 2 of people from the county who had visited the army base who either fell ill themselves or who had children that were stricken with influenza and pneumonia. The first soldier at the camp reported ill with influenza at sick call on March 4. Within three weeks, more than 1,100 soldiers at the camp, which held an average of 56,222 troops, required hospitalization, and thousands more required infirmary treatment. Meanwhile, Funston sent an uninterrupted stream of men to other American locations and to Europe, especially France. On March 18, influenza cases were reported in Camps Forrest and Greenleaf in Georgia. By the end of April, 24 of the 36 main Army camps suffered an influenza epidemic. Thirty of the 50 largest cities in the country also had a spike in excess mortality from influenza and pneumonia in April.

Also at the end of April, influenza erupted in France, beginning at Brest, the main port of disembarkation for American troops. After that, army operations proved to be the most influential factor in the spread of the epidemic elsewhere in the world. It seems likely that military policymakers either did not appreciate the role of their operations in spreading the epidemic or chose to regard it as an unfortunate but necessary consequence of war. Another lesson from this occurrence has been that a worldwide flu epidemic could potentially emerge anywhere, including a sparsely populated county in the United States, not only in a densely populated region in Asia.

Typhus Fever in World War I

As devastating as the 1918 flu pandemic was for the military and civilian populations alike during the latter part of World War I, it probably did not influence the course of the war and of history as much as the outbreak of typhus fever on the European Eastern Front during the first World War. Typhus fever is a louse-borne disease, and the lice that carry typhus fever are common in large aggregations of persons who do not bathe or change clothes with any regularity and are forced by circumstances to live in close quarters, which are also the situations that infantry, refugees, and prisoners are likely to encounter. In late November of 1914, typhus fever, which had been endemic in Serbia for centuries, began to appear among Serbian refugees fleeing the Austrian attack on Belgrade. Shortly afterwards, cases

were reported from the army and among the prisoners of war, but caused little alarm. However, this disease had played a decisive role earlier in European military history, when, in 1812, typhus fever shattered Napoleon's invasion of Russia, destroying the French army well before it reached Moscow.

The Austrian invasion was soon repulsed, but the devastation of Northern Serbia created ripe conditions for the spread of typhus. The first outbreak of cases occurred among Austrian prisoners at Valjevo, followed within a week by outbreaks throughout the rest of the country. The infection traveled with the refugee population, on prisoner of war trains, and with moving armies, and was rapidly disseminated to all parts of Serbia, resulting in a scene of horror reminiscent of the Black Death. At the start of World War I, Serbia numbered some three million people. Within six months, one in six Serbians developed typhus fever. Over 200,000 people, including 70,000 Serbian troops and half of the 60,000 Austrian prisoners, died from the disease. The outbreak spread beyond Serbia into Russia, as the famine and dislocation of the Russian revolution destroyed sanitation and social infrastructure, eventually resulting in 20 million cases in that country, half of whom died.

War and Forced Migration

A study carried out between January and March 2004, with Liberian refugee women staying at the United Nations refugee camp at a village in Nigeria, shows how forced migration contributes to increased incidence of communicable diseases. Liberia's civil war resulted in approximately 215,000 refugees at the end of 2001. During the civil war, according to some estimates, up to 40% of all Liberian women were raped. Loss of family exposed women to increased rape, prostitution, and increasing risk of HIV and other sexually transmitted infections. Lack of postwar shelter compounds other problems and increased exposure to mosquito-borne diseases. Lack of clean drinking water introduced risks of bacillary dysentery, cholera, diarrheal disease, typhoid, hepatitis A, and other diseases.

Recent War Experience: Operation Iraqi Freedom

In the spring of 2003, 83,000 United States Marines participated in the opening phase of Operation Iraqi Freedom. A Navy Preventive Medicine Department laboratory was set up to provide diagnostic support for Marine medical units during a period of repositioning in south-central Iraq. Specimen collection boxes were sent to more than 30 primary-care medical stations handling 500-900 personnel each. The laboratory had the capability to detect many different disease agents. By far the most common reason for infectious disease sick call visits was gastrointestinal illness; no other symptoms had equivalent impact. An enteropathogen was detected in 23% of stool samples, with norovirus detected in 30 stool samples obtained from 14 different battalion or similar-sized units; next in frequency were *Shigella flexneri* and *Shigella sonnei*, which were isolated from 26 stool samples (20%) obtained from 15 units. Ciprofloxacin was effective *in vitro* against most bacterial agents, but neither doxycycline (which was taken daily as the antimalarial prophylaxis dose) nor trimethoprim-sulfamethoxazole were effective. Otherwise, personnel remained free of infectious illness during this phase of the conflict, because other infectious agents were rare or absent.

War Wounds

Nothing is more basic to a discussion of war and infectious disease than the control of wound infections. Prior to contemporary efficient and airborne medevac procedures, military surgeons worked by a rule of thumb:

patch up and move on. Even today, at frontline dressing stations no time is wasted on the hopelessly injured. A seriously wounded soldier has to survive the stretcher trip through the field treatment station, hospital station, evacuation hospital to base hospital, sometimes in a different country, before he or she receives the medical luxuries of thorough surgical care, as when American combatants in contemporary Iraq are given definitive treatment in a hospital in Germany. It is a given in the military that "every wound is infected." For example, prior to World War I, tetanus, a great killer in all previous wars, was practically eliminated by routine injections of anti-tetanic serum to all wounded soldiers.

Penicillin was first tested for military use in the spring of 1943. By autumn, doctors were using the antibiotic in combat zones, where it was limited to American and Allied military and to patients with life-threatening infections. Flight crews of the Eighth Air Force stationed in Britain were the first to directly benefit from the drug. Rationing was necessary, as a single infection could require two million or more units of the drug. During the war, the armed forces received 85% of the nation's production. With the implementation of successful mass-production techniques, production of units tripled during 1944–1945. Penicillin became the war's wonder drug, and its remarkable medical effects on infectious disease made World War II different from any previous war.

The mass production of penicillin for military use gave impetus to the widespread use of antibiotics to fight infection on a wide scale in civil society after the war. Contemporary antibiotic-resistant bacterial strains pose an analogous threat to wounded troops. In spite of antibiotic treatment and better antiseptic practices under combat conditions, it is still necessary to debride wounds and amputate seriously damaged limbs under combat situations in order to prevent gangrene and other runaway infection. The first use of debridement, the surgical excision of necrotic (dead) or infected tissue and the removal of foreign bodies from contaminated wounds to forestall infection, was made by a French medical officer in 1914. Prior to the introduction of debridement, all but simple incised wounds were treated by surgically opening the wound, removing obvious foreign bodies, and then irrigating with sterile salt solution or oxidizers such as hydrogen peroxide in an attempt to sterilize the lesion. The wound was left open and freely drained or was packed with gauze, and immobilized by suitable splints if necessary. Discharge of pus was treated by drainage tubes made of glass or rubber.

War and Public Health Infrastructure Damage

Often the public health impact of war goes unmeasured, but efforts were made to gauge the effects of the Balkan wars in the early 1990s. A public health assessment in

Bosnia-Herzegovina and in the areas of Serbia and Montenegro hosting Bosnian refugees in 1993 revealed widespread disruption to basic health services, displacement of more than one million Bosnians, severe food shortages in Muslim enclaves, and extensive destruction of public water and sanitation systems. War-related violence was the most important public health risk in that nation. Civilians on all sides of the conflict were intentional targets of physical and sexual violence. The impact of the war on the health status of the population was difficult to document; however, in central Bosnia, perinatal and child mortality rates doubled between 1991 and 1993. The crude death rate in one Muslim enclave between April 1992 and March 1993 was four times the pre-war rate. Prevalence rates of severe malnutrition among both adults and children in central Bosnia increased steadily throughout the course of the conflict. Major epidemics of communicable diseases were not reported, however, but public health conditions were ripe for such epidemics. The lack of epidemics in this case is scientifically significant to infectious disease studies. It challenges many historical assertions and assumptions about public health in war time.

■ Impacts and Issues

The intentional release of biological agents by belligerents or terrorists is a possibility that has received urgent attention following the anthrax attacks in the United States in 2001, but which was under intensive study by the military prior to that time. Law enforcement agencies, military planners, public health officials, and clinicians are gaining an increasing awareness of this potential threat. From a military perspective, an important component of the protective pre-exposure resources against this threat is immunization. In addition, certain vaccines are an accepted component of post-exposure prophylaxis against potential bioterrorist threat agents. These vaccines might, therefore, be used to respond to a terrorist attack against civilians.

Biological warfare agents may be classified in several ways: (1) operationally, as lethal or incapacitating agents, and as agents with or without potential for secondary transmission; (2) according to intended target, as antipersonnel, antianimal, antiplant, or antimateriel; and (3) according to type, as replicating pathogens, toxins, or biomodulators. Among the greatest threats are both replicating pathogens (bacteria and viruses) and toxins.

Anthrax: Fortunately, few infectious agents possess characteristics suitable for effective large-scale employment. However, *Bacillus anthracis* has properties that are ideal for this purpose. It is omnipresent in soil and the ease with which it can be cultured makes anthrax readily available to armies and to terrorists. Its lethality, ability to form tough spores, and its affinity for aerosoli-

zation (production as a fine mist) combine to make anthrax one of the greatest biological threats. Anthrax was prominent in the biological weapons programs of Iraq and the former Soviet Union; the Aum Shinrikyo cult also stockpiled it. The World Health Organization (WHO) estimates that the release of 110 lb. (50 kg) of anthrax spores along a 1.2-mi (2-km) line upwind of a city of 500,000 people would produce 125,000 infections and 95,000 deaths, far more than with any other agent considered. Consequently, research programs at military laboratories have devoted considerable effort to improving on the anthrax vaccines that have been in use for decades.

Plague: One of the earliest recorded attempts at biological warfare was the effort of besieging Tatar warriors to catapult the corpses of their own plague victims over the city walls of Kaffa in the Crimea in order to initiate an epidemic within the city. The Japanese released millions of infected fleas over Manchurian cities, resulting in numerous human plague cases. During the Vietnam War, plague vaccine was routinely administered to members of the United States armed services, and only eight cases of plague were reported among this population, which corresponds to a rate of about one case per million person-years of exposure. The success of this vaccine is evident when compared with the 330-fold greater incidence of plague among the unvaccinated South Vietnamese civilian population.

Brucellosis: Brucellosis is considered to be an incapacitating agent likely to produce large numbers of casualties but little mortality. Nevertheless, brucellosis is highly infective. In the 1950s the United States chose *Brucella suis* as the first agent to be produced for its biological warfare program. Veterinary vaccines that have significant efficacy against brucellosis have been studied and employed. The vaccination of livestock in combination with the slaughter of infected animals is largely responsible for the declining incidence of human brucellosis. In the United States, the decline of human brucellosis cases reported to the CDC has paralleled the control of infections due to *Brucella abortus* in cattle.

Tularemia: *Francisella tularensis* is sometimes considered a lethal biological warfare agent, since high-dose aerosol dissemination would result in a disproportionate number of cases of the pneumonic form of tularemia. *F. tularensis* followed *B. suis* into the United States bioweapons program in 1955, and extensive testing of the weaponization potential of the agent was conducted in human volunteers at Fort Detrick. The organism was also thought to have been prominent in the biological arsenal of the Soviet Union. American and Russian collaboration has provided the seed stock for tularemia vaccines currently in use throughout the world.

Q fever: *Coxiella burnetii*, the causative agent of Q fever, is a gram-negative coccobacillus resistant to heat and dryness that grows easily in embryonated chicken eggs and is highly infectious by aerosol. This organism was cultivated by the United States bioweapons program as a potential incapacitating agent.

Smallpox: Although endemic smallpox was eradicated throughout the world in 1977, the virus remains a potential biological weapon in the eyes of many military planners. Concerns persist that clandestine stocks of virus may exist outside of CDC in Atlanta, Georgia, and Koltsovo in Russia, the two WHO-authorized repositories of the virus.

Botulism: Iraq chose to weaponize botulinum toxin during the Gulf War in 1991, although its usefulness as a weapon might be limited by its instability during storage and modest range upon aerosolization. Nonetheless, when delivered by aerosolization, botulinum toxins would be expected to produce cases of typical clinical botulism. Moreover, terrorists might also use botulinum toxins to sabotage food supplies. No licensed vaccine exists today.

Staphylococcal enterotoxin B (SEB) intoxication: SEB is one of several pyrogenic exotoxins produced by Staphylococcus aureus, and is considered a viable incapacitating agent by biological warfare planners. Although SEB is a cause of food-borne disease, its use in biological warfare would likely involve aerosolization, with which it would cause a systemic fever accompanied by pulmonary symptoms. No SEB vaccine is currently available for human use.

Although the United States Department of Defense has initiated an anthrax immunization campaign through-out the armed forces, it is likely that other anti-biological-warfare vaccines will eventually be employed to protect armed services personnel. In a civilian context, use of these vaccines is more problematic, because the nature of the threat is less well defined. Nonetheless, certain vaccines, such as anthrax and smallpox, may have applicability in the prevention and management of exposed civilian populations.

SEE ALSO *Anthrax; Bioterrorism; Influenza Pandemic of 1918; Plague, Early History; Plague, Modern History; Public Health and Infectious Disease.*

BIBLIOGRAPHY

Books

Barry, J.M. *The Great Influenza: The Epic Story of the Deadliest Plague in History.* New York: Viking, 2004.

Zinsser, Hans. *Rats, Lice and History.* Boston: Little, Brown & Company, 1935 (reprinted 1996).

Periodicals

Toole, M.J., S. Galson, and W. Brady. "Refugees, Forced Displacement, and War: Are War and Public Health Compatible?" *The Lancet* 341, 8854 (May 8, 1993): 1193–1196.

Web Sites

Jiang, X., et al. *Cabi.org.* "Gastroenteritis in U.S. Marines During Operation Iraqi Freedom." <http://www.cababstractsplus.org/google/abstract.asp?AcNo=20053058791> (accessed June 1, 2007).

U.S. Army Center for Health Promotion and Disease Prevention. "Medical Threats Briefing Homepage." <http://usachppm.apgea.army.mil/HIOMTB> (accessed June 1, 2007).

World Health Organization. "Global Atlas of Infectious Diseases." <http://gamapserver.who.int/GlobalAtlas/home.asp> (accessed June 1, 2007).

Kenneth LaPensee

Water-borne Disease

■ Introduction

Water-borne diseases are caused by water that is contaminated with microorganisms. The microbes—typically bacteria, viruses, protozoa, and parasites—are usually found in the intestinal tracts of humans and other creatures. In most cases, the water becomes contaminated by feces that carry the microbes.

Over 1 billion people worldwide do not have access to safe drinking water, and 3.4 million people die each year due to water-borne diseases, according to the World Health Organization (WHO). Indeed, water-borne diseases are the most common cause of disease and death in the world, according to the WHO. While this is largely a problem in developing and underdeveloped countries, developed nations, including the United States, are not immune. An estimated 900,000 water-borne-related illnesses and almost 1,000 deaths occur in the United States each year, according to the U.S. Centers for Disease Control and Prevention (CDC).

■ Disease History, Characteristics, and Transmission

As noted above, water-borne diseases are caused by a wide range of pathogens, including bacteria, viruses, parasites, and protozoa. Examples of bacteria that are important water-borne pathogenic organisms include *Vibrio cholerae* (the bacteria that causes cholera), various species *Campylobacter*, *Salmonella*, *Shigella*, and a type of *Escherichia coli* designated O157:H7.

An example of a pathogenic water-borne virus is the norovirus, which has become notorious in causing disease outbreaks on cruise ships, and in day care centers and universities. In the winter of 2007, classes were interrupted at two universities in the Canadian province of Nova Scotia because of simultaneous outbreaks of water-borne norovirus diarrhea. Viruses that normally dwell in the intestinal tract are also capable of causing disease if they contaminate water. Just one example is hepatitis (several forms of hepatitis are caused by several types of hepatitis virus).

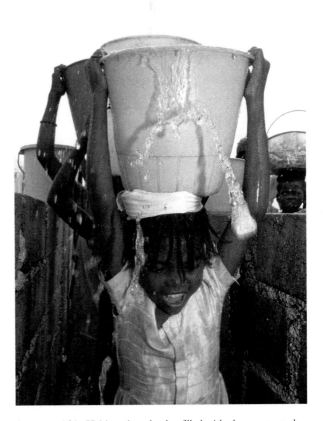

A young girl in Haiti carries a bucket filled with clean water to be used for cooking and cleaning. The water facility, which began operation in the early 1990s, provides water to the residents living in one of the country's poorest areas. The clean water helps to reduce diseases such as cholera, common in the slums. *AP Images.*

895

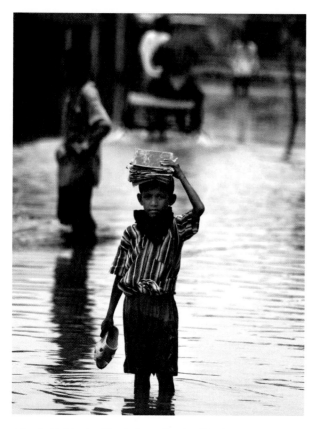

A boy holds his school books in one hand and his shoes in the other as he crosses knee-deep flood waters near Dhaka, Bangladesh, in 2002. Rain caused overflowing rivers to break through mud embankments, swamping villagers. Relief officials battled flood-related diseases, which killed more than 50 people. *AP Images.*

As occurred in the Nova Scotia incidents, water-borne diseases are often the result of drinking or bathing in contaminated freshwater. Saltwater-borne microbial diseases also exist, and bacteria, viruses, and algae are typically associated with these illnesses. Explosive growth of certain algal species in ocean water can lead to the accumulation of these algae in oysters and other shellfish that feed by filtering water. If people eat the affected shellfish, various diseases can result. Some of these can be serious, producing paralysis and death.

Amebiasis is a common water-borne disease that is caused by the parasite *Entamoeba histolytica*. This parasite is normally found in feces, and can cause disease when fecal-contaminated water is consumed. About one of every 10 people who consume *E. histolytica*—which translates to millions of people worldwide—becomes ill. Their symptoms can be mild (diarrhea, stomach ache, and cramping), but, in some people, a severe form of amebiasis called amebic dysentery develops. The destruction of cells lining the intestinal tract produces bloody diarrhea. More rarely, the parasite can spread to the liver, lungs, or the brain.

Cryptosporidiosis is another water-borne disease caused by a parasite. This illness is caused parasites of the genus *Cryptosporidium*, especially *C. parvum*. The organism's life cycle consists of a small, inert form and an actively growing form. The inert form can pass through the filters used in water treatment plants and can survive exposure to chlorine. Once inside a person, the resulting infection can persist for months despite treatment.

Once relatively rare, cryptosporidiosis increased in prevalence in the United States beginning in the 1980s, as expansion of urban areas brought more people into contact with the animals that naturally harbor the parasite in their intestinal tracts. Symptoms of cryptosporidiosis include dehydration, persistent stomach upset, weight loss, nausea, and vomiting. The parasite can be passed from person to person. As of 2007, cryptosporidiosis is one of the most common causes of water-borne disease in the United States. A well-known outbreak occurred in Milwaukee, Wisconsin, in 1993; over 200,000 people were sickened during this outbreak.

Yet another parasite-mediated water-borne disease is cyclosporiasis, which is caused by *Cyclospora cayetanensis*. A hallmark of this infection is the sudden and explosive diarrhea that repeatedly occurs. Other symptoms include weight loss, dehydration, stomach upset, and fatigue.

Giardiasis is a disease caused by an intestinal parasite called *Giardia lamblia* (sometimes called *Giardia intestinalis*). Over the past 20 years, this disease has become one of the most common water-borne human diseases in the United States. In North America, it is sometimes known as beaver fever, since the beaver is one of the animals that naturally harbor the parasite in their intestinal tracts. Symptoms of giardiasis include diarrhea, intestinal gas, stomach cramps, upset stomach, and nausea. The lingering intestinal upset of giardiasis can be debilitating.

■ Scope and Distribution

Water-borne diseases caused by microorganisms occur worldwide. Virtually every country experiences water-borne illnesses, although the diseases tend to be more prevalent in tropical countries where the warmer climate favors the persistence of bacteria and viruses that enter the water from the intestinal tract. water-borne diseases are especially problematic in developing and underdeveloped nations, where adequate water treatment facilities may be lacking and safe drinking water may be in short supply. For example, in 2000, about 140,000 cases of cholera were reported to the WHO, and these infections resulted in 5,000 deaths. About 87% of these cases occurred in Africa.

Treatment and Prevention

Drinking water can be treated to remove or destroy contaminating microorganisms. Chlorination, one well-known treatment, destroys pathogenic bacteria, nuisance bacteria, parasites, and other organisms. Others treatments include exposure of the water to ultraviolet light (which rearranges the microbes' genetic material so that they cannot reproduce) and ozone, and the passage of water through a filter whose openings are so small that even viruses are removed.

Water-borne diseases that are caused by bacteria, protozoa, and some parasites can be treated using compounds that kill the target organism. For example, antibiotics are effective against bacteria. Viruses are more problematic, since antibiotics are not effective.

The best strategy is not to treat an infection, but to avoid getting the infection. Sensible precautions include washing hands after having a bowel movement, never drinking water that has not been treated (if in doubt, do not drink), and avoiding bathing or swimming in water that is known to be polluted. In many North American and European communities, recreational water is monitored and notices are posted restricting swimming when the water is determined to be contaminated.

Impacts and Issues

The global impact of water-borne disease is huge. The U.S. Centers for Disease Control and Prevention (CDC) estimates that there are over 4 billion episodes of diarrhea due to the consumption of contaminated water, and more than 2 million deaths. Tragically, most of these deaths occur among children in developing and underdeveloped countries. The WHO estimates that 4,000 children die every day from water-borne diseases. According to the CDC and the WHO, more than 2 billion people living in poverty are especially susceptible to water-borne disease, mainly due to contaminated surface water or inadequately treated drinking water.

People whose immune systems are not operating efficiently can develop more severe or persistent forms of water-borne diseases, such as cryptosporidiosis. The latter has become a significant threat for people with acquired immunodeficiency syndrome (AIDS, also cited as acquired immune deficiency syndrome) and those who take immunosuppressive drugs to reduce the chance of rejection of a transplanted organ.

Aside from the human tragedy, this massive loss of life robs countries of the next generation of citizens and workers, which has serious consequences for the future population level and economic strength of these nations. For such nations, water treatment must be a priority. Analysts at the WHO and other agencies have estimated that for every dollar spent on water treatment, the economic return due to lower rates of death and disease

WORDS TO KNOW

CHLORINATION: Chlorination refers to a chemical process that is used primarily to disinfect drinking water and spills of microorganisms. The active agent in chlorination is the element chlorine, or a derivative of chlorine (e.g., chlorine dioxide). Chlorination is a swift and economical means of destroying many, but not all, microorganisms that are a health-threat in fluid such as drinking water.

DIARRHEA: To most individuals, diarrhea means an increased frequency or decreased consistency of bowel movements; however, the medical definition is more exact than this explanation. In many developed countries, the average number of bowel movements is three per day. However, researchers have found that diarrhea, which is not a disease, best correlates with an increase in stool weight; stool weights above 10.5 ounces (300 grams) per day generally indicates diarrhea. This is mainly due to excess water, which normally makes up 60 to 85% of fecal matter. In this way, true diarrhea is distinguished from diseases that cause only an increase in the number of bowel movements (hyperdefecation), or incontinence (involuntary loss of bowel contents). Diarrhea is also classified by physicians into acute, which lasts one to two weeks, and chronic, which continues for longer than four weeks. Viral and bacterial infections are the most common causes of acute diarrhea.

FECES: Solid waste of a living body.

NOROVIRUS: Norovirus is a type of virus that contain ribonucleic acid as the genetic material, and which causes an intestinal infection known as gastroenteritis. A well-known example is Norwalk-like virus.

PATHOGEN: A disease causing agent, such as a bacteria, virus, fungus, etc.

would be $3–$4 per country. The resulting economic boost could help lift some nations out of poverty.

The problem of water-borne disease is not confined to the poor regions of the globe, however. Even in developed countries, a breakdown of water treatment can lead to disease. A well-known recent example occurred in the Canadian community of Walkerton, Ontario, in the

IN CONTEXT: DISEASE IN DEVELOPING NATIONS

Contaminated clean water supplies are often a major factor in the spread of disease. Besides climate, the most common reasons for clean water shortages are caused primarily by human activity. Water pollution can occur from both industry and leaking of septic (waste) water into the water supply system. In both cases, the water may become dangerous for the health of the people and unusable for industry. Purification of industrial waste is expensive, and sometimes, economic interests may conflict with protecting the environment. Many developing countries cannot afford proper water purification because their main concern is survival rather than the quality of the environment. Pollution, however, is a global concern and affects people in other countries besides the source of the pollution.

summer of 2000. The accidental flooding of a community well with run-off from a cattle farm, combined with inadequate treatment of the drinking water led to an outbreak of *E. coli* O157:H7-mediated illness that sickened over 2,000 people and killed seven. Some of the survivors were left with permanent damage to their kidneys due to the destructive effects of a toxin produced by the bacteria.

In many countries, drinking water is monitored to ensure that it is free from pathogenic bacteria, viruses, and protozoa. In the United States, CDC surveillance programs detect water-borne outbreaks and help direct federal, state, and municipal responses to the outbreaks. Similar efforts in developing and underdeveloped countries have been far less successful, as population increases in these poorer countries have outstripped the economic capability of governments to put in place the necessary water treatment technologies. By 2015, the United Nations has set a goal of cutting the number of people without access to safe drinking water by 50%.

Despite the continuing challenges, some successes have occurred. Initiatives such as the CDC's Healthy Drinking Water Program, the United Nations International Decade for Action: Water for Life 2005–2015, and the WHO's household water treatment and safe storage network are bringing simple and relatively inexpensive water treatment methods to rural areas in Africa, Central America, and South America, and helping to safeguard water in the United States. As one example, a disease called drancunculiasis, which formerly affected almost 4 million people each year in African countries, has been almost eliminated. As of 2007, the disease is detectable in only 12 nations in Africa.

SEE ALSO *Amebiasis; Bacterial Disease;* Campylobacter *Infection; Cholera; Cryptosporidiosis; Cyclosporiasis; Dracunculiasis; Dysentery;* Escherichia coli *O157:H7; Giardiasis; Mosquito-Borne Diseases; Norovirus Infection;* Salmonella *Infection (Salmonellosis); Shigellosis; Viral Disease.*

BIBLIOGRAPHY

Books

Ewald, Paul. *Plague Time: The New Germ Theory of Disease.* New York: Anchor, 2002.

Percival, Steven, et al. *Microbiology of water-borne Diseases: Microbiological Aspects and Risks.* New York: Academic Press, 2004.

Powell, Michael, and Oliver Fischer. *101 Diseases You Don't Want to Get.* New York: Thunder's Mouth Press, 2005.

Web Sites

Centers for Disease Control and Prevention. "Water-borne Diseases." October 23, 2001. <http://www.cdc.gov/ncidod/diseases/list_water-borne.htm> (accessed April 19, 2007).

Brian Hoyle

West Nile

Introduction

The West Nile virus is a member of the Flaviviridae family. It causes an inflammation of the lining of nerve cells located in the spinal cord (meningitis) and the brain (encephalitis). Originally detected in Africa in the late 1930s, the virus did not spread to North America until 1999. Since that time, its North American prevalence and geographical distribution has increased.

Disease History, Characteristics, and Transmission

West Nile virus was first isolated in 1937 from a woman in the West Nile District of Uganda. The virus took its name from this location. During the 1950s, the ability of the virus to cause meningitis and encephalitis in humans and the resulting health threat of the virus was recognized. A decade later, the virus was linked to the development of encephalitis in horses.

Since the 1930s, the virus has been detected in humans, animals, and birds in Africa, the Middle East, Eastern Europe, and West Asia, but it did not arrive in North America until the end of the twentieth century. Scientists are not certain if West Nile virus spread from Africa to other regions of the world, such as North America, or if the virus was always present in North America, but was only revealed when tests for it were performed. However, the pattern of reported cases in North America is more consistent with the introduction of the virus from overseas and its subsequent spread. Assuming that the virus was, in fact, introduced to the North American continent, the way in which it was transported across the Atlantic Ocean to the East Coast of the United States is still unknown. Bird migration is one theory. Another theory suggests that a mosquito infected with the virus could have arrived in a shipment of goods.

Immediately after its appearance in North America, West Nile became noteworthy. In the summer of 1999, 62 cases of West Nile disease were reported in New York City. Seven people died as a result of the infection. The city experienced another outbreak the following summer, when 21 more cases and two deaths occurred. In the span of 1999–2000, the virus was also detected in other states along the coast of the northeastern United States. These early infections generated a great deal of

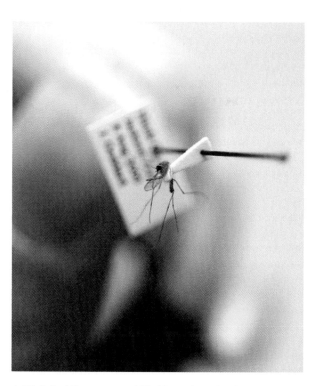

A Mississippi Department of Health employee holds one of the *Culex* mosquito species that has been identified as the primary carrier of the West Nile virus (WNV) in the South. The virus has been detected in all mainland states in the United States. *AP Images.*

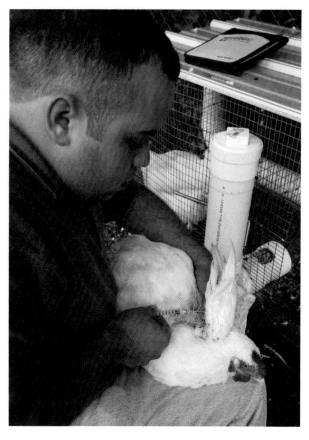

A health official takes a blood sample from a chicken in Monroe, Louisiana. The bird was tested to determine if it was infected with the West Nile virus. *Dan Currier/Getty Images.*

concern, since they raised the possibility of a looming epidemic. This proved not to be the case, although the geographical range of the virus began to expand.

West Nile is a vector-borne disease. It is spread from infected birds to humans, mainly by mosquitoes (most commonly, the mosquito species *Culex pipiens*). Robins, jays, and crows are the most common avian reservoirs of the virus. As with other mosquito-transmitted diseases, the virus is acquired by a mosquito when it feeds on the blood of an infected animal or bird. The virus remains in the salivary gland of the mosquito and, when the same mosquito subsequently seeks a blood meal from a person, transfer of the virus can occur. The cases in New York City in 1999, and especially in 2000, were probably caused by mosquitoes that were able to survive the cold winter months by seeking refuge in warm and damp pipes, abandoned tunnels, subway tunnels, or other locations such as root cellars, barns, and caves. In the spring, the mosquitoes re-emerged and a new round of infections began. Not only humans were affected, but in the springs of 2000 and 2001, many crows died from the viral infection. Indeed, for those who monitor the appearance of West Nile disease, bird die-offs in the

spring can be a signal that the infection is re-emerging, and that precautions are necessary to avoid human infection.

Research has shown that two populations of *Culex pipiens* exist in Europe; one seeks its blood meal exclusively from humans and the other from animals. The chance of a mosquito taking a blood meal from an infected bird and then feeding on a human are very low. However, in North America, the mosquito population has adapted to feed on both birds and humans, so the chance that a mosquito will seek blood meals from an animal and then from a human is greater. This is probably why West Nile disease has spread so much faster in North America than in Europe.

When the West Nile virus enters a human host via a mosquito bite, the virus replicates in the blood. Then, in a way that is still not clear, the virus is able to cross the blood brain barrier and enter the brain. Normally, passage into the brain is regulated by this very efficient blood brain barrier. The barrier is so efficient that some drugs are unable to cross it, but the barrier is not able to keep the virus out of the brain. Formation of new virus particles in the brain tissue stimulates an immune response that—along with the infection—can cause inflammation of the brain, a serious condition known as encephalitis.

Approximately 80% of infected individuals present no symptoms. Many individuals, however, can exhibit symptoms of West Nile that include: the development of fever, headache, muscle aches throughout the body (particularly in the back), loss of appetite, nausea with vomiting, diarrhea, swelling of the lymph nodes, and a skin rash. The infection tends to clear within a few weeks with no or mild complications.

In fewer than 1% of people who are infected with the virus, the infection becomes more serious. Inflammation of the nerve lining in the brain (encephalitis) and spinal cord (meningitis) develops. When meningitis or encephalitis develops, symptoms include a high fever, severe headache, stiff neck, mental disorientation, uncontrolled muscle spasms, loss of coordination, paralysis, and convulsions. A person can lapse into a coma and die. Survivors can be left with permanent damage, such as paralysis on one side of the body, similar to the paralysis seen in cases of polio. In severe cases, the paralysis affects the muscles used for breathing, and mechanical breathing assistance may be necessary.

The prospect that a serious disease can be acquired from a mosquito bite is alarming to many, since mosquitoes are often very common during spring and summer in North America and, despite precautions, can be hard to avoid. Fortunately, at least for now, the incidence of the virus in North American mosquito populations is very low. Scientists who have sampled mosquitoes for the presence of the virus have determined that typically only about 1% of mosquitoes harbor the virus, even in an

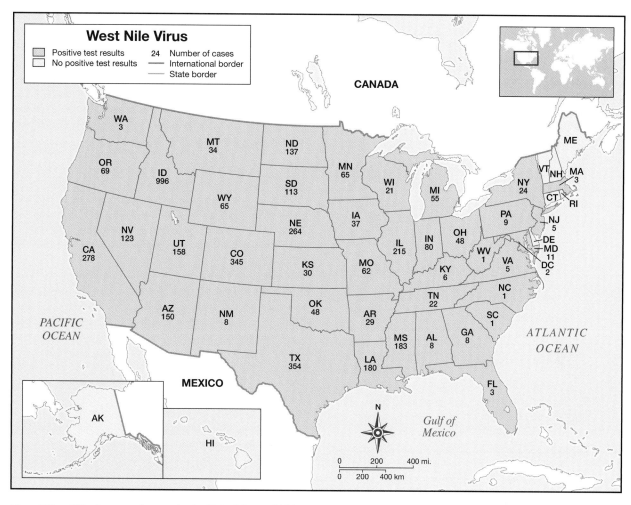

Map of West Nile virus cases by state in the United States, 2006. *Data courtesy of Centers for Disease Control.*

area that is a known hotspot of the disease. The risk of a person contracting West Nile disease is small, and can be minimized still further by taking some common-sense precautions.

A number of factors increase the risk of contracting West Nile disease. The time of year is one factor. In more northern climates, late spring to early fall is the peak season for mosquitoes and the risk of contracting the disease is higher during those seasons. In southern regions that are warmer year-round, the risk is more constant.

Another risk factor is geography. Certain areas of the United States and Canada have greater mosquito populations that other areas, and therefore are areas of higher risk. For example, in 2006, Texas—which has coastline on the Gulf of Mexico—reported 330 cases of West Nile disease, while the drier and more inland state of New Mexico reported only eight cases. More locally, areas that have more stagnant water are more apt to be a breeding ground for mosquitoes.

A third risk factor is occupation. Someone whose job or recreational activities takes them outdoors is more at

risk of exposure to mosquitoes than someone who spends more time indoors. Finally, people whose immune systems is not functioning efficiently—such as the elderly, the sick, and transplant patients whose immune systems have been deliberately supressed—are at higher risk, since they are less able to fight a viral infection.

■ Scope and Distribution

West Nile disease has occurred in Europe, Africa, the Middle East, parts of Asia, and North America. Outbreaks have occurred in all these regions, most recently in the United States and Canada from 1999–2003. The geographical distribution of the virus in North America has been steadily increasing since its appearance on the continent in 1999. By the summer of 2001, dead birds that tested positive for the virus were found in Toronto, Ontario (Canada), northern Florida, and Milwaukee, Wisconsin. A year later, over 300 cases and at least 14 deaths were reported and the virus was recovered from

WORDS TO KNOW

ENCEPHALITIS: A type of acute brain inflammation, most often due to infection by a virus.

MENINGITIS: Meningitis is an inflammation of the meninges—the three layers of protective membranes that line the spinal cord and the brain. Meningitis can occur when there is an infection near the brain or spinal cord, such as a respiratory infection in the sinuses, the mastoids, or the cavities around the ear. Disease organisms can also travel to the meninges through the bloodstream. The first signs may be a severe headache and neck stiffness followed by fever, vomiting, a rash, and, then, convulsions leading to loss of consciousness. Meningitis generally involves two types: non-bacterial meningitis, which is often called aseptic meningitis, and bacterial meningitis, which is referred to as purulent meningitis.

VECTOR: Any agent, living or otherwise, that carries and transmits parasites and diseases. Also, an organism or chemical used to transport a gene into a new host cell.

the Yukon. In 2005, the last full year for which data is available, there were 239 cases and 12 deaths in Canada.

While birds are involved in the transmission of West Nile disease to people, dogs and cats also can be infected with the virus. This has caused fears that many pet owners could be at risk of the disease. While it does mean that a pet owner could acquire the virus after a mosquito has bitten a cat or dog, there is no evidence of a direct transmission from either animal to people.

Squirrels may also be susceptible to infection with West Nile virus. While there is no evidence that the virus is transmitted to someone from a squirrel or from handling a squirrel carcass, the presence of a dead squirrel could be an indication that West Nile disease is present in an area. Sensible precautions, including the use of gloves when disposing of a squirrel carcass, will prevent infection.

There may also be a genetic component to West Nile virus susceptibility. Researchers have found that an alteration in a gene called CCR5, which affects the functioning of T cells (important immune system cells), can produce more serious symptoms of the disease. Several studies have found that the proportion of people possessing the gene mutation is much higher in those with West Nile disease than in the general population. Curiously, the gene mutation helps protect people infected with the human immunodeficiency virus (HIV) from developing acquired immunodeficiency syndrome (AIDS, also cited as acquired immune deficiency syndrome).

dead birds in more western states. By August 2002, West Nile virus was reported in 41 states and by 2003 only the states of Alaska, Hawaii, Washington, Oregon, and Maine had not reported cases of the disease. By 2006, the disease had spread to the states of Washington and Oregon, and into Mexico. As of early 2007, the hotspots for the disease are California, Illinois, Louisiana, Nebraska, South Dakota, and Texas.

The number of cases have been increasing as well. In 2002, 4,155 cases and 284 deaths were reported to the U.S. Centers for Disease Control and Prevention (CDC). The next year, 9,862 cases and 264 fatalities were reported. About 30% of these cases involved meningitis or encephalitis and required extensive hospital care. From 2004–2006, 9,758 cases and 380 deaths were reported. During these last three years, the number of cases and number of deaths increased each year.

In Canada in 2001, the virus was uncovered in dead birds and mosquitoes in the province of Ontario. In 2002, 10 deaths occurred among the 416 cases reported to Health Canada, and the disease had spread to the province of Quebec. The following year, the number of cases increased to 1,494 and 14 deaths were reported. By 2003, the virus had been detected all across the country from British Columbia to Nova Scotia and as far north as

■ Treatment and Prevention

West Nile disease is almost always acquired from a mosquito bite. While some species of ticks can harbor the virus, no tick-borne disease has been reported in a human. Furthermore, West Nile disease is not contagious—routine person-to-person transmission does not occur. In 2002, the CDC reported that it is possible to transmit West Nile virus via transfusion of virus-contaminated blood, transplant of a contaminated organ, and breast milk. Infection of a fetus by its mother prior to birth may also be possible. However, infections that do not involve mosquito bites are thought to be rare.

In Canada, all donated blood is screened year-round. Blood banks in the United States screen donated blood during peak infection periods. In addition, Britain's National Blood Service screens donated blood for the virus if the donor is known to have visited the United States or Canada in the previous month.

While there is no human vaccine effective against West Nile virus, a vaccine for horses is available. The vaccine has been used by some zoos to vaccinate birds; however, whether this strategy worked cannot be gauged until the birds are exposed to the virus. The equine vaccine, which contains weakened but intact West Nile virus, has not been studied in humans, and people should not use it. Veterinary vaccines are not subject to the same regulatory approvals as are human vaccines, and their safety for humans cannot be assured.

Prevention of infection focuses on minimizing the opportunity for contact with mosquitoes. Sensible precautions include using insect repellent sprays or creams that contain DEET (meta-dimethyl toluamide), wearing protective clothing such as long-sleeve shirts and long pants when outdoors, avoiding areas of stagnant water that can be breeding grounds for mosquitoes, and removing any objects that could contain stagnant water—birdbaths, clogged roof gutters, unused swimming pools, and disused tires—from a backyard. In addition, avoiding outdoor activity during the early morning and evening, when mosquitoes are most active, is a wise precaution.

DEET-containing insect repellents should not be used on infants or young children. For these youngsters and those who prefer not to be exposed to DEET, the CDC recommends oil of lemon eucalyptus. It is an efficient repellent, but does not retain its potency as long as DEET does.

■ Impacts and Issues

West Nile disease has quickly become a significant public health threat in North America. The possibilities of large outbreaks and the potential seriousness of the infection—one of every 150 people who contract the disease develops meningitis or encephalitis—has created near-panic in the public. Agencies, such as the CDC, have devoted significant effort to informing people about the disease and publicizing the common-sense preventative measures that can help protect people.

The economic consequences of West Nile disease can be great. For example, in 2002, it was estimated that about $200 million in health care costs were associated with the disease in the United States. There are other costs as well. For example, national, state, and local agencies have surveillance programs to monitor mosquito, bird, and even human populations for the virus, and they also conduct initiatives to increase awareness of the disease among the public and health care providers.

Spraying of mosquito breeding sites is a proven way of reducing the mosquito population. However, those opposed to such spraying are concerned that the possible environmental degradation from the chemical spray is a greater danger than any cases of West Nile that might develop. Those in favor of spraying maintain that the increasing spread of West Nile disease and the increasing number of deaths argues for intervention and control programs, including spraying.

■ Primary Source Connection

As part of an effort to combat West Nile Virus, the United States Food and Drug Administration (FDA) publishes information articles designed to alert the pub-

---

IN CONTEXT: REAL-WORLD RISKS

According to the National Institute for Occupational Safety and Health: "Workers at risk of exposure to WNV (West Nile Virus) include those working outdoors when mosquitoes are biting. Outdoor workers at risk include farmers, foresters, landscapers, groundskeepers and gardeners, painters, roofers, pavers, construction workers, laborers, mechanics, and other outdoor workers. Entomologists and other field workers are also at risk while conducting surveillance and other research outdoors."

"Although WNV is most often transmitted by the bite of infected mosquitoes, the virus can also be transmitted through contact with infected animals, their blood, or other tissues. Thus laboratory, field, and clinical workers who handle tissues or fluids infected with WNV or who perform necropsies are at risk of WNV exposure."

SOURCE: *National Institute for Occupational Safety and Health*

---

lic to potential dangers and to provide concrete steps to reduce risk. The recommendations were formulated by the Centers for Disease Control and Prevention (CDC).

This press release announced a new test designed to expedite diagnosis of West Nile virus along with a list of preventative steps recommended by the FDA in 2000—and that are current as of March 2007—to avoid risk of acquiring West Nile disease, especially until definitive treatment or vaccines are developed and tested.

First Test Approved to Help Detect West Nile Virus

The Food and Drug Administration has cleared the first test that will help physicians diagnose cases of potentially deadly West Nile virus earlier than with current methods.

The West Nile Virus IgM Capture ELISA test is intended to be used in people who have symptoms of viral encephalitis or meningitis, which are serious inflammatory conditions of the brain or spinal cord that may occur in people infected with the virus.

"The rapid review and approval of this blood test, which uses antibody levels to identify persons who were recently exposed to West Nile virus, reflects FDA's commitment to making safe and effective medical products available promptly," says FDA Commissioner Mark B. McClellan, MD, Ph.D. The new test works by detecting the levels of IgM, a particular type of antibody to West Nile virus, in blood serum. It is manufactured by PanBio Ltd. of Windsor, Australia.

West Nile virus is a mosquito-borne virus first detected in the United States in 1999. While it often causes a mild infection that clears without further treatment, some people, especially those over 50, develop severe infections resulting in neurological disease and even death. The virus is most prevalent during peak mosquito season, beginning in July and ending in October.

By 2002, West Nile virus had spread to most of the continental United States. The CDC reported this season's first human case of West Nile virus in the United States in early July. As of early August, three deaths in Texas and Alabama had been attributed to the virus. The CDC says that West Nile virus activity detected in humans began a "significant uptick" in early August 2003.

The new diagnostic test is a significant breakthrough in the detection of West Nile virus. However, it's important to know that it is not a donor screening test, but is one of several tools used by the physician to determine if the patient is infected. Results from the IgM Capture ELISA must be confirmed with other laboratory tests as part of a comprehensive evaluation. The test is designed to be used in cases when someone has symptoms of West Nile encephalitis or meningitis—headache, high fever, neck stiffness, stupor, disorientation, coma, tremors, convulsions, muscle weakness, and paralysis.

In addition to its usefulness for diagnosing individuals with the infection, the test has the potential to help monitor the scope and spread of the disease. The FDA has established guidance and procedures to avoid collection and use of blood that might be at risk for transmitting West Nile virus. The agency is cooperating with the country's blood organizations, both in the laboratory and in epidemiological investigations of the virus. In August 2002, prior to any actual report of transmission, the FDA alerted the blood industry to be vigilant in excluding symptomatic donors and then later that year provided guidance to blood establishments on procedures to protect the blood supply. The FDA updated this guidance in May 2003, based on experience with the 2002 outbreak.

Additionally, the agency is working with manufacturers to expedite development of necessary medical products, such as screening tests and additional diagnostic methods. Experimental donor screening tests have been put into place and have been available nationwide since July 1, 2003. These tests add a measure of safety and will prevent contaminated blood from entering the nation's blood supply.

Other federal efforts are ongoing to combat West Nile virus. The National Institutes of Health (NIH) is supporting ongoing research at universities and companies nationwide aimed at developing the public health tools to help fight the infection. Currently the NIH is funding four areas of research for West Nile virus: diagnosis, prevention, therapy, and basic research that look at the virus as it replicates in animals, humans, and mosquitoes.

In the area of prevention, the NIH is supporting three different approaches to vaccines, including a live vaccine made by mixing West Nile virus with the already established yellow fever vaccine Through its grants and contracts, the NIH is the largest supporter of infectious disease research in the United States.

For now, the CDC, the FDA and the NIH all agree that the most important message about the virus is that people need to be prepared and take the steps necessary to prevent mosquito bites and avoid exposure, especially until treatment or vaccines are available to add additional layers of protection.

Reduce the Risk of West Nile Virus

1. Avoid mosquito bites

- Cover up. Wear long-sleeved shirts, long pants, and socks sprayed with repellent while outdoors.
- Avoid mosquitoes, which often bite between dusk and dawn.
- Limit time outdoors during these hours.
- Spray insect repellent containing DEET (look for N, N-diethyl-m-toluamide) on exposed skin outdoors.
- Spray clothing with repellents containing DEET or permethrin.
- Don't spray repellent on skin under clothing.
- Don't use permethrin on skin.
- Use repellent carefully.
- Don't put repellent on kids' hands because it may get into their mouths or eyes.

2. Mosquito-proof your home

- Install or fix window and door screens.
- Drain standing water, where mosquitoes like to breed.
- Look around every week for possible mosquito breeding places.
- Empty water from buckets, cans, pool covers, flowerpots, and other items.
- Throw away or cover up stored tires and other items not being used.
- Clean outdoor pet water bowls weekly.
- Check to see if rain gutters are clogged.

3. Help your community

- Dead birds help health departments track West Nile virus.
- Check with your local or state health department to find out their policy for reporting dead birds.

RADOS, CAROL. "FIRST TEST APPROVED TO HELP DETECT WEST NILE VIRUS" *FDA CONSUMER* 37 (SEPTEMBER–OCTOBER 2003).

Sᴇᴇ Aʟsᴏ *Arthropod-borne Disease; Climate Change and Infectious Disease; Emerging Infectious Diseases; Encephalitis; Meningitis, Viral; Mosquito-borne Diseases; Vector-borne Disease.*

BIBLIOGRAPHY

Books

Sfakianos, Jeffrey N., and David Heymann. *West Nile Virus.* London: Chelsea House, 2005.

White, Dennis J., and Dale L. Morse. *West Nile Virus: Detection, Surveillance, and Control.* New York: New York Academy of Sciences, 2002.

Periodicals

Boyer, Jere, Thomas File, and William Franks. "West Nile Virus: The First Pandemic of the Twenty-first Century." *Ohio Journal of Science* 102 (2002): 98–102.

Web Sites

Centers for Disease Control and Prevention. "West Nile Virus." March 6, 2007. <http://www.cdc.gov/ncidod/dvbid/westnile/index.htm> (accessed March 23, 2007).

Brian Hoyle

Whipworm (Trichuriasis)

■ Introduction

Whipworm, or trichuriasis, is caused by an infestation of the helminth (parasitic worm) *Trichuris trichiura*. This roundworm infects human hosts and reproduces within the large intestine. Transmission of this parasite occurs when infective eggs are passed via the feces and contaminate food and soil. Humans ingest contaminated food or soil to become infected. Light infestations often cause no symptoms, or mild symptoms, while heavy infestations can cause more serious complications including anemia, rectal prolapse, appendicitis, and colitis.

Treatment for whipworm involves anti-parasitic medication containing either mebendazole or albendazole. In addition, treatment may be necessary for accompanying symptoms. Whipworm is a worldwide infection that is prevalent in tropical, densely populated countries, especially in regions with poor sanitation methods. Both adults and children can become infected, although children tend to have a higher infection rate. Whipworm can be prevented by avoiding consumption of contaminated foods, maintaining high sanitation practices, and washing hands after working or playing in soil.

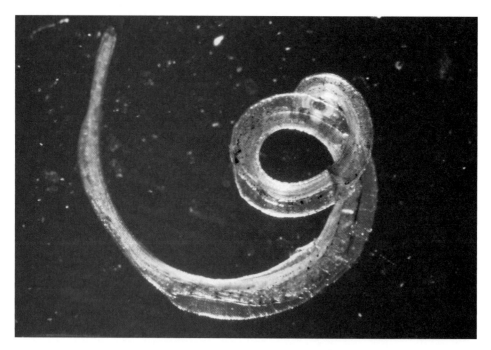

A light micrograph shows an adult male whipworm (*Trichuris trichiura*), a parasite in humans. The front of the worm (upper left) is narrow and pointed like a hair or whip. Adult worms live in the intestines with the front end buried in the intestinal wall. *CNRI/Photo Researchers, Inc.*

Disease History, Characteristics, and Transmission

Whipworm infection is a parasitic infection caused by ingestion of the whipworm, or roundworm, *Trichuris trichiura*. The life cycle of *T. trichiura* involves a human host for the maturation of worms and the production of eggs. Humans become infested after ingesting food or soil contaminated with embryonated (containing an embryo) whipworm eggs. The eggs hatch and mature in the small intestine before migrating to the large intestine. Here, the worms attach to the intestine walls, reach about 4 inches in length, and become sexually mature. The worms mate and two to three months after entering the body, females produce up to 20,000 eggs a day. These eggs pass out of the body with the feces and remain in moist, dark conditions until they are ingested by a new host. Without extremes in temperatures, the eggs can remain viable in soil for years.

In cases where infestation is low, that is, fewer than 100 worms, people usually suffer no symptoms, but some may experience flatulence, abdominal pain, constipation, or diarrhea. If heavily infested, symptoms include weight loss, abdominal pain, nausea, bloody stools, and diarrhea. In severe cases, gastrointestinal problems, anemia, and even rectal prolapse, where the rectum protrudes outside of the body, may occur. The disease is diagnosed when a stool ova and parasite exam reveals the presence of *T. trichiura* or their eggs.

Scope and Distribution

Whipworm occurs worldwide. According to the Centers for Disease Control and Prevention (CDC), this parasitic worm is the third most common roundworm to infect humans. The CDC estimates the prevalence of whipworm at approximately 800 million people worldwide. However, the majority of whipworm infections occur in regions with dense populations and a tropical climate. Poor sanitation levels also increase the likelihood of the disease. Whipworm is most common in areas of Southeast Asia, the Caribbean, and Central and South America. Although whipworm infestations can occur in the United States, Japan, Western Europe, or Australasia, it is not common.

Children are at the greatest risk of infection. This is generally thought to be a result of infrequent handwashing and their penchant for playing in soil. As soil may be contaminated with whipworm, failure to wash hands thoroughly before contact with the mouth or food increases their chance of infection.

Treatment and Prevention

As most cases of whipworm tend to be asymptomatic, and treatment usually involves removing the worms.

WORDS TO KNOW

HELMINTH: A representative of various phyla of worm-like animals.

HOST: Organism that serves as the habitat for a parasite, or possibly for a symbiont. A host may provide nutrition to the parasite or symbiont, or simply a place in which to live.

OVA: Mature female sex cells produced in the ovaries. (Singular: ovum.)

This is achieved through administration of medication containing either mebendazole, which is recommended by the CDC, or albendazole. For symptomatic cases, supportive treatment may be necessary in addition to the anti-parasitic medication. In some cases in which large blood loss occurs, there is a risk of anemia developing. Therefore, iron supplements may be necessary to prevent an iron deficiency.

Whipworm infection is prevented by avoiding contact with contaminated soil and contaminated food. This may involve wearing protective clothing while working in potentially contaminated soil, or washing hands thoroughly after touching soil. Food can be washed and cooked to remove parasites. In addition, crude sanitation, such as the collection of human feces for disposal or for use as fertilizer, is a common way for the infection to spread. Therefore, improved sanitation methods will decrease the likelihood of infections spreading.

Impacts and Issues

Whipworm infections are most likely to occur in developing countries, or countries with dense populations, tropical weather, or poor sanitation methods. In economically depressed countries, 95% of children with protein deficiency and anemia also have whipworm infection. It is in these same countries that medical infrastructure is often limited and seldom able to deliver the repeated anti-helminth medication that successful treatment whipworm infection requires.

Another issue related to whipworm infections involves the potential complications that can arise following heavy whipworm infestations. Anemia, a complication that results in a low transfer of oxygen to body tissues, directly affects tissue development. As children are commonly infected, this complication could affect their growth and overall health. Girls with whipworm infection are particularly vulnerable to anemia caused by whipworm infestation, as they experience additional blood loss with menstruation and often begin childbearing at a relatively young age in countries where whipworm is endemic.

The World Health Organization has identified several key strategies in reducing whipworm infestation in people living in developing countries. Rather than reduce the number of whipworm infections in people (the old strategy), health authorities now work to reduce the number of worms residing in each person. This strategy recognizes the fact that re-infection will probably occur, and focuses on lessening the severity of the disease. Drugs are also now delivered to schools and other long-standing facilities, where minimally trained local citizens can administer them. This strategy is showing more success in delivering repeated treatments than relying on mobile medical teams.

SEE ALSO *Handwashing; Helminth Disease; Hookworm (Ancylostoma) Infection; Parasitic Diseases; Pinworm (Enterobius vermicularis) Infection; Roundworm (Ascariasis) infection; Sanitation.*

BIBLIOGRAPHY

Books

Bush, A.O., J.C. Fernandez, G.W. Esch, and J.R. Seed. *Parasitism: The Diversity and Ecology of Animal Parasites.* New York: Cambridge University Press, 2001.

Mandell, G.L., J.E. Bennett, and R. Dolin. *Principles and Practice of Infectious Diseases. vol. 2.* Philadelphia, PA: Elsevier, 2005.

Web Sites

Centers for Disease Control (CDC). "Trichuriasis." July 27, 2004 <http://www.dpd.cdc.gov/DPDx/HTML/Trichuriasis.htm> (accessed March 9, 2007).

National Institute of Allergy and Infectious Diseases. "Parasitic Roundworm Diseases." March 8, 2005 <http://www.niaid.nih.gov/factsheets/roundwor.htm> (accessed March 9, 2007).

Whooping Cough (Pertussis)

■ Introduction

Whooping cough is also known as pertussis, a word that means "intense cough." It is caused by the bacterium *Bordetella pertussis*, which is a pathogen (disease-causing organism) with a propensity for lung tissue. Whooping cough was once the leading cause of death in children under five in the United States. In 1945, it caused more deaths than diphtheria, scarlet fever, measles, and polio combined. Since the introduction of an effective vaccine in the late 1940s, the number of cases of whooping cough has decreased sharply, although there have been increases in recent years.

Whooping cough is no ordinary cough. The disease is marked by bouts of severe spasmodic coughing that end with a characteristic "whooping" sound and vomiting. Complications from secondary bacterial infection include pneumonia and ear infection. Mortality is greatest among infants, especially those who are born prematurely. Whooping cough is a highly contagious disease, so it is important that children be vaccinated against it.

■ Disease History, Characteristics, and Transmission

The causative agent of whooping cough is *B. pertussis*, which is a Gram-negative coccus (a short, rod-shaped

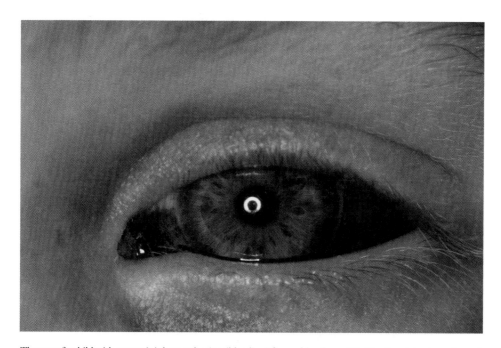

The eye of a child with pertussis is hemorrhaging (bleeding) from a blood vessel that has burst due to prolonged coughing. The blood has pooled beneath the conjunctiva, the membrane that covers the front of the eye. Vision is not affected; the blood is eventually absorbed into the body.   *Dr. M.A. Ansary/Photo Researchers, Inc.*

WORDS TO KNOW

ANTIBIOTIC RESISTANCE: The ability of bacteria to resist the actions of antibiotic drugs.

GRAM-NEGATIVE BACTERIA: All types of bacteria identified and classified as a group that does not retain crystal-violet dye during Gram's method of staining.

PAROXYSM: In medicine, a paroxysm may be a fit, convulsion, or seizure. It may also be a sudden worsening or recurrence of disease symptoms.

PATHOGEN: A disease causing agent, such as a bacteria, virus, fungus, etc.

PNEUMONIA: Pneumonia is inflammation of the lung accompanied by filling of some air sacs with fluid (consolidation). It can be caused by a number of infectious agents, including bacteria, viruses, and fungi.

VACCINE: A substance that is introduced to stimulate antibody production and thus provide immunity to a particular disease.

bacterium). The term Gram-negative refers to the way the microbe reacts with Gram stain, which is used to prepare samples for microscopy. *B. pertussis* specifically infects the tissue of the lung, and its incubation period is 6–20 days.

Whooping cough may last for several weeks and is divided into three distinct stages. The catarrhal stage involves non-specific symptoms, such as a runny nose, a mild cough, and a mild fever, which may easily be mistaken for a cold. This stage may continue for a week or so, before the second, so-called paroxysmal stage sets in. This is marked by paroxysms—or attacks—of severe, repetitive coughing ending in a 'whooping' sound and vomiting, usually accompanied by exhaustion. The coughing has a choking quality, and the patient's face may look congested. There may be between two and 50 attacks a day, occurring more frequently at night. Between attacks the patient does not usually cough at all.

The whooping sound comes from the larynx or voice box, as the patient finally takes a proper breath in after an attack. Complications of this stage of whooping cough include convulsions and seizures arising from a reduced supply of oxygen to the brain. This is thought to occur either because of the coughing itself or due to a toxin released by *B. pertussis*. This stage lasts for one to four weeks, during which time secondary bacterial infec-

tions like otitis media—an infection of the middle ear—and pneumonia may set in. The latter is the most common and deadly complication of whooping cough.

The final stage of whooping cough is convalescence and is characterized by a fading away of the cough, in both frequency and intensity. Surveillance data in the United States from 1980 to 1989 suggest that the clinical course of whooping cough is complicated by pneumonia in about 22% of cases, by seizures in 3% of cases and by encephalopathy (a swelling of the brain) in about 1% of cases. Mortality in infants aged less than one month was 1.3% and among infants aged 2–11 months was 0.3%. A case of whooping cough usually gives a patient lifelong immunity to further attacks.

Whooping cough is a highly contagious disease, particularly in the catarrhal stage and up to three weeks after the start of the paroxysmal stage. Adults and adolescents, who may have a milder form of the disease, act as a reservoir of infection. The disease is transmitted through coughing and sneezing, which exposes people to infected respiratory secretions.

■ Scope and Distribution

Whooping cough has been known as a childhood disease for several hundred years. According to the World Health Organization (WHO) there were 39 million cases of whooping cough around the world in the year 2000, with 297,000 deaths. In many countries, regular epidemics occur every three to five years. Those who have not been fully immunized, either because they are too young or for some other reason, are most at risk of dying from whooping cough.

Before the introduction of the whooping cough vaccine, the disease was the leading cause of death from infectious disease in the under-fives in the United States. Outbreaks tend to occur in the United States between July and October, with about one-third of cases being in infants less than six months old and 60% of the total being in the under-five age group. Premature babies are particularly at risk of whooping cough and are more likely to develop complications than older children.

The whooping cough vaccine reduced the number of whooping cough cases 100-fold by 1970, compared to figures for 1945. But there has been an increase since then, with several states reporting epidemics. The increases have been higher among adolescents and adults than among children, suggesting some waning of immunity in the older age groups. In 1996, the year of the last major outbreak, the Centers for Disease Control and Prevention (CDC) reported nearly 8,000 cases, which was the highest number since 1967. Around 5,000–7,000 cases of whooping cough are reported each year to the CDC, and this number is probably fewer than the actual number of cases. In 2003, there were 13 deaths from whooping cough in the United States.

■ Treatment and Prevention

Antibiotics will shorten the course of whooping cough, if given in the early stages of the disease, but do not tend to shorten the paroxysmal stage. However, antibiotic treatment does help prevent the transmission of the disease. Erythromycin is the antibiotic that is usually recommended for the treatment of whooping cough. A major concern is the emergence of strains of *B. pertussis* that are resistant to antibiotics. Patients with whooping cough readily become dehydrated and should be given plenty of fluids.

The pertussis vaccine is generally given in combination with vaccines against diphtheria and tetanus (the DTP vaccine). The WHO recommends three injection of DTP be given at the ages of six, ten and 14 weeks, with a booster injection between 18 months and six years. Up to half of children receiving the vaccine will become feverish immediately afterwards for up to 24 hours and may have soreness and redness at the site of the injection.

■ Impacts and Issues

Whooping cough remains a serious health threat for children around the world, which is why joint efforts of the WHO and other agencies are aimed toward universal vaccination for children. As with other diseases, such as diphtheria and polio, the lives of many children around the world are at risk because they have not been vaccinated. In countries where the health infrastructure is weak or lacking, because of socioeconomic and political problems or geographical factors, access to vaccination may be patchy or non-existent. For example, several children died during two outbreaks of whooping cough in 2003 in Badakhshan, a northeastern province of Afghanistan. An emergency team from the Afghan Health Ministry and the WHO mounted a mass distribution of erthyromycin. Badakhshan is mountainous, isolated, and has few health workers. Many children who live there are malnourished. These factors put them at risk of whooping cough and many other infections.

SEE ALSO *Childhood Infectious Diseases, Immunization Impacts.*

BIBLIOGRAPHY

Books

Wilson, Walter R., and Merle A. Sande. *Current Diagnosis & Treatment in Infectious Diseases.* New York: McGraw Hill, 2001.

Web Sites

Centers for Disease Control and Prevention. "Pertussis." October 13, 2005. <http://www.cdc.gov/ncidod/dbmd/diseaseinfo/pertussis_t.htm> (accessed May 3, 2007).

Whoopingcough.net. "Whooping Cough Information." <http://www.whoopingcough.net/> (accessed May 3, 2007).

World Health Organization. "Pertussis." <http://www.who.int/immunization/topics/pertussis/en/index.html> (accessed May 3, 2007).

Women, Minorities, and Infectious Disease

■ Introduction

Infectious disease research and programs for women examine a host of factors, including social class, income, religious factors, geographic location, access to medical care and transportation, and other demographic and environmental issues. While women in developed countries often have life spans that are longer than those of men, in developing countries the average woman who reaches age sixty-five lives only three-fourths as long as her female counterparts in developed countries. Poverty, infectious disease, and lack of access to health care all feed into this disparity.

Research into infectious disease issues and gender often focuses on mother-child transmission of certain diseases, such as HIV/AIDS; prevention includes behavioral and pharmaceutical interventions. Malaria, schistosomiasis, group B streptococcus (GBS), hepatitis B (HBV), human papillomavirus (HPV), and all forms of sexually transmitted diseases disproportionately affect women. Repeated pregnancies and breastfeeding can leave women in lower economic conditions chronically malnourished, with weakened immune systems.

Minority populations also experience higher rates of infectious disease and higher morbidity and mortality rates overall. Minority women, in particular, have lower rates of health care service use, increased rates of infectious disease, increased disability rates, and shorter life spans on average than non-minority women. In the United States, persons in minority populations, such as Hispanic men, tend to seek services for infectious disease such as HIV/AIDS at much later stages in the disease course than their non-minority counterparts.

Cultural expectations, socioeconomic status, age, and education level all affect disease transmission rates (maternal-child transmission, transmission to and from sexual partners, or transmission within the family and community) and the progression of disease in women. Because women often act as the gatekeepers for health care in their families, reaching women to promote public health initiatives and reduce infectious disease transmission has become a major component of public health programs.

■ History and Scientific Foundations

Medical research studies historically focused on male participants and applied results to women. The assumption that the male body and the female body were similar with the exception of the reproductive system led to lower rates of female research study participants, and a "one-size-fits-all" approach when applying the results from studies that examined men only. Assumptions about infectious disease transmission and progression in women based on such research proved to be incorrect in many instances.

Research on TB rates in developed countries noted that in the 1930s through the 1950s, infection rates for women 15–34 were higher than those of men in the same age range. For women of childbearing years, the time from infection to disease itself is swifter than for similarly aged males, but as prevention and treatment options became more prevalent, infection among women decreased.

In 2004 a study of tuberculosis rates among men and women in Bangladesh showed that the female to male ratio of TB infections there stood at 0.33 to 1, even when women's lower rate of access to health care is factored out. Previous research had questioned whether TB is underreported among women in developing countries. The 2004 findings confirmed a previous study from 2000, but many women's public health researchers questioned the prevailing concept that women consistently underreport or are underrepresented in research studies. In such cases, studying women's rates of tuberculosis along with those of men demonstrated that studying only men could lead to erroneous assumptions that impacted women's health.

In the developing world, women often face discrimination or cultural shame for contracting sexually transmitted disease, but also for contracting other infections such as malaria and TB. A mother diagnosed with TB is less likely to complete a drug protocol for many reasons, including lack of time to complete appointments with health-care workers, devotion of financial resources to children rather than self, or lack of access to appropriate health-care providers (i.e., female physicians for female patients, as required by some religions). By not following treatment protocols, the mother puts her children, partners, and other families at greater transmission risk. In addition, pregnancy and childbirth can make women especially vulnerable to infectious diseases, such as malaria, because pregnant women experience decreased immunity and increased susceptibility. Pregnancy can also lead to malnutrition and chronic anemia in women of childbearing years. In areas where birth control is unavailable or a violation of cultural practices, closely-spaced pregnancies weaken women and compromise overall health, leaving women vulnerable to infectious disease.

Over the past two decades HIV/AIDS prevention and treatment has dominated public health issues related to minority populations and women. More than 50% of all new identified HIV cases in the United States are African American, although only 12–13% of the population is African American. In addition, black women account for more than 70% of all female cases, Hispanic women 8–9%, Caucasian women 18–19%, and the rest a mixture of various racial and ethnic groups. Minority women have become the focus of HIV/AIDS public health efforts in the United States in terms of behavioral and drug-based approaches to prevention and treatment.

■ Applications and Research

HIV/AIDS and tuberculosis have converged in many developing countries. Immunocompromised (persons with a weakened immune system) patients are vulnerable to TB, and the two infectious diseases have posed a challenge to public health workers. Pregnant women face even greater obstacles, since their lowered immunity makes them more susceptible to infectious disease, and treatment can be limited by concerns about fetal exposure to certain drugs.

In addition, women often seek treatment when the disease is more advanced. Human papillomavirus (HPV), for example, is highly treatable in early stages, but in later stages some strains of the virus can lead to cervical cancer. Routine pap smears can detect pre-cancerous changes in cervical tissue, but women in developing nations and minority women in the United States receive such preventive care at lower rates. Advanced cervical cancer can be difficult to treat. In the United States, more than one-third of women diagnosed with invasive cervical

WORDS TO KNOW

IMMUNOCOMPROMISED: A reduction of the ability of the immune system to recognize and respond to the presence of foreign material.

MICROBICIDE: A microbicide is a compound that kills microorganisms such as bacteria, fungi, and protozoa.

MORBIDITY: The term "morbidity" comes from the Latin word "morbus," which means sick. In medicine it refers not just to the state of being ill, but also to the severity of the illness. A serious disease is said to have a high morbidity.

MORTALITY: Mortality is the condition of being susceptible to death. The term "mortality" comes from the Latin word *mors*, which means "death." Mortality can also refer to the rate of deaths caused by an illness or injury, i.e., "Rabies has a high mortality."

cancer will die from the disease. In the developing world, fewer than 5% of all women undergo a pap smear every five years. Condom use, which aids in reducing HPV and other STD transmission, is lower for minority women and women in developing nations engaged in sexual intercourse. A new vaccine that protects against most of the HPV strains that lead to cervical cancer is expensive, and rarely available for women in the developing world.

HIV/AIDS research and programs for prevention and treatment in developing nations focus a significant amount of resources on sub-Saharan Africa. Seventy-seven percent of all women living with HIV/AIDS worldwide live in this region. Fifty-seven percent of all HIV/AIDs cases in sub-Saharan Africa are women, according to United Nations Population Fund data, and in those African countries with the highest HIV/AIDS rates, women of childbearing years (ages 15–49) account for 75% of all HIV/AIDS patients.

Women and minorities in higher-income countries are affected by HIV/AIDS trends as well. Data from the Centers for Disease Control and Prevention (CDC), released in 2004, show that HIV/AIDS is the leading cause of death for African American women between the ages of 25 and 34, and the fourth leading cause of death for Hispanic women of the same ages. The data also show that North America experienced one of the largest increases in HIV/AIDS female patients in the world.

The CDC initiated a new campaign in 2003, targeted at female minorities, called Advancing HIV Prevention.

According to the CDC: "This initiative comprises four strategies: making HIV testing a routine part of medical care, implementing new models for diagnosing HIV infections outside medical settings, preventing new infections by working with HIV-infected persons and their partners, and further decreasing perinatal HIV transmission."

The same four points are applied to women in the developing world, although women in North America have easier access to regular, stable medical care and to antiretroviral medications that help control HIV/AIDS and reduce transmission rates during pregnancy and childbirth. The 1994 introduction of zidovudine (AZT) during pregnancy and in the antenatal period led to a dramatic drop in maternal-child transmission rates. The use of AZT in the developing world has been controversial, since cost, access to medical facilities, and cultural myths about the transmission path of HIV/AIDS present obstacles to public health efforts.

■ Impacts and Issues

Female reproductive health and roles continue to dominate research and public health programming in the area of infectious diseases, such as HIV/AIDS, HPV, HBV, and other STDs. Creating safe and consistent medical care facilities for women in developing nations is as significant as creating such health-care settings for women and minorities in lower socioeconomic levels in developed countries such as the United States.

Women experience higher infection rates of various STDs, including HIV/AIDS, from vaginal intercourse than do men. In addition, sexual violence leaves women worldwide vulnerable to disease transmission. Microbicidal gels, inserted into the vagina prior to sexual intercourse, are a promising area of research. As of late 2006, trials were underway to test gels that had shown some effectiveness in preventing the spread of HIV in animal tests.

A vaginal microbicide that does not need to be refrigerated, is highly portable, and affords women control over the use of the product could be a powerful tool in public health efforts according to researchers. Many men in areas of the world where HIV/AIDS is prevalent refuse to use condoms as a cultural matter. A microbicidal gel could be undetected and used by women as a form of protection against infection via sexual violence. Public health officials note that prostitutes, who are key transmission points and can often infect hundreds of men, could use the gel to help protect themselves and their clients. While worldwide and U.S. campaigns to promote condom use have had limited success due to cultural bias against condoms, the gels or creams represent a workaround that takes into account issues unique to women and sexuality.

SEE ALSO *HIV; Sexually Transmitted Diseases; United Nations Millennium Goals and Infectious Disease; World Health Organization (WHO).*

BIBLIOGRAPHY

Books

Faro, Sebastian, and David Soper. *Infectious Diseases in Women.* Saunders, 2001.

Periodicals

Holmes, C.B., H. Hausler, and P. Nunn. "A Review of Sex Differences in the Epidemiology of Tuberculosis." *The International Journal of Tuberculosis and Lung Disease* 2 (1998): 96–104.

Katz, Ingrid T., and Alexi A. Wright. "Preventing Cervical Cancer in the Developing World." *New England Journal of Medicine* 354 (March 16, 2006): 1110.

Kelley, C.F., et al. "Clinical, Epidemiologic Characteristics of Foreign-born Latinos with HIV/AIDS at an Urban HIV Clinic." *The AIDS Reader* 17 (February 2007): 73–74, 78–80, 85–88.

Perrino, T., et al. "Main Partner's Resistance to Condoms and HIV Protection Among Disadvantaged, Minority Women." *Women & Health* 42, no. 3 (2005): 37–56.

Salim, M.A., et al. "Gender Differences in Tuberculosis: A Prevalence Survey Done in Bangladesh." *The International Journal of Tuberculosis and Lung Disease* 8 (August 2004): 952–957.

Thorne, C., and M.L. Newell. "Safety of Agents Used to Prevent Mother-to-Child Transmission of HIV: Is There Any Cause for Concern?" *Drug Safety* 30, no. 3 (2007): 203–213.

Weber, J., et al. "The Development of Vaginal Microbicides for the Prevention of HIV Transmission." *Public Library of Science Medicine* 2 (May 2005): e142.

Web Sites

National Center for Infectious Diseases. Centers for Disease Control and Prevention. "Office of Minority and Women's Health." February 5, 2004. <http://www.cdc.gov/ncidod/omwh/infectious.htm> (accessed March 13, 2007).

Women's Health.gov. "Minority Women's Health." November 2006. <http://www.4woman.gov/minority/> (accessed March 13, 2007).

World Health Organization. "Women, Ageing, and Health." June 2000. <http://www.who.int/mediacentre/factsheets/fs252/en/> (accessed March 13, 2007).

Melanie Barton Zoltán

World Health Organization (WHO)

Introduction

The World Health Organization, as part of the United Nations (UN), has expertise to coordinate international public health matters. Within its constitution, its mission "is the attainment by all peoples of the highest possible level of health." With health as its prime concern, the WHO defines health as "a state of complete physical, mental, and social well-being and not merely the absence of disease or infirmity." Its prime concern is to, generally, promote the health of all peoples of the world and to, specifically, combat diseases—especially critical infectious diseases.

The public widely recognizes some work performed by WHO. The WHO responds to natural and human-made disasters by providing emergency aid, funds medical research, conducts immunization campaigns against fatal diseases, and improves housing, nutrition, sanitation, and working conditions in developing countries.

The WHO is probably best known for its immunization programs and smallpox eradication. Currently, it is working with other health organizations to treat tuberculosis, malaria, SARS (severe acute respiratory syndrome), and HIV/AIDS (human immunodeficiency virus/acquired immunodeficiency deficiency syndrome).

However, the WHO also performs work that is less familiar to the public. It charts statistical health trends and issues warnings about possible health problems. The WHO is also responsible for assigning a common international name to drugs. WHO standards are used for measuring air and water pollution. WHO personnel work with agencies, foundations, governments, non-governmental organizations, and private sector groups to address the world's health needs.

Headquartered in Geneva, Switzerland, the WHO consists of one hundred ninety three Member States (along with two associate Member States). It is governed through representatives within its World Health Assembly. A thirty-four-member Executive Board, elected by the World Health Assembly, supports the WHO. In addition, six regional committees focus on health concerns within Southeast Asia, the Eastern Mediterranean, the Americas, Africa, the Western Pacific, and Europe.

History and Scientific Foundations

Chinese physician Szeming Sze, Norse physician Karl Evang, and Brazilian physician Geraldo de Paula Souze proposed the formation of an international health organization in 1945 at the United Nations (UN) Conference on International Organization (San Francisco, California). The constitution for the international health organization was approved in 1946. The UN approved its charter and the World Health Organization was established on April 7, 1948. It became the successor organization of the Health Organization, which was an agency of the League of Nations.

The priorities for the fledgling organization were to deal with cholera, malaria, maternal and child health, mental health, nutrition and environmental sanitation, parasitic diseases, plague, smallpox, venereal diseases, yellow fever, and viral diseases. It also expanded immunization programs for diphtheria, measles, polio, whooping cough, tetanus, and tuberculosis.

The WHO provided health programs for food, food safety, and nutrition; health education; immunizations; prevention and control of endemic diseases; essential drugs; safe water and sanitation; and treatment of diseases and injuries.

Applications and Research

Three of the WHO's largest programs called for the global eradication of smallpox, polio, and leprosy (Hansen's disease). The worldwide campaign to eliminate smallpox began in 1967 as the WHO held vaccination programs in developing countries. By 1972, only a few countries in Africa and southern Asia reported any

WORDS TO KNOW

ENDEMIC: Present in a particular area or among a particular group of people.

ERADICATION: The process of destroying or eliminating a microorgan or disease.

MULTIBACILLARY: The more severe form of leprosy (Hansen's disease) is called multibacillary leprosy. It is defined as the presence of more than 5 skin lesions on the patient with a positive skin-smear test. The less severe form of leprosy is called paucibacillary leprosy.

PAUCIBACILLARY: Paucibacillary refers to an infectious condition, such as a certain form of leprosy, characterized by few, rather than many, bacilli, which are a rod-shaped type of bacterium.

incidence of smallpox. In 1979, the WHO reported that smallpox was eradicated throughout the world.

In the 1980s, the WHO led programs to eliminate polio and leprosy. Today, the Global Polio Eradication Initiative (GPEI) is a partnership among the World Health Organization, Rotary International, the Centers for Disease Control and Prevention (CDC), and the United Nations Children's Fund (UNICEF) to eliminate polio. The WHO provides strategic planning; technical direction; and monitoring, evaluation, and certification for the coordinating and planning of the Initiative.

As of May 1, 2007, according to the GPEI, the number of polio cases worldwide is 130 (107 in endemic countries and 23 in non-endemic countries). In 2006, 1,997 cases (1,869 in endemic countries and 128 in non-endemic countries) of polio were reported.

The WHO has been instrumental in reducing the number of leprosy cases around the world. The key to this success is a campaign to deliver information, diagnoses, and treatment to endemic countries. The WHO has recommended two types of multi-drug therapy (MDT) since 1993: a two-year treatment for multibacillary cases using clofazimine, dapsone, and rifampicin; and a six-month treatment for paucibacillary cases using dapsone and rifampicin. Free packs of MDT have been supplied by the WHO to all endemic countries since 1995, and this process has been extended into 2010.

According to WHO statistics, as of early 2006, approximately 219,826 cases of leprosy are known to exist in 115 countries/territories. In the previous four years, the number of new cases has steadily declined by about 20% annually. Areas where leprosy are still preva-

lent include Angola, Brazil, Central African Republic, the Congo, India, Madagascar, Mozambique, Nepal, and Tanzania.

■ Impacts and Issues

The WHO estimates that over one billion people worldwide do not have access to clean drinking water. Contaminated water is a source of infectious disease and parasites. The United Nations announced the "Water for Life" Decade, a cooperative initiative between several UN agencies and local governments to increase access to clean water and promote sanitation. By 2015, their goal is to reduce by half the number of people living without clean water and to aggressively treat or eradicate waterborne diseases and parasites in areas where they have been endemic.

At the United Nations Millennium Summit in 2000, 189 governments adopted a set of goals, most aimed at improving the quality of life for people worldwide. The Millennium Development Goals (or Millennium Goals) seek to reduce poverty, protect the environment, fight infectious disease, and promote health. The WHO is a key organization in the Millennium Goals project.

Several of the Millennium Goals directly address infectious disease. Goals to reduce infant mortality and promote maternal wellness both involve projects to combat infectious disease. Goal Six specifically seeks to combat HIV/AIDS, malaria, and other diseases. In response to the Millennium Goals challenge, the WHO, along with UNAIDS and other organizations, launched the "3 by 5 Initiative" with the aim of treating 3 million HIV/AIDS infected persons with antiretroviral therapy. To combat malaria, the WHO has partnered with private organizations to provide mosquito netting and preventative medications.

The WHO's disease-based approach has been criticized by some as being too simple and narrow for society's changing needs in the 2000s. Critics tell of the poorest of countries desperately in need of health assistance, but not receiving any from the WHO. Some public health officials find that its Member States withhold funds to receive support for their own agendas. The WHO has been criticized for not doing more to reduce the escalating cost for drugs used in developing countries. In addition, more organizations are competing with the WHO, such as the World Bank, which makes it more difficult for the WHO to garner financial support. In contrast, the entire 2005 budget of the WHO was about the same amount as public health expenditures in the state of California in 2005.

SEE ALSO *CDC (Centers for Disease Control and Prevention); Malaria; Polio (Poliomyelitis); Polio Eradication Campaign; Smallpox; Smallpox Eradication And Storage; Tuberculosis.*

BIBLIOGRAPHY

Books

Burci, Gian Luca. *World Health Organization.* Hague, Netherlands: Kluwer Law International, 2004.

Sze, Seming. *The Origins of the World Health Organization: A Personal Memoir 1945–1948.* Boca Raton, FL: LISZ, 1982.

Web Sites

BBC News. "World Health Organization: a profile." April 25, 2003 <http://news.bbc.co.uk/1/hi/health/2975139.stm> (accessed May 8, 2007).

Global Polio Eradication Initiative (GPEI). "Home website of GPEI." <http://www.polioeradication.org/> (accessed May 7, 2007).

World Health Organization (WHO). <http://www.who.int/en/> (accessed May 8, 2007).

World Health Organization. "The World Health Report 2006—Working Together for Health." <http://www.who.int/whr/2006/en/> (accessed May 7, 2007).

William Arthur Atkins

World Trade and Infectious Disease

■ Introduction

World trade impacts the epidemiology of infectious diseases in numerous ways, including commercial travel by air and rail, shipping of contaminated goods, transportation of disease vectors with shipped goods or via commercial transportation, and the consumption of translocated plants and animals that have been infected with non-native pathogens.

The globalization of world commerce has brought about unprecedented contact between populations and exposure to foreign pathogenic organisms that is radically changing the distribution of communicable diseases worldwide. Consequently, the urgency of international collaboration on public health information and disease control has risen to a point where an outbreak of a serious communicable disease anywhere in the world raises alarms and spawns defensive activity everywhere. The limiting of the SARS outbreak in 2004 through quarantine and restriction of wild animal markets and social interaction provides an example of how such collective defense measures can be effective. However, lessons taken from that outbreak and sober reflection on the potential virulence of certain pathogens such as avian influenza, anthrax and tuberculosis have revealed gaps in international cooperation and preparedness for the consequences of possible pandemics that world trade could facilitate. The future of disease control and local public health will increasingly depend on the processes of globalization and their impact on the distribution of pathogens and on environmental change, which can create new ecological niches for pathogenic organisms.

■ History and Scientific Foundations

The Impact of Globalization

Human travel and movement have been the main source of epidemics throughout recorded history. Trade cara-vans, religious pilgrimages, and military maneuvers facilitated the spread of many diseases, including plague and smallpox. Smallpox is presumed to have spread from Egypt or India along historical trade routes, where it was first thought to have become adapted to humans sometime before 1000 BC. For most of history, human populations were relatively isolated. Only in recent centuries has there been extensive contact between the peoples, flora, and fauna of the Old and New Worlds. Contact between the European colonists and native American populations during trade and exploration led to the transmission of measles, influenza, mumps, smallpox, tuberculosis, and other infections from the crowded urban centers of Europe, which caused the suddenly exposed native American populations to drop by at least one-third.

Intensifying global trade, which entails deregulated trade and investment, can have a mixed impact on public health. When global trade brings economic growth and disseminates technologies such as antibiotics and other medications that enhance life expectancy, there are broad benefits to public health. However, some aspects of globalization erode public health infrastructure and jeopardize health by causing the deterioration of social and environmental conditions, undermining the livelihoods of certain population groups, and sowing some unhealthful lifestyle patterns. Global environmental changes, related to population growth and intensified economic activity, include air pollution, deforestation and desertification, depletion of terrestrial aquifers and ocean fisheries, and decreased biodiversity. Some of these processes pose public health risks.

On the positive side, improvements in the public health of industrializing countries have resulted from widespread social, nutritional, and material changes such as improved sanitation and other deliberate public-health interventions, including vaccination and disease vector eradication programs. Health gains have begun more recently in developing nations in the wake of population control efforts, application of knowledge about sanitation and vaccination, improved nutrition, vector control, and gradually improved treatment of infectious diseases. However, shifts in the ecology of local habitats brought about by environmental change related to globalization can have a profound impact on the distribution of infectious diseases.

Globalization and the Ecology of Infectious Disease

The main reason for the adverse effects of globalization is the disruption of traditional and largely self-contained agricultural societies that produce, consume, and trade on a local basis, using technologies that have a low impact on the environment. The social and environmental determinants of public health for these societies are predominantly local. Over the past century, industrialization and modernization have changed the amount of contact, influence, and trade between societies; created new hierarchical business associations; and have increased the impact of technology on the environment. The former balance between local populations and the pathogens in their environments is often disturbed and new pathogens are introduced into local regions, increasing the probability of serious disease outbreaks for which local people either lack herd immunity or the means for effective treatment.

Globalization of commerce and culture has also spurred an increase in human mobility. Much of this travel is voluntary, connected with business, tourism, and movement of labor. Some of this mobility is involuntary, caused by war (which is often connected with trade advantage or resource access issues), social breakdown, and natural disasters. A recent study found that the number of environmental and political refugees has increased about tenfold since 1980. The increased transnational movement of labor generally brings economic benefits to both developed and less developed economies, but also increases the transmission of ideas, values, and microbiological agents that affect disease patterns.

The globalization of world trade thus fundamentally changes the ecological context of infectious disease epidemiology by opening new opportunities for transmission and environmental niches for pathogens while also increasing the need for transnational public health information sharing and cooperation for disease prevention and treatment. Perhaps more than any other current trend, world trade brings home the importance of viewing epidemiology as more than the analysis of risk factors for disease, but rather as the study of ecological systems that mediate disease distribution and causation.

Global Trade and Travel

Global trade necessitates greatly increased travel for transactions, and travel is a major force in disease emergence and spread. According to the Centers for Disease Control (CDC), the current volume, speed, and reach of travel are unprecedented. Travel and trade facilitate the

WORDS TO KNOW

BUSHMEAT: The meat of terrestrial wild and exotic animals, typically those that live in parts of Africa, Asia, and the Americas; also known as wild meat.

ENDEMIC: Present in a particular area or among a particular group of people.

EPIDEMIOLOGY: Epidemiology is the study of various factors that influence the occurrence, distribution, prevention, and control of disease, injury, and other health-related events in a defined human population. By the application of various analytical techniques including mathematical analysis of the data, the probable cause of an infectious outbreak can be pinpointed.

GLOBALIZATION: The integration of national and local systems into a global economy through increased trade, manufacturing, communications, and migration.

HERD IMMUNITY: Herd immunity is a resistance to disease that occurs in a population when a proportion of them have been immunized against it. The theory is that it is less likely that an infectious disease will spread in a group where some individuals are less likely to contract it.

PATHOGENIC: Something causing or capable of causing disease.

VECTOR: Any agent, living or otherwise, that carries and transmits parasites and diseases. Also, an organism or chemical used to transport a gene into a new host cell.

ZOONOTIC: A zoonotic disease is a disease that can be transmitted between animals and humans. Examples of zoonotic diseases are anthrax, plague, and Q-fever.

mixing of diverse genetic pools and harbored microorganisms at rates and in combinations unknown. Such massive mobility and other concomitant changes in social, political, climatic, environmental, and technologic factors have converged to favor the emergence of infectious diseases.

Disease emergence or reemergence generally requires several simultaneous events. Travel introduces a potentially pathogenic microbe into a new geographic region. However, in order to become established and cause disease a microorganism must survive, proliferate, and find a way to enter a vulnerable host.

Global travel, changing patterns of resistance and susceptibility, and the emergence of infectious diseases also affect plants, animals, and insect vectors. Infectious diseases are dynamic. Most new infections are not caused by genuinely new pathogens. Agents involved in new and reemergent infections include viruses, bacteria, fungi, protozoa, and helminths. Human activities that provide new opportunities for the proliferation of these microbes are the most potent factors driving infectious disease emergence.

Travel is relevant in the emergence of disease if it changes an ecosystem in ways that promote the transmission of disease by introducing new organisms or by altering the ecosystem in ways that facilitate the proliferation of new or endemic pathogens. Travel introduces such organisms by transporting pathogens (in or on travelers' bodies, including microbiologic flora or disease vectors) and carrying dormant infections that have been controlled by the travelers' immune systems and genetic makeup but to which native populations are not immune. Pathogens are also introduced to new ecosystems by luggage and whatever it contains. Direct change of native ecosystems in ways that favor disease emergence can occur when trade brings about changes in cultural preferences, customs, behavioral patterns, and local technology.

■ Applications and Research

Trade in Wildlife—An Infectious Disease "Time Bomb"

Worldwide trade in wildlife creates opportunities for infectious disease transmission that cause outbreaks in both humans and livestock. In turn, these outbreaks threaten international trade, agriculture, native wildlife populations, and the integrity of local ecosystems. Disease outbreaks resulting from wildlife trade have caused hundreds of billions of dollars of economic destruction globally.

According to the CDC, estimating the volume of the global wildlife trade is extremely difficult because it encompasses activities ranging from local barter to major international commerce via ships, rail, and aircraft. A significant proportion of this trade is conducted either informally or illegally. It is estimated that 40,000 live primates, four million live birds, 640,000 live reptiles, and 350 million live tropical fish are traded globally each year. Guangzhou, China, has live wildlife markets that trade in masked palm civets, ferret badgers, barking deer, wild boars, hedgehogs, foxes, squirrels, bamboo rats, gerbils, snakes, and endangered leopards, as well as domesticated dogs, cats, and rabbits. Lacking precise

trade data, the CDC conservatively estimates that in East and Southeast Asia, tens of millions of wild animals are shipped annually, both within the region and from around the world for food or use in traditional medicine.

The estimate for trade and regional consumption of wild animal meat in Central Africa is more than 2.2 billion lb (1 billion kg) per year, and estimates for consumption in the Amazon Basin are in the range of 220 million lb (100 million kg) annually. For mammals, this amounts to 6.4 million to 15.8 million individual animals. In Central Africa, estimates range over 500 million mammals.

Hunters, brokers/distributors, and consumers have some degree of contact as each animal is traded. Other wildlife in the trade is exposed, as are domestic animals and wild scavengers in villages and market areas that consume the remnants and wastes from the traded wildlife. The CDC calculates that multiple billions of direct and indirect contacts among wildlife, humans, and domestic animals result from the wildlife trade annually. The global scope of this trade, together with rapid modern transportation and the role of markets as network hubs rather than as final destinations, dramatically increases the movement and potential cross-species transmission of communicable pathogens that every animal naturally hosts. Since trade in wildlife functions as networks with the markets as major hubs, these markets provide control opportunities to maximize the effects of public health and other regulatory efforts.

Far from being a peripheral public health risk, trade in wild animals presents one of the most severe health threats facing modern society. Perhaps the most significant human disease outbreak in the past several years directly attributable to wildlife trade (specifically, trade in civet cats) was the epidemic of severe acute respiratory syndrome (SARS) in 2003. Control efforts in Guangzhou involved the confiscation of a reported 838,500 wild animals from the markets. A study of antibody evidence of exposure to the SARS Coronavirus demonstrated a dramatic rise from low or zero prevalence of civets at farms to an approximately 80% prevalence in civets tested in markets.

Since 1980, more than 35 new infectious diseases have emerged in humans, approximately one every eight months. The origin of HIV is likely linked to human consumption of nonhuman primates. Recent Ebola hemorrhagic fever outbreaks have been traced to index patient contact with infected great apes that are hunted for food.

The collateral transmission of infectious agents due to the wildlife trade is not limited to human pathogens but also involves pathogens of domestic animals and native wildlife. Ominously, H5N1 Type-A Influenza virus was recently isolated from two mountain hawk eagles illegally imported to Belgium from Thailand. Monkeypox was transmitted to a native rodent species and then to humans in the United States by imported wild African rodents for the United States pet trade. Chytridiomycosis, a fungal disease now identified as a major cause of the extinction of 30% of amphibian species worldwide, has been spread by the international trade in African clawed frogs.

Many domestic animal diseases are transmitted through the same species of parasites carried by imported animals. Ticks have been removed from nearly 100 shipments of wild animals inspected by the U.S. Department of Agriculture. Ticks carry many diseases that threaten livestock and human health, including heartwater disease, Lyme disease, and babesiosis.

CDC examination of epidemiological data indicates that the possibility of emerging infectious diseases spreading between persons and animals is rising due to human activities ranging from the handling of bushmeat and the trade in exotic animals to the destruction or disturbance of wild habitat. The majority (61%) of listed human pathogens is known to be zoonotic, and multiple host pathogens are twice as likely to be associated with an emerging human infectious disease. More than three-quarters of pathogens found in livestock are shared with other host species.

The sudden increase of emerging or reemerging livestock disease outbreaks around the world since the mid 1990s, including bovine spongiform encephalopathy (BSE), foot-and-mouth disease, avian influenza, and swine fever, has cost the world economy $80 billion. In early 2003, the United Nations reported that more than one third of the global meat trade was embargoed as a result of mad cow disease, avian influenza, and other livestock disease outbreaks. Efforts to control the spread of avian influenza in Asian countries since 2003 have required the culling of more than 140 million chickens.

Any attempt to eradicate the trade in wild species is doomed to failure. However, the experience of slowing the spread of SARS by regulating the market in Guangzhou shows that focusing efforts at wildlife markets to regulate, reduce, or in some cases, eliminate the trade in particular wildlife species could provide a cost-effective approach to decreasing the risks of disease for humans, domestic animals, wildlife, and ecosystems.

■ Impacts and Issues

Updating International Health Regulations

The International Health Regulations (IHR) are the only existing global regulations for infectious disease control. These regulations have not been appreciably changed since their original issuance in 1951. The World Health Organization (WHO) is currently attempting to modernize the IHR, in view of the many emerging global public health threats posed by international trade, travel, and other worldwide human activity.

In an article published in the *Journal of the American Medical Association* in 2004, Lawrence Gostin recommended IHR revisions to improve global health, including:

1. Adopting a robust mission, emphasizing the WHO's core public health purposes, functions, and essential services

2. Assuming a broad scope, flexibly covering various health threats

3. Taking responsibility for global surveillance, developing information networks of official and informal data sources

4. Evaluating the adequacy of national public health systems, setting performance criteria, measuring outcomes, and holding states accountable for public protection

5. Ensuring the protection of human rights, setting science-based standards and fair procedures

6. Promoting good governance, adopting the principles of fairness, objectivity, and transparency

Overall, recommendations are for according the WHO with sweeping responsibility for enforcing health norms and ensuring state compliance while providing generous economic and technical assistance to poorer countries. Enforcement options for the WHO remain unclear, but there is an implicit reliance in the recommendations upon the power of world public opinion, possibly backed up by sanctions imposed by influential countries against those that withhold cooperation. Given the intimacy with which the world is now connected in the struggle against infectious disease, the rich and poor nations have an equal stake in assuring that all nations have the tools to combat emerging and reemerging diseases that result from global trade.

SEE ALSO *Public Health and Infectious Disease; Travel and Infectious Disease.*

BIBLIOGRAPHY

Books

Myers, N., and J. Kent. *Environmental Exodus: An Emergent Crisis in the Global Arena.* New York: Climate Institute, 1995.

Periodicals

Gostin, L.O. "International Infectious Disease Law: Revision of the World Health Organization's International Health Regulations." *Journal of the American Medical Association* 291 (2004): 2623-2627. (Also available at <http://jama.ama-assn.org/cgi/content/full/291/21/2623>; accessed May 26, 2007).
Karesh, W.B., R.A. Cook, E.L. Bennett, and J. Newcomb. "Wildlife Trade and Global Disease

Emergence." *Emerging Infectious Diseases* 11, 7 (July 2005). Available at <http://www.cdc.gov/ eid> (accessed May 26, 2007).

McMichael A., and R. Beaglehole. "The Changing Global Context of Public Health." *The Lancet* 356, 9228 (August 2000): 495–499.

Kenneth T. LaPensee

Yaws

■ Introduction

Yaws is a chronic infection, which primarily affects the skin, bones, and cartilage of its victims. Yaws is nearly unknown in developed countries. A spiral shaped bacterium called *Treponema pertenue* causes yaws. These bacteria, called spirochetes, are closely related to the bacteria that causes syphilis. The spirochetes spread from person to person by direct contact of skin with infectious yaws sores. Crowding, poor sanitation, and dirty water all contribute to spreading yaws, and the disease primarily affects the poor in tropical areas of Africa, Asia, and Latin America.

■ Disease History, Characteristics, and Transmission

The initial lesion of yaws appears where the bacteria enter the skin, and soon a red bump called a papule develops. The papule, measuring 0.8–2 in (2–5 cm) in diameter, is painless but often itchy. Scratching results in an open, ulcerated sore. This first sore takes three to six months to heal, and meanwhile, the spirochetes spread to other parts of the body through the lymph system or the blood stream.

Soon more red papules similar to the initial sore develop and eventually, the infected individual has multiple sores spread over the body. During the wet season in the tropics, these sores may get quite large resembling fleshy red wartlike growths. They eventually heal, but often scars develop at the sites of the sores. The disease is not fatal, but relapses are common up to 10 years after the initial infection.

Other problems caused by the yaws bacteria include enlarged lymph nodes in the armpits, neck, or groin. Sores may develop on the feet (making walking quite difficult) or the palms. The bones, particularly the bones of the fingers and the long bones in the arms and legs, may be affected, as well as the skin. Pain from the affected bones makes sleeping difficult.

The disease may seem to go away after a few years, but the bacteria are alive and well in the skin and bones. The latent (dormant) period may persist, but in about 10% of those afflicted, the sores reappear after 5–10 years.

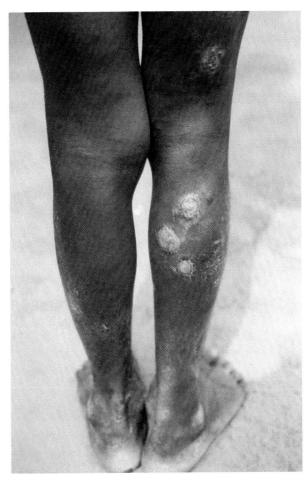

A 14-year-old girl with yaws displays ulcerations on her legs. *Centers for Disease Control/Dr. Peter Perine.*

WORDS TO KNOW

INCIDENCE: The number of new cases of a disease or injury that occur in a population during a specified period of time.

LATENT INFECTION: An infection already established in the body but not yet causing symptoms, or having ceased to cause symptoms after an active period, is a latent infection.

PAPULE: A papule is a small, solid bump on the skin.

RE-EMERGING INFECTIOUS DISEASE: Re-emerging infectious diseases are illnesses such as malaria, diphtheria, tuberculosis, and polio that were once nearly absent from the world but are starting to cause greater numbers of infections once again. These illnesses are reappearing for many reasons. Malaria and other mosquito-borne illnesses increase when mosquito-control measures decrease. Other diseases are spreading because people have stopped being vaccinated, as happened with diphtheria after the collapse of the Soviet Union. A few diseases are reemerging because drugs to treat them have become less available or drug-resistant strains have developed.

When yaws reappears, the individual suffers marked thickening of the skin on the palms and soles as well as hard nodules under the skin around the joints. Particularly disfiguring are bony growths in the bone of the upper jaw and nose. The skin and membranes of the nose and upper mouth can be involved, and result in the destruction of the upper mouth and nasal passages. Where the mouth and nose were, a gaping hole develops.

■ Scope and Distribution

Yaws occurs mostly in children under age 15, and mostly in tropical areas of Africa, Asia, and Latin America. The World Health Organization estimates that up to 500,000 people have yaws in either its latent or active form.

■ Treatment and Prevention

Yaws is a disease with a cure. At a cost of about 32 (U.S.) cents, a single injection of long-acting penicillin given in the muscle rapidly destroys the yaws bacteria. Relapses after treatment appear to be rare, and yaws bacteria have not become resistant to penicillin. For those with penicillin allergies, tetracycline or erythromycin is the drug of choice.

■ Impacts and Issues

Children are most often afflicted, yet current pediatric textbooks devote less than a page to the description and treatment of yaws. Children need not suffer the disability and disfigurement of yaws, and eliminating yaws from the globe is a possibility. Yaws can be defeated because it only occurs in humans and only occurs in specific areas making surveillance efforts easier. Additionally, an inexpensive drug cures yaws. In the 1950s, the World Health Organization mounted a campaign to eliminate yaws, and after more than 300 million people received treatment, the global incidence of yaws dropped more than 95 percent. Unfortunately, interest waned, and with reduced surveillance, yaws has made a comeback, re-emerging in the twenty-first century.

In early 2007, the World Health Organization convened a meeting to revive interest in eliminating yaws. The strategy developed at the meeting involves identifying the people at risk for yaws, actively treating all infected people and their close contacts, and most importantly a renewed surveillance effort. Participants in the meeting announced the goal of eliminating yaws in South-East Asia by 2012.

Archeologists found evidence of yaws in the bones of human ancient ancestors. Modern medicine has the ability to ensure this disease disappears from the historical record, and no more children suffer the disfigurement of yaws.

SEE ALSO *Re-emerging Infectious Diseases.*

BIBLIOGRAPHY

Web Sites

World Health Organization. "Yaws." <http://www.searo.who.int/en/Section10/Section2134.htm> (accessed May 2, 2007).

World Health Organization. "Yaws Elimination in India: A Step Towards Eradication." <http://www.whoindia.org/EN/Section210/Section424.htm> (accessed May 2, 2007).

L. S. Clements

Yellow Fever

■ Introduction

Yellow fever is an acute viral disease that is spread by mosquitoes and occurs in Africa and South America. Although a vaccine is available to prevent the disease, the incidence of yellow fever is growing, especially in South America. In this article, the virologist Jack Woodall discusses yellow fever and relates his first-hand experience in studying the disease. Woodall is the director of the Nucleus for the Investigation of Emerging Infectious Diseases at the Federal University of Rio de Janeiro in Brazil.

■ Disease History, Characteristics, and Transmission

From the seventeenth to the beginning of the twentieth century, the major ports of the United States suffered from periodic epidemics of yellow fever. New York was afflicted in 1668, Boston in 1691, and Philadelphia in 1793, where one in ten of its inhabitants died. Work on digging the Panama Canal was stalled because of the huge toll of yellow fever and malaria on the workers. The U.S. Army decided to do something about this.

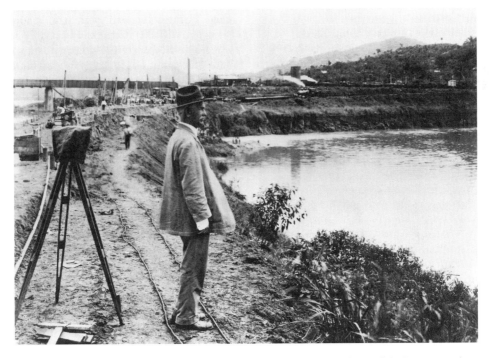

U.S. Army surgeon William Crawford Gorgas (1854–1920) surveys the building of the Panama canal, c. 1910. Gorgas was given the task of suppressing yellow fever and malaria in Cuba and the Canal Zone. Controlling the mosquitoes that caused epidemics of these diseases meant that construction workers were no longer succumbing to these illnesses and were finally able to finish the canal. © Bettmann/Corbis.

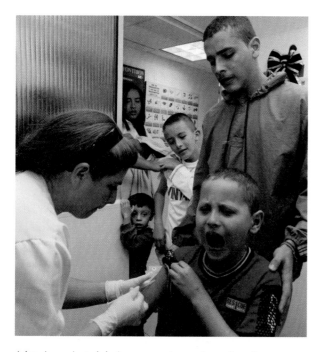

A boy is vaccinated during a campaign against yellow fever at an airport in Bogotá, Colombia. All those traveling to northern Colombia, as well as tropical regions of neighboring countries, required vaccination against yellow fever during a 2004 outbreak of the disease. *AP Images.*

It set up a Yellow Fever Commission in Cuba, which was having an epidemic, and was at the time under U.S. control.

Jesse Lazear was a handsome young U.S. Army physician with a Vandyke beard, stationed in Baltimore at the start of the twentieth century. He and a colleague joined the Commission, and both volunteered to test a new theory, that the disease was transmitted by mosquitoes. They allowed themselves to be bitten by local mosquitoes; both came down with yellow fever, but only one survived; Jesse died of it.

Other soldiers, whose names have not gone down in history, volunteered to sleep in the sheets stained by the blood and vomit of yellow fever victims. Those who did so in mosquito-proofed huts did not get the disease, whereas others sleeping in clean sheets, but without mosquito netting became ill and some died. So without even knowing that yellow fever was caused by a virus, a control program could be put in place. U.S. Army General William C. Gorgas, who had himself survived yellow fever he caught in Texas, implemented mosquito control, and eradicated yellow fever from Havana, Cuba, and the Brazilian ports of Rio de Janeiro and Santos, and the Panama Canal was completed.

Before the isolation of the yellow fever virus, no vaccine could be made, and before the advent of the vaccine, yellow fever research was a hazardous undertaking. The International Health Division of the Rockefeller Foundation established yellow fever research laboratories in East and West Africa and South America to try to delimit the areas endemic (areas where the disease naturally occurs) for the disease. Six of their scientists died of yellow fever.

There are some basic things you need to know about yellow fever. First, it is the classic viral hemorrhagic fever, with sudden onset of fever, chills, headache, backache, nausea and vomiting, causing damage to the liver, kidneys and heart, and hemorrhage, with a death rate of 20–50 percent in severe cases. The liver damage produces the yellow jaundice that gives the disease its name. It is endemic in the jungles of Africa and South America, but every so often breaks out in the cities, especially in West Africa, for example in Nigeria between 1986 and 1991. The World Health Organization estimates that it still causes around 200 thousand cases with 30 thousand deaths every year.

Second, as it is a virus disease, antibiotics have no effect on it. The antiviral drug ribavirin, given within the first five days of infection, improved survival in hamsters, so might do the same for humans. Otherwise, there is only supportive treatment, and you either recover or you don't. Laboratory diagnosis is done by isolation of the virus in tissue culture from blood taken within the first five days of illness; this test takes a few days to produce a result. Rapid tests for specific components of the virus in blood samples take only hours. If these tests fail, diagnosis can still be made by finding specific antibodies in the serum later in the course of the illness. In Brazil in the days before these tests were available, a small block of tissue was removed from the liver of a victim's corpse using a steel punch to pierce the abdomen. The specimen was placed in formalin to preserve it and examined at the lab, often after days of canoe travel down the Amazon, under the microscope for characteristic stained spots inside the cells called Councilman bodies. Nowadays, we know that some other jungle viruses also produce Councilman bodies, but certainly in the majority of cases their presence proved that the victim had died of yellow fever.

Following the example of General Gorgas, other great public health figures such as Fred Soper of the Rockefeller Foundation, Cuba's Carlos Finlay and Brazil's Oswaldo Cruz spread the gospel, and by the end of 1924 yellow fever had been eradicated from the cities of Mexico, Central America, and Ecuador. In fact, there was hope that it could be eradicated from the Americas altogether, until researchers made the unwelcome discovery of an outbreak in a rural area of Brazil where the urban vector mosquito, *Aedes aegypti*, did not exist. The virus was cycling between monkeys and tree-top mosquito species, and infecting people who ventured into the forest to hunt, collect timber, or cut it down to make plantations.

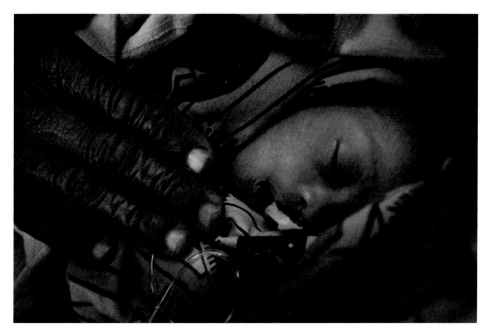

A week-old baby is treated for yellow fever at a hospital in Malawi, Africa, in 2002. The World Food Programme estimates that 3.2 million people in Malawi suffer from a variety of health problems made worse by malnutrition due to a continuing food crisis. *Ami Vitale/Getty Images.*

This discovery ended the hope of continent-wide eradication. Even if you could kill every monkey in the jungle—and who would want to do that?—the virus would survive because it has been found that it is passed down by mosquitoes through their eggs, generation after generation. Some people have dreamed of replacing the vector (transmitter) mosquitoes in nature with the same species genetically engineered to be resistant to the virus, but the probability that this could be done is around zero. So in rural areas, yellow fever only gets into a human by accident, when an infected mosquito mistakes him for a monkey. But when it does, he goes back to his hut, runs a fever, and infects the *Aedes aegypti* there. After a few days incubation, the infected mosquitoes then transmit yellow fever to his family and neighbors.

The next thing that happens is that one of the people who falls ill in the village seeks hospital care in the nearest town. There he infects the local *A. aegypti* and starts an urban epidemic. Infected townspeople in turn carry the yellow fever to the country's capital and major ports. In the days of sailing ships, fresh water was carried on deck in open barrels, in which the mosquito bred. Passengers and crew coming on board after having been bitten by infected mosquitoes ashore would fall ill at sea, and the water-barrel mosquitoes would start an epidemic that would continue until the ship reached the U.S., Canada (Halifax in 1861), even Europe—Spain, France, England and Italy in the 1800s. There, it would be taken ashore by disembarking passengers, crew and mosquitoes, to start an epidemic.

The last outbreak of yellow fever in the United States was in 1905, when New Orleans and other Southern ports were affected. But since the demise of sailing ships, the last urban yellow fever epidemic in the western hemisphere occurred in Trinidad, West Indies, in 1954, unless you count some more recent cases on the outskirts of the town of Santa Cruz, Bolivia, which could actually have been contracted in the countryside.

A puzzling question is, why has yellow fever never spread to Asia? Its cities are full of dengue, which is carried there by the same mosquito species as in Africa and the Americas, and their jungles and temples are full of monkeys that are highly susceptible to it—the virus was first isolated by injecting the blood of a sick African into an Asian rhesus macaque. Passengers incubating the disease have jetted home from the jungles of Africa or South America to fall ill in the USA and Europe, where fortunately they did not spread the disease—but the same could occur with passengers to India or China; what a mess that would create. There is not enough vaccine in the world to cope with a wide-spread epidemic in either of those countries.

Explanations for Asia's exemption are not convincing. There is a theory that immunity against dengue, which is endemic in Asia, and related viruses, cross-protects against yellow fever. But there is plenty of dengue and related viruses in South America and Africa, and it doesn't seem to cross-protect on those continents. It was thought that the Asian strains of *A. aegypti* might not be as efficient in carrying the virus, but lab experiments have proved that they are.

World Health Organization

Recent data:

The yellow fever situation in Africa and South America in 2004 Weekly Epidemiological Record. Vol. 80, 29,2005

Yellow fever epidemiological data in Africa, 2004

Country	Cases	Deaths	Lethality (percentage)
Cote d'Ivoire	92	4	4%
Burkina Faso	14	6	43%
Guinea	6	0	0%
Cameroon	6	0	0%
Liberia	5	5	100%
Senegal	2	0	0%
Mali	2	1	50%
Ghana	1	0	0%

(Source : WHO, 2005)

Yellow fever epidemiological data in South America, 2004

Country	Cases	Deaths	Lethality (percentage)
Peru	61	31	51%
Colombia	30	11	37%
Bolivia	10	4	40%
Brazil	5	3	60%
Venezuela	5	3	60%

(Source: WHO, 2005)

So, yellow fever cannot be eradicated, and there is no cure. Fortunately, there is a vaccine, possibly the most successful vaccine ever developed; one painless shot and you are protected for life, although it is best to get a booster every ten years. I was privileged to know the vaccine's developer, Max Theiler, a long-faced South African with bruised-looking eyes who worked at the Rockefeller Foundation Virus Laboratory on New York City's Upper East Side, and was an ardent baseball fan. He passed the yellow fever virus through lab animals and then embryonated chicken eggs until it lost the ability to attack the nervous system. The attenuated strain, code-named 17D, was field-tested in Brazil in 1937, and had since protected many millions of people, saving countless lives. It won him the Nobel Prize many years later. The French also developed a vaccine in the brains of mice, which had side effects, but did protect millions in their West African colonies. Theiler's 17D vaccine or derivatives are now routinely incorporated in the childhood vaccination schedule of many endemic countries.

■ Impacts and Issues

Where are we now, at the start of a new century? The big cities of Brazil suffer dengue outbreaks every year, which as mentioned above is spread by the same mosquito that carries yellow fever. Mosquito control has not been successful, since it is not pursued as rigorously as in the days of Oswaldo Cruz, 100 years earlier.

Since the *A. aegypti* mosquito breeds in domestic and peridomestic containers holding water—water jars, rain-water barrels, drums, discarded tires, cans and plastic containers, drinking vessels for domestic animals, flower vases—getting rid of those should be easy. All you have to do is to throw out those that you can, empty out the water from those you cannot, or change the water in your pet's dish and flower vases every three days, before any mosquito larvae in there can turn into adults. But in places where trash collection is intermittent or non-existent, and the public is apathetic, this just doesn't happen. People like to see trucks and sanitary agents going through the streets with insecticide fogging machines, but all that does is knock out that day's mosquitoes—plenty more will hatch tomorrow.

At the end of 1999, hundreds of Brazilian tourists went to celebrate the New Year at a popular resort at the edge of the jungle called Chapada de Veadeiros. Not all had been vaccinated against yellow fever. Some were bitten by infected jungle mosquitoes and returned home only to be hospitalized with the disease in the major cities of Rio de Janeiro, Sao Paulo, Brasilia, and Goiania. By some miracle, there was no epidemic, but we might not be so lucky next time.

So even if you have no plans to travel outside the cities of countries in the yellow fever belts of Africa or South America, it is prudent to get vaccinated, no matter what it costs. The only exceptions would be infants less than nine months old, pregnant women, those with egg allergy (since the vaccine is made in eggs), and people who are immunosuppressed for any reason (for example, those undergoing cancer therapy or organ transplants, carriers of HIV). Also if you are over 65 you should consult your doctor before getting the shot, because you are at higher risk of rare side effects of the vaccine. He or she will probably tell you not to have it if you promise to stay in the cities, and if an epidemic breaks out to come straight home, where, if you should get a fever within two weeks of returning, you should inform your doctor that you may have been exposed to yellow fever.

But I really worry about Asia.

WORDS TO KNOW

ATTENUATED STRAIN: A bacterium or virus that has been weakened, often used as the basis of a vaccine against the specific disease caused by the bacterium or virus.

ENDEMIC: Present in a particular area or among a particular group of people.

HEMORRHAGIC FEVER: A hemorrhagic fever is caused by viral infection and features a high fever and a high volume of (copious) bleeding. The bleeding is caused by the formation of tiny blood clots throughout the bloodstream. These blood clots—also called microthrombi—deplete platelets and fibrinogen in the bloodstream. When bleeding begins, the factors needed for the clotting of the blood are scarce. Thus, uncontrolled bleeding (hemorrhage) ensues.

VECTOR: Any agent, living or otherwise, that carries and transmits parasites and diseases. Also, an organism or chemical used to transport a gene into a new host cell.

■ Primary Source Connection

Dr. Carlos Finlay began studying yellow fever in the 1870s and in 1881 was the first to assert that the *Aedes* mosquito was the vector of disease for yellow fever. Finlay's research was largely ignored for decades until a team of United States researchers posited a substantially similar theory in 1900. The following article from the *New York Times* discusses the scientific community's belated recognition of Finlay's contributions to yellow fever research.

Dr. Finlay Gets Full Credit Now

HAVANA PHYSICIAN WHO SOLVED THE YELLOW FEVER PROBLEM IS EXTOLLED HERE AND ABROAD

Said Mosquitos Carried It

And Allowed a Contaminated Insect to Sting Him to Prove It—Theory Ridiculed at First   Reversing the usual order of things, scientists are determined that the rest of the world shall recognize in his lifetime the inestimable boon that Dr. Charles (or Carlos) J. Finlay of Havana conferred upon mankind when he formed the correct idea of how yellow fever is transmitted, proved his theory by self-inoculation, and forced it upon enlightened physicians and sanitarians after it had been rejected by contemporaries who regarded him as a nuisance.

Thousands of physicians who are well acquainted with the experiments of Reed, Carroll, and Lazear, who lost their lives in yellow fever investigations, never heard of Finlay. And yet he was their inspiration, and his experiments antedated theirs by a score of years. They succumbed, willing martyrs to the great cause; but he still lives and labors, revered by those working in the higher plains of science, regarded with something akin to awe by those who hear of him casually for the first time, and now, it seems, about to receive full credit, belated though it is, from the wide world.

It is now just thirty years and two weeks since Dr. Finlay read a paper before the Royal Academy of Havana, in which he propounded the novel theory that yellow fever was propagated by through the agency of mosquitos. And it is just six weeks ago that a physician in Edinburgh, commenting on Dr. Finlay and his discover, in the course of a letter wrote:

"Considering the times, it will eventually be considered one of the most wonderful pieces of constructive work in the history of medicine, but, like every other advance, it was rejected by contemporaries. Unlike nearly all other great medical discoverers, however, he has lived to see the acceptance of his facts and has not had to die of a broken heart; but it has been enough to break any one's heart to see himself so utterly ignored while the world has been singing the praises of the men upon whom he forced his ideas."

Further along the same physician writes:

"No doubt Reed himself, if alive, would blush at the methods used, and would continue to insist upon giving Finlay full credit for the great conception. Too high praise cannot be given also to Lazear and Carroll for their bravery, but Finlay did the self-same inoculation twenty years earlier. Finlay, indeed, used these Americans as one would a tool, and he had to force them, for they, too, laughed at him.

"It seems to me that the credit for initiating the experiments confirming Finlay's discovery is due to Leonard Wood, who, as Governor, forced the matter along in the very city where Spanish generals had positively prohibited such work."

History of the Discovery

The Medical Record, which has all the facts in its possession, has undertaken to establish the brilliant work of Dr. Finlay in such a manner that all may know of it. The editor has written an article embodying the history of the discovery. After relating that Dr. Finlay's theory, was received with incredulity and more or less good-natured ridicule, he says;

"Nothing daunted, however, with true grit he continued his observations on the remarkable coincidence between the prevalence of yellow fever and the temporary increase in the number of mosquitos—studied the anatomy, the manner of breeding, and the habits of the mosquitos, and also continued his inoculation experiments. These were begun in July, 1881, at which time he obtained a well-marked attack of yellow fever following a bite by a contaminated mosquito.

"In a paper published in The American Journal of the Medical Sciences in October, 1886, Finlay describes the mosquito which he regarded as the agent in the spread of yellow fever. It had a dark-colored body with ventral surface coated thick skin and marked with gray or white rings; on each side of the abdomen was a double row of white spots; its most striking feature was five white rings on the hind legs, present but less marked on the anterior and middle legs; white spots were visible on the side of the thorax and front of the head, while the corselet presented a combination of white lines in the figure of a two-stringed lyre; the wings when closed did not cover the body."

Dr. Finlay made further close observations of this mosquito, which is now known to science as Stegomyia calopus (the yellow-fever mosquito,) finding that it did its flying and biting between between 9 and 10 o'clock in the morning.

"In the same article," continues the writer, "Finlay argues with much acuteness in support of his theory, and he concludes with the passage, which we quote at length, since it sets forth so clearly the views as to the spread of yellow fever that are universally held to-day.

Dr. Finlay's Argument

"'From the evidence adduced in the preceding pages,' he writes, 'I conclude that while yellow fever is incapable of propagation by its own unaided efforts, it might be artificially communicated by inoculation, and only becomes epidemic when such inoculation can be verified by some external natural agent, such as the mosquito.'"

"'The history and etiology of yellow fever exclude from our consideration as possibly agents of transmission other blood-sucking insects such as fleas &c., the habits and geographical distribution of which in no wise agree with the course of that disease; whereas a careful study of the habits and a natural history of the mosquito shows a remarkable agreement with the circumstances that favor or impede the transmission of yellow fever.'"

"So far as my information goes this disease appears incapable of propagation wherever tropical do not or are not likely to exist, ceasing to be epidemic at the time limits of temperature and altitude which are incompatible with the functional activity of these insects; while, on the other hand, it spreads readily wherever they abound. From these considerations, taken in connection with my successful attempts in producing experimental yellow fever by means of the mosquito's sting, it is to be inferred that these insects are the habitual agents of transmission.'"

In an article running through several numbers of The Edinburgh Medical Journal in 1894, Dr. Finlay again set forth his mosquito theory, and once more in The Medical Record, on May 27, 1899, before the United States Army Commission had proved its correctness in such a manner that there could be no denial. In the latter article he asks:

"Why should not the houses in yellow fever countries be provided with mosquito blinds, such as are used in the United States as a matter of comfort, while here it might be a question of life or death?"

He next went on to tell how the larvae might be destroyed and the mosquitos exterminated, and described ideal sanitary measures and hospital construction. In brief, he foreshadowed conditions which afterward became realities and converted hot-beds of yellow fever into delightful health resorts.

"There can be not doubt that yellow fever might be stamped out from Cuba and Puerto Rico," he said, "and malaria reduced to a minimum. It would then be the business of the port and quarantine officers to prevent the introduction of fresh germs."

His Dreams Realized "When the United States Army occupied Havana," the writer continues, "Finlay saw his opportunity, and went to the sanitary authorities with his mosquito and his theory, and urged them to investigate the subject and prove the theory which he knew to be a fact. He was received with polite toleration, but without great enthusiasm. He persisted, nevertheless, in season and out of season, and in fact made such a nuisance of himself that an investigation was finally decided upon, his confidence arousing a suspicion that he might, after all, be on the right track.

"The results of this investigation are well known. Major Reed and his associates, Agramonte, Carroll, and Lazear, took Finlay's mosquito and his data and by a series of experiments, the equal of any in the annals of scientific investigation, established beyond cavil the mosquito doctrine of yellow fever transmission.

"Some of his views were found to be erroneous, which is not surprising when one considers the disadvantages under which he labored single-handed, but his basic idea was found to be absolutely correct. Making a practical application of this doctrine and perfecting the measures outlines by Finlay in his Medical Record article, the genius of Gorgas converted the two notorious pestholes, Havana and Panama, into health resorts.

"This is all ancient history, but for that very reason it is in danger of being forgotten. Even such a master of medical history as Osler forgot it in an address on the transmission of disease through the agency of blood-sucking insects, which he delivered before the London School of Tropical Medicine last Spring. In this address he omitted all mention of Finlay's work, and only when he was reminded of it by a letter from Guiteras of Havana in The Lancet did her apparently recall the great part which this pioneer has taken in the establishment of the mosquito doctrine."

Dr. Finlay was born in Cuba and has devoted his life to the inhabitants of that island, although his work has extended to a wide sphere, but the Scotch really claim and are justly proud of him and his achievements.

"DR. FINLAY GETS FULL CREDIT NOW: HAVANA PHYSICIAN WHO SOLVED THE YELLOW FEVER PROBLEM IS EXTOLLED HERE AND ABROAD," *NEW YORK TIMES*, SEPTEMBER 3, 1911.

SEE ALSO *Arthropod-borne Disease; Hemorrhagic Fevers; Host and Vector; Tropical Infectious Diseases.*

BIBLIOGRAPHY

Books

Dickerson, James L. *Yellow Fever: A Deadly Disease Poised to Kill Again.* New York: Prometheus, 2006.

Periodicals

Woodall, Jack. "Why Mosquitoes Trump Birds." *The Scientist.* (January 2006).

Web Sites

Centers for Disease Control and Prevention (CDC). "Yellow Fever - Disease and Vaccine." <http://www.cdc.gov/ncidod/dvbid/yellowfever/index.htm> (accessed June 13, 2007).

World Health Organization. "Togo: Yellow Fever Vaccination Campaign Protects 1.3 Million People." <http://www.who.int/features/2007/yellow_fever/en/index.html> (accessed June 13, 2007).

Jack Woodall

Yersiniosis

Introduction

Yersiniosis is an intestinal disease found mostly in children and young adults that is caused by bacteria in the genus *Yersinia*. In the United States, the rod-shaped bacterium *Yersinia enterocolitica* causes the most illness from yersiniosis, primarily in young children. This bacterium is found in the feces of infected humans and animals and in some foods. The infectious disease is characterized by intestinal pain and by symptoms that resemble appendicitis.

According to the Foodborne Diseases Active Surveillance Network (FoodNet), as monitored by the Centers for Disease Control and Prevention (CDC), about one *Y. enterocolitica* infection occurs for every 100,000 persons annually in the United States. Children are infected at higher rates than adults. The infection is more common in the colder months of the year because the bacteria prefer cooler temperatures.

Disease History, Characteristics, and Transmission

Adults most often acquire yersiniosis when they don't practice proper hygiene, especially handwashing. Other activities that can lead to transmission of *Y. enterocolitica* include eating contaminated foods, such as undercooked or raw pork (especially chitterlings, which are made from the large intestines of pigs). Sometimes, humans contract the disease after coming in contact with the feces or urine of infected animals. Handling contaminated soil or contaminated human feces can also cause the infection. Although commonly assumed, yersiniosis does not originate from the mouths of infected humans.

Children can acquire the infection from drinking contaminated milk that is not pasteurized or untreated water. Babies acquire the infection when adults carelessly handle raw pork and do not wash their hands before handling the baby or objects in contract with the baby, such as bottles, clothing, and toys.

Infants are especially susceptible to yersiniosis. A medical professional should be consulted as soon as symptoms appear in an infant in order to assure that health complications do not result. It is especially important that infants younger than three months be immediately treated if suspected of being infected with yersiniosis because bacteremia (a blood infection) can result. An infant with bacteremia is often treated in a hospital or major medical facility due to the seriousness of this condition.

Yersiniosis can cause numerous symptoms, which primarily depend on the age of the patient. Most symptoms appear within three to seven days of being infected. They often last one to three weeks, but sometimes longer. In young children, common symptoms include abdominal pain, watery diarrhea often containing blood or mucus, and fever. In older children and adults, common symptoms include abdominal pain on the right portion of the body (similar to symptoms reported for appendicitis) and fever. Other symptoms include nausea and vomiting. Some people do not have noticeable symptoms, but they still excrete the bacteria in their stool and can infect others. Complications from yersiniosis can include joint pain, skin rashes, and spread of the bacteria into the bloodstream.

Scope and Distribution

Yersiniosis is found worldwide, but it more prevalent in areas where wild or domesticated animals, primarily pigs, are found. The bacterium that causes yersiniosis is found worldwide, however, the infection itself is more likely to be found in areas with poor sanitary conditions and among people with poor personal hygiene. For the most part, yersiniosis is a relatively uncommon bacterial infection in the United States.

Treatment and Prevention

Diagnosis of yersiniosis is generally performed through detection of the organism in the stools (feces) of infected people. The organism can also be detected through culture samples taken from the bile, blood, joint fluid, lymph nodes, or urine of patients. Stool samples can also distinguish between yersiniosis and appendicitis.

Treatment is usually not necessary when cases are uncomplicated. However, treatment is needed when cases become complicated, such as when severe symptoms occur or bacteria enter in the bloodstream. Then, antibiotics, such as aminoglycosides, fluoroquinolones, or tirmethoprim/sulfamethoxazole, are often prescribed.

Long-term problems caused by lack of treatment can result. Joint pain in the ankles, knees, or wrists sometimes occurs. Such pain often develops about one month after diarrhea occurs. A skin rash sometimes appears on the legs and trunk; women more frequently develop this complication than do men.

Yersiniosis can be prevented by eating only thoroughly cooked meats and, especially, and by staying away from raw or undercooked pork. Pork and other meats should be cooked to an internal temperature of at least 150°F (66°C). In addition, people should only consume pasteurized milk and milk products to avoid yersiniosis.

Prevention can be maximized by washing hands after handling raw meat, going to the bathroom, changing diapers (and promptly throwing away soiled diapers), and touching animals. Hands should be washed thoroughly with soap and water before playing with infants or touching their toys, bottles, or other such objects. Kitchen countertops, cutting boards, and other utensils should be cleaned regularly, especially after raw meat is prepared. Animal and human feces should be disposed of in a sanitary manner. Water supplies should be protected from human and animal wastes.

Impacts and Issues

Chitterlings (pig intestines) is a traditional holiday food in some parts of the world, such as the United States. The preparation of chitterlings is a long and messy process that is a primary source of yersiniosis infection. Fecal matter is sometimes contained in the pork intestines, posing a health concern to those in direct contact with the contaminated intestines, and to children and infants who may be exposed to *Y. enterocolitica* by adult caregivers who have handled the contaminated intestines. The CDC states that public awareness campaigns are mounted each year in an attempt to eliminate such contamination. However, for the most part, these campaigns have been unsuccessful. Measures are continuing to be developed and implemented to prevent this disease among people who perform what the CDC considers a high-risk health activity.

Several U.S. federal agencies are involved in the control and prevention of yersiniosis. The CDC monitors yersiniosis through its FoodNet and also conducts surveillance and investigations whenever outbreaks of the disease occur. This agency also uses public awareness campaigns to publicize the dangers associated with yersiniosis. The U.S. Food and Drug Administration (FDA) inspects food and milk processing plants and restaurants in order to assure safe products are consumed by all U.S. citizens.

The United States Department of Agriculture (USDA) monitors the health of domesticated animals raised for food. It inspects food slaughtering and processing plants to ensure that the human food supply is not contaminated. The U.S. Environmental Protection Agency (EPA) monitors and regulates the safety of U.S. drinking water to prevent the transmission of yersiniosis and other infectious diseases through the water supply.

SEE ALSO *Bacterial Disease; Food-borne Disease and Food Safety; Handwashing; Parasitic Diseases.*

BIBLIOGRAPHY

Books

Bannister, Barbara A. *Infection: Microbiology and Management.* Malden, MA: Blackwell Publishing, 2006.

WORDS TO KNOW

BACTEREMIA: Bacteremia occurs when bacteria enter the bloodstream. This condition may occur through a wound or infection, or through a surgical procedure or injection. Bacteremia may cause no symptoms and resolve without treatment, or it may produce fever and other symptoms of infection. In some cases, bacteremia leads to septic shock, a potentially life-threatening condition.

PASTEURIZATION: Pasteurization is a process where fluids such as wine and milk are heated for a predetermined time at a temperature that is below the boiling point of the liquid. The treatment kills any microorganisms that are in the fluid but does not alter the taste, appearance, or nutritive value of the fluid.

SURVEILLANCE: The systematic analysis, collection, evaluation, interpretation, and dissemination of data. In public health, it assists in the identification of health threats and the planning, implementation, and evaluation of responses to those threats.

Cohen, Jonathan, and William G. Powderly, eds. *Infectious Diseases.* New York: Mosby, 2004.

Ryan, Kenneth J., and C. George Ray, eds. *Sherris Medical Microbiology: An Introduction to Infectious Diseases.* New York: McGraw Hill, 2004.

Web Sites

Centers for Disease Control and Prevention. "Yersinia enterocolitica." October 25, 2005. <http://www.cdc.gov/ncidod/dbmd/diseaseinfo/yersinia_g.htm> (accessed April 7, 2007).

Food Safety and Inspection Service, U.S. Department of Agriculture. "Yersiniosis and Chitterlings: Tips to Protect You and Those You Care for from Foodborne Illness." February 2, 2007. <http://www.fsis.usda.gov/Fact_Sheets/Yersiniosis_and_Chitterlings/index.asp> (accessed April 9, 2007).

Zoonoses

Introduction

A zoonosis (pronounced ZOO-oh-NO-sis) is a disease that can be transmitted from animals to humans under natural conditions. Some zoonoses, after being transmitted from animals to humans, can be transmitted from human to human. There are hundreds of zoonoses, including some of the most deadly diseases known. For example, avian influenza (flu) pandemics begin as zoonoses transmitted from birds, and malaria is transmitted by mosquitoes and kills about a million people annually. New zoonoses have been emerging in recent years with increased frequency due partly to the incursion of increasing human populations into animal habitats. The World Health Organization (WHO) said in 2007 that 75% of new communicable human diseases that have emerged over the last 10 years are zoonoses caused by pathogens found in animals or animal products. Zoonoses are found in all societies, but are most common and most deadly in poorer countries.

Disease History, Characteristics, and Transmission

Many zoonoses have afflicted human beings throughout their history. Before the development of agriculture in approximately 8,000 BC, people lived in small nomadic groups. Because their diet included wild game, they were prone to parasitic zoonotic diseases, such as hookworm. However, members of such groups who survived to adulthood tended to be healthy. Because of the relative mutual isolation of these groups, epidemic disease was rare.

After the domestication of plants and food animals, people began to live in larger groups and in closer contact with a variety of animals, including sheep, pigs, cattle, goats, and chickens. This made the transmission of diseases from animals to humans more likely, as well as the transmission of diseases from person to person. Tuberculosis, measles, smallpox, and influenza first entered human populations through agricultural contact with animals and animal products, and new influenza strains still are transmitted to human populations from domesticated pig and bird populations in Asia.

The development of global trade routes allowed the spread of epidemic diseases that had lost all connection with their original animal hosts, as well as of diseases that remained zoonotic, such as bubonic plague. Bubonic plague, which is caused by the bacterium *Yersinia pestis*, first appeared in Europe in 542 AD, but it only devastated the European population after 1346, when flea-infested furs were brought from China over recently opened trade routes. In a few years this zoonosis killed approximately one-third of the population of Europe and about 75 million people worldwide. Bubonic plague is maintained in rodent populations and transmitted to humans by flea and rodent bites.

Since the development of powered transportation in the nineteenth century, a whole new set of opportunities has arisen for zoonoses to travel the world. Migrant workers, political and economic refugees, tourists, and military personnel move quickly and in large numbers from one part of the world to another. Animals and animal products are moved globally by airplane and ship, sometimes inadvertently, as when rats and insect eggs are transported along with cargo. The tiger mosquito may have hitchhiked from Asia to the United States in worn tires shipped from the United States to Japan for retreading and then returned to the United States. Some experts warn that these mosquitoes may contribute to increased zoonotic transmission of North American viruses, including the LaCrosse virus, as they spread. The West Nile virus, which produced a notorious outbreak in 1999 and is transmitted to humans through mosquito bites, was apparently brought to the United States from Israel on an airplane, either by a stowaway mosquito or an infected human traveler.

Zoonoses can be transmitted to humans by bites, scratches, saliva, dander (skin flakes, similar to dandruff), droppings, and blood. Certain zoonoses, such as

WORDS TO KNOW

EMERGING INFECTIOUS DISEASE: New infectious diseases such as SARS and West Nile virus, as well as previously known diseases such as malaria, tuberculosis, and bacterial pneumonias that are appearing in forms that are resistant to drug treatments, are termed emerging infectious diseases.

HOST: Organism that serves as the habitat for a parasite, or possibly for a symbiont. A host may provide nutrition to the parasite or symbiont, or simply a place in which to live.

RE-EMERGING INFECTIOUS DISEASE: Re-emerging infectious diseases are illnesses such as malaria, diphtheria, tuberculosis, and polio that were once nearly absent from the world but are starting to cause greater numbers of infections once again. These illnesses are reappearing for many reasons. Malaria and other mosquito-borne illnesses increase when mosquito-control measures decrease. Other diseases are spreading because people have stopped being vaccinated, as happened with diphtheria after the collapse of the Soviet Union. A few diseases are reemerging because drugs to treat them have become less available or drug-resistant strains have developed.

RESERVOIR: The animal or organism in which the virus or parasite normally resides.

VECTOR: Any agent, living or otherwise, that carries and transmits parasites and diseases. Also, an organism or chemical used to transport a gene into a new host cell.

of invertebrate animals including insects. For example, birds are a natural reservoir of West Nile virus, and the disease is transmitted to humans by a mosquito vector.

Some experts reserve the term "zoonosis" for a disease that is transmitted to humans from vertebrate animals, that is, animals with spinal columns, such as cattle, dogs, cats, and rats. By this definition, diseases spread to humans by insect bites are not zoonoses, but disease or death cause by the bites of venomous snakes and fishes are. Snake bites kill over 30,000 people per year worldwide, mostly in Asia.

■ Scope and Distribution

The geographical distribution of any given zoonosis depends on the geographical distribution of its host animal or animals. All parts of the world are affected by zoonotic diseases. While most zoonoses are most common in less developed countries in Asia, Africa, and South America, a few, such as Lyme disease and trichinellosis, are more common in North American and Europe. Millions of people get sick each year from food-borne bacterial zoonoses, such as *E. coli*, salmonellosis, campylobacteriosis, anthrax, and brucellosis. Cystericercosis, a zoonosis caused by a parasite that lives in pigs, can cause headache and epilepsy and infects approximately one out of every 1,000 inhabitants of Latin America. Viral zoonoses include rabies, which kills about 55,000 people every year worldwide (mostly from dog bites). Avian influenza, a viral zoonosis that derives its name from the fact that the animal reservoir for the virus is birds, could infect a large part of the human population if it combined with other viruses or mutated in such a way as to become transmissible directly between humans. Experts fear that tens or hundreds of millions of people could die in an pandemic outbreak of such a virus, as occurred in 1918, when between 50 and 100 million people died during the Spanish influenza pandemic.

■ Treatment and Prevention

Treatment of zoonoses varies by infection type. Zoonoses can be caused by viruses, bacteria, parasites, and fungi. Bacterial infections can usually be combated with antibiotics; antifungals, antiparasitics, and antivirals may be used against other infections, but options are generally more limited for fighting non-bacterial infections. For example, there is no available treatment for West Nile virus, which can cause fatal encephalitis in some victims. Treatment of West Nile is supportive, that is, directed at relieving symptoms and helping the patient's own immune system fight off the infection, if it can.

Prevention of zoonoses is primarily aimed at reducing the incidence of the zoonosis in the animal population from which it is transmitted to humans. For

trichinellosis, are transmitted when humans eat the flesh of certain animals. Dog and bat bites can transmit rabies, cat bites can transmit cat-scratch fever, monkey bites can transmit hepatitis B, and rat bites can transmit leptospirosis, bubonic plague, salmonellosis, and rat-bite fever.

Animals serve as the natural reservoir of some zoonotic diseases, and the vector of others. A reservoir is a long-term host organism that maintains an infective agent, usually a virus, bacteria, or parasite. The reservoir is usually not affected by the agent or is without symptoms, and can then pass on the infectious agent either by direct contact, or through a vector. A vector transfers an infectious agent from an infected host to an uninfected animal or human. Vectors are often arthropods, a group

example, destroying rabid dogs decreases the incidence of rabies in humans. Spraying DDT to keep down mosquito populations that can transmit malaria and other diseases has a similar effect. Veterinary medicine and human medicine must cooperate in many of these measures designed to reduce zoonotic disease.

Humans can also decrease the likelihood of contracting a zoonotic disease by avoiding contact with infected animals and their feces and infected food products. Food products may be rendered safe by excluding infected animals from the food supply, as in the case of anthrax or trichinellosis, or by improved food preparation (e.g., pasteurizing, thorough cooking, slaughterhouse sanitation).

■ Impacts and Issues

Over 200 zoonoses are known, and more are emerging all the time. As long as an expanding human population continues to encroach on animal habitats, the likelihood that more zoonotic diseases will appear remains high. As noted earlier, 75% of recently emerging or re-emerging diseases are zoonoses. These include unconventional diseases such as prion diseases (transmissible spongiform encephalopathies), which are caused not by viruses or living organisms but by deformed proteins that, when ingested, cause similar protein deformation in the animal or human that has eaten the meat. These deformed proteins can accumulate in the central nervous system and cause mental degeneration and death. However, an emergent pathogen need not be unknown or unusual. A disease is considered emerging if it appears in an area where it has not previously been reported, as, for example, West Nile virus appearing in the United States.

SEE ALSO *Animal Importation; Arthropod-borne Disease; Bovine Spongiform Encephalopathy ("Mad Cow" Disease); Brucellosis; Cat Scratch Disease; Dengue and Dengue Hemorrhagic Fever; Ebola; Emerging Infectious Diseases; Giardiasis; Hantavrus; Lyme Disease; Malaria; Prion Disease; Rat-Bite Fever; Ringworm; Trichinellosis.*

BIBLIOGRAPHY

Books

Krauss, Hartmut. *Zoonoses: Infectious Diseases Transmissible from Animals to Humans.* Washington, DC: ASM Press, 2003.

Torrey, E. Fuller, and Robert H. Yolken. *The Beasts of the Earth: Animals, Humans, and Disease.* Piscataway, NJ: Rutgers University Press, 2005.

Periodicals

Chomel, Bruno B., et al. "Wildlife, Exotic Pets, and Emerging Zoonoses." *Emerging Infectious Diseases* 13 (January 2007): 6–11. Also available online at: <http://www.cdc.gov/ncidod/eid/13/1/6.htm> (accessed May 11, 2007).

Meslin, F.-X. "Global Aspects of Emerging and Potential Zoonoses: a WHO Perspective." *Emerging Infectious Diseases* 3 (April-June 1997): 223–228. Also available online at: <http://www.cdc.gov/ncidod/eid/vol3no2/meslin.htm> (accessed May 11, 2007).

O'Brien, Sarah J. "Foodborne Zoonoses." *British Medical Journal* 331 (November 26, 2005): 1217–1218. Also available online at: <http://www.bmj.com/cgi/content/full/331/7527/1217> (accessed May 11, 2007).

Web Sites

San Diego Natural History Museum. "Zoonoses: Animal-borne Diseases." <http://www.sdnhm.org/fieldguide/zoonoses/index.html> (accessed February 27, 2007).

World Health Organization. "Report of the WHO/FAO/OIE Joint Consultation on Emerging Zoonotic Diseases." 2004. <http://whqlibdoc.who.int/hq/2004/WHO_CDS_CPE_ZFK_2004.9.pdf> (accessed February 28, 2007).

Sources Consulted

BOOKS

Achord, James L. *Understanding Hepatitis.* Oxford, MS: University of Mississippi Press, 2002.

Adler, Michael, et al. *ABC of Sexually Transmitted Diseases.* London: BMJ, 2004.

Adley, Catherine C., ed. *Food-borne Pathogens: Methods and Protocols.* Totowa, NJ: Humana Press, 2006.

Al-Doory, Yousef, and Arthur F. DiSalvo, eds. *Blastomycosis.* New York: Plenum, 1992.

American Academy of Orthopedic Surgeons. *Bloodborne Pathogens.* 5th ed. New York: Jones and Bartlett, 2007.

Arguin, P.M., P.E. Kozarsky, and A.W. Navin. *Health Information for International Travel 2005–2006.* Washington, DC: U.S. Department of Health and Human Services, 2005.

Askari, Fred. *Hepatitis C: The Silent Epidemic.* Cambridge, MA: Da Capo, 2005.

Atkinson, William, et al., eds. *Epidemiology and Prevention of Vaccine-preventable Diseases.* Atlanta: U.S. Centers for Disease Control and Prevention, 2002.

Bankston, John. *Joseph Lister and the Story of Antiseptics.* Hockessin, DE: Mitchell Lane Publishers, 2004.

Bannister, Barbara A. *Infection: Microbiology and Management.* Malden, MA: Blackwell Publishing, 2006.

Barry, John M. *The Great Influenza: The Epic Story of the Deadliest Plague In History.* New York: Viking, 2004.

Beers, M.H. *The Merck Manual of Diagnosis and Therapy.* 18th ed. Whitehouse Station, NJ: Merck, 2006.

Belkin, Shimshon S., and Rita R. Colwell. *Oceans and Health: Pathogens in the Marine Environment.* New York: Springer, 2005.

Bellenir, Karen, ed. *Infectious Diseases Sourcebook.* Detroit, MI: Omnigraphics, 2004.

Bennenson, A.S., ed. *Control of Communicable Diseases Manual.* 16th ed. Washington, DC: American Public Health Association, 1995.

Berger, Stephen A., Charles A. Calisher, J.S. Keystone. *Exotic Viral Diseases: A Global Guide.* Hamilton, ON: BC Decker, 2003.

Bertolotti, Dan. *Hope in Hell: Inside the World of Doctors Without Borders.* Tonawanda, NY: Firefly Books, 2004.

Bethe, Marilyn R. *Global Spread of the Avian Flu: Issues And Actions.* Hauppauge, NY: Nova Science, 2007.

Betsy, Tom, and James Keogh. *Microbiology Demystified.* New York: McGraw-Hill Professional, 2005.

Black, Jacquelyn G. *Microbiology: Principles and Explorations.* New York: John Wiley & Sons, 2004.

Black, Jacquelyn G. *Pigeons: The Fascinating Saga of the World's Most Revered and Reviled Bird.* New York: Grove Press, 2006.

Blechman, Andrew D. *Microbiology: Principles and Explorations.* New York: John Wiley & Sons, 2004.

Bloch, Marc. *The Royal Touch. Sacred Monarchy and Scrofula in England and France.* London: Routledge and Kegan Paul; Montreal: McGill-Queen's University Press, 1973.

Bloom, Barry R., and Paul-Henri Lambert. *The Vaccine Book.* Oxford: Academic Press, 2002.

Bloom, Ona, and Jennifer Morgan. *Encephalitis.* London: Chelsea House Publications, 2005.

Bluestone, Charles D. *Targeting Therapies in Otitis Media and Otitis Externa.* Hamilton, Ontario, Canada: Decker DTC, 2004.

Boccaccio, Giovanni. *The Decameron*. Mark Musa, trans. New York: Signet, 1992.

Bollet, Alfred J. *Plagues and Poxes: The Impact of Human History on Epidemic Disease*. New York: Demos Medical Publishing, 2004.

Booss, John, and Margaret M. Esiri. *Viral Encephalitis in Humans*. Washington, DC: ASM Press, 2003.

Brock, David. *Infectious Fungi*. Philadelphia: Chelsea House Publishers, 2006.

Brock, Thomas D. *Robert Koch, A Life in Medicine and Bacteriology*. Madison, WI: Science Tech Publishers, 1988.

Brower, Jennifer, and Peter Chalk. *The Global Threat of New and Reemerging Infectious Diseases: Reconciling U.S. National Security and Public Health Policy*. Santa Monica, CA: Rand, 2003.

Brunelle, Lynn, and Barbara Ravage. *Bacteria*. Milwaukee: Gareth Stevens, 2003.

Burci, Gian Luca. *World Health Organization*. Hague, Netherlands: Kluwer Law International, 2004.

Bush, A.O., et al. *Parasitism: The Diversity and Ecology of Animal Parasites*. New York: Cambridge University Press, 2001.

Cane, Patricia, ed. *Respiratory Syncytial Virus*. Volume 14 of *Perspectives in Medical Virology*. New York: Elsevier Science, 2006.

Carmichael, Anne G. *Plague and the Poor in Renaissance Florence*. Cambridge: Cambridge University Press, 1986.

Carrell, Jennifer Lee. *The Speckled Monster: A Historical Tale of Battling the Smallpox Epidemic*. New York: Dutton, 2003.

Centers for Disease Control and Prevention. *Protecting the Nation's Health in an Era of Globalization*. Atlanta: Office of Health Communication, National Center for Infectious Disease, Centers for Disease Control and Prevention, 2002.

Centers for Disease Control. *Tuberculosis Statistics: States and Cities, 1984*. Atlanta: Centers for Disease Control, 1985.

Cheng, Liang, and David G. Bostwick, eds. *Essentials of Anatomic Pathology*. Totowa, NJ: Humana Press, 2006.

Clark, David P. *Molecular Biology Made Simple and Fun*. 3rd ed. St. Louis: Cache River Press, 2005.

Clark, Robert P. *Global Life Systems: Population, Food, and Disease in the Process of Globalization*. Lanham, MD: Rowman and Littlefield, 2000.

Cohen, Jonathan, and William G. Powderly, eds. *Infectious Diseases*. New York: Mosby, 2004.

Cole, Leonard A. *The Eleventh Plague: The Politics of Biological and Chemical Warfare*. New York: WH Freeman and Company, 1996.

Collier, Leslie, and John Oxford. *Human Virology*. New York: Oxford University Press, 2006.

Committee on Climate, Ecosystems, Infectious Diseases, and Human Health, Board on Atmospheric Sciences and Climate, National Research Council (U.S.A.). *Under the Weather: Climate, Ecosystems, and Infectious Disease*. Washington, DC: National Academy Press, 2001.

Committee on Infectious Diseases of Mice and Rats, Institute of Laboratory Animal Resources, Commission on Life Sciences, National Research Council. *Infectious Diseases of Mice and Rats*. Washington, DC: National Academy of Sciences, 1991.

Connolly, M.A. *Communicable Disease Control in Emergencies: A Field Manual*. Geneva: World Health Organization, 2006.

Corsby, Alfred W. *America's Forgotten Pandemic*. New York: Cambridge University Press, 2003.

Crompton, D.W.T., A. Montresor, and M.C. Nesheim. *Controlling Disease Due to Helminth Infections*. Geneva: World Health Organization, 2004.

Dale, Jeremy W., and Simon F. Park. *Molecular Genetics of Bacteria*. New York: John Wiley, 2004.

Daly, D.J., and J. Gani. *Epidemic Modeling: An Introduction*. New York, Cambridge, 2001.

Daniel Thomas M. *Captain of Death: The Story of Tuberculosis*. Rochester, NY: University of Rochester Press, 2005.

DeGregori, Thomas R. *Bountiful Harvest: Technology, Food Safety, and the Environment*. Washington, Cato Institute, 2002.

Demaitre, Luke. *Leprosy in Premodern Medicine: A Malady of the Whole Body*. Baltimore, MD: Johns Hopkins University Press, 2007.

Despommier, Dickson D., et al. *Parasitic Diseases*. 5th ed. New York: Apple Trees Productions, 2005.

Dickerson, James L. *Yellow Fever: A Deadly Disease Poised to Kill Again*. New York: Prometheus, 2006.

DiClaudio, Dennis. *The Hypochondriac's Pocket Guide to Horrible Diseases You Probably Already Have*. New York: Bloomsbury, 2005.

Dismukes, W.E., P.G. Pappas, and J.D. Sobel. *Clinical Mycology*. New York: Oxford University Press, 2003.

Douglas, Ann. *The Mother of All Toddler Books.* New York: John Wiley & Sons, 2004.

Dowell, Scott F. *Protecting the Nation's Health in an Era of Globalization: CDC's Global Infectious Disease Strategy.* Atlanta, GA: Department of Health and Human Services, Centers for Disease Control, 2002.

Drexler, Madeline. *Secret Agents: The Menace of Emerging Infections.* New York: Penguin, 2003.

Driscoll, John S. *Antiviral Drugs.* New York: Wiley, 2005.

Duncan, K. *Hunting the 1918 Flu: One Scientist's Search for a Killer Virus.* Toronto: University of Toronto Press, 2003.

Edlow, Jonathan A. *Bull's Eye: Unraveling the Medical Mystery of Lyme Disease.* New Haven, CT: Yale University Press, 2004.

Edlow, Jonathan A., ed. *Tick-borne Diseases.* Philadelphia, PA: W.B. Saunders Company, 2002.

Ergonul, Onder, and Chris C. Whitehouse, eds. *Crimean-Congo Hemorrhagic Fever: A Global Perspective.* New York: Springer, 2007.

Ericsson, Charles D. *Traveler's Diarrhea.* Hamilton, ON, Canada: BC Decker, 2003.

Erlandsen, Stanley, and Ernest Meyer. *Giardia and Giardiasis, Biology Pathogenesis, and Epidemiology.* New York: Springer, 2001.

Ernest, Paul H. *How to Have Healthy Eyes for Life.* New York: Hudson Mills Press, 2003.

Ewald, Paul. *Plague Time: The New Germ Theory of Disease.* New York: Anchor, 2002.

Farb, Daniel. *Bioterrorism Hemorrhagic Viruses.* Los Angeles: University of Health Care, 2004.

Faro, Sebastian, and David Soper. *Infectious Diseases in Women.* Saunders, 2001.

Ferreiros, C. *Emerging Strategies in the Fight against Meningitis.* Oxford: Garland Science, 2002.

Fidler, David P. *International Law and Infectious Diseases.* Oxford: Clarendon Press, 1999.

Fields, Denise, and Ari Brown. *Toddler 411: Clear Answers and Smart Advice for Your Toddler.* Boulder: Windsor Peak Press, 2006.

Fluss, Sev S. "International Public Health Law: An Overview," *Oxford Textbook of Public Health.* 3rd ed. Roger Detels, Walter W. Holland, James McEwen, and Gilbert S. Omenn, eds. Oxford: Oxford University Press, 1997.

Fong, I.W., and K. Alibek. *Bioterrorism and Infectious Agents: A New Dilemma for the 21st Century.* New York: Springer Science, 2005.

Fong, I.W., and Karl Drlica, eds. *Reemergence of Established Pathogens in the 21st Century.* New York: Springer, 2003.

Freeman-Cook, Lisa, and Kevin D. Freeman-Cook. *Staphylococcus aureus Infections.* London: Chelsea House, 2005.

Friedman, Ellen M., and James P. Barassi. *My Ear Hurts!: A Complete Guide to Understanding and Treating Your Child's Ear Infections.* Darby, PA: Diane Publishing Company, 2004.

Gandy, Matthew, and Alimuddin Zumla. *The Return of the White Plague: Global Poverty and the "New" Tuberculosis.* New York: Verso, 2003.

Garrett, Laurie. *The Coming Plague: Newly Emerging Diseases in a World out of Balance.* London: Virago Press, 1995.

Gates, Robert H. *Infectious Disease Secrets.* 2nd ed. Philadelphia: Hanley and Beltus, 2003.

Gillespie S., and K. Bamford. *Medical Microbiology and Infection at a Glance.* Malden, UK: Blackwell, 2000.

Gladwin, Mark, and Bill Trattler. *Clinical Microbiology Made Ridiculously Simple.* 3rd ed. Miami: Medmaster, 2003.

Glynn, Ian, and Jennifer Glynn. *Life and Death of Smallpox.* London: Profile Books, 2005.

Goldsmith, Connie. *Influenza: The Next Pandemic?* Brookfield, CT: Twenty-first Century Books, 2006.

Goodman, Jesse L., David T. Dennis, and Daniel E. Sonenshine. *Tick-borne Diseases of Humans.* Washington, DC: ASM Press, 2005.

Gould, Tony. *A Disease Apart: Leprosy in the Modern World.* New York: St. Martin's Press, 2005.

Gould, Tony. *A Summer Plague: Polio and Its Survivors.* New Haven: Yale University Press, 1997.

Graunt, J. *Natural and Political Observations Made upon the Bills of Mortality.* London, 1662. Reprinted by Johns Hopkins Press, 1939.

Guerrant, Richard I., David H. Walker, and Peter F. Weller. *Tropical Infectious Diseases: Principles, Pathogens & Practice.* Oxford: Churchill Livingstone, 2005.

Harper, David R., and Andrea S. Meyer. *Of Mice, Men, and Microbes: Hantavirus.* Burlington, MA: Academic Press, 1999.

Hart, Tony. *Microterrors: The Complete Guide to Bacterial, Viral and Fungal Infections that Threaten Our Health.* Tonawanda: Firefly Books, 2004.

Hays, J.N. *The Burdens of Disease: Epidemics and Human Response in Western History.* New Brunswick, New Jersey: Rutgers University Press, 1998.

Hennekens, C.H., and J.E. Buring. *Epidemiology in Medicine.* Boston: Little, Brown, 1987.

Heymann, David L. *Control of Communicable Diseases Manual,* 18th ed. Washington, DC: American Public Health Association, 2004, pp. 700.

Hoffman, Gretchen. *Mononucleosis.* New York: Benchmark Books, 2006.

Holland, Celia V., and Malcolm W. Kennedy, eds. *The Geohelminths: Ascaris, Trichuris, and Hookworm.* Boston, MA: Kluwer Academic Publishers, 2002.

Honigsbaum, Mark. *The Fever Trail: In Search of the Cure for Malaria.* New York: Picador, 2003.

Hoppe, Kirk. *Lords of the Fly: Sleeping Sickness Control in British East Africa, 1900-1960.* Westport, Conn.: Praeger, 2003.

Howard, D.H. *Pathogenic Fungi in Humans and Animals.* New York: Marcel Dekker, 2003.

Iannini, Paul B. *Contemporary Diagnosis and Management of Urinary Tract Infections.* Newtown, PA: Handbooks in Health Care, 2003.

ICON Health Publications. *Necrotizing Fasciitis.* San Diego, CA: ICON Health Publications, 2004.

Jacqueline Wolf, *Don't Kill Your Baby: Public Health and the Decline of Breastfeeding in the 19th and 20th Centuries.* Columbus: Ohio University Press, 2001.

James, Jenny Lynd. *Microbial Hazard Indentification in Fresh Fruits and Vegetables.* New York: Wiley-Interscience, 2006.

Jamison, Dean T., ed., et al. *Disease and Mortality in Sub-Saharan Africa.* New York: World Bank Publications, 2006.

Janse, Allison. *The Germ Freak's Guide to Outwitting Colds and Flu: Guerilla Tactics to Keep Yourself Healthy at Home, at Work and in the World.* Deerfield Beach: HCI, 2005.

Johanson, Paula. *HIV and AIDS (Coping in a Changing World).* New York: Rosen, 2007.

Joynson, David H.M., and Tim G. Wreghitt. *Toxoplasmosis.* Cambridge: Cambridge University Press, 2005.

Ketley, Julian. *Campylobacter.* New York: Taylor & Francis, 2005.

Koff, R.S, and Wu, G.Y. *Chronic Viral Hepatitis.* Totowa: Humana Press, 2002.

Kolata, Gina. *Flu: The Story of the Great Influenza Pandemic of 1918 & the Search for the Virus That Caused It.* Upland, PA: Diane Pub. Co., 2001.

Koplow, David. *Smallpox: The Fight to Eradicate a Global Scourge.* Berkeley, CA: University of California Press, 2004.

Korting, H. C., ed. *Mycoses: Diagnosis, Therapy and Prophylaxis of Fungal Diseases.* Berlin, Germany: Blackwell Science, 2005.

Krauss, Hartmut. *Zoonoses: Infectious Diseases Transmissible from Animals to Humans.* Washington, DC: ASM Press, 2003.

Kruel, Donald. *Trypanosomiasis.* London: Chelsea House, 2007.

Kumara, Vinay, Nelso Fausto, and Abul Abbas. *Robbins and Cotran Pathologic Basis of Disease.* 7th ed. Philadelphia: Saunders, 2004.

Lawrence, Jean, and Dee May. *Infection Control in the Community.* New York: Churchill Livingstone, 2003.

Lax, Alister. *Toxin: The Cunning of Bacterial Poisons.* Oxford: Oxford University Press, 2005.

Lee, Bok Y., ed. *The Wound Management Manual.* New York: McGraw Hill, 2005.

Leuenroth, Stephanie J. *Hantavirus Pulmonary Syndrome (Deadly Diseases and Epidemics).* New York: Chelsea House, 2006.

Levy, Stuart B. *The Antibiotic Paradox: How the Misuse of Antibiotics Destroys Their Curative Powers.* New York: Harper Collins, 2002.

Lindsay, David S., and Louis M. Weiss. *Opportunistic Infections: Toxoplasma, Sarcocystis, and Microsporidia (World Class Parasites).* New York: Springer, 2004.

Lock, Stephen, Stephen Last, and George Dunea. *The Oxford Illustrated Companion to Medicine.* Oxford: Oxford University Press, 2001.

Lopez, Alan, Colin Mathers, and Majid Ezzati. *Global Burden of Disease and Risk Factors.* World Bank Group. 2006.

Lyon, Maureen, and Lawrence J. D'Angelo. *Teenagers, HIV, and AIDS: Insights from Youths Living with the Virus.* Washington, DC: Praeger Publishers, 2006.

Mackenzie, J.S., et al. *Japanese Encephalitis and West Nile Viruses.* New York: Springer, 2002.

Maddocks, Steven. *UNICEF.* Chicago, IL: Raintree, 2004.

Mandell, G.L., J.E. Bennett, and R. Dolin. *Principles and Practice of Infectious Diseases.* 6th ed. Philadelphia, PA: Elsevier, 2004.

Margulies, Phillip. *West Nile Virus.* New York: Rosen Publishing Group, 2003.

Marquardt, William H. *Biology of Disease Vectors.* 2nd ed. New York: Academic Press, 2004.

Maule, Aaron G., and Nikki J. Marks, eds. *Parasitic Flatworms: Molecular Biology, Biochemistry,*

Immunology and Physiology. Wallingford, UK: CABI Publishing, 2006.

Mayer, Kenneth H., and H.F. Pizer. *The AIDS Pandemic: Impact on Science and Society.* San Diego: Academic Press, 2004.

Mayho, Paul, and Richard Coker. *The Tuberculosis Survival Handbook.* West Palm Beach, FL: Merit Publishing International, 2006.

McCoy, William F. *Preventing Legionellosis.* London: IWA Publishing, 2006.

McDonnell, Gerald E. *Antisepsis, Disinfection, and Sterilization: Types, Action, and Resistance.* Washington, DC: ASM Press, 2007.

McMichael, A.J., et al. *Climate Change and Human Health: Risks and Responses,* Geneva, Switzerland: World Health Organization, 2003.

McNeill, William Hardy. *Plagues and Peoples.* New York: Doubleday, 1998.

Médecins Sans Frontières, eds. *In the Shadow of Just Wars: Violence, Politics, and Humanitarian Action.* Translated by Fabrice Weissman and Doctors Without Borders. Ithaca, NY: Cornell University Press, 2004.

Miller, Judith, et al. *Germs: Biological Weapons and America's Secret War.* New York: Simon & Schuster, 2002.

Mims, C., et al. *Medical Microbiology.* St. Louis, MO: Mosby, 2004.

Murray, Patrick, Ken Rosenthal, and Michael Pfaller. *Medical Microbiology.* 5th ed. Philadelphia: Elsevier, 2005.

Myers, N., and J. Kent. *Environmental Exodus: An Emergent Crisis in the Global Arena.* New York: Climate Institute, 1995.

Nelson, Kenrad E., and Carolyn F. Masters Williams. *Infectious Disease Epidemiology: Theory and Practice.* 2nd ed. Sudbury, MA: Jones & Bartlett, 2007.

Nestle, Marion. *What to Eat.* New York: North Point Press, 2006.

Nuland, S.B. *The Doctors' Plague: Germs, Childbed Fever, and the Strange Story of Ignàc Semmelweis.* New York: W.W. Norton & Company, 2004.

Oshinsky, David. *Polio: An American Story.* New York: Oxford University Press, 2006.

Palladino, Michael A., and Stuart Hill. *Emerging Infectious Diseases.* New York: Benjamin Cummings, 2005.

Palladino, Michael A., and David Wesner. *HIV and AIDS (Special Topics in Biology Series).* San Francisco: Benjamin Cummings, 2005.

Parker, James N. *The Official Patient's Sourcebook on Trachoma.* San Diego, CA: Icon Health Publications, 2002.

Parker, James N., and Philip M. Parker. *The Official Patient's Sourcebook on Giardiasis.* San Diego, CA: Icon Health Publications, 2002.

Parker, James N., and Philip M. Parker, eds. *The Official Patient's Sourcebook on Anisakiasis: A Revised and Updated Directory for the Internet Age.* San Diego, CA: Icon Health Publications, 2002.

Pelis, Kim. *Charles Nicolle, Pasteur's Imperial Missionary: Typhus and Tunisia.* Rochester: University of Rochester, 2006.

Pelton, Robert Young. *Robert Young Pelton's The World's Most Dangerous Places.* 5th ed. New York: Collins, 2003.

Percival, Steven, et al. *Microbiology of Water-borne Diseases: Microbiological Aspects and Risks.* New York: Academic Press, 2004.

Persing, David H., et al, eds. *Molecular Microbiology: Diagnostic Principles and Practice.* Seattle: Corixa Corp, 2003.

Peters, C.J., and Mark Olshaker. *Virus Hunter: Thirty Years of Battling Hot Viruses around the World.* New York: Anchor, 1998.

Peters, Wallace, and Geoffrey Pasvol. *Tropical Medicine and Parasitology.* 5th ed. London: Mosby, 2002.

Pierce, John R., and James V. Writer. *Yellow Jack: How Yellow Fever Ravaged America and Walter Reed Discovered Its Deadly Secrets.* Hoboken, NJ: John Wiley & Sons, 2005.

Porter Roy, ed. *Cambridge Illustrated History of Medicine.* Cambridge: Cambridge University Press, 1996.

Powell, Michael, and Oliver Fischer. *101 Diseases You Don't Want to Get.* New York: Thunder's Mouth Press, 2005.

Prescott, Lansing M., John P. Harley, and Donald A. Klein. *Microbiology.* New York: McGraw Hill, 2004.

Procopius, *History of the Wars,* vol. I, H.B. Dewing, trans. Cambridge, MA: Harvard University Press, 1914, pp. 451–473.

Regis, Ed. *Virus Ground Zero: Stalking the Killer Viruses with the Centers for Disease Control.* New York: Pocket Books, 2003.

Richardson, Malcolm, and Elizabeth Johnson. *Pocket Guide to Fungal Infection.* Boston: Blackwell, 2006.

Richardson, V.C.G. *Diseases of Small Domestic Rodents.* Oxford, UK, and Malden, MA: Blackwell Publishing, 2003.

Ridley, R.M, and H.F. Baker. *Fatal Protein: The Story of CJD, BSE and Other Prion Diseases.* Oxford: Oxford University Press, 1998.

Rodriguez, Ana Maria. *Edward Jenner: Conqueror of Smallpox.* Springfield, NJ: Enslow, 2006.

Roemer, Ruth. "Comparative National Public Health Legislation, " *Oxford Textbook of Public Health.* 3rd ed. Roger Detels, Walter W. Holland, James McEwen, and Gilbert S. Omenn, eds. Oxford: Oxford University Press, 1997.

Roemmele, Jacqueline A., and Donna Batdorff. *Surviving the Flesh-eating Bacteria: Understanding, Preventing, Treating, and Living with Necrotizing Fascitis.* New York: Avery, 2003.

Rosaler, Maxine. *Listeriosis (Epidemics).* New York: Rosen Publishing Group, 2003.

Rothstein, Mark A. *Quarantine And Isolation: Lessons Learned from Sars: A Report to the CDC.* Darby PA: Diane Publishing, 2003.

Rudolph, Collin D. et al., eds. *Rudolph's Pediatrics.* New York: McGraw-Hill, 2003.

Ryan, Kenneth J., and C. George Ray, eds. *Sherris Medical Microbiology: An Introduction to Infectious Diseases.* New York: McGraw Hill, 2004.

Ryser, Elliot T., and Elmer H. Marth. *Listeria, Listeriosis, and Food Safety.* 3rd ed. Boca Raton: CRC, 2007.

Salyers, Abigail A., and Dixie D. Whitt. *Revenge of the Microbes: How Bacterial Resistance Is Undermining the Antibiotic Miracle.* Washington, DC: ASM Press, 2005.

Samuel, William M., et al., eds. *Parasitic Diseases of Wild Mammals.* Ames, IA: Iowa State University Press, 2001.

Sarasin, Philipp, and Giselle Weiss. *Anthrax: Bioterror as Fact and Fantasy.* Cambridge, MA: Harvard University Press, 2006.

Scheld, W. Michael, et al. *Emerging Infections.* Washington, DC: ASM, 2006.

Schmidt, Michael A. *Childhood Ear Infections: A Parent's Guide to Alternative Treatments.* Berkeley, CA: North Atlantic Books, 2004.

Schneider, Mary Jane. *Introduction to Public Health.* 2nd ed. Boston: Jones & Bartlett Publishers, 2005.

Schopf, J. William. *Life's Origin: The Beginnings of Biological Evolution.* Berkeley: University of California Press, 2002.

Sears, William, and Martha Sears. *The Baby Book: Everything You Need to Know About Your Baby from Birth to Age Two.* 2nd ed. New York: Little, Brown, 2003.

Seifert, H. Steven, and Victor J. Dirta, eds. *Evolution of Microbial Pathogens.* Washington, DC: ASM Press, 2006.

Sfakianos, Jeffrey N., and David Heymann. *West Nile Virus.* London: Chelsea House, 2005.

Shephard, David A.E. *John Snow: Anaesthetist to a Queen and Epidemiologist to a Nation.* Cornwall, Prince Edward Island, Canada: York Point, 1995.

Shnayersen, Michael, and Mark J. Plotkin. *The Killers Within: the Deadly Rise of Drug-Resistant Bacteria.* Boston: Back Bay, 2003.

Sindermann, Carl J. *Coastal Pollution: Effects on Living Resources and Humans.* Boca Raton: CRC, 2005.

Singh G., and S. Prabhakar, eds. *Taenia Solium Cysticercosis: From Basic to Clinical Science.* Chandigarh, India: CABI Publishing, 2002.

Smith, Tara. *Ebola.* London: Chelsea House Publications, 2005.

Smith, Tara, and Edward Alcamo. *Streptococcus (Group A) (Deadly Diseases and Epidemics).* Philadelphia, PA: Chelsea House Publications, 2004.

Sobel, Jack D. *Contemporary Diagnosis and Management of Fungal Infections.* Newtown, PA: Handbooks in Health Care, 2003.

Speilman, Andrew, and Michael D'Antonio. *Mosquito: A Natural History of Our Most Persistent and Deadly Foe.* New York: Hyperion, 2001.

Swabe, Joanna. *Animals, Disease, and Human Society: Human-Animal Relations and the Rise of Veterinary Medicine.* London: Routledge, 1999.

Sze, Seming. *The Origins of the World Health Organization: A Personal Memoir 1945–1948.* Boca Raton, FL: LISZ, 1982.

Szklo, M., and F. Javier Nieto. *Epidemiology: Beyond the Basics.* Boston: Jones & Bartlett Publishers, 2006.

Tabor, Edward. *Emerging Viruses in Human Populations.* New York: Elsevier, 2007.

Tamparo, Carol D. *Diseases of the Human Body.* Philadelphia: F.A. Davis Co., 2005.

Tan, J. *Expert Guide to Infectious Diseases.* Philadelphia: American College of Physicians, 2002.

Tan, James. *Expert Guide to Infectious Diseases.* Philadephia: American College of Physicians, 2002.

Thompson, Kimberly, and Debra Fulghum. *Overkill: Repairing the Damage Caused by Our Unhealthy*

INFECTIOUS DISEASES: IN CONTEXT

Obsession with Germs, Antibiotics, and Antibacterial Products. New York: Rodale Books, 2002.

Tierno, Philip M. *The Secret Life of Germs: What They Are, Why We Need Them, and How We Can Protect Ourselves Against Them.* New York: Atria, 2004.

Torrence, Paul F. *Antiviral Drug Discovery for Emerging Diseases and Bioterrorism Threats.* New York: Wiley-Interscience, 2005.

Torrey, E. Fuller, and Robert H. Yolken. *The Beasts of the Earth: Animals, Humans, and Disease.* Piscataway, NJ: Rutgers University Press, 2005.

Tortora, Gerard J., Berell R. Funke, and Christine L. Case. *Microbiology: An Introduction.* New York: Benjamin Cummings, 2006.

Tselis, Alex, and Hal B. Jenson. *Epstein-Barr Virus.* London: Informa Healthcare, 2006.

Turnock, Bernard J. *Public Health, What It Is and How It Works.* 3rd ed. Boston: Jones & Bartlett Publishers, 2004.

Tyler, Kevin M., and Michael A. Miles. *American Trypanosomiasis.* New York: Springer, 2006.

Tyrrell, David, and Michael Fielder. *Cold Wars: The Fight Against the Common Cold.* New York: Oxford University Press, 2002.

U.S. Department of Health and Human Services *2006 Guide to Surviving Bird Flu: Common Sense Strategies and Preparedness Plans—Avian Flu and H5N1 Threat.* Progressive Management, 2006.

U.S. Food and Drug Administration Center for Food Safety and Applied Nutrition. *Bad Bug Book: Foodborne Pathogenic Microorganisms and Natural Toxins Handbook.* McLean, VA: International Medical Publishing, Inc., 2004.

Umar, C.S. *New Developments in Epstein-Barr Virus Research.* New York: Nova Science Publishers, 2006.

UNICEF. *1946–2006: Sixty Years for Children.* New York: UNICEF, 2006.

USAMRIID *USAMRIID's Medical Management of Biological Casualties Handbook,* 6th ed. Fort Detrick, MD: U.S. Army Medical research Institute of Infectious Diseases, 2005.

Van Der Merwe, Jacob I.T. *Survival of the Cleanest: A Common Sense Guide to Preventing Infectious Disease.* Victoria, BC: Spicers Publishing, 2005.

Vanderhoof-Forschner, Karen. *Everything You Need to Know About Lyme Disease and Other Tick-Borne Disorders.* 2nd ed. New York: Wiley, 2003.

Waller, John. *The Discovery of the Germ: Twenty Years That Transformed the Way We Think About Disease.* New York: Columbia University Press, 2003.

Walsh, Christopher. *Antibiotics: Actions, Origins, Resistance.* Herndon, VA: ASM Press, 2003.

Wamala, Sarah P., and Ichiro Kawachi. *Globalization and Health.* New York: Oxford University Press, 2006.

Webber, R. *Communicable Disease Epidemiology and Control.* New York: CABI Publishing, 2005.

Weizer, Jennifer S., and Sharon Fekrat. *All About Your Eyes.* Raleigh: Duke University Press, 2006.

Wenzel, Richard P. *Prevention and Control of Nosocomial Infections.* Philadelphia: Lippincott Williams & Wilkins, 2003.

White, Dennis J., and Dale L. Morse. *West Nile Virus: Detection, Surveillance, and Control.* New York: New York Academy of Sciences, 2002.

Whiteside, Alan. *HIV/AIDS: A Very Short Introduction.* Oxford: Oxford University Press, 2007.

Wilks, David, Mark Farrington, and David Rubenstein. *The Infectious Disease.* 2nd ed. Malden: Blackwell, 2003.

Wilson, Walter R., and Merle A. Sande. *Current Diagnosis & Treatment in Infectious Diseases.* New York: McGraw Hill, 2001.

Wobeser, Gary A. *Essentials of Disease in Wild Animals.* Boston: Blackwell Publishing Professional, 2005.

World Health Organization. *Human Leptospirosis: Guidance for Diagnosis, Surveillance and Control.* Malta: World Health Organization, 2003.

World Health Organization. *International Health Regulations 2005.* 4th ed (annot.). New York: WHO, 2005.

World Health Organization. *Preventing HIV/AIDS in Young People.* Geneva: WHO, 2006.

Wrigley, E.A., and R.S. Scofield. *The Population History of England, 1541–1871: A Reconstruction.* Cambridge, MA: Harvard University Press, 1984.

Yosipovitch, Gil, et al., eds. *Itch: Basic Mechanisms and Therapy.* Oxford: Taylor & Francis, 2004.

Zhai, Hongho, and Howard I. Maibach. *Dermatotoxicology.* New York: CRC Press, 2004.

Zimmerman, Barry E., and David J. Zimmerman. *Killer Germs.* New York: McGraw-Hill, 2002.

Zinsser, Hans. *Rats, Lice and History.* Boston: Little, Brown & Company, 1935 (reprinted 1996).

PERIODICALS

Adler, Nancy E., and Joan M. Ostrove. "Socioeconomic Status and Health: What We Know and What We Don't," *Ann N Y Acad Sci.* 1999; 896:3-15.

Allen, Arthur. "Bucking the Herd: Parents Who Refuse Vaccinations for Their Children May Be Putting Entire Communities at Risk." *Atlantic Monthly* 290, 2 (September 2002).

Allingham, J.S., et al. "Structures of Microfilament Destabilizing Toxins Bound to Actin Provide Insight into Toxin Design and Activity." *Proceedings of the National Academy of Science* 102 (2005): 14527–14532.

Altman, Lawrence K. "Flu Samples, Released in Error, Are Mostly Destroyed, U.S. Says." *New York Times* April 22, 2005.

Anderson, Alicia D. "Q Fever and the U.S. Military." *Emerging Infectious Diseases* 11: 1320–1323 (2005).

Andraws, R., J.S. Berger, and D.L Brown. "Effects of Antibiotic Therapy on Outcomes of Patients with Coronary Artery Disease: A Meta-analysis of Randomized Controlled Trials." *Journal of the American Medical Association* no. 293 (2005): 2641–2647.

Aufderheide, A.C., et al. "A 9,000-year Record of Chagas' Disease." *Proceedings of the National Academy of Sciences of the United States of America* 101 (2004): 2034–2039.

Baker, Russell, "Memoir of a Small-Town Boyhood." *The New York Times* September 12, 1982.

Barlow, Frank. "The King's Evil," *The English Historical Review*, 95, 374 (January 1980), pp. 3-27.

Barnes, Denise, "Time's Up on School Shots; 434 Students Sent to Court." *The Washington Times* (October 2, 2003).

Barry, John M. "The Site of Origin of the 1918 Influenza Pandemic and its Public Health Implications." *Journal of Translational Medicine* 2004.

Beers, S., and T. Abramo. "Otitis Externa Review." *Pediatric Emergency Care* 20 (April 2004): 250–256.

Belongia, Edward A., and Allison L. Naleway. "Smallpox Vaccine: The Good, the Bad, and the Ugly." *Clinical Medicine and Research* 1, 2 (2003): 87-92.

Benitz, Willem E., et al. "Risk Factors for Early-onset Group B Streptococcal Sepsis: Estimation of Odds Ratios by Critical Literature Review." *Pediatrics* 103 (1999): 1–14.

Berg, Paul., et al. "Summary Statement of the Asilomar Conference on Recombinant DNA Molecules." *Proceedings of the National Academy of Sciences of the United States of America* 72 (1975): 1981–1984.

Booth, Timothy F., et al. "Detection of Airborne Severe Acute Respiratory Syndrome (SARS) Coronavirus and Environmental Contamination in SARS Outbreak Units." *Journal of Infectious Diseases* 191 (2005): 1472–1477.

Boseley, S. "Can You Catch Cancer?" *The Guardian* (January 24, 2006).

Boyer, Jere, Thomas File, and William Franks. "West Nile Virus: The First Pandemic of the Twenty-First Century." *Ohio Journal of Science* 102 (2002): 98–102.

Bradley T. Smith, Thomas V. Inglesby, and Tara O'Toole. "Biodefense R&D: Anticipating Future Threats, Establishing a Strategic Environment." *Biosecurity & Bioterrorism.* 1 (3): 193–202, 2003.

Bradsher, Keith. "Carrier of SARS Made Seven Flights Before Treatment." *New York Times* (April 10, 2003).

Broad, William J. "Anthrax Not Weapons Grade, Official Says." *New York Times* (September 26, 2006).

Brouqui, Phillipe, and Didier Raoult. "Arthropod-borne diseases in homeless." *Ann N Y Acad Sci.* (October 2006, 1078: 223-35) Brouqui, Phillipe, Andreas Stein, et al. "Ectoparasitism and Vector-borne Diseases in 930 Homeless People from Marseilles." *Medicine* (Baltimore). (2005 Jan; 84(1): 61-8).

Bruschi, F., and K.D. Murrel. "New Aspects of Human Trichinellosis: The Impact of New Trichinella Species." *Postgraduate Medical Journal* 78 (2002): 15–23.

Buenz, Eric J. "Disrupted Spatial Memory is a Consequence of Picornavirus Infection." *Neurobiology of Disease* 24 (2006): 266–273.

Butler, D. "Fatal Fruit Bat Virus Sparks Epidemics in Southern Asia." *Nature* 429 (May 6, 2004): 7.

Cairncross, S., Muller, R., and Zagaria, N. "Dracunculiasis (Guinea Worm Disease) and the Eradication Initiative." *Clinical Microbiology Reviews* 15, 2 (2002): 223–246.

Case, Anne, and Francis Wilson. "Health and Well-being in South Africa: Evidence from the Langeberg Survey." Princeton University, 2001.

Casemore, David P. "Foodborne Illness: Foodborne Protozoal Infection." *Lancet* 336 (1990): 1427–1433.

Centers for Disease Control and Prevention. "Interim Pre-pandemic Planning Guidance: Community Strategy for Pandemic Influenza Mitigation in the United States." Washington, DC: U.S. Department of Health and Human Services, February 2007, page 8. Also available online at <http://www2a.cdc.gov/phlp/docs/community_mitigation.pdf>

Chamany, S., et al. "A Large Histoplasmosis Outbreak Among High School Students in Indiana, 2001." *Pediatric Infectious Disease Journal* vol. 23, no. 10 (2004): 909–914.

Chan, K.P., K.T. Goh, C.Y. Chong. "Epidemic Hand, Foot and Mouth Disease caused by Human Enterovirus 71, Singapore." *Emerging Infectious Diseases* 9, 1 (2003): 78–85.

Chang, Douglas C., et al. "Multistate Outbreak of *Fusarium* Keratitis Associated with Use of a Contact Lens Solution." *Journal of the American Medical Association* 296 (2006): 953–963.

Check, Erika. "Heightened Security After Flu Scare Sparks Biosafety Debate." *Nature* 432 (2005): 943.

Cheng, Allen C., and Bart J. Currie. "Melioidosis: Epidemiology, Pathophysiology, and Management." *Clinical Microbiology Reviews* 18 (April 2005): 383–416. Also available online at: <http://cmr.asm.org/cgi/content/full/18/2/383>.

Chomel, Bruno B., et al. "Wildlife, Exotic Pets, and Emerging Zoonoses." *Emerging Infectious Diseases* 13 (January 2007): 6–11. Also available online at: <http://www.cdc.gov/ncidod/eid/13/1/6.htm> (accessed May 11, 2007).

Cohen, H.W., R.M. Gould, and V.W. Sidel. "The Pitfalls of Bioterrorism Preparedness: The Anthrax and Smallpox Experiences." *Am J Public Health* (2004): 94:1667–1671.

Cohen, Jon. "Fulfilling Koch's Postulates." *Science* 266 (1994):1647.

Cohen, Jon. "Leaks Produce a Torrent of Denials." *Science* 298 (November 15, 2002): 1313–1315.

Cohen, Stuart A. "On the Precipice: Private-Sector Vaccine Delivery." *Pediatric News* 40 (April 1, 2006).

Coles F.B., et al. "A Multistate Outbreak of Sporotrichosis Associated with Sphagnum Moss." *American Journal of Epidemiology* (1992): 136, 475–487.

Cook, H., et al. "Heterosexual Transmission of Community-associated Methicillin-resistant *Staphylococcus aureus*." *Clinical & Infectious Disease* (2007) 44: 410–413.

Corbett, E., et al. "The Growing Burden of Tuberculosis: Global Trends and Interactions with the HIV Epidemic." *Archives of Internal Medicine* 163, 9 (May 12, 2003): 1009–1021.

Cowan, George. "Rickettsial Diseases: The Typhus Group of Fevers - A Review." *Postgraduate Medical Journal* 76 (2000): 269–272.

Cowley, Geoffrey. "The Life of a Virus Hunter." *Newsweek* (May 15, 2006).

Cox, F.E.G. "History of Human Parasitology." *Clinical Microbiology Reviews* vol. 15, no. 4 (2002): 595-612.

Crawford, D.H. "An Introduction to Viruses and Cancer." *Microbiology Today* 56 (2005): 110–112.

Cunha, Burke A. "Effective Antibiotic-Resistance Control Strategies." *The Lancet.* 357 (2001): 1307.

Cunningham, Madeleine W. "Pathogenesis of Group A Streptococcal Infections." *Clinical Microbiology Reviews* 13 (2000): 470-511.

DaSilva, E., "Biological Warfare, Terrorism, and the Biological Toxin Weapons Convention." *Electronic Journal of Biotechnology* 3 (1999): 1–17

Davies. M., et al. "Outbreaks of *Escherichia coli* O157:H7 Associated with Petting Zoos—North Carolina, Florida, and Arizona, 2004 and 2005." *Morbidity and Mortality Weekly* 54: 1277–1281 (2005).

Day, Troy, Andrew Park, Neal Madras, Abba Gumel, and Jianhong Wu. "When is Quarantine a Useful Control Strategy for Emerging Infectious Diseases?" *American Journal of Epidemiology* 163: 479-485 (2006).

De Vincenzi, I. "A Longitudinal Study of Human Immunodeficiency Virus Transmission by Heterosexual Partners." *New England Journal of Medicine* 331 (August 11, 1994): 341–346.

Diep, Binh An, et al. "Complete Genome Sequence of USA300, An Epidemic Clone of Community-Acquired Methicillin-Resistant *Staphylococcus aureus*." *The Lancet* 367 (March 4, 2006): 731–740.

Dire, D.J., and T.W. McGovern. "CBRNE - Biological Warfare Agents." *eMedicine Journal* 4 (2002): 1–39.

Donta, Sam. "Late and Chronic Lyme Disease: Symptom Overlap with Chronic Fatigue Syndrome and Fibromyalgia." *Medical Clinics of North America* 86 (2002): 341–349.

Drancourt, M., and D. Raoult. "Molecular Insights into the History of Plague." *Microbes and Infection* 4 (January 2002): 105–109.

Dunne, E.F., et al. "Prevalence of HPV Infection Among Females in the United States." *Journal of the American Medical Association* 297 (February 28, 2007): 813–819.

Durham, Sharon. "Finding Solutions to *Campylobacter* in Poultry Production." *Agricultural Research* 54 (2006): 10–11.

Editorial. "Following Koch's Example." *Nature Reviews Microbiology* 3 (2005): 906.

Elliott, S.P. "Rat Bite Fever and *Streptobacillus moniliformis.*" *Clinical Microbiology Reviews* January 1, 2007: 20 (1): 13–22.

Elston, Dirk M. "Drugs Used in the Treatment of Pediculosis." *Journal of Drugs in Dermatology* 4.2 (March-April 2005): 207–211.

Enserink, Martin, and Jocelyn Kaiser. "Accidental Anthrax Shipment Spurs Debate Over Safety." *Nature* 304 (2004): 1726–1727.

Enserink, Martin. "WHA Gives Yellow Light for Variola Studies." *Science* 308 (May 27, 2005): 1235.

Esposito, Joseph J., et al. "Genome Sequence Diversity and Clues to the Evolution of Variola (Smallpox) Virus." *Science* 313 (2006): 807–812.

Facklam, Richard. "What Happened to the Streptococci: Overview of Taxonomic and Nomenclature Changes." *Clinical Microbiology Reviews* 15 (2002): 613-630.

Factor, Stephanie H., et al. "Invasive Group A Streptococcal Disease: Risk Factors for Adults." *Emerging Infectious Diseases* 9 (2003): 970–977.

Faden, Ruth R., Patrick S. Duggan, and Ruth Karron. *New York Times Online* "Who Pays to Stop a Pandemic?" February 9, 2007. <http://www.nytimes.com/2007/02/09/opinion/09faden.html?_r=1&oref=slogin&pagewanted= print>.

Falsey, A.R., et al. "The 'Common Cold' in Frail Older Persons: Impact of Rhinovirus and Coronavirus in a Senior Daycare Center." J Am Geriatr Soc (June 1997): 45 (6): 706–712

Farmer, P. "Social Inequalities and Emerging Infectious Diseases." *Emerging Infectious Diseases* Vol. 2, No. 4. October-December, 1996.

Fauci, Anthony S. *Milbank Memorial Fund.* 2005 Robert H. Ebert Memorial Lecture. "Emerging and Re-emerging Infectious Diseases: The Perpetual Challenge." <http://www.milbank.org/reports/0601fauci/0601Fauci.pdf>

Felitti, Vincent J. "GIDEON: Global Infectious Diseases and Epidemiology Online Network." *JAMA.* (2005): 293: 1674–1675.

Fendrick, A. Mark, et al. "The Economic Burden of Non-Influenza-Related Viral Respiratory Tract Infection in the United States." *Archives of Internal Medicine* 163 (2003): 487–494.

Ferguson, Neil M. "Ecological and Immunological Determinants of Influenza Evolution." *Nature* 4222 (2003): 428-433.

Finn, Robert. "Fever of Unknown Origin? Consider Cat Scratch Disease." *Family Practice News* 35 (September 1, 2005): 67.

Frederickson, Donald S. "The First Twenty-Five Years After Asilomar." *Perspectives in Biology and Medicine* 44 (2001): 170–182.

Gips, Michael A. "Open Border, Insert Foot and Mouth." *Security Management* 45, 6 (2001): 14.

Glaser, Vicki. "A Career Path in Arbovirology—An Interview with Robert E. Shope, M.D." *Vectorbone and Zoonotic Diseases* 3, 1 (March 2003): 53-56.

Glass T.A., and M. Schoch-Spana. "Bioterrorism and the People: How to Vaccinate a City against Panic." *Clinical Infectious Diseases* (2002) 34: 217–23.

Goldmann, Donald. "System Failure versus Personal Accountability—The Case for Clean Hands." *NEJM* (July 13, 2006): 355: 121–123.

Gompper, Matthew E. and Amber N. Wright. "Altered Prevalence of Raccoon Roundworm (*Baylisascaris procyonis*) Owing to Manipulated Contact Rates of Hosts." *Journal of Zoology* (2005), 266: 215–219.

Gorman C. "The Avian Flu: How Scared Should We Be?" *Time* October 17, 2005, page 30.

Gostin L.O., J.W. Sapsin, S.B. Teret, et al. "The Model State Emergency Health Powers Act: Planning for and Response to Bioterrorism and Naturally Occurring Infectious Diseases." *JAMA* (2002): 288:622–628.

Gostin, L.O. "International Infectious Disease Law: Revision of the World Health Organization's International Health Regulations." *Journal of the American Medical Association* 291 (2004): 2623-2627. (Also available at <http://jama.ama-assn.org/cgi/content/full/291/21/2623>.

Gottlieb, M.S., et.al. "*Pneumocystis* Pneumonia—Los Angeles" Morbidity and Mortality Weekly Report (June 5, 1981): (30) 21, 1–3. Available online at <http://www.cdc.gov/mmwr/preview/mmwrhtml/june_5.htm>.

Greenfeld, Karl Taro. "The Virus Hunters: When the Deadly SARS Virus Struck China Three Years Ago, Beijing Responded with a Massive Coverup. If It Weren't for the Persistence of Two Young Reporters and One Doctor Who Had Seen Enough, SARS Might Have Killed Thousands More. There's No Guarantee the World Will Be

So Lucky Next Time." *Foreign Policy* (March, April 2006): 153, 42.

Greenwald, Jeffrey L., Gale R. Burstein, Jonathan Pincus, and Richard Branson. "A Rapid Review of Rapid HIV Antibody Tests." *Current Infectious Disease Reports* 8 (2006): 125–131.

Grischow, Jeff D. "K.R.S. Morris and Tsetse Eradication in the Gold Coast, 1928-51." *Africa* 76, 3 (2006): 381-409.

Gross, C.P., and K.A. Sepkowitz. "The Myth of the Medical Breakthrough: Smallpox, Vaccination, and Jenner Reconsidered." *International Journal of Infectious Disease* 3 (1998), 54–60.

Gross, Ludwick. "How Charles Nicolle of the Pasteur Institute Discovered that Epidemic Typhus Is Transmitted by Lice: Reminiscences from My Years at the Pasteur Institute in Paris." *Proceedings of the National Academy of Sciences of the United States of America* (October 1996): vol. 93, 10539–10540.

Haines, A., et al. "Climate Change and Human Health: Impacts, Vulnerability, and Mitigation." *The Lancet* 367 (2006): 2101-2110.

Halloran, M. Elizabeth, et al. "Containing Bioterrorist Smallpox." *Science* 298 (November 15, 2002): 1428–1432.

Handel, A., I.M. Longini, Jr., and R. Antia. "What is the best control strategy for multiple infectious disease outbreaks?" *Proceedings of the Royal Society of London. Biological sciences* 22; 274 (1611) March 2007: 833-7.

Harries, Anthony, and Dermot Maher. *TB/HIV: A Clinical Manual* World Health Organization, 1996.

Hawralek, Jason. "Giardiasis: Pathophysiology and Management." *Alternative Medicine Review* 8.2 (2003): 129–143.

Hawryluck, Laura, et al. "SARS Control and Psychological Effects of Quarantine, Toronto, Canada." *Emerging Infectious Diseases* 10 (2004): 1206–1212.

Hayes, Edward B., and Joseph Piesman. "How Can We Prevent Lyme Disease?" *New England Journal of Medicine* 348 (2003): 2424–2429.

Health Protection Agency. "Scarlet Fever Outbreak in Two Nurseries in South West England." *CDR Weekly* 16 (March 2, 2006): 1–2.

Hecht, R., et al. "Putting It Together: AIDS and the Millennium Development Goals." *PLoS Medicine* 3, 11 (2006).

Hector, R., and R. Laniado-Laborin. "Coccidioidomycosis—A Fungal Disease of the Americas." *PloS Medicine* January 25 2005. <http://medicine.plos journals.org/perlserv/?request=get-document&doi=10.1371/journal.pmed.0020002>.

Hellard, M.E., and C.E. Aitken. "HIV in Prison: What are the Risks and What Can Be Done?" *Sexual Health* 1 (2004): 107–113.

Herwaldt, B.L., et al. "Endemic Babesiosis in Another Eastern State: New Jersey." *Emerging Infectious Diseases* 9 (February 2003): 184–188.

Hill, C.A., et al. "Arthropod-borne Diseases: Vector Control in the Genomics Era." *Nature Reviews Microbiology* 3 (March 2005): 262–268.

Hilts, Philip J. "'79 Anthrax Traced to Soviet Military." *New York Times* (November 18, 1994).

Hochedez P. et al. "Chikungunya Infection in Travelers." *Emerging Infectious Diseases* vol. 12, no. 10 (2006): 1565–1567.

Hoffman, Michelle. "New Medicine for Old Mummies: Diagnosing Disease in Some Very Old 'Patients'." *American Scientist* 86 (May-June 1998).

Holmes, C.B., H. Hausler, and P. Nunn. "A Review of Sex Differences in the Epidemiology of Tuberculosis." *The International Journal of Tuberculosis and Lung Disease* 2 (1998): 96–104.

Holmes, Edward C. "1918 and All That." *Nature* 303 (2004): 1787–1788.

Hopkins, D.R. et al. "Dracunculiasis Eradication: The Final Inch." *The American Journal of Tropical Medicine and Hygiene* 73, 4 (2005): 669–675.

Hoque, M. Ekramul, et al. "Nappy Handling and Risk of Giardiasis." *Lancet* 357(2001): 1017.

Hotez, Peter J., et al. "Hookworm Infection." *New England Journal of Medicine* August 19, 2004, vol. 351:799-807, number 8.

Hotez, Peter. "Dark Winters Ahead." *Foreign Policy* (November-December 2001): 84.

Huff, Jennifer L., and Peter A. Barry. "B-Virus (*Cercopithecine herpesvirus* 1) Infection in Humans and Macaques: Potential for Zoonotic Disease." *Emerging Infectious Diseases* 9 (February 2003): 246–250. Also available online at: <http://oacu.od.nih.gov/UsefulResources/resources/emergindis2003.pdf>.

Huhn, G.D., et al. "Monkeypox in the Western Hemisphere." *New England Journal of Medicine* 350 (April 22, 2004): 1790–1791.

Hymes, K.B., J.B. Greene, A. Marcus, et al. "Kaposi's Sarcoma in Homosexual Men: A Report of Eight Cases." *Lancet* 2 (1981): 598–600.

Irwin, R.S., and J.M. Madison. "Primary Care: The Diagnosis and Treatment of Cough." *New England Journal of Medicine* 343 (2000): 1715–1721.

Jackson, Patricia L. "Healthy People 2010 Objective: Reduce Number and Frequency of Courses of Antibiotics for Ear Infections in Young Children." *Pediatric Nursing* 27 (2000): 591–595.

Jansen, A., et al. "Leptospirosis in Germany, 1962–2003." *Emerging Infectious Diseases* 11 (2005): 1048–1054.

Jernigan, D. B., et al. "Investigation of Bioterrorism-Related Anthrax, United States, 2001: Epidemiologic Findings." *Emerging Infectious Diseases* 8 (2002): 1019–1028.

Johnson, Niall P.A.S. "Updating the Accounts: Global Mortality of the 1918–1920 "'Spanish' Influenza Pandemic." *Bulletin of the History of Medicine* 76 (2002): 105–115.

Kaiser, Jocelyn. "Quick Save for Infectious-Disease Grants at NIAID." *Science* 303 (2004): 941.

Kaiser, Jocelyn. "Resurrected Influenza Virus Yields Secrets of Deadly 1918 Pandemic." *Science* 310 (2005): 28029.

Kaplan, Edward L., et al. "Reduced Ability of Penicillin to Eradicate Ingested Group A Streptococci from Epithelial Cells: Clinical and Pathogenic Implications." *Clinical Infectious Diseases* 43 (2006): 1398–1406.

Karesh, W.B., R.A. Cook, E.L. Bennett, and J. Newcomb. "Wildlife Trade and Global Disease Emergence." *Emerging Infectious Diseases* 11, 7 (July 2005). Available at <http://www.cdc.gov/eid>.

Katz, Ingrid T., and Alexi A. Wright. "Preventing Cervical Cancer in the Developing World." *New England Journal of Medicine* 354 (March 16, 2006): 1110.

Kelley, C.F., et al. "Clinical, Epidemiologic Characteristics of Foreign-born Latinos with HIV/AIDS at an Urban HIV Clinic." *The AIDS Reader* 17 (February 2007): 73–74, 78–80, 85–88.

Kimberlin, D.W., and R.J. Whitley. "Varicella-Zoster Vaccine for the Prevention of Herpes Zoster." *New England Journal of Medicine* 356 (March 29, 2007): 1338–1343.

Kirkland, T.N., and J. Fierer. "Coccidioidomycosis: A Reemerging Infectious Disease." *Emerging Infectious Diseases* 2, 3 (July-September 1996).

Kochi, Arata. "WHO Malaria Head to Environmentalists: "Help Save African Babies as You Are Helping to Save the Environment." World Health Organization Press Statement. September 15, 2006.

Koelle, Katia, et al. "Epochal Evolution Shapes the Phylodynamics of Interpandemic Influenza A (H3N2) in Humans." *Science* 314 (2006): 1898–1903.

Kohn, Marek. "Why an Unequal Society is an Unhealthy Society: Poor Relationships and Low Status Don't Just Make People Envious. They also Interfere with the Immune System and Damage Health." *New Statesman* (1996) 133.4698 (July 26, 2004): 30 (2).

Kolata, Gina. "A Dangerous Form of Strep Stirs Concern in Resurgence." *New York Times* (June 8, 1994).

Koopman, Jim. "Controlling Smallpox." *Science* 298 (2002): 1342–1344.

Kozukeev, Turatbek, B., S. Ajeilat, M. Favorov. "Risk Factors for Brucellosis - Leylek and Kadamjay Districts, Batken Oblast, Kyrgyzstan, January - November, 2003." *Morbidity and Mortality Weekly* 55 (SUP01): 31–34 (2006).

Kreeger, Karen Young. "Stalking the Deadly Hantavirus: A Study in Teamwork." *The Scientist* vol. 8, 14.

Kristof, Nicholas D. "At 12, a Mother of Two." *The New York Times* May 28, 2006.

Ksiazek T.G., et al. "A Novel Coronavirus Associated with Severe Acute Respiratory Syndrome." *New England Journal of Medicine* 10.1056. April 10, 2003.

Laver, Graeme and Elspeth Garman. "The Origin and Control of Pandemic Influenza." *Science* 293 (2001): 1776–1777.

Leibovich, Mark. "In Clean Politics, Flesh Is Pressed, Then Sanitized." *New York Times* October 28, 2006. <http://www.nytimes.com/2006/10/28/us/politics/28dirty.html?_r=1&th&emc=th&oref=slogin>.

Leroy, E.M., et al. "Fruits Bats as Reservoirs of Ebola Virus." *Nature* 438 (December 1, 2005): 575–576.

Lester, Robert S., et al. "Novel Cases of Blastomycosis Acquired in Toronto, Ontario." *Canadian Medical Association Journal* 163 (November 14, 2000): 1309–1312.

Lewis, Katharine Kranz. "The Pandemic Threat: Is Massachusetts Prepared? Findings from the Forum on Pandemic Flu, sponsored by the Massachusetts Health Policy Forum," June 2006. Policy Brief. The Massachusetts Policy Forum, August, 2006.

Lipsitch, Marc, and Matthew H. Samore. "Antimicrobial Use and Antimicrobial Resistance: A Population Perspective." *Emerging Infectious Diseases* 8 (2002): 347-354.

Lipton, Eric. "Bid to Stockpile Bioterror Drugs Stymied by Setbacks." *New York Times* (September 18, 2006).

Littman, R.J., and M.L. Littman. "Galen and the Antonine Plague." *The American Journal of Philology* 94, 3 (Autumn 1973), pp. 243–255.

Lomax, Elisabeth. "Hereditary of Acquired Disease? Early Nineteenth Century Debates on the Cause of Infantile Scrofula and Tuberculosis," *Journal of the History of Medicine and Allied Sciences* October 1977, pp. 356-374.

Loo, Yueh-Ming, and Michael Gale Jr. "Fatal Immunity and the 1918 Virus." *Nature* 445 (2007): 18–19.

Mabey, D.C., A. Foster, and A.W. Solomon. "Trachoma." *Lancet* (July 2003): 362 (9379): 223–229.

Margolis, Todd P., and J.P. Whitcher. "Fusarium—A New Culprit in the Contact Lens Case." *Journal of the American Medical Association* 296 (2006): 985–987.

Marshall, S. "Scarlet Fever: the Disease in the UK." *The Pharmaceutical Journal* 277 (July 22, 2006): 115–116.

Martens, Pim, and Susanne C. Moser. "Health Impacts of Climate Change." *Science* 292 (2001): 1065-1066.

Maunula, Leena. "Norovirus Outbreaks from Drinking Water." *Emerging Infectious Diseases* 11: 1716–1722 (2005).

McKinney, Maureen. "Travel Advisories: Wait 'Til You Hear What They Say about Us." *Daily Herald* (Arlington Heights, IL) March 21, 2005.

McMichael A., and R. Beaglehole. "The Changing Global Context of Public Health." *The Lancet* 356, 9228 (August 2000): 495-499.

McMichael, A.J., Rosale E. Woodruff, and Simon Hales. "Climate Change and Human Health: Present and Future Risks." *The Lancet* 367 (2006): 859-861.

McMinn, P.C. "An Overview of the Evolution of Enterovirus 71 and its Clinical and Public Health Significance." *FEMS Microbiology Reviews* 26, 1 (2002): 91–107.

McNeil Jr., Donald G. "Worrisome New Link: AIDS Drugs and Leprosy." *New York Times* October 24, 2006.

Meng, Tze-Chiang, et al. "Inhibition of *Giardia lamblia* Excystation by Antibodies against Cyst Walls and by Wheat Germ Agglutinin." *Infection and Immunity* 64 (1996): 2151-2157.

Meningococcal Disease and College Students." *Morbidity and Mortality Weekly Reports* 49 (June 30, 2000): 11–20.

Meslin, F.-X. "Global Aspects of Emerging and Potential Zoonoses: a WHO Perspective." *Emerging Infectious Diseases* 3 (April-June 1997): 223–228. Also available online at: <http://www.cdc.gov/ncidod/eid/vol3no2/meslin.htm>.

Miller, Laurie C. "Internationally Adopted Children–Immigration Status." Letter to the Editor. *Pediatrics* 103.5 (May 1999): 1078(1).

Mills, Christina E., James M. Robins, and March Lipsitch. "Transmissibility of 1918 Pandemic Influenza." *Science* 432 (2004): 904–906.

Mira, Marcelo, et al. "Susceptibility to Leprosy is Associated with *PARK2* and *PACRG*." *Nature* 427 (2004): 636-40.

Monot, Marc, et al. "On the Origin of Leprosy." *Science* 308 (2005): 1040–1042.

Monto, Arnold S. "Vaccines and Antiviral Drugs in Pandemic Preparedness." *Emerging Infectious Diseases* 12 (January 2006): 55–61.

Moorhead, Andrew. "Trichinellosis in the United States, 1991–1996: Declining but not Gone." *Journal of the American Medical Association* 281 (1999): 1472.

Morbidity and Mortality Weekly Report. "Guidelines for Prevention of Herpesvirus Simiae (B Virus) Infection in Monkey Handlers." October 23, 1987. <http://www.cdc.gov/mmwr/preview/mmwr html/00015936.htm>.

Morgan, Thomas E. "Plague or Poetry? Thucydides on the Epidemic at Athens." *Transactions of the American Philological Association* 124 (1994), pp. 197–209.

Musher, Daniel M., et al. "Trends in Bacteremic Infection Due to *Streptococcus pyogenes* (Group A Streptococcus), 1986–1995." *Emerging Infectious Diseases* 2 (1996): 54–56.

Normile, Dennis. "WHO Gives a Cautious Green Light to Smallpox Experiments." *Science* 306 (November 19, 2004): 1270–1271.

O'Brien, Sarah J. "Foodborne Zoonoses." *British Medical Journal* 331 (November 26, 2005): 1217–1218. Also available online at: <http://www.bmj.com/cgi/content/full/331/7527/1217>.

Osrin, David, et al. "Serious Bacterial Infections in Newborn Infants in Developing Countries." *Pediatric and Neonatal Infections* 17 (2004): 217-224.

Palacio, H., et al. "Norovirus Outbreak among Evacuees from Hurricane Katrina - Houston, Texas, September 2005." *Morbidity and Mortality Weekly* 54: 1016–1019 (2005).

Palacios, Gustavo, et al. "Masstag Polymerase Chain Reaction for Differential Diagnosis of Viral Hemorrhagic Fevers." *Emerging Infectious Diseases* 12 (2006): 692–695.

Parola, P., C.D. Paddock, and D. Raoult. "Tick-Borne Rickettsioses Around the World: Emerging Diseases Challenging Old Concepts." *Clinical Microbiology Reviews* 18 (October 2005): 719–756. Also available online at <http://cmr.asm.org/cgi/content/full/18/4/719>.

Pemberton M.N. et al. "Recurrent Kawasaki Disease." *British Dental Journal* 186 (1999): 6, 270–271.

Peplies, Jorg, Frank Oliver Glockner, and Rudolf Amann. "Optimization Strategies for DNA Microarray-Based Detection of Bacteria with 16S rRNA-Targeting Oligonucleotide Probes." *Applied and Environmental Microbiology* 69 (2003): 1397–1407.

Perrino, T., et al. "Main Partner's Resistance to Condoms and HIV Protection Among Disadvantaged, Minority Women." *Women & Health* 42, no. 3 (2005): 37–56.

Peters, C.J., and J.W. Leduc. "An Introduction to Ebola: The Virus and the Disease." *Journal of Infectious Diseases* Supp.1 (1999): 179-187.

Pittet, Didier, et al. "Effectiveness of a Hospital-Wide Programme to Improve Compliance with Hand Hygiene." *The Lancet* 356 (October 14, 2000): 1307–1312.

Pollack, Andrew. "Vaccines Are Good Business for Drug Makers." *The New York Times* October 29, 2004.

Porter, Mark. "Doctor Who Sparked the MMR Debate Faces Misconduct Charge." *The Evening Standard* June 12, 2006.

Potera, Carol. "In Disaster's Wake: Tsunami Lung." *Environmental Health Perspectives* 113 (2005): 11, 734.

Pramodh, Nathaniel. "Limiting the Spread of Communicable Diseases Caused by Human Population Movement." *Journal of Rural and Remote Environmental Health* (2003): 2(1), 23–32.

Price, Lance B. et al. "Fluoroquinolone-resistant *Campylobacter* Isolates from Conventional and Antibiotic-free Chicken Products." *Environmental Health Perspectives* 113 (2005): 557–561.

Pulliam, J.R., H.E. Field, and K.J. Olival. "Nipah Virus Strain Variation." *Emerging Infectious Diseases* 11 (December 2005): 1978–1979.

Quasem, Himaya, and Heather Greenaway. "Nurseries Told to Clean Up Their Act; Exclusive the E Coli Crisis." *Sunday Mail* May 14, 2006. p.5.

Rados, Carol. "First Test Approved to Help Detect West Nile Virus." *FDA Consumer* 37 (September–October 2003).

Raja, N.S., M.Z. Ahmed, and N.N. Singh. "Melioidosis: An Emerging Infectious Disease." *Journal of Postgraduate Medicine* 51 (2005): 140–145. Also available online at: <http://www.jpgmonline.com/article.asp?issn=0022-3859;year=2005;volume=51;issue=2;spage=140; epage=145;aulast=Raja>.

Ramamoorthi, Nandhini, et al. "The Lyme Disease Agent Exploits a Tick Protein to Infect the Mammalian Host." *Nature* 436 (July 28, 2005): 573–577.

Raoult, Didier, and Véronique Roux. "The Body Louse as a Vector of Reemerging Human Diseases." *Clinical Infectious Diseases* 29 (1999): 888–911.

Read, Timothy R., et al. "Comparative Genome Sequencing for Discovery of Novel Polymorphisms in *Bacillus anthracis.*" *Science.* 296 (2002): 2028–2033.

Reiner, David S., et al. "Identification and Localization of Cyst-Specific Antigens of *Giardia lamblia.*" *Infection and Immunity.* 57 (1989): 963-968.

Rice, Amy L., et al. "Malnutrition as an Underlying Cause of Childhood Deaths Associated with Infectious Diseases in Developing Countries." *Bulletin of the World Health Organization* 78 (2000): 1207-1218.

Rice, L.B. "Emergence of Vancomycin-resistant Enterococci." *Emerging Infectious Diseases,* (March-April 2001): 7 (2) 183–87.

Rosenthal, E. "From China's Provinces, a Crafty Germ Spreads." *New York Times* April 27, 2003.

Rosovitz, M.J., and Stephen H. Leppla. "Virus Deals Anthrax a Killer Blow." *Nature* 418 (2002): 825–826.

Ross, John J., and Douglas N. Keeling. "Cutaneous Blastomycosis in New Brunswick: Case Report." *Canadian Medical Association Journal* 163 (November 14, 2000): 1303–1305.

Ross, Ronald. "This Day Relenting God." in *Memoirs with a Full Account of the Great Malaria Problem and Its Solution* London: John Murray, 1923.

Russell, Josiah C. "That Earlier Plague." *Demography* 5, 1 (1968), 174–184.

Salim, M.A., et al. "Gender Differences in Tuberculosis: A Prevalence Survey Done in Bangladesh." *The International Journal of Tuberculosis and Lung Disease* 8 (August 2004): 952–957.

Sawitri, Adisti Sukma. "Officials Blame Poor Hygiene on Dengue Rise." *Jakarta Post* (January 26, 2007).

Schwebke, J.R., and D. Burgess. "Trichomoniasis Is a Common Infection Whose Prevention Has Not Been a Priority." *Clinical Microbiology Review* 17 (2004): 794–803.

Sempere J.M., V. Soriano, and J.M. Benito. "T Regulatory Cells and HIV Infection." *AIDS Rev.* (Jan-March 2007): 9 (1): 54–60.

Seppa, N. "Hepatitis E Vaccine Passes Critical Test." *Science News* 171 (March 3, 2007): 9, 131.

Shapin, Steven. "SICK CITY." *The New Yorker* Nov 6, 2006.

Shea, Katherine M. "Antibiotic Resistance: What is the Impact of Agricultural Uses of Antibiotics on Children's Health?" *Pediatrics.* 112 (2003): 253-258.

Sheldon, Tony. "The Virus Hunter." *BMJ* 327 (October 25, 2003): 950.

Silbergeld, Ellen K., and Polly Walker. "What If Cipro Stopped Working?" *New York Times* (November 3, 2001). Available online at <http://query.nytimes.com/gst/fullpage.html?sec=health&res=9C0DEED91F30F930A35752C1A9679C8B63>.

Simon, Harvey B. "Old Bugs Learn Some New Tricks; As More Drugs Are Created to Fight Infection, Bacteria Mutate and Strike in Another Form." *Newsweek* (Dec 11, 2006): 74.

Smith, David L., et al. "Agricultural Antibiotics and Human Health." *PloS Medicine* 2 (2005): 731-735.

Smith, J.P. "Healthy Bodies and Thick Wallets: The Dual Relationship between Health and Economic Status." *Journal of Economic Perspectives* 13(2), 1999: 145-66.

Smith, Kerri. "Concern as Revived 1918 Flu Virus Kills Monkeys." *Nature* 445 (2007): 237.

Sorvillo, Frank, et al. "*Baylisascaris procyonis*: An Emerging Helminthic Zoonosis." *Emerging Infectious Diseases* (April 2002), 8, 4: 355–359.

Splete, Heidi. "Raspberries Implicated in Norovirus Outbreaks." *Family Practice News* (2006) 36: 23-24.

Squires, Sally. "Must You Be Such a Drip?" *Washington Post* (January 30, 2007).

Sréter, Tamás et al. "Echinococcus Multilocularis: An Emerging Pathogen in Hungary and Central Eastern Europe?" *Emerging Infectious Diseases* 9 (2003): 384–386.

Steere, Allen C. "Lyme Disease." *New England Journal of Medicine* 345 (2001): 115–123.

Steinbrook R. "Global Health: The AIDS Epidemic in 2004." *New England Journal of Medicine* 2004; 351: 115–117, Jul 8, 2004.

Steinbrook R. "HIV in India—A Complex Epidemic." *New England Journal of Medicine* 2007; 356: 1089–1093, Mar 15, 2007.

Steinbrook R. "HIV in India—The Challenges Ahead." *New England Journal of Medicine* 2007; 356: 1197–1201, Mar 22, 2007.

Stevens, Dennis L. "Streptococcal Toxic-Shock Syndrome: Spectrum of Disease, Pathogenesis, and New Concepts in Treatment." *Emerging Infectious Diseases* 1 (1995): 69–76.

Stone L., R. Olinky, and A. Huppert. "Seasonal Dynamics of Recurrent Epidemics." *Nature* 2007 Mar 29; 446 (7135): 533–6.

Strausbaugh L.J., S.R. Sukumar, and C.L. Joseph. "Infectious Disease Outbreaks in Nursing Homes: An Unappreciated Hazard for Frail Elderly Persons." *Clinical Infectious Diseases* 36 (2003): 870–876.

Struck, Doug. "Climate Change Drives Disease to New Territory: Viruses Moving North to Areas Unprepared for Them, Experts Say." *Washington Post* (May 5, 2006).

Thorne, C., and M.L. Newell. "Safety of Agents Used to Prevent Mother-to-Child Transmission of HIV: Is There Any Cause for Concern?" *Drug Safety* 30, no. 3 (2007): 203–213.

Toole, M.J., S. Galson, and W. Brady. "Refugees, Forced Displacement, and War: Are War and Public Health Compatible?" *The Lancet* 341, 8854 (May 8, 1993): 1193–1196.

Tumpey, Terrence M., et al. "Characterization of the Reconstructed 1918 Spanish Influenza Pandemic Virus." *Science* 310 (2005): 77–80.

Turner, Ronald B., et al. "An Evaluation of *Echinacea augustifolia* in Experimental Rhinovirus Infections." *New England Journal of Medicine* 353 (2005): 341–348.

Vacomo, V., et al. "Natural History of *Bartonella* Infections (An Exception to Koch's Postulate)." *Clinical and Diagnostic Laboratory Immunology* 9 (2002): 8–18.

Van Lieshout, M., et al. "Climate Change and Malaria: Analysis of the SRES Climate and Socio-Economic Scenarios." *Global Environmental Change* 14 (2004): 87-99.

Verbrugge, L.M., et al. "Prospective Study of Swimmer's Itch Incidence and Severity." *Journal of Parasitology* (2004) 90: 697–704.

Vincent, Jean-Louis. "Nosocomial Infections in Adult Intensive-care Units." *The Lancet* 361 (June 14, 2003): 2068–2077.

Vitek, C.R., and M. Wharton. "Diphtheria in the Fomer Soviet Union: Reemergence of a

Pandemic Disease." *Emerging Infectious Diseases* 4 (October-December 1998). This article is available online <http://www.cdc.gov/ncidod/eid/vol4no4/vitek.htm>

Vogel, Gretchen. "Searching for Living Relics of the Cell's Early Days." *Science* 277 (1997): 1604.

Wade, Nicholas. "What a Story Lice Can Tell." *New York Times* (October 5, 2004).

Wald, A., and L. Corey. "How Does Herpes Simplex Virus Type 2 Influence Human Immunodeficiency Virus Infection and Pathogenesis?" *The Journal of Infectious Diseases* 187 (2003): 1519–1512.

Wang, J., et al. "Platensimycin Is a Selective FabF Inhibitor with Potent Antibiotic Properties." *Nature* (2006) 441: 358–363.

Weber, J., et al. "The Development of Vaginal Microbicides for the Prevention of HIV Transmission." *Public Library of Science Medicine* 2 (May 2005): e142.

Webster, R.G. and E.J. Walker. "The World is Teetering on the Edge of a Pandemic that Could Kill a Large Fraction of the Human Population." *American Scientist* 91 (2003): 122.

Weinstein, A. "Topical Treatment of Common Superficial Tinea Infections." *American Family Physician* 65 (May 15, 2002): 2095–2102.

Weinstock H., et al. "Sexually Transmitted Diseases Among American Youth: Incidence and Prevalence Estimates, 2000." *Perspectives on Sexual and Reproductive Health* 2004; 36 (1): 6–10.

Wheeler, Susan. "Henry IV of France Touching for Scrofula by Pierre Firens." *Journal of the History of Medicine and Allied Sciences* 58 (2003), pp. 79-81.

Wickens, Hayley, and Paul Wade. "Understanding Antibiotic Resistance." *The Pharmaceutical Journal* 274 (2005): 501–504.

Willis, Judith Levine. "Mono: Tough for Teens and Twenty-Somethings." *FDA Consumer* (May, June 1998): 32,3.

Wilson-Clark, Samantha D., S. Squires, and S. Deeksi "Bacterial Meningitis among Cochlear Implant Recipients—Canada 2002." *Morbidity and Mortality Weekly* 55: S20-S25 (2006).

Witkowski, Joseph A., and Lawrence Charles Parish. "Pediculosis and Resistance: The Perennial Problem." *Clinics in Dermatology* 20 (2002): 87–92.

Witt, Kristine L., et al. "Elevated Frequencies of Micronucleated Erythrocytes in Infants Exposed to Zidovudine in Utero and Postpartum to Prevent Mother-to-Child Transmission of HIV." *Environmental and Molecular Mutagenesis* 48 (April-May 2007): 322–329.

Woodall, Jack. "Why Mosquitoes Trump Birds." *The Scientist* (January 2006).

World Health Organization (WHO). "Economic Costs Of Malaria Are Many Times Higher Than Previously Estimated." Press Release. April 25, 2000.

World Health Organization (WHO), Epidemic and Pandemic Alert and Response (EPR). "Avian Influenza—Necessary Precautions to Prevent Human Infection of H5N1, Need for Virus Sharing." *Disease Outbreak News* July 16, 2004.

World Health Organization (WHO). "Rotavirus Vaccines." *Weekly Epidemiological Record* 81 (January 6, 2006): 8 Also available online at: <http://www.who.int/wer/2006/wer8101.pdf>.

Wormser, Gary P. "Early Lyme Disease." *New England Journal of Medicine* 354 (2006): 2794–2800.

The Writing Committee of the World Health Organization Consultation on Human Influenza A/H5. "Avian Influenza A (H5N1) Infection in Humans." *New England Journal of Medicine* 353 (September 29, 2005): 1374–1385.

Yu, Ignatius T.S. et al. "Temporal-spatial Analysis of Severe Acute Respiratory Syndrome among Hospital Inpatients." *Clinical Infectious Diseases* 40 (2005): 1237–1243.

Zezima, Katie. "School is Shut After Outbreak of Encephalitis Kills a Pupil." *New York Times* (January 4, 2007): A14(L).

Zoler, Mitchel L. "Long-term, Acute Care Hospitals Breed Antibiotic Resistance." *Internal Medicine News* 37 (September 15, 2004): 51–52.

WEB SITES

AIDSinfo. <http://aidsinfo.nih.gov> (accessed April 9, 2007).

American Academy of Dermatology. "Researchers Urge Soldiers and Civilians Returning from Iraq to Be Aware of 'Baghdad Boil.'" June 30, 2005. <http://www.aad.org/aad/Newsroom/Researchers+Urge+Soldiers+and+civilians+returning.htm> (accessed February 26, 2007).

American Cancer Society. "Frequently Asked Questions About Human Papilloma Virus (HPV) Vaccines." <http://www.cancer.org/docroot/CRI/content/CRI_2_6x_FAQ_HPV_Vaccines.asp> (accessed February 25, 2007).

American Cancer Society. "Infectious Agents and Cancer." October 17, 2006. <http://www.cancer.org/docroot/PED/content/PED_1_3X_Infectious_Agents_and_Cancer.asp?sitearea=PED> (accessed February 19, 2007).

American Lung Association. "Pneumonia Fact Sheet." April 2006. <http://www.lungusa.org/site/apps/nl/content3.asp?c=dvLUK9O0E&b=2060321&content_id={08C669B0-E845-4C9C-8B1E-285348BC83BD}&notoc=1> (accessed March 25, 2007).

American Lyme Disease Foundation. "Home Page." September 22, 2006. <http://www.aldf.com/> (accessed February 7, 2007).

American Museum of Natural History. "Some Facts about Psittacosis." 2003. <http://research.amnh.org/users/nyneve/psittacosis.html#hist> (accessed Mar. 7, 2007).

American Red Cross. "Blood Donation Eligibility Guidelines." March 21, 2005. <http://www.redcross.org/services/biomed/0,1082,0_557_,00.html> (accessed January 16, 2007).

American Society for Microbiology. "Don't Get Caught Dirty Handed." <http://www.washup.org/> (accessed June 10, 2007).

American Society for Microbiology. "Gross...You Didn't Wash Your Hands?" <http://www.microbeworld.org/know/wash.aspx> (accessed June 10, 2007).

Armed Forces Institute of Pathology. "Buruli Ulcer." February 4, 2004. <http://www.afip.org/Departments/infectious/bu/> (accessed April 24, 2007).

Australian Government. "Cryptosporidiosis." April 2006 <http://www.healthinsite.gov.au/topics/Cryptosporidiosis> (accessed Jan. 29, 2007).

Avert: Averting HIV and AIDS. "Providing Drug Treatment for Millions." April 19, 2007. <http://www.avert.org/drugtreatment.htm> (accessed May 26, 2007).

Baylor College of Medicine. "Potential Bioterrorism Agents." July 5, 2006. <http://www.bcm.edu/molvir/eidbt/eidbt-mvm-pbt.htm> (accessed March 12, 2007).

Bill & Melinda Gates Foundation. "Malaria Vaccine Initiative: Solving the Malaria Vaccine Puzzle." September 2005.<http://www.gatesfoundation.org/StoryGallery/GlobalHealth/SGGHMalariaMVI-011019.htm> (accessed January 31, 2007).

Bill & Melinda Gates Foundation. <http://www.gatesfoundation.org/default.htm> (accessed May 31, 2007).

The BSE Inquiry Report. "Home Page." <http://www.bseinquiry.gov.uk/index.htm> (accessed May 15, 2007).

Cambridge University. "Fasciola hepatica: The Liver Fluke." October 5, 1998 <http://www.path.cam.ac.uk/~schisto/OtherFlukes/Fasciola.html#minorFasc> (accessed February 23, 2007).

Cambridge University. "Helminth Infections of Man." October 5, 1998 <http://www.path.cam.ac.uk/~schisto/General_Parasitology/Hm.helminths.html> (accessed February 23, 2007).

Cambridge University. "Opisthorchis sinensis: The Chinese Liver Fluke." Oct. 5, 1998 <http://www.path.cam.ac.uk/~schisto/OtherFlukes/Opisthorchis.egg.html> (accessed February 23, 2007).

Campaign for Access to Essential Medecines. "Companies Not Selling New AIDS Drugs in Africa." <http://www.accessmed-msf.org/index.asp> (accessed May 15, 2007).

Canadian Medical Association. "Blastomycosis." November 4, 2000. <http://www.cmaj.ca/cgi/content/full/163/10/1231> (accessed March 11, 2007).

Cancer Research UK. "Cervical Cancer. International Statistics." <http://info.cancerresearchuk.org/cancerstats/types/cervix/international/> (accessed February 25, 2007).

CDC (Centers for Disease Control and Prevention). "CDCSite Index A-Z." <http://www.cdc.gov/flu/avian/> (accessed May 21, 2007).

Center for Food Safety and Applied Nutrition, Federal Food and Drug Administration. "Anisakis simplex and related worms." <http://www.cfsan.fda.gov/~mow/chap25.html> (accessed March 1, 2007).

Commoncold, Inc. "The Common Cold." 2005. <http://www.commoncold.org/> (accessed January 31, 2007).

Commonwealth Scientific and Industrial Research Organisation (CSIRO). "Fighting Nipah Virus." May 23, 2006 <http://www.csiro.au/science/ps1so.html> (accessed March 28, 2007).

Cutler, Sally J., Veterinary Laboratories Agency (Surrey, United Kingdom), U.S. Centers for Disease Control and Prevention. "Possibilities for Relapsing Fever Reemergence." March 2006 <http://www.cdc.gov/ncidod/eid/vol12no03/05-0899.htm> (accessed April 27, 2007).

Department for Environment, Food and Rural Affairs. "BSE: Frequently Asked Questions." October 3, 2006 <http://www.defra.gov.uk/animalh/bse/faq.html> (accessed January 26, 2007).

Department of Health and Human Services, Centers for Disease Control and Prevention. "Parasitic Diseases." February 16, 2007 <http://www.cdc.gov/ncidod/dpd/index.htm> (accessed April 30, 2007).

Department of Health, New York State. "Sporotrichosis." June 2004 <http://www.health.state.ny.

us/diseases/communicable/sporotrichosis/fact_sheet.htm> (accessed Mar. 12, 2007).

Department of Health, Western Australia. "Cryptosporidiosis: Environmental Health Guide." 2006 <http://www.health.wa.gov.au/envirohealth/water/docs/Cryptospordiosis_EH_Guide.pdf> (accessed Jan. 29, 2007).

Deployment Health Clinical Center. "Leishmaniasis." June 21, 2004 <http://www.pdhealth.mil/leish.asp> (accessed February 26, 2007).

Directors of Health Promotion and Education (DHPE). "Chagas Disease." <http://www.dhpe.org/infect/Chagas.html> (accessed January 31, 2007).

Directors of Health Promotion and Education (DHPE). "Lymphatic Filariasis." 2005 <http://www.dhpe.org/infect/Lymphfil.html> (accessed March 5, 2007).

Division of Parasitic Diseases, U.S. Centers for Disease Control and Prevention (CDC). "Hookworm Infection." <http://www.cdc.gov/ncidod/dpd/parasites/hookworm/factsht_hookworm.htm> (accessed March 14, 2007).

Division of Parasitic Diseases, U.S. Centers for Disease Control and Prevention. "Taeniasis." November 29, 2006 <http://www.dpd.cdc.gov/dpdx/Default.htm> (accessed March 27, 2007).

Epidemiology and Disease Control Program (EDCP). "Cyclosporiasis Fact Sheet." <http://edcp.org/factsheets/cyclospor.html> (accessed March 8, 2007).

Food Standards Agency. "BSE." <http://www.food.gov.uk/bse> (accessed January 26, 2007).

Georgia State University. "National B Virus Resource Center." <http://www2.gsu.edu/~wwwvir/> (accessed April 17, 2007).

GIDEON. "GIDEON Content- Outbreaks." <http://www.gideononline.com/content/outbreaks. htm> (accessed May 1, 2007).

Global Polio Eradication Initiative (GPEI). "Home website of GPEI." <http://www.polioeradication.org/> (accessed May 7, 2007).

Harvard Medical School Center for Health and the Global Environment. "Climate Change Futures: Health, Ecological and Economic Dimensions." 2005 <http://chge.med.harvard.edu> (accessed May 26, 2007).

Health Protection Agency. "Clostridium Difficile." <http://www.hpa.org.uk/infections/topics_az/clostridium_difficile/default.htm> (accessed January 30, 2007).

Health Protection Agency. "Diphtheria." February 2, 2006. <http://www.hpa.org.uk/infections/topics_az/diphtheria/gen_info.htm> (accessed February 16, 2007).

Health Protection Agency. "Impetigo: Factsheet for Schools." <http://www.hpa.org.uk/infections/topics_az/wfhfactsheets/WFHImpetigo.htm> (accessed March 6, 2007).

Helicobacter Foundation. "H. pylori." <http://www.helico.com/h_general.html> (accessed May 30, 2007).

Illinois Department of Public Health. "Monkeypox." <http://www.idph.state.il.us/health/infect/monkeypox.htm> (accessed March 6, 2007).

Illinois Department of Public Health. "Rocky Mountain Spotted Fever." <http://www. idph.state.il.us/public/hb/hbrmsf.htm> (accessed March 6, 2007).

Infectious Diseases Society of America. "Tularemia: Current, Comprehensive Information on Pathogenesis, Microbiology, Epidemiology, Diagnosis, Treatment, and Prophylaxis." March 5, 2007. <http://www.cidrap.umn.edu/idsa/bt/tularemia/biofacts/tularemiafactsheet.html#_Agent> (accessed April 5, 2007).

INRUD. "International Network for the Rational Use of Drugs." <http://www.inrud.org> (accessed May 26, 2007).

International Leprosy Association. "Global Project on the History of Leprosy." October 10, 2003 <http://www.leprosyhistory.org/english/englishhome.htm> (accessed February 6, 2007).

International Panel on Climate Change (United Nations). "Climate Change 2007: Impacts, Adaptation and Vulnerability." 2007 <http://www.ipcc.ch/SPM13apr07.pdf> (accessed May 26, 2007).

International Panel on Climate Change (United Nations). "Climate Change 2007: The Physical Science Basis." 2007 <http://ipcc-wg1.ucar.edu/wg1/docs/WG1AR4_SPM_PlenaryApproved.pdf> (accessed May 26, 2007).

International Society for Infectious Diseases. "Angiostrongylus Meningitis—China (04)." Oct. 1, 2006 <http://www.promedmail.org/pls/promed/f?p=2400:1202:1604187183216986886::NO::F2400_P1202_CHECK_DISPLAY,F2400_P1202_PUB_MAIL_ID:X,34650> (accessed Jan. 25, 2007).

International Society of Infectious Diseases. "ProMED." <http://www.promedmail.org> (accessed June 5, 2007).

International Society for Infectious Diseases. "ProMed Mail: Mitten Crab—USA and Canada." August 1, 1999. <http://www.promedmail.org/pls/promed/f?p=2400:1000> (accessed May 26, 2007).

International Trachoma Initiative. "Trachoma is a hidden disease." 2005 <http http://www.trachoma.org/trachoma.php> (accessed April 2, 2007).

Internet Modern History Sourcebook. "Oliver Wendell Holmes: Contagiousness of Puerperal Fever, 1843." August 1998 <http://www.fordham.edu/halsall/mod/1843holmes-fever.html> (accessed March 8, 2007).

Journal of Young Investigators. "Smallpox: Historical Review of a Potential Bioterrorist Tool." September 2002. <http://www.jyi.org/volumes/volume6/issue3/features/bourzac.html> (accessed February 21, 2007).

Kaiser Family Foundation. "The Global HIV-AIDS Timeline." <http://www.kff.org/hivaids/timeline/hivtimeline.cfm> (accessed February 19, 2007).

Kawasaki Disease Foundation. "Kawasaki Disease Foundation: Caring for Precious Hearts." <http://www.kdfoundation.org/> (accessed February 28, 2007).

KidsHealth for Parents. "Infections: Pinworm." April 2005. <http://www.kidshealth.org/parent/infections/parasitic/pinworm.html> (accessed March 16, 2007).

KidsHealth for Parents. "Infections: Swimmer's Ear." March 2006 <http://www.kidshealth.org/parent/infections/ear/swimmer_ear.html> (accessed March 27, 2007).

Ledford, Heidi. "Jetsetters are Key Clues to Epidemics." *nature.com* January 29, 2007 <http://www.nature.com/news/2007/070129/full/070129-5.html> (accessed May 18, 2007).

Médecins Sans Frontièrs/Doctors Without Borders. "About Us." <http://www.doctorswithoutborders.org/aboutus/index.cfm> (accessed May 15, 2007).

Médicins Sans Frontières. "Campaign for Access to Essential Medicines." <http://www.accessmedmsf.org> (accessed May 26, 2007).

Marshall, Barry J. Nobelprize.org. "Nobel Lecture: Helicobacter Connections." 1995. <http://nobelprize.org/nobel_prizes/medicine/laureates/2005/marshall-lecture.html/b> (accessed June 3, 2007).

Maryland Department of Health and Mental Hygiene. "Kawasaki Disease Fact Sheet." May 2002 <http://edcp.org/factsheets/kawasaki.html> (accessed February 28, 2007).

MayoClinic.com. "Pneumonia." May 12, 2005. <http://www.mayoclinic.com/health/pneumo nia/DS00135> (accessed March 25, 2007).

MayoClinic.com. "Ringworm of the Body." October 4, 2006. <http://www.mayoclinic.com/health/ringworm/DS00489/DSECTION=1> (accessed March 22, 2007).

MayoClinic.com. "Strep throat." November 3, 2006. <http://www.mayoclinic.com/health/strepthroat/DS00260> (accessed May 1, 2007).

MayoClinic.com. "Tetanus." December 29, 2006. <http://www.mayoclinic.com/health/tetanus/DS00227/DSECTION=7> (accessed March 27, 2007).

McCulloch, J. Huston, and James R. Meginniss. Ohio State University. "A Statistical Model of Smallpox Vaccine Dilution." May 17, 2002. <http://www. econ.ohio-state.edu/jhm/smallpox.htm> (accessed June 14, 2007).

McKnight, Jake. Médicins Sans Frontières. "Isaac." June 13, 2007. <http://www.uk2.msf.org/UKNews/Letters/jakemcknightisaac.htm> (accessed June 11, 2007).

The Measles Initiative. "Home Page." March 16, 2007. <http://www.measlesinitiative.org/index3. asp> (accessed March 20, 2007).

Meat and Livestock Commission. "Beef Information." October 2005 <http://www.meatmatters.com/sections/britishmeat/beef_information.php> (accessed January 26, 2007).

Meat Promotion Wales. "Liver Fluke." <http://www.hybucigcymru.org.uk/content.php?nID=206&lID=1> (accessed February 23, 2007).

Medline Plus. "Encephalitis." <http://www.nlm.nih.gov/medlineplus/encephalitis.html> (accessed March 20, 2007).

Medline Plus. "Impetigo." February 26, 2007 <http://www.nlm.nih.gov/medlineplus/ency/article/0008 60.htm> (accessed March 6, 2007).

Medline Plus. "Urinary Tract Infection." <http://www.nlm.nih.gov/medlineplus/ency/article/0005 21.htm> (accessed March 20, 2007).

MedlinePlus. "Ascariasis." October 9, 2006. <http://www.nlm.nih.gov/medlineplus/ency/article/000628.htm> (accessed May 21, 2007).

MedlinePlus. "Ringworm." June 16, 2005 <http://www.nlm.nih.gov/medlineplus/ency/article/0014 39.htm> (accessed March 28, 2007).

The Meningitis Trust. "Viral Meningitis: The Facts." <http://www.meningitis-trust.org/disease_info/Viral-Meningitis.pdf> (accessed May 3, 2007).

Molecular Expressions(TM). "Optical Microscopy Primer." March 6, 2005 <http://micro. magnet.fsu.edu/primer/index.html> (accessed May 8, 2007).

National Center for Biotechnology Information. "Diseases of the Immune System." <http://www.ncbi.nlm.

nih.gov/disease/Immune.html> (accessed June 13, 2007).

National Center for Biotechnology Information. "Microbiologic Examination." in *Medical Microbiology,* 4th ed., Samuel Baron, ed. <http://www.ncbi.nlm.nih.gov/books/bv.fcgi?rid=mmed.section.5451> (accessed April 2, 2007).

National Center for Infectious Diseases. Centers for Disease Control and Prevention. "Office of Minority and Women's Health." February 5, 2004 <http://www.cdc.gov/ncidod/omwh/infectious.htm> (accessed March 13, 2007).

National Eye Institute. "Histoplasmosis." December 2006 <http://www.nei.nih.gov/health/histoplasmosis/index.asp> (accessed February 23, 2007).

National Food Service Management Institute. "Wash Your Hands." <http://www.nfsmi.org/Information/ handsindex.html>. (accessed June 10, 2007).

National Guideline Clearinghouse. "Hemorrhagic Fever Viruses as Biological Weapons: Medical and Public Health Management." March 5, 2007 <http://www.guideline.gov/summary/summary.aspx?ss=15&doc_id=3224&nbr=2450> (accessed March 11, 2007).

National Institute of Allergy and Infectious Disease (NIAID). "Rotavirus Vaccine: Preventing Severe Diarrheal Disease in Infants." May 25, 1999 <http://www.niaid.nih.gov/Publications/discovery/rotav.htm> (accessed March 12, 2007).

National Institute of Allergy and Infectious Diseases. "HIV/AIDS: Koch's Postulates Fulfilled." September 1995 <http://www.niaid.nih.gov/Publications/hivaids/12.htm> (accessed February 1, 2007).

National Institute of Allergy and Infectious Diseases. "Understanding the Immune System." <http://health.nih.gov/viewPublication.asp?disease_id=63&publication_id=2841&pdf=yes> (accessed June 13, 2007).

National Institute of Allergy and Infectious Diseases. "Emerging Infectious Diseases." <http://www.niaid.nih.gov/dmid/eid/> (accessed May 25, 2007).

National Institute of Allergy and Infectious Diseases. "Gonorrhea." August 2006 <http://www.niaid.nih.gov/factsheets/stdgon.htm> (accessed February 23, 2007).

National Institute of Allergy and Infectious Diseases. "Group A Streptococcal Infections." November 2005. <http://www.niaid.nih.gov/factsheets/strep.htm> (accessed February 14, 2007).

National Institute of Allergy and Infectious Diseases. "Parasitic Roundworm Diseases." March 8, 2005 <http://www.niaid.nih.gov/factsheets/roundwor.htm> (accessed Mar 9, 2007).

National Institute of Allergy and Infectious Diseases. <http://www3.niaid.nih.gov/> (accessed February 9, 2007).

National Institute on Deafness and Other Communication Disorders. "Otitis Media (Ear Infection)." July 2002. <http://www.nidcd. nih.gov/health/hearing/otitism.asp> (accessed April 10, 2007).

National Institute of Neurological Disorders and Stroke. "Kuru Information Page." February 14, 2007. <http:// www.ninds.nih.gov/disorders/kuru/kuru.htm> (accessed March 19, 2007).

National Institutes of Health. "List of Cancer-Causing Agents Grows." January 31, 2005 <http://www.nih.gov/news/pr/jan2005/niehs-31.htm> (accessed February 19, 2007).

National Library of Medicine, National Institutes of Health. "Trachoma." September 22, 2006 <http://www.nlm.nih.gov/medlineplus/ency/article/001486.htm> (accessed April 2, 2007).

National Necrotizing Fasciitis Foundation. "Home Page." January 28, 2007 <http://www.nnff.org/> (accessed February 14, 2007).

The National Pediculosis Association. "Welcome to Headlice.org." 2007 <http://www. headlice.org/> (accessed January 22, 2007).

National Vaccine Program Office, United States Department of Health and Human Services. "Pandemics and Pandemic Scares in the 20th Century." <http://www.hhs.gov/nvpo/pandemics/flu3.htm#10> (accessed January 23, 2007).

Network for Good. "Doctors Without Borders USA." <http://partners.guidestar.org/controller/searchResults.gs?action_gsReport=1&partner=networkforgood&ein=13-3433452> (accessed May 20, 2007).

New York State Department of Health. "Babesiosis." June 2004 <http://www.health.state.ny.us/diseases /communicable/babesiosis/fact_sheet.htm> (accessed February 1, 2007).

New York State Department of Health. "Cryptosporidiosis." June 2004 <http://www.health.state.ny.us/diseases/communicable/cryptosporidiosis/fact_sheet.htm> (accessed Jan. 29, 2007).

New York State Department of Health. "Shigellosis." June 2004 <http://www.health.state.ny.us/diseases/communicable/shigellosis/fact_sheet.htm> (accessed March 12, 2007).

New York State Department of Health. "Vancomycin Resistant Enterococcus (VRE)." <http://www.

health.state.ny.us/diseases/communicablevanco mycin_resistant_enterococcus/fact_sheet.htm> (accessed May 21, 2007).

NHS Direct. "Sexually Transmitted Infections." <http:// www.nhsdirect.nhs.uk/articles/> (accessed May 16, 2007).

NIH Vaccine Research Center. "Become an HIV Vaccine Study Volunteer." <http://www.niaid.nih.gov/ vrc/clintrials/clin_steps.htm%20%20%20> (accessed April 9, 2007).

Nobelprize.org, Nobel Foundation. "The Nobel Peace Price 1965." <http://nobelprize.org/nobel_ prizes/peace/laureates/1965/> (accessed June 17, 2007).

Nobelprize.org, Nobel Foundation. "The Nobel Prize in Physiology or Medicine 2005." Press Release, October 3, 2005 <http://nobelprize.org/nobel_ prizes/medicine/laureat> (accessed June 7, 2007).

Nobelprize.org, Nobel Foundation. "The Nobel Peace Prize 1999: Médecins Sans Frontières." <http://nobelprize.org/peace/laureates/1999/ index.html> (accessed May 20, 2007).

NSW Health Department. "Psittacosis: Questions and Answers." 2002 <http://www.health.nsw. gov.au/public-health/pdf/PsittacosisQA.pdf> (accessed March 7, 2007).

Office of Laboratory Security, Public Health Agency of Canada. "Ascaris lumbricoides." January 23, 2001 <http://www.phac-aspc.gc.ca/msds-ftss/ msds9e.html> (accessed May 21, 2007).

Pan American Health Organization. "Chagas Disease (American Trypanosomiasis)." <http://www.paho. org/english/ad/dpc/cd/chagas.htm> (accessed January 31, 2007).

Pan American Health Organization. "The Common Cold." <http://www.paho.org/English/AD/DPC/ CD/AIEPI-1-3.9.pdf> (accessed January 31, 2007).

PLoS Medicine, Public Library of Science. "Rapid-Impact Interventions: How a Policy of Integrated Control for Africa's Neglected Tropical Diseases Could Benefit the Poor." October 11, 2005 <http:// medicine.plosjour nals.org/perlserv/?request=get document &doi=10.1371/journal.pmed.0020336# JOURNAL-PMED-0020336-T001> (accessed May 21, 2007).

ProMED Mail, International Society for Infectious Diseases. "Anisakiasis—Israel: suspected." <http://www. promedmail.org/pls/promed/f?p=2400:1202: 16245428003054921509::NO::F2400_P1202_ CHECK_DISPLAY,F2400_P1202_PUB_MAIL_ ID:X,23022> (accessed March 1, 2007).

ProMED Mail. "Food-borne Parasitic Infections Increase in China." May 18, 2005 <http://www.promedmail. org/pls/promed/f?p=2400:1202:99765310568 9672184::NO::F2400_P1202_CHECK_DISP LAY,F2400_P1202_PUB_MAIL_ID:X,28969> (accessed February 23, 2007).

Public Health Agency of Canada. "Material Safety Data Sheet—Infectious Substances." April 23, 2001 <http://www.phac-aspc.gc.ca/msds-ftss/ msds172e.html> (accessed February 8, 2007).

Rotavirus Vaccine Program (RVP). "About RVP." 2007 <http://www.rotavirusvaccine.org/about.htm> (accessed March 12, 2007).

Royal College of Obstetricians and Gynaecologists (United Kingdom). "Prevention of Early Onset Neonatal Group B Streptococcal Disease." November 2003 <http://www.rcog.org.uk/ index.asp? PageID=520> (accessed February 2, 2007).

San Diego Natural History Museum. "Zoonoses: Animal-borne Diseases." <http://www.sdnhm.org/ fieldguide/zoonoses/index.html> (accessed February 27, 2007).

SkinCareGuide Network. "Herpes Guide—from Cold Sores to Genital Herpes." Feb 21, 2007 <http:// www.herpesguide.ca> (accessed Feb 22, 2007).

Southern Illinois University. "Mycotic Infections." <http://www.cehs.siu.edu/fix/medmicro/mycotic. htm> (accessed March 6, 2007).

Stanford University. "Hepatitis D virus." March 2004 <http://www.stanford.edu/group/virus/ delta/ 2004hammon/Deltavirus.htm> (accessed March 5, 2007).

Stanford University. "History [of Babesiosis]." May 24, 2006 <http://www.stanford.edu/class/humbio103 /ParaSites2006/Babesiosis/history.html> (accessed February 1, 2007).

Stanford University. "Lassa Fever Virus." 2005 <http:// www.stanford.edu/group/virus/arena /2005/ LassaFeverVirus.htm> (accessed February 22, 2007).

Stanford University. "Monkeypox." Winter 2000 <http://www.stanford.edu/group/virus/pox/ 2000/monkeypox_virus.html> (accessed March 6, 2007).

Stanford University. "The Parasite: Balantidium coli. The Disease: Balantidiasis." May 23, 2003 <http://www.stanford.edu/class/humbio103/ ParaSites2003/Balantidium dium_coli _ParaSite .htm> (accessed February 2, 2007).

Todar's Online Textbook of Bacteriology. "Diphtheria." <http://textbookofbacteriology.net/diphtheria. html> (accessed February 16, 2007).

The Toxic Shock Information Service. "Toxic Shock Syndrome: The Facts." <http://www.toxicshock.com> (accessed May 2, 2007).

Tropical Medicine Central Resource. "Shigellosis." <http://tmcr.usuhs.mil/tmcr/chapter19/intro.htm> (accessed).

U.K. Creutzfeldt-Jakob Disease Surveillance Unit. "National Creutzfeldt-Jakob Disease Surveillance Unit." February 5, 2007 <http://www.cjd.ed.ac.uk> (accessed February 21, 2007).

U.S. Army Center for Health Promotion and Disease Prevention. "Medical Threats Briefing Homepage." <http://usachppm.apgea.army.mil/HIOMTB> (accessed June 1, 2007).

U.S. Centers for Disease Control and Prevention (CDC). "Home Website of the CDC." May 4, 2007 <http://www.cdc.gov/> (accessed May 4, 2007).

U.S. Department of Health and Human Services. "FDA Licenses Chickenpox Vaccine." March 17, 2005 <http://www.fda.gov/bbs/topics/NEWS/NEW00509.html> (accessed March 8, 2007).

U.S. Department of Health and Human Services. "Medical Privacy—National Standards to Protect the Privacy of Personal Health Information." <http://www.hhs.gov/ocr/hipaa/> (accessed June 8, 2007).

U.S. Department of Health and Human Services. "Pandemic Flu.gov." April 26, 2007 <http://www.pandemicflu.gov/index.html> (accessed April 28, 2007).

U.S. Department of Health and Human Services. "Shingles: An Unwelcome Encore." June 2005. <http://www.fda.gov/FDAC/features/2001/301_pox.html> (accessed March 7, 2007).

U.S. Department of Labor Occupational Safety & Health Administration. "Bloodborne Pathogens and Needlestick Prevention OSHA Standards." <http://www.osha.gov/SLTC/bloodbornepathogens.standards.html> (accessed February 8, 2007).

U.S. Department of State. "Parties and Signatories of the Biological Weapons Convention" <http://www.state.gov/t/ac/bw/fs/2002/8026.htm> (May 25, 2007)

U.S. Food and Drug Administration (FDA). "Commonly Asked Questions about BSE in Products Regulated by FDA's Center for Food Safety and Applied Nutrition (CFSAN)." September 14, 2005 <http://www.cfsan.fda.gov/~comm/bsefaq.html> (accessed January 26, 2007).

U.S. Food and Drug Administration (FDA). "Clostridium botulinum." <http://www.cfsan.fda.gov/~mow/chap2.html> (accessed March 1, 2007).

UCLA. Department of Epidemiology. School of Public Health. "John Snow." <http://www.ph.ucla.edu/epi/snow.html> (accessed March 30, 2007).

UNICEF. "Home website of UNICEF." <http://www.unicef.org/> (accessed June 17, 2007).

UNICEF. "A Promise to Children." <http://www.unicef.org/wsc/> (accessed June 17, 2007).

United Nations Cyber School Bus. "Declaration of the Rights of the Child (1959)." <http://www.un.org/cyberschoolbus/humanrights/resources/child.asp> (accessed June 17, 2007).

United Nations Economic and Social Council (ECOSOC). "Home website of ECOSOC." <http://www.un.org/ecosoc/> (accessed June 17, 2007).

United Nations. "Millennium Development Goals Report 2006." Sections 2.10–11 (Child Mortality from Infectious Disease), Sections 2.14–15 (Malaria and AIDS Goals) <http://unstats.un.org/unsd/mdg/Resources/Static/Products/Prog ress2006/MDGReport2006.pdf> (accessed March 11, 2007).

United Nations. "Progress towards the Millennium Development Goals, 1990–2005." <http://mdgs.un.org/unsd/mdg/Host.aspx?Content=Products/Progress2005.htm> (accessed March 11, 2007).

United Nations. "Secretary General's Report on the Work of the Organization." <http://mdgs.un.org/unsd/mdg/Resources/Static/Products/SGReports/61_1/a_61_1_e.pdf> (accessed March 11, 2007).

United Nations. "UN Development Group National Monitoring Reports." <http://www.undg.org/index.cfm?P=87> (accessed March 11, 2007).

United States General Accounting Office. "Infectious Disease Outbreaks." April 9, 2003 <http://www.gao.gov/new.items/d03654t.pdf> (accessed May 12, 2007).

University of Alabama. "History of Monkeypox." May 25, 2005 <http://www.bioterrorism.uab.edu/EI/monkeypox/history.html> (accessed March 6, 2007).

University of Arizona: The Biology Project. "Immunology and HIV. Immune System's Response to HIV." <http://www.biology.arizona.edu/immunology/tutorials/AIDS> (accessed June 8, 2007).

University of California, Los Angeles. School of Public Health. Department of Epidemiology. "John Snow." <http://www.ph.ucla.edu/epi/snow.html> (accessed February 13, 2007).

University of Virginia Health System. "Yellow Fever and the Walter Reed Commission." <http://www.healthsystem.virginia.edu/internet/library/historical/medical_history/yellow_fever/index.cfm> (accessed June 1, 2007).

University of Virginia Health System. "What is Microbiology?" <http://www.healthsystem. virginia. edu/uvahealth/adult_path/micro.cfm> (accessed April 2, 2007).

Valley Fever Connections. "Valley Fever." <http:// www.valley-fever.org> (accessed March 8, 2007).

Virginia Bioinformatics Institute, Virginia Tech. "Burkholderia mallei." May 15, 2004. <http://path port .vbi.vt.edu/pathinfo/pathogens/Burkholderia _mallei.html> (accessed April 26, 2007).

The White House (U.S. Government). "National Strategy for Pandemic Influenza." November 1, 2005 <http://www.whitehouse.gov/homeland /pandemic-influenza.html> (accessed January 23, 2007).

Whoopingcough.net. "Whooping Cough Information." <http://www.whoopingcough. net/> (accessed May 3, 2007).

Women's Health.gov. "Minority Women's Health." November 2006. <http://www.4woman.gov/ minority/> (accessed March 13, 2007).

The World Bank. "Defeating Onchocerciasis (Riverblindness) in Africa." <http://www. worldbank.org /afr/gper/defeating.htm> (accessed April 22, 2007).

World Care Council. "The Patients' Charter for Tuberculosis Care." 2006. Available online at <http:// www.who.int/tb/publications/2006/istc_charter. pdf> (accessed April 10, 2007)

World Health Organization. "Health Adaptation to Climate Change." 2005 <http://www.who. int/globalchange/climate/gefproject/en/index. html> (accessed May 26, 2007).

World Health Organization. "Dracunculiasis eradication." 2007 <http://www.who.int/dra cunculiasis/en/> (accessed February 22, 2007).

World Health Organization. "Lymphatic Filariasis." September 2000 <http://www.who.int/mediacentre/factsheets/fs102/en/> (accessed March 5, 2007).

World Health Organization. "Maternal Deaths Disproportionately High in Developing Countries." October 20, 2003 <http://www.who.int/ mediacentre/news/releases/2003/pr77/en/index. html> (accessed March 8, 2007).

World Health Organization. "A Review of the Technical Basis for the Control of Associated with Group A Streptococcal Infections." 2005 <http:// www.who.int/child-adolescent-health/New_Publi cations/CHILD_HEALTH/DP/WHO_FCH_CA H _05.08.pdf> (accessed February 2, 2007).

World Health Organization. "Rift Valley Fever." September 2000 <http://www.who.int/mediacentre/ factsheets/fs207/en/> (accessed March 9, 2007).

World Health Organization. <http://www.who. int/en/> (accessed May 8, 2007).

World Health Organization Epidemic and Pandemic Alert and Response. "Global Outbreak Alert & Response Network." <http://www.who.int/csr/ outbreaknetwork/en> (accessed May 12, 2007).

World Health Organization Initiative for Vaccine Research (IVR). "Sexually Transmitted Diseases." <http://www.who.int/vaccine_research/diseases/ soa_std/en/index.html> (accessed January 28, 2007).

World Health Organization Prevention of Blindness and Visual Impairment. "Trachoma." <http:// www.who.int/blindness/causes/priority/en/ index2.html> (accessed February 14, 2007).

World Health Organization Western Pacific Region. "Investigation into China's recent SARS Outbreak Yields Important Lessons for Global Public Health." July 2, 2004 <http://www.wpro.who. int/sars/docs/update/update_07022004.asp> (accessed May 12, 2007).

World Health Organization, Epidemic and Pandemic Alert and Response (EPR), Disease Outbreak News "Accidental exposure to smallpox vaccine in the Russian Federation: 20 June, 2000." <http://www.who.int/csr/don/2000_06_20e/ en/index.html> (accessed April 12, 2007)

World Health Organization. Global Polio Eradication Initiative. "2005 Annual Report." May 2006. <http://www.polioeradication.org/content/publi cations/annualreport2005.asp> (accessed March 25, 2007).

World Health Organization. Initiative for Vaccine Research. "Typhoid." <http://www.who.int/vaccine _research/diseases/typhoid/en/index.html> (accessed May 2, 2007).

World Health Organization. "Togo: Yellow Fever Vaccination Campaign Protects 1.3 Million People." <http://www.who.int/features/2007 /yellow_ fever/en/index.html> (accessed June 13, 2007).

World Health Organization. "Avian Influenza." <http:// www.who.int/csr/disease/avian_influenza/en/ index.html> (accessed May 10, 2007).

World Health Organization. "Blood Transfusion Safety." <http://www.who.int/bloodsafety/en/> (accessed January 16, 2007).

World Health Organization. "Crimean-Congo Hemorrhagic Fever." <http://who.int/mediacentre/ factsheets/fs208/en/> (accessed March 8, 2007).

World Health Organization. "Dengue and Dengue Hemorrhagic Fever." <http://www.who.int/media centre/factsheets/fs117/en/> (accessed May 25, 2007).

World Health Organization. "Global Patient Safety Challenge 2005–2006: Clean Care is Safer Care." 2005 <http://www.who.int/entity/patientsafety/events/05/GPSC_Launch_ENGL ISH_FINAL.pdf> (accessed February 20, 2007).

World Health Organization. "International Health Regulations." <http://www.who.int/csr/ihr/voluntarycompliancemay06EN%20.pdf> (accessed April 21, 2007).

World Health Organization. "Magnitude and Causes of Visual Impairment." November 2004. <http://www.who.int/mediacentre/factsheets/fs282/en/> (accessed April 22, 2007).

World Health Organization. "Malaria." May 2007 <http://www.who.int/topics/malaria/en> (accessed May 9, 2007).

World Health Organization. "Meningitis in Africa: Hundreds of Thousands Vaccinated." <http://www.who.int/mediacentre/news/notes/2007/np12/en/index.html> (accessed May 25, 2007).

World Health Organization. "Neglected Tropical Diseases." <http://www.who.int/neglected _diseases/en/> (accessed May 17, 2007).

World Health Organization. "Partners for Parasite Control (PPC)." <http://www.who.int/wormcontrol/en/> (accessed March 14, 2007).

World Health Organization. "Report of the WHO/FAO/OIE Joint Consultation on Emerging Zoonotic Diseases." 2004 <http://whqlibdoc.who.int/hq/2004/WHO_CDS_CPE_ZFK_2004.9.pdf> (accessed February 28, 2007).

World Health Organization. "Sexually Transmitted Infections." <http://www.who.int/reproduct ive-health/stis/docs/sti_factsheet_2004.pdf> (accessed May 1, 2007).

World Health Organization. "Tuberculosis and Air Travel: Guidelines for Prevention and Control." 2006 <: http://www.who.int/tb/publications/2006/who_htm_tb_2006_363.pdf> (accessed May 17, 2007).

World Health Organization. "WHO Announces End of Ebola Outbreak in Southern Sudan." Press Release, August 7, 2004 Available online at <http://www.who.int/csr/don/2004_08_07/en/index.html>

World Health Organization. "WHO Model List of Essential Medicines." April 2007 <http://www.who.int/medicines/publications/EML15. pdf> (accessed May 26, 2007).

World Health Organization. "Women, Ageing, and Health." June 2000 <http://www.who.int/mediacentre/factsheets/fs252/en/> (accessed March 13, 2007).

World Health Organization. "The World Health Report 2004—Changing History." <http://www.who.int/whr/2004/en/> (accessed June 4, 2007).

World Health Organization. "The World Health Report 2006—Working Together for Health." <http://www.who.int/whr/2006/en/> (accessed May 7, 2007).

World Health Organization. "World TB Day—March 24th." <http://www.stoptb.org/events/world_tb_day/> (accessed April 10, 2007).

World Health Organization. "Yaws Elimination in India: A Step Towards Eradication." <http://www.whoindia.org/EN/Section210/Section424.htm> (accessed May 2, 2007).

Yale-New Haven Hospital. "Contact Precautions." <http://www.med.yale.edu/ynhh/infection/contact/contact.html> (accessed May 27, 2007).

Yale-New Haven Hospital. "YNHH Infection Control; Introduction. "<http://www.med.yale.edu/ynhh/infection/precautions/intro.html> (accessed June 13, 2007).

General Index

Page numbers in **boldface** indicate the main essay for a topic, and primary source page numbers are in ***boldface and italics***. An *italicized* page number indicates a photo or illustration. An *s* following a page number indicates the use of the term in a sidebar, and *t* indicates a table.

South America
  Buruli ulcer, 1:130
  cancer-infectious disease link,
    1:137
  Chagas disease, 1:149, 150, 151
  Eastern equine encephalitis,
    1:265, 266
  filariasis, 1:316
  hantaviruses, 1:364
  leishmaniasis, 1:484
  leprosy, 1:488, 490
  lung fluke infections, 1:506
  malaria, 2:517, 566
  river blindness, 2:716
  Rocky Mountain spotted fever,
    2:720
  smallpox, 2:770, 771
  St. Louis encephalitis, 2:731
  taeniasis, 2:812
  tapeworm infections, 2:814
  tick-borne relapsing fever, 2:695
  tropical diseases, 2:835
  typhoid fever, 2:850
  typhus, 2:855
  whipworm, 2:907
  yellow fever, 2:566, 926, 928t
  See also specific countries
South Korea, avian flu outbreak, 1:74
Southeast Asia
  bilharzia, 1:94
  Burkholderia-related diseases,
    1:127
  cancer-infectious disease link,
    1:137
  chikungunya, 1:157, 158
  dengue fever, 1:234
  diphtheria, 1:244
  early plague, 2:632
  filariasis, 1:315
  malaria, 2:517
  plague, 2:637
  roundworm infections, 2:725
  syphilis, 2:805
  tropical diseases, 2:835
  tuberculosis, 2:841
  typhoid fever, 2:850
  whipworm, 2:907
  wildlife trade, 2:920
  See also specific countries
Southeast Poultry Research Laboratory, 1:441
Southern blot analysis, 1:325
Southwark and Vauxhall Company,
  1:295
Southwestern United States
  coccidioidomycosis, 1:194
  hantaviruses, 1:148, 364–365
  plague, 2:637
Souza, Geraldo de Paula, 2:915
Soviet Union and biological weapons,
  1:43–44, 97; 2:774
  See also Russia
Spa safety, 1:411–412

Space research and bacteria, 2:789
Spain, disease outbreaks in, 1:245;
  2:695
Spanish flu pandemic. *See* Influenza
  pandemic of 1918
Speaker, Andrew, 1:343, 419, 481;
  2:840
Special Program for Research and
  Training in Tropical Diseases, 1:4
Species identification, 1:325
Spectroscopy, for pathogen identification, 1:103–104
Spencer, Charles, 2:553
Spinal polio, 2:649
Spirillum minus infections,
  2:687–688
Spirochetes, mode of locomotion,
  1:509
Spleen enlargement and mononucleosis, 2:559, 563–564
Spontaneous antibiotic resistance,
  1:52
Spontaneous generation hypothesis,
  1:329–330, 331
Sporadic Creutzfeldt-Jakob disease,
  2:657
Sporanox. *See* Itraconazole
Spore forms
  anthrax, 1:44–45
  bacterial diseases, 1:84–85
  Clostridium botulinum, 1:115,
    116
  Cryptococcus neoformans, 1:215
  food safety and, 1:318
  histoplasmosis, 1:399
  resistance to disinfectants, 1:251
  sterilization resistance, 2:788, 789
Sporotrichosis, 2:780–781
Sporozoites, 2:517, 615
Spotted fevers, 2:852, 853, 854
  See also Rocky Mountain spotted
    fever
Spraying programs
  dengue fever, 1:234; 2:569
  Eastern equine encephalitis, 1:266
  leishmaniasis, 1:484, 486
  malaria, 2:516, 520–521, 878
  mosquito-borne disease, 1:266,
    408–409
  relapsing fever, 2:695
  West Nile virus, 2:903, 904
Squirrels
  plague, 2:636
  typhus, 2:855
  West Nile virus, 2:902
Sri Lanka, malaria in, 2:519
St. Louis encephalitis, 1:287, 372;
  2:731–732
St. Louis University Hospital, 2:870

Stages 1-3 of Lyme disease,
  1:510–511
Staining techniques, 1:221; 2:554
Standard precautions, 2:782–784
  handwashing and, 1:359; 2:782,
    783
  infection control and, 1:431
  purpose, 1:114
  See also Airborne precautions;
    Contact precautions
Stapes bones, 2:803
Staphylococcal enterotoxin B (SEB),
  as biological weapon, 2:894
Staphylococcus aureus infections,
  2:785–787
  antibiotic resistance, 1:49–50, 51;
    2:549
  as bacterial meningitis cause,
    2:540
  Haemophilus influenzae culturing
    and, 1:352
  impetigo and, 1:428, 428–430
  nosocomial infections and, 2:598
  petri dish culture, 2:785
  toxic shock from, 2:819
  See also MRSa
State level infrastructure
  field level response and, 2:608
  isolation and quarantine policies,
    2:745–746
  Model State Emergency Health
    Powers Act and, 1:103, 481
  overview, 2:665
  reporting systems, 1:298, 299;
    2:600
State Research Center of Virology
  and Biotechnology (Russia), 2:774,
  777
Statistical analysis and epidemiology,
  1:297
Status (social) and health, 1:425
STDs. *See* Sexually transmitted
  diseases
Steam sterilization (autoclaving),
  2:783, 788–789
Steer, Allen, 1:508
Stein, Andreas, 1:65
Steiner, Rudolf, 1:164
Sterilants, regulation of, 1:57
Sterilization, 2:788–790
  vs. disinfection, 1:57
  vs. sanitization, 1:431
Sternberg, George, 1:308, 309
Stewart, William, 1:51
Stinear, Tim, 1:130
Stockpiling of drugs
  antiviral drugs, 1:454, 455
  as infection control measure,
    2:669
  influenza vaccine, 2:873